Encyclopedia of Pediatrics

Encyclopedia of Pediatrics

Edited by Vanessa Stevens

hayle
medical

New York

Hayle Medical,
750 Third Avenue, 9th Floor,
New York, NY 10017, USA

Visit us on the World Wide Web at:
www.haylemedical.com

ISBN: 978-1-63241-731-2

Cataloging-in-Publication Data

Encyclopedia of pediatrics / edited by Vanessa Stevens.
    p. cm.
Includes bibliographical references and index.
ISBN 978-1-63241-731-2
1. Pediatrics--Encyclopedias. 2. Children--Diseases--Encyclopedias.
3. Children--Health and hygiene--Encyclopedias. I. Stevens, Vanessa.
RJ45 .E53 2019
618.92--dc23

Table of Contents

Permissions

List of Contributors

Index

Preface

The branch of medicine concerned with the care of infants, children and adolescents is known as pediatrics. A specialist in this field is called a pediatrician. Hebiatrics is a subfield covered under pediatrics. It focuses on the care of those who are going through the adolescent phase of development in their life. The adolescent phase begins with puberty, which occurs at around the age of 10-11 in girls, and 11-12 in boys. Some of the common issues associated with adolescents, which are covered under the field of hebiatrics include sexually transmitted disease, substance abuse, acne, eating disorders, unintended pregnancy, among others. This book provides comprehensive insights into the field of pediatrics. It strives to provide a fair idea about this discipline and to help develop a better understanding of the latest advances within this field. For someone with an interest and eye for detail, this book covers the most significant aspects of pediatrics.

This book unites the global concepts and researches in an organized manner for a comprehensive understanding of the subject. It is a ripe text for all researchers, students, scientists or anyone else who is interested in acquiring a better knowledge of this dynamic field.

I extend my sincere thanks to the contributors for such eloquent research chapters. Finally, I thank my family for being a source of support and help.

Editor

Practice and outcomes of neonatal resuscitation for newborns with birth asphyxia at Kakamega County General Hospital, Kenya: a direct observation study

Duncan N. Shikuku[1*], Benson Milimo[2], Elizabeth Ayebare[1], Peter Gisore[3] and Gorrette Nalwadda[1]

Abstract

Background: About three – quarters of all neonatal deaths occur during the first week of life, with over half of these occurring within the first 24 h after birth. The first minutes after birth are critical to reducing neonatal mortality. Successful neonatal resuscitation (NR) has the potential to prevent these perinatal mortalities related to birth asphyxia. This study described the practice of NR and outcomes of newborns with birth asphyxia in a busy referral hospital.

Methods: Direct observations of 138 NRs by 28 healthcare providers (HCPs) were conducted using a predetermined checklist adapted from the national pediatric resuscitation protocol. Descriptive statistics were computed and chi – square tests were used to test associations between the newborn outcome at 1 h and the NR processes for the observed newborns. Logistic regression models assessed the relationship between the survival status at 1 h versus the NR processes and newborn characteristics.

Results: Nurses performed 72.5% of the NRs. A warm environment was maintained in 71% of the resuscitations. Airway was checked for almost all newborns (98%) who did not initiate spontaneous breathing after stimulation. However, only 40% of newborns were correctly cared for in case of meconium presence in airway. Bag and mask ventilation (BMV) was initiated in 100% of newborns who did not respond to stimulation and airway maintenance. About 86.2% of resuscitated newborns survived after 1 h. Removing wet cloth ($P = 0.035$, OR = 2.90, CI = 1.08–7.76), keeping baby warm ($P = 0.018$, OR = 3.30, CI = 1.22–8.88), meconium in airway ($P = 0.042$, OR = 0.34, CI = 0.12–0.96) and gestation age ($P = 0.007$, OR = 1.38, CI = 1.10–1.75) were associated with newborn outcome at 1 h.

Conclusions: Mentorship and regular cost – effective NR trainings with focus on maintaining the warm chain during NR, airway maintenance in meconium presence, BMV and care for premature babies are needed for HCPs providing NR.

Keywords: Birth asphyxia, Neonatal resuscitation, Newborn, Kenya

* Correspondence: dnshikuku@yahoo.com
[1]Department of Nursing, Makerere University, School of Health Sciences, Kampala, Uganda
Full list of author information is available at the end of the article

Background

Globally, approximately 4 million deaths occur in neonates with 99% of them occurring in low and middle income countries [1]. Birth asphyxia, defined as the failure to initiate and sustain breathing at birth by WHO, causes about a quarter of all the neonatal deaths [2]. Approximately three – quarters of all neonatal deaths occur during the first week of life, with a million babies dying on the day they are born [3]. Conspicuously, over half of these neonatal deaths occur within the first 24 h after birth [4, 5]. However, morbidity and mortality from birth asphyxia is mostly preventable and treatable [6]. Effective resuscitation at birth can prevent a large proportion – approximately 30% - of these deaths [7]. Furthermore, resuscitation may avert 5–10% of deaths due to complications of preterm birth [8].

Evidence around the world also show that the risk of death increases by 16% for every 30 s delay in initiating ventilation up to six minutes and every 6% for every minute of delay of applied bag and mask ventilation [5]. Therefore, it is clear that the first minutes after birth are critical to reducing neonatal mortality. Evidence suggests that successful neonatal resuscitation by well – trained HCPs to provide appropriate and adequate resuscitation has the potential to prevent perinatal mortality caused by intrapartum related asphyxia for almost two million babies annually [3]. Newborns with birth asphyxia can suffer from short- to long-term neurological complications. Severe asphyxia has been linked to cerebral palsy, mental retardation, epilepsy and learning disabilities [9]. Therefore, there is need for urgent referral of complicated birth asphyxia cases to higher well specialized facilities in order to assist prevent some of these complications if anticipated early enough [6].

Neonatal mortality in Kenya is still high at 21 per 1000 live births [10] with Kenya aiming to achieve the global SDG target of neonatal mortality to at least as low as 12 per 1000 live births by 2030 [11]. Birth asphyxia is the leading cause of neonatal mortality contributing to 29% of the deaths in the country [12]. The ministry of health (Kenya) recognizes the importance of neonatal resuscitation (NR) as part of the basic emergency obstetric and newborn care (BEmONC) from level 2 health facilities [13]. National guidelines in the form of protocols have been developed and reviewed over time to standardize the performance of NR for newborns with birth asphyxia [14].

However, despite the HCPs' pre – service and in – service training, guidelines and job aids with adequate equipment in NR, practices of HCPs with regard to NR are still reported to be poor [15–17]. Ineffective or wrong resuscitation practices are linked to the persistently high neonatal deaths from birth asphyxia in the first 1–24 h [18]. Kakamega county region is the second most populated region in the country with a high neonatal mortality rate of 28 per 1000 live births [19]. To better describe the healthcare practice and outcomes, the three Donabedian domains of healthcare assessment: structures/resources, process and outcomes are used [20]. This study aimed to describe the practice of NR and outcomes of newborns with birth asphyxia in a busy main regional referral hospital.

Methods

This was a cross - sectional study employing direct observations of NR in labour ward and maternity theatre between April and June 2016 at the regional Kakamega County General Hospital. This method is non – intrusive, where the HCPs do what they normally do (resuscitation) without being interrupted or disturbed by the observer [21, 22]. This allowed the HCPs to be observed in their natural fashion providing NR without interfering in their process of care. However, the newborn unit was excluded as newborns are only referred here after stabilizing from the initial resuscitation done in labor ward or maternity theatre immediately after delivery.

All the HCPs who were involved in resuscitating a newborn and voluntarily consented to participate in the study were observed during resuscitation sessions. The HCPs should have been working in the labor ward and/ or the maternity theatre and providing direct NR services. Trainee nursing and medical students were excluded (unlicensed to practice). Newborns with birth asphyxia who met the inclusion criteria based on the WHO and the American Academy of Pediatrics were recruited [2, 23]. The criteria included: failure to initiate spontaneous respirations at birth/within 1 min of delivery and/or gasping breathing at 30 s after birth and/or baby is floppy and/or bluish or has central cyanosis (blue tongue). Stillbirths (birth of a baby who shows no signs of life [no gasping, breathing, heartbeat or movement]) and those with congenital abnormalities incompatible with life were excluded. Consecutive sampling was used to select all the newborns that required NR immediately after birth and met the inclusion criteria until the required sample size was achieved. It is estimated that about 1 in 10 babies needs help to breathe immediately after birth and therefore, a quick assessment immediately after birth remains the best way to know if a baby needs help to breathe [24]. The Kish Leslie formula ($n = Z^2 \, pq/e^2$) for cross – sectional studies was used to calculate the sample size of the NRs to be observed [25]. The Z (variate from normal distribution that represents the level of confidence) was 1.96; p (estimated proportion of attribute present in a population) was set at 10% as the number of newborns who require resuscitation to breathe at birth [24]; and $q = 1 - p$. The desired level of precision (e) was set at 95% (minimum acceptable errors at 5%) giving a total of 138 as the desired newborn resuscitations to be observed. Each HCP was observed for between three to five times providing NR care.

Study procedures

The hospital's labor ward and theatre had a common central resuscitation area where all NRs were performed. Four research assistants (RAs) (one for day shift, one for evening shift and two for night shifts) were recruited and observed the NRs. The RAs were nurses recruited from among the hospital nurses from the antenatal ward with experience and formal NR training. This was to minimize the Hawthorne effect associated with observation studies [26]. This was on the assumption that the HCPs were less likely to change their practices when being observed by another HCP in the same unit as opposed to an observer from outside the hospital. Thus, they were not given any formal NR training by the primary investigator but were given a two day instruction/ training on how to observe resuscitations against a predetermined checklist. Two practical observations were done with the principal investigator to ensure that all the RAs used the checklist in a similar manner.

Preparation phase

Significance of the study was explained to HCPs and written informed consent from HCPs was sought with emphasis on voluntary participation. The HCPs were sensitized once on the researcher's intent to observe the actual resuscitation without subsequent reminders during the actual procedure. Upon consenting, HCP's biodata details were completed in the structured direct observation checklist.

Data collection

All the three shifts (morning, evening and night duty) were covered in order not to miss out on the resuscitations. A research assistant was present at the resuscitation area every time a delivery was being conducted either in theatre or delivery room. In case of two resuscitations occurring at the same time, the observer went to the delivery that began first. However, this situation only occurred twice. The observer strategically positioned herself near the resuscitaire in order to have a clear view of the resuscitation process from the start to end.

First, information was collected about the availability, functionality and accessibility of the essential NR equipment at the resuscitaire. Once a newborn was delivered, the observer included the resuscitation only if two criteria were fulfilled. First, the HCP receiving the newborn had consented to participate in the study and the newborn delivered required resuscitation (met the eligibility criteria). The RA observed the actual NR as conducted by the HCP on the ward against the

predetermined checklist to assess the skills of the HCP under observation (See structured observation checklist in Additional file 1).

The assessment of the skill focused on the following areas: preparation, the Airway, Breathing and Circulation. Being a direct observation study, the researchers tried their best not interfere in the NR process as it is non – intrusive [21, 22]. The study focused on the HCPs NR techniques as routinely done by HCPs individually. However, in case of practices deemed to be harmful or compromising resuscitation and likely to lead to irreparable damage/death of the neonate, the observer assisted by calling for help from the other HCP to intervene so as to ensure that the neonate would be given the greatest chance of survival as recommended [2, 24]. The RAs then recorded any inappropriate or harmful NR practices observed including holding the neonate upside down, shaking the neonate vigorously, hard patting/slapping of neonate on back, flicking foot of the neonate, vigorously wiping neonate and squeezing chest of neonate.

At the end of the NR, infection prevention practices were observed. This included decontamination and disinfection of the resuscitation equipment such as suction device, mask and oxygen tubing for next use.

Stepwise immediate and at 5 min, 10 min and 1 h outcomes for the resuscitated babies were monitored and documented. This included outcomes after drying/ stimulation, clearing of airway and adequate bag and mask ventilation. Other outcomes e.g. death were captured indirectly under the "others" since they may be attributed to other factors (confounders) not directly related to NR. This helped us assess the specific intervention for each newborn resuscitated differently during the resuscitation process based on the outcome at each step of resuscitation undertaken.

Data quality control and management

The structured observation checklist was pretested first at the Mulago Hospital labor ward of Uganda to ensure reliability and validity in the data collected. Random visits by primary investigator were conducted to ensure that observations were being carried out as instructed and checklists were being filled in on site. At the end of the shifts, forms and checklists were checked by the primary investigator for completeness and errors before leaving the study area/site. The data collected was be kept strictly confidential.

Variables and measurements

The primary outcome was the newborn's outcome status at 1 h. This was a binary outcome: alive or dead. The independent variables influencing the newborn outcome focused on the Donabedian domains of structures and processes. The independent process variables expected to influence the newborn outcome were also constructed as binary with "yes = 1" and "no = 0." Process variables/items were broadly classified under the 3 principle areas of NR process. They were: drying/stimulation [three items], airway maintenance [four items], bag and mask ventilation [seven items] including the optional cardiopulmonary resuscitation [two items] (Table 3). Structural/input factors were measured by NR equipment availability, HCP cadre, training/qualifications and experience, support staff supervision and NR trainings.

Data were captured using the Microsoft Office Excel 2013 software and exported to STATA version 13 for analysis. The unit of analysis was the resuscitated neonate. All the data from HCPs who had 3–5 observations were analyzed. This was a representative and appropriate comparison that eliminated the early initial fears of the HCP of being observed during the practice [26].

For process indicators, descriptive statistics were used and where proportions were calculated, 95%CI were computed. Pearson's chi – square tests were used to test the associations between the newborn outcome at 1 h and the NR processes and newborn characteristics. Logistic regression models were used to assess the association between the process indicators (NR steps) and the primary outcome (survival at 1 h). However, since the NR steps are dependent, the regression was done independently for each NR step performed. Newborn characteristics that were significant in the bivariate analysis were retained as predictors in the final model. With a 95% confidence interval, P – values ≤0.05 were considered statistically significant.

Results
Health care providers background characteristics
Twenty eight HCPs with a median age of 30 years (range 24–50) participated in the study. Nurses/midwives were the majority cadre (71.4%) providing newborn resuscitation. Two thirds of nurses/midwives (65%) were registered diploma holders and one third (35%) were bachelor degree nurses. Most of the HCPs (89.3%) had worked in the maternity ward providing NR care for more than a year. Eighteen HCPs (64.3%) reported ever attending a NR training. Most HCPs (66.7%) had such trainings over 12 months prior to this study. Importantly, all the HCPs who participated in the study had at least undergone either a formal NR training or a non – specific NR induction training (the initial orientation offered to new staffs joining the maternity unit on a number of emergency obstetrics and neonatal care skills e.g. neonatal resuscitation, manual removal of the placenta, maternal resuscitation etc. at the hospital). More than half ($n = 17$, 60.7%) of the HCPs had attended the Basic Emergency Obstetrics and Neonatal Care (BEmONC) training that has a component on NR with at least half ($n = 9$, 52.9%) of them completing the training within

the past six months prior to the study. Support supervision in NR was reported by most HCPs (89.3%). Over half of the HCPs (60%) reported having received the supervision within the past year prior to this study by the maternity unit manager and/or the labour ward in – charge.

Nurses provided NR for the majority of the newborn babies (72.5%). Majority of the newborn babies (63.8%) were cared for by HCPs who had undergone a NR training. The HCPs with over a year experience working in maternity performed most of the NRs (89.1%) (See Table 1).

Health facility characteristics
Helping Babies Breathe (HBB) NR action plans and guidelines were displayed at the resuscitation area. No immediate newborn care and warm chain charts were observed in the unit. All the basic NR equipment: two resuscitaires equipped with electric warmers; oxygen source (two oxygen cylinders, oxygen flow meters and oxygen tubing); suction devices (electric suction machine & colored suction bulbs); ambubags; term face masks (size 1) and the wall clock were available, functional and accessible at the common resuscitation station. However, only one functional preterm mask (size 0) was available and occasionally shareable between the labor ward and the newborn unit. A clean dry towel for drying the newborn was present in each delivery pack.

Infection prevention practices
In 97.8% ($n = 135$) resuscitation cases, equipment used (suction devices and face masks) were well processed with the HCPs adhering to recommended infection prevention practices. These were cleaning of ventilating face mask and the suction device, decontamination in 0.5% sodium hypochlorite solution for 10 min (although occasionally some stayed longer than the 10 min), washing with soap and water and rinsed well and aired to dry until next use.

Processes of care
General characteristics of newborns resuscitated
A total of 1569 deliveries were conducted at the hospital during the study period. Observations of 138 NRs performed by 28 HCPs were done by the RAs. Majority of the deliveries ($n = 82$, 59.4%) were by spontaneous vertex delivery (SVD) and cesarean section ($n = 49$, 35.5%). The mean birth weight was 3211.2 g (SD ± 936.0); lowest had 900 g and highest had 5000 g. Thirty (21.7%) newborns had low birth weight (< 2500 g) while 51 (37.0%) of the newborns were preterm births with gestational ages less than 37 weeks. Fifty seven (41.3%) newborns had meconium present in their airway at delivery (See Table 2).

Overall neonatal resuscitation processes performed
Nearly all ($n = 122$, 88%) the newborns were dried gently by rubbing the back with the dry towel. However, the

Table 1 Background characteristics of HCPs with the distribution of newborns resuscitated at KCGH

HCP Characteristics	Frequency ($n = 28$)	Percentage (%)	Newborns resuscitated ($n = 138$)	Percentage (%)
Age (years)				
< 25 years	3	10.7	15	10.9
> 25–50 years	25	89.3	123	89.1
Sex				
Male	8	28.6	38	27.5
Female	20	71.4	100	72.5
Professional Cadre				
Nurses/midwives	20	71.4	100	72.5
Medical officers	4	14.3	20	14.5
Anesthetists	3	10.7	13	9.4
Clinical officers	1	3.6	5	3.6
Qualification				
Diploma	15	53.6	73	52.9
Bachelor degree	13	46.4	65	47.1
Previous training in NR				
Yes	18	64.3	88	63.8
No	10	35.7	50	36.2
Period since the last NR training ($n = 18$)[a]			($n = 88$)	
< 6 months	6	33.3	30	34.1
≥ Over 12 months	12	66.7	58	65.9
Support supervision in NR				
Yes	25	89.3	123	89.1
No	3	10.7	15	10.9
Period since last support supervision in NR ($n = 25$)			(n = 123)	
Past 6 months	9	36.0	45	32.6
> 6–12 months	6	24.0	30	21.7
> 12 months	10	40.0	48	34.8
Period working in maternity				
< 1 year	3	10.7	15	10.9
> 1 year – 5 years	17	60.7	83	60.1
≥ 5 years	8	28.6	40	29.0

[a]no HCP trained within last 6–12 months

wet towel was not removed in a third of the newborns (31%) resuscitated. A few inappropriate stimulation practices observed during the resuscitations included: vigorously rubbing the baby's back and chest ($n = 11$, 8%), flicking the baby's feet ($n = 3$, 2.2%) and patting the baby's back ($n = 1$, 0.7%).

The airway was checked and cleared for all ($n = 123$) newborns who did not respond to stimulation with any form of airway secretions. Meconium was present in the airway in 57 (46%) of the newborns. Suctioning of airway before stimulation in presence of meconium as per the national guidelines was only correctly done in 23 (40%) of the newborns. Inappropriate head positioning (head not in neutral position to facilitate airway opening) to clear the airway was observed in 21 (17%) cases and 11 (7.2%) of the newborns were turned upside down and back patted. A few ($n = 6$, 4.9%) newborns required prolonged suctioning with a bulb suction device for over 10 min to open the airway.

Bag and mask ventilation (BMV) was initiated for all the newborns who did not initiate breathing after airway clearance ($n = 66$, 100%). Ventilation was initiated within the Golden minute in just over half ($n = 36$, 54.6%) of the newborns who required help. The mean time for initiation of bag valve and mask ventilation was 69. 2 s (SD ± 19.6). Less than half ($n = 30$, 45.5%) of the newborns did not respond after the initial BMV for a minute and required advanced/subsequent BMV.

Table 2 Characteristics of the resuscitated newborns

Characteristic	Frequency ($n = 138$)	Percentage (%)
Mode of delivery		
SVD	82	59.4
C/S	49	35.5
Breech extraction	6	4.4
Others[a]	1	0.7
Birth weight (grams)		
< 2500 g	30	21.7
≥ 2500 g	108	78.3
Gestational age (weeks)		
< 37 weeks	51	37.0
≥ 37 weeks	87	63.0
Meconium present		
Yes	57	41.3
No	81	58.7

[a]Others included assisted delivery by vacuum extraction

Chest compressions with effective breaths and supplemental oxygen were provided for the newborns who did not initiate spontaneous breathing after the advanced BMV as per the national guidelines (See Table 3). Outside the national guidelines, administration of intravenous 10% dextrose through the newborn's umbilical vein was observed in nine (6.5%) cases who needed ventilation support.

Neonatal outcomes
General neonatal outcomes after resuscitation

All the newborns ($n = 138$, 100%) resuscitated were followed up from 1, 5, 10 min and at 1 h. The mean APGAR scores were 5.9 (SD ±1.3) at 1 min, 6.9 (SD ± 2.0) at 5 min and 8.1 (SD ± 2.9) at 10 min for the 138 newborns resuscitated. More than half ($n = 73$, 52.9%) of the newborns had APGAR scores less than 6 at 1 min with the remainder ($n = 65$, 47.1%) having APGAR scores of 7 at 1 min. Overall, majority of the neonates ($n = 119$, 86.2%) survived. Of the 19 (13.8%) who died, a third (n = 6, 31.6%) died before 10 min after birth with the remaining deaths ($n = 13$, 68.4%) occurring within the first hour of life.

Over half ($n = 72$, 52.2%) of the newborns initiated spontaneous breathing after the initial drying and airway suction stimulation. Less than half ($n = 66$, 47.8%) of the newborns required bag and mask ventilation to initiate spontaneous breathing (See Fig. 1).

Type of care post neonatal resuscitation at 1 h

Of the neonates who were breathing at 1 h, 85 (71.4%) were under normal routine care with the mother and the

Table 3 Neonatal resuscitation performance at the Kakamega County General Hospital

NR step performance	Number	Percent	95% CI
Drying/Stimulation ($n = 138$)			
Baby dried thoroughly by gently rubbing the back	122	88	83–94
Wet cloth removed	95	69	61–77
Baby kept warm	98	71	63–79
Airway clearance ($n = 123$)			
Checked airway	121	98	96–100
Meconium ©	57	46	37–55
If meconium, suctioning done before stimulation	23	40	27–53
Airway cleared with suction bulb if unresponsive	123	100	
Baby's head in neutral position	102	83	76–90
Bag and mask ventilation for breathing ($n = 66$)			
Initial BMV initiated within the Golden minute	36	55	42–67
Subsequent BMV (n = 30)			
HCP call for help	26	87	74–100
Correct mask size used during BMV	25	83	69–97
Chest movements observed with each ventilation	19	63	45–82
BMV rate within 30–50 breaths/minute	18	60	41–79
Baby's HR checked at 1 min	22	73	56–90
Cardiopulmonary resuscitation ($n = 24$)			
Chest compressions	20	83	67–99
Supportive oxygen	21	88	73–102

Meconium © meconium present in airway, *BMV* Bag and mask ventilation, *HCP* Healthcare provider, *HR* Heart rate). Percentages rounded off to the nearest whole number

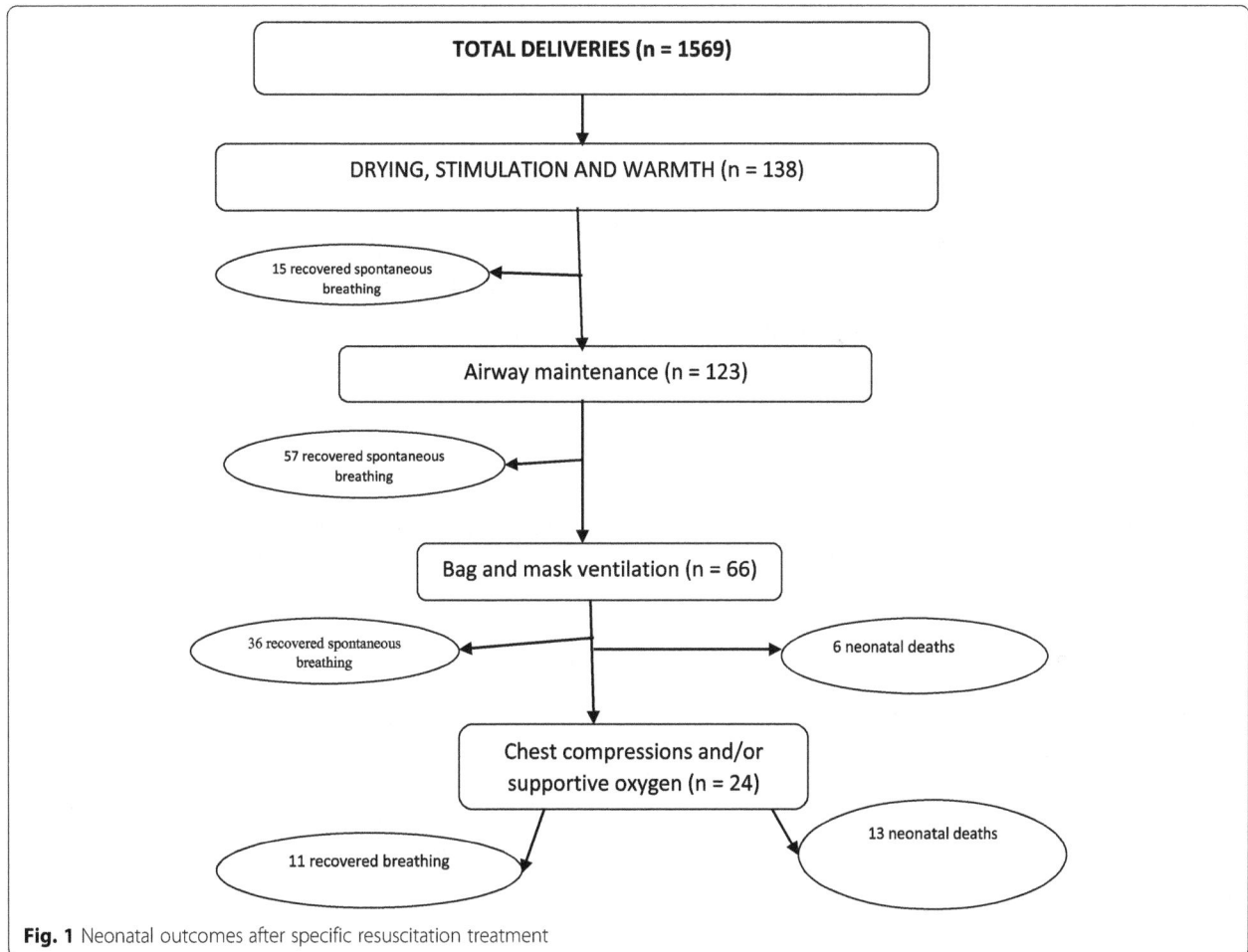

Fig. 1 Neonatal outcomes after specific resuscitation treatment

remaining 34 (28.6%) were in special newborn care unit for supportive oxygen and/or other specific management for the newborns at risk after birth (See Fig. 2). Unstable newborns after the standard bag and mask ventilation with room air were referred to the facility's newborn unit for positive pressure ventilation – oxygen administration via the nasal cannulae and intravenous fluids administration. Other care included antibiotics administration, nasogastric tube feeding and kangaroo mother care as per the national guidelines on essential newborn care. Newborns requiring specialized positive pressure ventilation - Continuous Positive Airway Pressure (CPAP) are usually referred to the nearby national teaching and referral hospital's newborn intensive care unit. No newborns were transferred for this specialized care during the period.

Association between the neonatal resuscitation practices and neonatal outcomes

Pearson's chi – square tests for removing wet cloth (X^2 = 4.7359, P = 0.030), keeping the baby warm (X^2 = 5.9852, P = 0.014), meconium presence in airway (X^2 = 4.4055, P = 0.036), suctioning before stimulation in meconium presence (X^2 = 4.3613, P = 0.037) and chest movements

with each bag and mask ventilation (X^2 = 4.6355, P = 0.031) showed statistically significant associations with the neonate's survival at 1 h. In addition, neonate's gestation age (X^2 = 12.76, P < 0.001) and birth weight (X^2 = 16.93, P = 0.001) were significantly associated with the neonate's survival or death (See Table 4).

Relationship between the newborn resuscitation processes and neonatal outcomes

The processes of NR are dependent and follow a specified order for every newborn. A logistic regression model performed independently for each NR process showed that removing the wet cloth after drying the newborn (OR = 2.90, p = 0.035, CI = 1.08–4.23) and keeping the baby warm after stimulation (OR = 3.30, p = 0.018, CI = 1.22–8.88) were significantly associated with survival of the newborn. Newborns with meconium presence in airway were 66% more likely not to survive past 1 h after resuscitation (OR = 0.34, p = 0.042, CI = 0.12–0.96). Gestation age ≥ 37 weeks was significantly associated with increased survival at 1 h post NR (OR = 1.38, p = 0.007, CI = 1.10–1.75) (See Table 5).

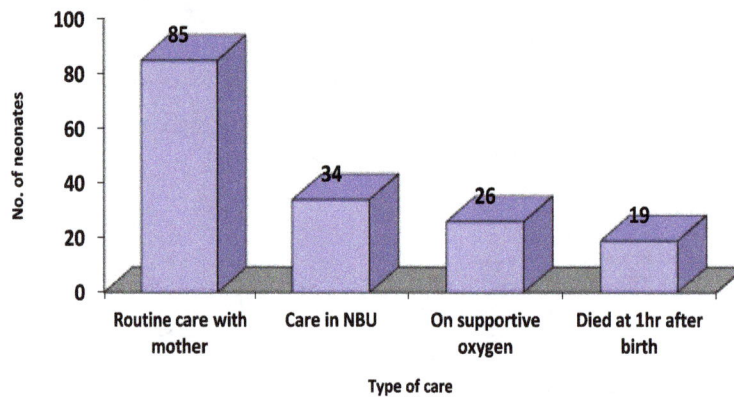

Fig. 2 Type of care post neonatal resuscitation at 1 h

Discussion

HCPs working with newborns must be well equipped with NR knowledge and skills in order to reduce neonatal mortality related to birth asphyxia. Our findings showed that most HCPs had undergone formal NR trainings over a year ago before this study. Supportive supervision was equally conducted for most HCPs by either the unit manager or ward in – charge at least over 6 months prior to this study. Absence of frequent monitoring of NR skills and refresher trainings every 6 months

Table 4 Association between neonatal resuscitation processes, newborn characteristics and neonatal outcomes

NR process		Neonate's Outcome at 1 h., n (%)		X^2	P value
		Alive	Died		
Baby dried by gently rubbing the back		105 (86%)	17 (14%)	0.0245	0.876
Wet cloth removed		86 (90.5%)	9 (9.5%)	4.7359	**0.030***
Baby kept warm		89 (90.8%)	9 (9.2%)	5.9852	**0.014***
Looked into airway		103 (85.1%)	18 (14.9%)	1.8584	0.173
Meconium		44 (77.2%)	13 (22.8%)	4.4055	**0.036***
Suctioning before drying in meconium		21 (91.3%)	2 (8.7%)	4.3613	**0.037***
Head in neutral position		89 (87.2%)	13 (12.8%)	3.3396	**0.068**
BMV within Golden minute		26 (72.2%)	10 (27.8%)	0.0394	0.843
Call for help		44 (73.3%)	16 (26.7%)	1.4486	0.229
Correct mask size during BMV		43 (72.9%)	16 (27.1%)	0.7561	0.385
Chest movements with BMV		39 (78.0%)	11 (22.0%)	4.6355	**0.031***
BMV within 30 - 50b/min		34 (75.6%)	11 (24.4%)	1.3015	0.254
HR checked		38 (74.5%)	13 (25.5%)	1.1904	0.275
Effective breath/chest compressions		8 (40.0%)	12 (60.0%)	1.6448	0.200
Supportive oxygen		11 (52.4%)	10 (47.6%)	2.9011	**0.089**
Newborn characteristics					
Gestation age (weeks)	**< 37**	37 (72.6%)	14 (27.5%)		
	≥37	82 (94.3%)	5 (5.8%)	12.76	**< 0.001***
Birth weight	< 2500 g	19 (63.3%)	11 (36.7%)		
	≥2500 g	100 (92.6%)	8 (7.4%)	16.93	**0.001***
Mode of delivery	SVD	68 (82.9%)	14 (17.1%)		
	C/S	44 (89.8%)	5 (10.2%)		
	Breech	6 (100%)	0 (0%)		
	Others	1 (100%)	0 (0%)	2.40	0.494

*$P \leq 0.05$ statistically significant

Table 5 Relationship between the NR processes, newborn characteristics and the neonatal outcomes

NR process	OR	P - value	95% CI
Drying/stimulation ($n = 138$)			
Dried thoroughly	0.88	0.876	0.18–4.23
Wet cloth removed	2.90	**0.035***	1.08–7.76
Baby kept warm	3.30	**0.018***	1.22–8.88
Airway clearance ($n = 123$)			
Checked airway	5.72	0.225	0.34–95.68
Meconium present in airway	0.34	**0.042***	0.12–0.96
Suctioning airway before stimulation in meconium presence ($n = 57$)	5.02	0.051	1.00–25.34
Head in neutral position	2.74	0.076	0.90–8.32
Bag and Mask Ventilation ($n = 66$)			
BMV within the Golden minute	1.11	0.843	0.38–3.24
Call for help ($n = 30$)	1.88	0.607	0.17–20.61
Correct mask for BMV ($n = 30$)	0.84	0.866	0.12–6.03
Chest movements on BMV ($n = 30$)	1.94	0.420	0.39–9.70
BMV within 30–50 b/min ($n = 30$)	1.27	0.757	0.28–5.87
HR checked at 1 min ($n = 30$)	2.08	0.429	0.34–12.72
Newborn characteristic			
Gestation age (weeks)	1.38	**0.007***	1.10–1.75
Birth weight (grams)	1.00	0.448	0.99–1.00

*$p \leq 0.05$ statistically significant

for HCPs make NR skills to decline rapidly over time as shown by a recent multi – country study on Helping Babies Breathe [27]. Elsewhere, there is evidence that HCPs with over two years of experience working in maternity unit had better NR skills compared to those with less in the same unit [15]. It is expected that those with more years of experience working in the unit help impart the same knowledge and skills to the new HCPs who join the service along the continuum.

Our findings revealed that HCPs were skilled in key critical NR steps in airway maintenance to initiate spontaneous breathing. This finding is reported in other studies conducted in other health facilities in the country [16, 17]. This could be explained by the availability of NR guidelines and action plans in NR, formal and/or informal trainings in NR and the necessary equipment to provide care in the hospital. However, a few newborns miss out on the most important step: being kept warm adequately and this could result in further neonatal deaths precipitated by hypothermia. Immediate essential newborn care after birth will reduce the neonatal morbidity and mortality that are most prevalent at this critical first hour after birth [6].

Bag and mask ventilation was initiated for all newborns who did not establish breathing after drying and airway clearance (with secretions). Our study finding show that HCPs clearly recognize the indication for bag and ventilation in newborns without or gasping respirations as

recommended [2, 24]. However, BMV intervention was not initiated within the golden minute for most resuscitations after failed stimulation and airway clearance to initiate breathing as recommended by the national and international guidelines [14, 24]. When breathing is delayed, the window of opportunity to reverse the consequences of asphyxia (reductions in important blood pressure & cerebral blood flow and cardiac arrest) is small. Our finding showed that HCPs' understanding of the importance of initiating BMV within the Golden minute after birth was poor. Evidence indicates that there is significant improvement in myocardial function and cerebral oxygenation when BMV is initiated within the Golden minute [2].

There is evidence that most resuscitated newborns will initiate spontaneous breathing after simple stimulation with very few going through the advanced NR steps involving chest compressions and drugs [8]. This implies that even in resource limited settings, many babies with birth asphyxia only require simple interventions to be able to initiate spontaneous breathing without difficulties. Good NR skills in drying/stimulating and airway clearance in cases of airway obstruction due to secretions and ensuring that the babies are kept warm may be all that is required to avert most of the neonatal deaths due to birth asphyxia.

Secretions obstruct the airway worsening the asphyxia. Our findings showed that newborns born with meconium – stained amniotic fluid in the airway who did not start breathing on their own had reduced chances of survival in the first hour after birth. Similarly, HCPs' NR skills were poor in airway clearance in presence of meconium in babies who did not start breathing on their own. Healthcare providers dried/stimulated newborns before airway clearance in presence of meconium in non – breathing newborns contrary to both the international and national guidelines on the management of meconium presence in the airway [2, 14, 24]. Clearing airway in meconium presence in newborns not breathing should be done before drying the baby thoroughly as meconium inhaled into the lungs can cause breathing problems [24]. Other studies done in Kenya also demonstrated that meconium presence was a predictor of birth asphyxia and yet this study found that clearing meconium before stimulation was poorly performed by majority of health workers observed [16, 17, 28]. This is despite the most recent national updates on NR guidelines revised in 2013 being available [14]. This indicates that there is a knowledge deficit and/or lack of regular updates on the part of the HCPs on the significance of meconium in the airway. As a result, many newborns born through meconium may suffer both short term and long term sequelae ranging from birth asphyxia and eventual early neonatal death.

Bag and mask ventilation with room air and subsequent transfer to positive pressure ventilation using the nasal cannulae for unstable newborns was the standard practice on oxygen use during resuscitation. This is to ensure that asphyxiated newborns are given the highest quality of care to improve their chances of survival as recommended [24]. This is critical as in cases where there is no oxygen, HCPs may tend to give priority to sourcing for oxygen instead of starting ventilation using bag and mask with room air and may cause loss of critical seconds/minutes in the first hour after birth. This is similar from other global findings where only a small number of newborns (less than 1%) may fail to respond to the initial treatment and thus require advanced resuscitation [29].

Potentially harmful/inappropriate NR practices are still prevalent in the labor wards. This finding is widely reported in the most recent studies on adherence of HCPs to the national NR guidelines in Kenya [16, 17, 28, 30]. This can be explained by the fact that most HCPs had undergone NR trainings to improve their knowledge and skills more than a year ago before this study. Recent evidence in Helping Babies Breathe training in Kenya and India has shown that NR skills decline more than knowledge over time [27].

Prematurity is among the top three causes of neonatal mortality in Kenya [12] and the leading cause globally [3]. Resuscitated newborns delivered at gestation age ≥ 37 weeks had increased chances of survival in our study. Absence of sophisticated equipment and personnel for specialized intensive newborn care for preterm babies at the facility could explain this disparity. This include the recommended pulse oximetry for deciding on the need for supplemental oxygen and to monitor the needed concentration of oxygen related to its benefits on mortality [2]. Healthcare providers need the evidence – based training required for urgent specialized care for premature birthing mothers and their premature babies to improve the perinatal outcomes. Sophisticated equipment and personnel with the special skill set for caring for preterm babies at the regional referral facility will benefit clients seeking care at the regional referral facilities.

This study did not consider possible maternal factors that could have led to the deaths of the resuscitated newborns. The Hawthorn's effect is a major drawback in direct observation studies; however, this helps to observe the 'where' and 'when' of the ongoing process/situation/behavior wanted. Multiple resuscitations per HCP were observed on the assumption that after a few minutes, the HCP would become accustomed to our presence and function in a more natural fashion. The small number of observations for the NR steps after failed initial stimulation and airway maintenance entails that our results should be interpreted in light of the small sample size.

Conclusions

The hospital is prepared with the basic equipment to provide NR with nurses/midwives being the primary providers of NR services. In addition, training in neonatal resuscitation for HCPs is poorly spaced allowing deterioration of key skills. Nurses/midwives and other HCPs providing NR need regular cost – effective NR trainings with focus on maintaining the warm chain for the newborns, airway clearance in meconium – stained amniotic fluid in airways of newborns not breathing, bag and mask ventilation and care for premature babies focusing on the knowledge and practical skills at least after every 6 months. Besides, mentorship programs for the new HCPs in the maternity unit by the more experienced HCPs in the maternity can help to pass knowledge and skills to the new staff joining the unit [31].

Abbreviations
BEmONC: Basic Emergency Obstetric and Newborn Care; BMV: Bag and Mask Ventilation; CI: Confidence Interval; CPAP: Continuous Positive Airway Pressure; HBB: Helping Babies Breathe; HCP: Health care provider; NR: Neonatal Resuscitation; OR: Odds Ratio; RA: Research Assistant; WHO: World Health Organization

Acknowledgements
The authors sincerely thank the mothers and newborns, administration, staff and research assistants at Kakamega County General Hospital for allowing and participating in the study and Prof. Dan Kaye for his oversight and expert guidance on data analysis and interpretation.

Authors' contributions
DNS: conceived the idea, developed the proposal, participated in data collection, analysis, report writing and drafted the manuscript. BM: involved in proposal development, review of data collection instruments, final report and the manuscript. EA: involved in proposal development, review of data collection instruments, final report and the manuscript. PG: involved in proposal development, review of data collection instruments and the manuscript. GN: involved in proposal development, review of methods and data collection instruments, supervised the analysis plan and final report and reviewed the manuscript. All authors read and approved the final manuscript.

Competing interests
The authors declare that they have no competing interests.

Author details
[1]Department of Nursing, Makerere University, School of Health Sciences, Kampala, Uganda. [2]Department of Midwifery and Gender, Moi University, School of Nursing, Eldoret, Kenya. [3]Department of Child Health & Pediatrics, Moi University, School of Medicine, Eldoret, Kenya.

References
1. Singhal N, Lockyer J, Fidler H, Keenan W, Little G, Bucher S, et al. Helping babies breathe: global neonatal resuscitation program development and formative educational evaluation. Resuscitation. 2012;83(1):90–6.
2. WHO. Guidelines on basic newborn resuscitation: World Health Organization; 2012.
3. Lawn JE, Blencowe H, Oza S, You D, Lee AC, Waiswa P, et al. Every newborn: progress, priorities, and potential beyond survival. Lancet. 2014;384(9938):189–205.
4. Bang A, Bellad R, Gisore P, Hibberd P, Patel A, Goudar S, et al. Implementation and evaluation of the helping babies breathe curriculum in three resource limited settings: does helping babies breathe save lives? A study protocol. BMC pregnancy and childbirth. 2014;14(1):116.
5. Ersdal HL, Mduma E, Svensen E, Perlman J. Birth asphyxia: a major cause of early neonatal mortality in a Tanzanian rural hospital. Pediatrics. 2012;129(5):e1238–e43.
6. Every Newborn Action Plan. Every newborn: an action plan to end preventable deaths. Every Newborn Action Plan. 2014;
7. Little GA, Keenan WJ, Niermeyer S, Singhal N, Lawn JE. Neonatal nursing and helping babies breathe: an effective intervention to decrease global neonatal mortality. Newborn Infant Nurs Rev. 2011;11(2):82–7.
8. Wall SN, Lee AC, Niermeyer S, English M, Keenan WJ, Carlo W, et al. Neonatal resuscitation in low-resource settings: what, who, and how to overcome challenges to scale up? Int J Gynecol Obstet. 2009;107:S47–64.
9. Morales P, Bustamante D, Espina-Marchant P, Neira-Peña T, Gutiérrez-Hernández MA, Allende-Castro C, et al. Pathophysiology of perinatal asphyxia: can we predict and improve individual outcomes? EPMA J. 2011;2(2):211.
10. KNBS and ICF. In: KNBoSal M, editor. Kenya demographics and health survey 2014. Calverton, Maryland: KNBS and ICF Macro; 2015.
11. United Nations. Transforming our world: the 2030 agenda for sustainable development goals. 2015.
12. MOH. National Guidelines for quality obstetrics and perinatal care. Kenya: Ministry of Public Health and Sanitation and Ministry of Medical Services, Division of Reproductive Health; 2012.
13. MOH. The Kenya health sector strategic and investment plan - KHSSP July 2012–June 2017: Government of Kenya; 2013.
14. MOH. Basic Paediatric protocols for ages upto 5 years - revised (Republic of Kenya): Government of Kenya; 2013. p. 38–9.
15. Alwar TO. Newborn resuscitation: knowledge and practice among midwives in Kenyatta National Hospital labour ward and maternity theatre [MMED dissertation]: University Of Nairobi; 2010.
16. Otido S. Adherence to newborn resuscitation guidelines in Garissa provincial general hospital [MMED dissertation]: University of Nairobi; 2013.
17. Bhurji JK. Determination of the adherence of nurses to national neonatal resuscitation guidelines at Pumwani maternity [MMED dissertation]: University of Nairobi; 2014.
18. Opiyo N, English M. In-service training for health professionals to improve care of seriously ill newborns and children in low-income countries. Cochrane Database Syst Rev. 2015;(5):Cd007071.
19. Health Sector Annual Performance Report and Priorities. Kakamega County: Annual Performance Report and Plan for Implementation of Health Services. Financial Year for Report: 2015–2016.
20. Donabedian A. The quality of care: how can it be assessed? JAMA. 1988;260(12):1743–8.
21. Tools UF. Tools and techniques: direct observation. User Fit Tools. 2015:33–44.
22. CDC. Data collection methods for program evaluation: observation. Centre for Disease Control and Prevention Evaluation Briefs. 2008;16(16):1-2.
23. American Academy of Pediatrics. Neonatal resuscitation program (NRP) 2012 [cited 2016 1st August]. Available from: http://www2.aap.org/nrp/about.html.
24. American Academy of Pediatrics. American Academy of Pediatrics: Helping Babies Breathe-The Golden Minute. Learner Workbook. 2010:11.
25. Kish L. Survey sampling John Wiley and Sons. New York: Inc; 1965.
26. Polit DF, Beck CT. Nursing research: principles and methods: Lippincott Williams & Wilkins; 2004.
27. Bang A, Patel A, Bellad R, Gisore P, Goudar SS, Esamai F, et al. Helping babies breathe (HBB) training: what happens to knowledge and skills over time? BMC Pregnancy Childbirth. 2016;16(1):364.
28. Gichogo DM. Prevalence of asphyxia, readiness for neonatal resuscitation and associated factors in Naivasha district hospital [MMED dissertation]: University of Nairobi; 2014.
29. Wall SN, Lee AC, Carlo W, Goldenberg R, Niermeyer S, Darmstadt GL, et al. Reducing intrapartum-related neonatal deaths in low-and middle income countries—what works? Seminars in perinatology: Elsevier; 2010.
30. Opiyo N. Improving clinical care for newborns in Kenyan hospitals [PhD dissertation]: University of Oslo; 2013.
31. Murila F, Obimbo MM, Musoke R. Assessment of knowledge on neonatal resuscitation amongst health care providers in Kenya. Pan African Medical Journal. 2012;11(1):78.

2

The cut-off levels of procalcitonin and C-reactive protein and the kinetics of mean platelet volume in preterm neonates with sepsis

C. Aydemir[1], H. Aydemir[2]* , F. Kokturk[3], C. Kulah[4] and A. G. Mungan[5]

Abstract

Background: Sepsis is a leading cause of morbidity and mortality among newborns. C-reactive protein (CRP) and procalcitonin (PCT) have some limitations in the diagnosis of preterm neonatal sepsis. In this study, the cut-offs of PCT and CRP, and the efficacy of mean platelet volume (MPV) were investigated.

Methods: We identified key demographic details and compared laboratory values between preterm infants with early onset and late onset neonatal sepsis (EONS/LONS) retrospectively. Blood samples were collected within the first few hours of the onset of clinical sepsis (CRP 1, PCT 1, MPV 1) and were repeated after 24 h (CRP 2, PCT 2, MPV 2). The optimal cut-offs for CRP, PCT and MPV were determined using receiver operating characteristic (ROC) analysis. Furthermore, pairwise comparisons of ROC curves were made to evaluate the performances of these tests.

Results: In EONS, the cut-off of CRP 1 was 2.6 mg/L, the sensitivity, specificity, PPV and NPV were 80.6, 83.0, 67.5 and 90.7%, respectively ($p < 0.001$). At a PCT 1 cut-off of 1.1 ng/mL, the sensitivity, specificity, PPV and NPV were 78.6, 81.2, 64.7 and 89.6%, respectively ($p < 0.001$). The sensitivity, specificity, PPV, and NPV of the CRP 1 cut-off of 3.6 mg/L for LONS were 78.3, 87.4, 74.8, and 89.4%, respectively. At a PCT 1 cut-off of 5.2 ng/mL, the sensitivity, specificity, PPV and NPV were 58.5, 95.5, 86.1, and 82.9% respectively. For proven sepsis, the cut-off of CRP 1 was 7.0 mg/L with a 76.5% sensitivity, 98.2% specificity, 94.9% PPV and 90.5% NPV ($p < 0.001$). At a PCT 1 cut-off of 1.36 ng/mL, the sensitivity, specificity, PPV and NPV were 90.8, 83.4, 70.6 and 94.4%, respectively ($p < 0.001$). In each subgroup, other than EONS, the performances of CRP 1 and PCT 1 measurements were found to be statistically higher than MPV 1. CRP 2 cut-off levels of LONS group and proven sepsis group were found to be lower than the initial values.

Conclusions: Optimal cut-off levels of CRP 1 and PCT 1 may differ in preterm sepsis subgroups. The diagnostic performances of CRP 1 and PCT 1 didn't differ however, they were more efficacious than MPV.

Keywords: Neonatal sepsis, Procalcitonin, CRP, MPV

* Correspondence: drhaydemir@yahoo.com
[2]Department of Infectious Diseases and Clinical Microbiology, Medical Faculty, Bulent Ecevit University, 67600 Zonguldak, Turkey
Full list of author information is available at the end of the article

Background

Sepsis is a major source of morbidity and mortality in the neonatal population and preterm infants are disproportionally affected [1]. Although positive blood culture is the gold standard used for definitive diagnosis of infection, this test is limited by the length of time it takes to grow microorganisms and potential for interference due to contamination [2, 3]. As clinical signs and symptoms can be very subtle and may mimic non-infectious conditions, there is a need to establish a range of effective biomarkers to aid in prompt decision making [1]. For the rapid identification of microorganisms causing sepsis, novel laboratory methods, such as cytokine and molecular analyses, have been developed; however, it is unlikely that these methods will be useful in the near future because they are not very cost effective [3, 4]. Serum C-reactive protein (CRP) and procalcitonin (PCT) are two of the most thoroughly investigated laboratory markers used to diagnose neonatal sepsis. They have proven to be helpful in the early diagnosis of bacterial invasion; however, they may also be affected by maternal and fetal non-infectious conditions [4]. PCT was suggested to increase physiologically in healthy preterm neonates during the early neonatal period [5, 6]. Gestational age was found to be one of the independent factors that influence the concentration of PCT [6]. Thrombocytopenia has been used as an early but nonspecific marker for sepsis [7, 8]. It has also been associated with prolonged hospitalization and reduced survival rates in previous studies [9–11]. The mean platelet volume (MPV) is another marker that has been available since the 1970s [12]. Although MPV measurements in healthy populations showed an inverse relationship with the platelet count, the clinical meaning of this relationship in neonates with sepsis has not been thoroughly investigated [13]. The objectives of this study were to evaluate the kinetics of MPV measurements, and PCT and CRP levels in preterm newborn sepsis. We also aimed to determine the most appropriate cut-off values for CRP, PCT and MPV using receiver operating characteristic (ROC) curves and identify the diagnostic sensitivity, specificity, positive predictive value (PPV), and negative predictive value (NPV) of each cut-off in early-onset preterm neonatal sepsis (EONS), late-onset preterm neonatal sepsis (LONS), proven and clinical preterm neonatal sepsis. Furthermore, we identified the differences in cut-offs between sepsis subgroups. Because immediate start of antibiotic therapy influences the final outcome in preterm septic neonates, we believe the cut-off levels of these parameters and the performances of these tests are important in the diagnosis of sepsis, especially for prematures.

Methods

Patients

Bulent Ecevit Teaching and Research Hospital is a 600-bed tertiary care hospital in Zonguldak, Turkey. The hospital contains a 20-bed neonatology intensive care unit. This unit offers level-3 neonatal intensive care, except for neonatal surgery, for West Blacksea region of Turkey (approximately 450 newborn hospitalizations per year, 60% of them are preterms). Newborns with at least two clinical symptoms and at least two laboratory signs regarding clinical, hemodynamic, tissue perfusion or inflammatory variables (from the Table 1) in presence of a result of suspected or proven infection (positive culture) and for whom there was no other reason to explain these findings other than infection were diagnosed with sepsis. Patients who fulfilled these criteria within 3 days of life were defined as having EONS. If the diagnosis of sepsis was made after 3 days of life, it was defined as LONS [14]. Proven sepsis was defined if the causative microorganism was isolated from the blood. Demographic findings, including prenatal, natal and postnatal histories, maternal age, gestational age, intrapartum maternal fever, presence of preterm and or prolonged rupture of membranes, chorioamnionitis, antibiotic treatment, clinical features, laboratory results and outcomes were recorded. Our retrospective study population consisted of 204 preterm septic newborns with a gestational age between 23 and 36 weeks hospitalized between January 2013 and December 2016. Fifteen newborns who had one of the following conditions were excluded from the study: chromosomal abnormality, major congenital malformation, multi-organ failure as a result of noninfectious conditions, malignancy, perinatal hypoxia, and asphyxia.

Control group

They had no clinical signs of sepsis. The platelet, MPV measurements, CRP, and PCT levels were obtained from these newborns at the moment of hospitalization. The control group was admitted to the hospital for perinatal conditions other than infection, such as hypoglycemia, indirect hyperbilirubinemia, or intrauterine growth restriction. They did not have treated with an antibiotic regimen. They had no diagnosis of sepsis during the hospitalization period. As a result, 223 infants fulfilled the inclusion criteria for the control group and therefore became the control population for the study.

Blood sampling, isolation and identification of microorganisms from cultures

Blood samples were obtained within the first few hours of the onset of clinical sepsis. The variables included hemoglobin, hematocrit, platelet count, MPV 1, leucocyte count, CRP 1, PCT 1, and blood culture. Blood

Table 1 Clinical and laboratory signs for sepsis diagnosis [33]

Clinical signs	Laboratory signs

Modified body temperature:
  1-Core temperature greater than 38,5 °C or less than 36 °C and/or
  2-Temperature instability
	Leucocyte count:
	  1- < 4000/mm^3 or
	  2- > 20,000/mm^3

Cardiovascular Instability:
  1-Bradycardia
  2-Tachycardia
  3-Rhythm instability:
  4-Reduced urinary output (less than 1 ml/kg/h),
  5-Hypotension
  6-Mottled skin,
  7-İmpaired peripheral perfusion
	Immature to total neutrophil ratio: ≥0.2

Skin and subcutaneous lesions:
  1-petechial rash
  2-sclerema
	Platelet count
	< 100,000 /mm^3

Respiratory instability:
  1-Apnoea or
  2-Tacypnoea or
  3-Requirement of ventilation support
	CRP > 15 mg/L or PCT ≥ 2 ng/mL.

Gastrointestinal:
  1-Feeding intolerance
  2-Poor sucking
  3-Abdominal distention
	Glucose intolerance confirmed at least 2 times:
	  1-Hyperglycaemia (blood glucose > 180 mg/dL or 10 mmol/L) or
	  2-Hypoglycaemia (glycaemia< 45 mg/dL or 2.5 mmol/L)

Nonspesific:
  1-Irritability
  2-Lethargy
  3-Hypotonia
	Metabolic acidosis:
	  1-Base excess (BE) < − 10 mEq/L or
	  2-Serum lactate > 2 mmol/L

CRP C-reactive protein, *PCT* Procalcitonin

sampling was repeated after 24 h including MPV 2, CRP 2, PCT 2. This blood sampling time interval for measurement of these parameters is a part of our hospital's neonatal sepsis protocol. Peripheral blood cultures were obtained before antibiotic treatment or before switching the antibiotic for clinical sepsis diagnosis. Urine and cerebrospinal fluid were cultured only when clinically indicated. Two positive blood cultures were required to confirm *Staphylococcus epidermidis* sepsis. Blood cultures were not routinely taken from the control preterm patients.

Blood cultures were performed in the BACTEC 9120 blood culture system (Becton Dickinson, USA). Isolates were identified using conventional methods, and when required, the results were confirmed by semi-automated API systems (bioMe'rieux, Marcyl'Etoile, France). Antibiotic susceptibility tests were performed by the Kirby–Bauer disk diffusion method according to the guidelines of the Clinical and Laboratory Standards Institute (CLSI) standards M100-S20–25.

Blood for complete blood counts was obtained via venipuncture, arterial puncture or a central catheter. The platelet count and MPV were determined using an automated hematology analyzer (UniCel DxH 800, Beckman Coulter), and quantitative determination of CRP in human serum was performed via high sensitive immunonephelometry implemented on an automatic analyzer (Beckman Coulter) according to the manufacturer's instructions.

The measurement of the PCT levels was performed using the ECLIA (electrochemiluminescence immunoassay) sandwich principle method (Cobas e 411, Elecsys BRAHMS PCT test, Roche Diagnostics GmbH, Mannheim, Germany). The measuring range was 0.02–100 ng/mL. Samples in the measurement range were diluted 1:4 with negative human serum. The concentration of the diluted sample was > 1.0 ng/mL. The functional sensitivity was 0.05 ng/mL, the analytical sensitivity was < 0.02 ng/mL, and the detection limit was < 0.02 ng/mL. The levels of PCT were measured to have an intra-assay of coefficient of variation (CV) < 2.7% and an interassay CV of < 5.0%.

Statistical analyses

Statistical analyses were performed with SPSS 19.0 software (SPSS Inc., Chicago, IL, USA). The distribution of the data was determined by the Shapiro-Wilk test. Continuous variables are expressed as median (min-max), and categorical variables are expressed as frequency and percent. A Pearson Chi-square test was used to determine differences between groups for categorical variables. Continuous variables were compared with the Mann-Whitney U test for two groups. Repeated measures were evaluated with the Friedman test. Dunn's test was used for the post hoc test after the Friedman test. A receiver operating characteristic (ROC) analysis was constructed to determine the best cut-off value to predict the outcome. The probability was calculated using a logistic regression model, and the estimated probabilities were used in a ROC analysis to calculate the area under curve (AUC) for different models. A p value of < 0.05 was considered statistically significant for all tests. At the planning stage of our study, the sepsis group included 240 patients. A preliminary power analysis was performed, and to achieve a 5% type I error probability and 80% prior power with 0.60 effect size, the sample size for control group was determined to be 240 patients. In sepsis group and control group, 36 and 17 of patients were full-term respectively. Because of making a comparison between preterm infants and full-terms were not possible statistically, full-term neonates were excluded from the study. In the study period, 204 preterm newborns who fulfilled the criteria of sepsis group, 223 preterm newborns who fulfilled the criteria of control group included the study.

Results
A total of 427 premature newborns (207 boys/48.5%, 220 girls/51.5%) were involved in this study. There were 204 newborns in the sepsis group and 223 newborns in the control group. Of the 204 infants with sepsis, 98 (48.0%) were diagnosed with proven sepsis. The remaining 106 infants (52.0%) had clinical sepsis. 98 (48.0%) of the patients were diagnosed with EONS, whereas 106 (52.0%) of the newborns were diagnosed with LONS. A total of 42 septic newborns (20.6%) (34 had proven sepsis and 8 had clinical sepsis) died during the observation period.

The pathogens isolated from the blood were approximately equally divided among Gram-negative ($n = 50$, 51%) and Gram-positive ($n = 48$, 49%) organisms. The two most common Gram-negative pathogens responsible for sepsis were *Escherichia coli* (22/98, 22,4%), and *Klebsiella pneumoniae* (20/98, 20,4%). Extended-spectrum beta-lactamase (ESBL) production was detected in 13 *E. coli/K. pneumoniae* isolates. *S. epidermidis* was the most commonly isolated Gram-positive pathogen (32/50, 64%). Methicillin resistance was detected in 36 of 42 (82%) *S. aureus/epidermidis* isolates. In EONS sepsis, Gram-positive bacteria were more common (27/46, 58.7%), whereas Gram-negative pathogens (30/52, 57.7%) were more commonly isolated from the blood of the infants with LONS. The most common pathogens isolated from the infants with EONS were *E.coli* (16/46, 34.8%), methicillin-resistant *S. epidermidis* (14/46, 30.4%) and methicillin-sensitive *S. epidermidis* (8/46, 17.9%). In the infants with LONS, *K. pneumoniae* (20/52, 38.5%) and methicillin-resistant *S. epidermidis* (15/52, 28.8%) were more common detected pathogens.

The differences between the gestational age, birth weight, male gender, and vaginal delivery rate and comparisons of the markers of sepsis are shown in Table 2. CRP 1 ($p < 0.001$), PCT 1 ($p < 0.001$) and MPV 1 ($p < 0.001$) measurements were significantly higher in the infected preterm infants versus the control group. Platelet counts for the initial diagnosis of sepsis were significantly lower in the infected infants ($p = 0.001$) when compared to infants in the control group (Table 2). The differences in the

Table 2 Demographical characteristics and laboratory values for the sepsis and control patients

	Sepsis $n = 204$	Control group $n = 223$	p
Gender, male n (%)	92 (45.1)	115 (51.6)	0.181
Vaginal delivery, n (%)	21.0 (10.3)	15.0 (6.7)	0.250
Age of mother (years) med (min-max)	29.0 (16.0–40.0)	29.0 (19.0–43.0)	0.592
Birth weight med (min-max)	1330.0 (550.0–2830.0)	1500.0 (640.0–2960.0)	0.025
Chorioamnionitis, n (%)	21.0 (10.3)	0.0 (0.0)	< 0.001
Early membrane rupture, n (%)	24.0 (11.8)	0.0 (0.0)	< 0.001
Thrombocytopenia, n (%)	71.0 (34.8)	7.0 (3.1)	< 0.001
Mortality, n (%)	42.0 (20.6)	0.0 (0.0)	< 0.001
Platelet 1 ($\times 10^3/mm^3$) med (min-max)	225.0 (23–601)	250.0 (93–705)	0.001
CRP 1 mg/L med (min-max)	15.0 (0.0–200.0)	1.5 (0.0–13.0)	< 0.001
PCT 1 ng/mL med (min-max)	10.1 (0.0–200.0)	0.2 (0.0–11.0)	< 0.001
MPV 1 fL med (min-max)	8.4 (5.9–12.1)	7.8 (6.0–11.2)	< 0.001

CRP C-reactive protein, *PCT* Procalcitonin, *MPV* Mean platelet volume

measurements of the platelet, MPV, CRP and PCT levels of the premature sepsis patients are presented in Table 3. The median second-day platelet measurement was significantly lower ($p = 0.008$) in the patients with EONS. The median MPV 1 ($p < 0.001$) and the MPV 2 ($p = 0.012$) levels were significantly higher in LONS group than the neonates with EONS. The median PCT 1 ($p < 0.001$) and PCT 2 measurements ($p < 0.001$), the CRP 1 level ($p < 0.001$), and the MPV 2 ($p < 0.001$) measurement were significantly higher in the proven sepsis group than the neonates with clinical sepsis (Table 3).

The optimum cut-off values for CRP, PCT and MPV were identified by drawing ROC curves. The cut-off values are shown in Table 4. For EONS, the cut-off of the CRP 1 was found to be 2.6 mg/L, the sensitivity, specificity, PPV and NPV were 80.6, 83.0, 67.5 and 90.7%, respectively ($p < 0.001$). For the diagnosis of the same group, at a PCT 1 cut-off level of 1.1 ng/mL, the sensitivity, specificity, PPV and NPV were 78.6, 81.2, 64.7 and 89.6%, respectively ($p < 0.001$).The optimum cut-off value of the CRP 1 was 3.6 mg/L for the diagnosis of LONS ($p < 0.001$). The sensitivity, specificity, PPV, and NPV of the CRP 1 cut-off for LONS were 78.3, 87.4, 74.8, and 89.4%, respectively. For the diagnosis of LONS, at a PCT 1 cut-off value of 5.2 ng/mL, the sensitivity, spesificity, PPV and NPV were 58.5, 95.5, 86.1 and 82.9% respectively. For proven sepsis, the cut-off level of the CRP 1 was 7.0 mg/L with 76.5% sensitivity, 98.2% specificity, 94.9% PPV and 90.5% NPV according to the ROC curves ($p < 0.001$). For proven sepsis, at a PCT 1 cut-off level of 1.36 ng/mL, the sensitivity, specificity, PPV and NPV were 90.8, 83.4, 70.6 and 94.4%, respectively ($p < 0.001$). After sepsis diagnosis, the second day cut-off values were shown in the same table (Table 4). The significant CRP 2 cut-off levels of LONS group and

proven sepsis group were found to be lower than the initial values. For the patients with LONS, at a cut-off level of 2.4 mg/L for CRP 2, the sensitivity, specificity, PPV and NPV were 69.8, 80.3, 62.7 and 84.8% respectively. For proven sepsis, the cut-off level of CRP was found to be 2.6 mg/L with 70.4% sensitivity, 83.0% specificity, 64.5% PPV and 86.4% NPV (Table 4).

Table 5 shows the pairwise comparison of ROC curves of CRP, PCT and MPV for the diagnosis of sepsis subgroups (Table 5). Pairwise comparisons were made if the cut-off level of the study parameter (CRP, PCT, MPV) was found to be statistically significant (Figs. 1, 2, 3, 4, 5 and 6). At the time of suspicion of sepsis, in each sepsis subgroup, other than EONS, the comparison of ROC curves of CRP and MPV and the comparison of ROC curves of PCT and MPV ($p < 0.001$) were found to be statistically significant. Area under curve (AUC) of PCT and AUC of CRP were higher than AUC of MPV in the study sepsis subgroups (Table 5). In each group, no statistically significant difference was found between the comparison of ROC curves of CRP 1 and PCT 1.

The ROC curves of CRP 1 and PCT 1 were combined in order to test whether this improves the diagnostic accuracy. The combinations were found statistically significant for EONS and LONS groups. For patients with EONS, the combination of CRP 1 (> 2.6 mg/L) and PCT 1(> 1.1 ng/mL) had 92.2% sensitivity, 41.9% specificity, 62.1% PPV, and 83.9% NPV. Thus, where sensitivity of the combination was higher, specificity was lower. For the diagnosis of LONS group, the combination of CRP 1 (> 3.6 mg/L) and PCT 1(> 5.2 ng/mL) had sensitivity, specificity, PPV, and NPV of 74.1, 80.0, 83.3, and 69.6%, respectively. According to the ROC curves, whereas the sensitivity of this combination was higher than the sensitivity of PCT 1 alone, the specificity was lower than

Table 3 Sepsis patients' laboratory values

	EONS $n = 98$	LONS $n = 106$	p	Proven sepsis $n = 98$	Clinical sepsis $n = 106$	p
Platelet $1 \times 10^3/mm^3$ med (min-max)	227.0 (40.0–442.0)	220.0 (23.0–601.0)	0.473	234.0 (23.0–498.0)	221.0 (40.0–601.0)	0.435
Platelet $2 \times 10^3/mm^3$ med (min-max)	192.0 (13.0–649.0)	223.0 (13.0–661.0)	0.008	209.5 (13.0–661.0)	212.5 (27.0–649.0)	0.036
CRP 1 mg/L med (min-max)	10.6 (0.0–200.0)	20.5 (0.0–170.0)	0.113	20.5 (0.6–170.0)	8.25 (10.0–200.0)	0.001
CRP 2 mg/L med (min-max)	3.6 (0.0–203.0)	6.2 (0.0–219.0)	0.075	5.4 (0.0–219.0)	3.8 (0.0–203.0)	0.103
PCT 1 ng/ml med (min-max)	9.6 (0.0–200.0)	10.1 (0.1–109.5)	0.107	18.0 (0.0–200.0)	1.6 0.0–200.0)	< 0.001
PCT 2 ng/ml med (min-max)	2.5 (0.1–200.0)	1.8 (0.1–200.0)	0.131	8.8 (0.1–120.0)	1.2 (0.1–120.0)	< 0.001
MPV 1 fL med (min-max)	8.0 (6.5–11.9)	8.9 (5.9–12.1)	< 0.001	8.5 (6.6–12.1)	8.3 (5.9–11.9)	0.239
MPV 2 fL med (min-max)	8.9 (6.7–11.2)	9.4 (6.3–13.5)	0.012	9.5 (6.7–11.8)	8.7 (6.3–13.5)	< 0.001

EONS Early neonatal sepsis, *LONS* Late onset neonatal sepsis, *CRP* C-reactive protein, *PCT* Procalcitonin, *MPV* Mean platelet volume

Table 4 Cut-off levels for procalcitonin, C-reactive protein and mean platelet volume in preterm neonatal sepsis subgroups

	Cut-off	Sensitivity % (95% CI)	Specificity % (95% CI)	PPV %	NPV%	AUC	p
EONS PCT 1 ng/mL	1.1	78.6 (69.1–86.2)	81.2 (75.4–86.1)	64.7	89.6	0.832	< 0.001
EONS PCT 2 ng/mL	0.48	83.7 (74.8–90.4)	67.3 (60.7–73.4)	52.9	90.4	0.801	< 0.001
EONS CRP 1 mg/L	2.6	80.6 (71.4–87.9)	83.0 (77.4–87.6)	67.5	90.7	0.838	< 0.001
EONS CRP 2 mg/L	2.6	59.2 (48.8–69.0)	83.0 (77.4–87.6)	60.4	82.2	0.696	< 0.001
EONS MPV 1 fL	7.9	61.2 (50.8–70.9)	54.3 (47.5–60.9)	37.0	76.1	0.563	0.073
EONS MPV 2 fL	8.2	69.4 (59.3–78.3)	66.4 (59.8–72.5)	47.6	83.1	0.704	< 0.001
LONS PCT 1 ng/mL	5.2	58.5 (48.5–68.0)	95.5 (91.9–97.8)	86.1	82.9	0.820	< 0.001
LONS PCT 2 ng/mL	1.1	60.4 (50.4–69.7)	81.2 (75.4–86.1)	60.4	81.2	0.745	< 0.001
LONS CRP 1 mg/L	3.6	78.3 (69.2–85.7)	87.4 (82.4–91.5)	74.8	89.4	0.856	< 0.001
LONS CRP 2 mg/L	2.4	69.8 (60.1–78.3)	80.3 (74.4–85.3)	62.7	84.8	0.791	< 0.001
LONS MPV 1 fL	8.4	60.4 (50.4–69.7)	72.2 (65.8–78.0)	50.8	79.3	0.689	< 0.001
LONS MPV 2 fL	8.4	75.5 (66.2–83.3)	72.2 (65.8–78.0)	56.3	86.1	0.786	< 0.001
Proven sepsis PCT 1 ng/mL	1.4	90.8 (83.3–95.7)	83.4 (77.9–88.0)	70.6	94.4	0.936	< 0.001
Proven sepsis PCT 2 ng/mL	1.1	75.5 (65.8–83.6)	81.2 (75.4–86.1)	63.8	88.3	0.829	< 0.001
Proven sepsis CRP 1 mg/L	7.0	76.5 (66.9–84.5)	98.2 (95.5–99.5)	94.9	90.5	0.922	< 0.001
Proven sepsis CRP 2 mg/L	2.6	70.4 (60.3–79.2)	83.0 (77.4–87.6)	64.5	86.4	0.771	< 0.001
Proven sepsis MPV 1 fL	7.9	73.5 (63.6–81.9)	54.3 (47.5–60.9)	41.4	82.3	0.653	< 0.001
Proven sepsis MPV 2 fL	8.9	71.4 (61.4–80.1)	82.5 (76.9–87.3)	64.2	86.8	0.811	< 0.001
Clinical sepsis PCT 1 ng/mL	1.2	57.6 (47.6–67.1)	82.1 (76.4–86.9)	60.4	80.3	0.724	< 0.001
Clinical sepsis PCT 2 ng/mL	0.5	67.9 (58.2–76.7)	67.3 (60.7–73.4)	49.7	81.5	0.720	< 0.001
Clinical sepsis CRP 1 mg/L	2.6	73.6 (64.1–81.7)	83.0 (77.4–87.6)	67.2	86.9	0.779	< 0.001
Clinical sepsis CRP 2 mg/L	2.4	59.4 (49.5–68.9)	80.3 (74.4–85.3)	58.9	80.6	0.722	< 0.001
Clinical sepsis MPV 1 fL	9.1	30.2 (21.7–39.9)	88.3 (83.4–92.2)	55.2	72.7	0.034	0.002
Clinical sepsis MPV 2 fL	8.1	72.6 (63.1–80.8)	62.3 (55.6–68.7)	47.8	82.7	0.686	< 0.001

EONS Early onset neonatal sepsis, *LONS* Late onset neonatal sepsis, *PPV* Positive predictive value, *NPV* Negative predictive value, *AUC* Area under curve, *PCT* Procalcitonin, *CRP* C-reactive protein, *MPV* Mean platelet volume

PCT 1. The sensitivity and the specificity of the combination of ROC curves were similar to the sensitivity and the specificity of CRP 1.

Discussion

Sepsis is a complex syndrome with significant morbidity and mortality. Despite recent advances in diagnosis, establishing definitive diagnostic criteria may be difficult. Developmental differences between children and adults lead to distinct variations in the epidemiology, pathophysiology, diagnosis and management in children compared with adults [15]. In addition to the clinical signs of sepsis, many laboratory biomarkers are under investigation to enable a rapid diagnosis of sepsis. Elevated PCT levels are nearly pathognomonic for sepsis and may be used to guide management, however the cut-off levels of PCT may vary and should not be used alone in the diagnosis of neonatal sepsis [16]. MPV values increase as a result of increased platelet production and/or increased platelet destruction in sepsis [17]. Although a substantial number of studies have focused on the relationship between sepsis and thrombocytopenia, few studies have investigated MPV kinetics.

CRP is one of the most studied and utilized laboratory markers for newborn sepsis. Because of the delay in synthesis, it may be low early in infection [18]. Moreover, non-infectious factors may influence CRP kinetics, for example; complications at delivery have been associated with non-specific elevations of CRP in the early perinatal period [18, 19]. In previous studies, the range of CRP sensitivity and specificity has been reported as 35–94% and 60–96%, respectively [19]. In a recently published study, CRP measurements were compared between EONS and LONS. The CRP levels of EONS were significantly lower than the levels of LONS. Moreover, CRP had 75% sensitivity and 76.3% specificity for proven sepsis with a cut-off of 0.16 mg/dL [2]. From previously published studies CRP was reported to have low sensitivity during the first hours of sepsis [18]. In our study, the median CRP 1 level was significantly higher in the patients with LONS than the patients with EONS. The optimum cut-off value in the diagnosis of LONS was

Table 5 Pairwise comparison of receiving operating characteristic curves in preterm neonatal sepsis subgroups at the time of clinical suspicion of sepsis

	95% CI	P
EONS CRP 1 -EONS PCT 1 AUC CRP 1 = 0.838 AUC PCT 1 = 0.832	−0.061-0.074	0.851
LONS CRP 1- LONS PCT 1 AUC CRP 1 = 0.856 AUC PCT 1 = 0.820	−0.027-0.099	0.260
LONS MPV1- LONS CRP 1 AUC MPV 1 = 0.689 AUC CRP 1 = 0.856	0.091–0.243	< 0.001
LONS MPV1- LONS PCT 1 AUC MPV 1 = 0.689 AUC PCT 1 = 0.820	0.055–0.207	0.001
Clinical sepsis CRP 1- Clinical sepsis PCT 1 AUC CRP 1 = 0.779 AUC PCT 1 = 0.724	−0.021-0.131	0.155
Clinical sepsis CRP 1- Clinical sepsis MPV 1 AUC CRP 1 = 0.779 AUC MPV 1 = 0.606	0.086–0.259	< 0.001
Clinical sepsis PCT 1- Clinical sepsis MPV 1 AUC PCT 1 = 0.724 AUC MPV 1 = 0.606	0.033–0.202	0.006
Proven sepsis CRP 1-Proven sepsis PCT 1 AUC CRP 1 = 0.922 AUC PCT 1 = 0.939	−0.034-0.063	0.556
Proven sepsis CRP 1-Proven sepsis MPV 1 AUC CRP 1 = 0.922 AUC MPV 1 = 0.653	0.196–0.343	< 0.001
Proven sepsis MPV 1-Proven sepsis PCT 1 AUC MPV 1 = 0.606 AUC PCT 1 = 0.939	0.212–0.355	< 0.001

EONS Early onset neonatal sepsis, *LONS* Late onset neonatal sepsis, *AUC* Area under curve: *CRP* C-reactive protein, *PCT* Procalcitonin, *MPV* Mean platelet volume

3.6 mg/L for CRP 1 in this study. The sensitivity, specificity, PPV, and NPV of the CRP 1 cut-off for the diagnosis of LONS were 78.3, 87.4, 74.8, and 89.4%, respectively. In EONS, we found the cut-off level of CRP 1 for the diagnosis of sepsis to be 2.6 mg/L with a 80.6% sensitivity, 83.0% specificity, 67.5% PPV and 90.7% NPV. Chiesa et al. investigated the reference interval of CRP in preterm newborns with EONS. They found the predicted CRP to be 0.1 mg/L at birth and the level increased to 1.7 at 27–36 h. Their birth cut-off level of CRP was lower than our cut-off level [5]. In another published study, the CRP and IL-6 cut-off levels were investigated in newborns. No significant difference was reported in the CRP levels between the proven and clinical sepsis groups; however, the authors identified a significant difference between the septic newborns and the control group. The cut-offs of CRP were determined to be 0.58 mg/dL and 0.48 mg/dL for proven sepsis and all sepsis, respectively. For proven sepsis, the sensitivity, specificity, PPV and NPV were 71, 97, 99 and 49%, respectively. The authors noted that the combination of CRP and IL6 may be more helpful with higher sensitivity and specificity [20]. In our study, it was striking that the median CRP 2 levels for all types of sepsis were found to be lower than the initial values. We found significant cut-offs of CRP 2 levels to be lower than the initial values in LONS and proven sepsis groups. We think it may be due to the response to antibiotics that were given promptly when the sepsis diagnosis was established. We also investigated the combination of CRP 1

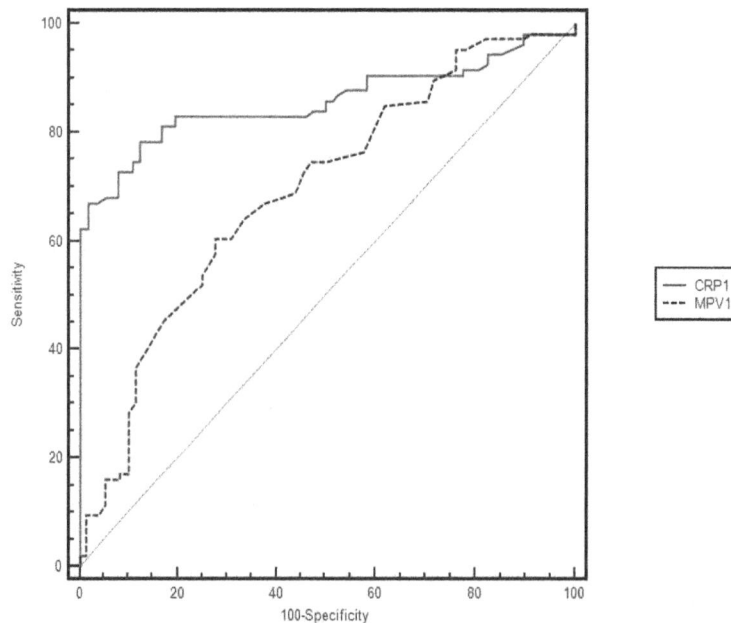

Fig. 1 Pairwise comparison of receiver operating characteristic (ROC) curves of C-reactive protein (CRP 1) and mean platelet volume (MPV 1) level on the first day of sepsis diagnosis in late onset preterm neonatal sepsis (LONS)

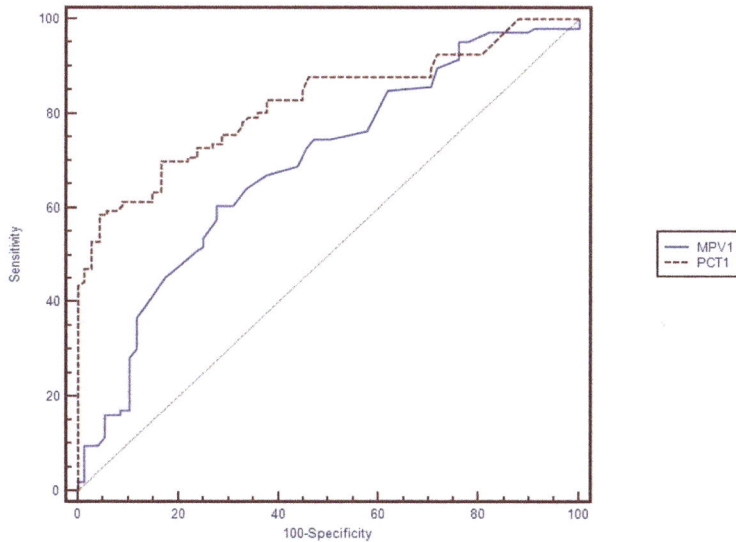

Fig. 2 Pairwise comparison of receiver operating characteristic (ROC) curves of mean platelet volume (MPV 1) and procalcitonin (PCT 1) level on the first day of sepsis diagnosis in late onset preterm neonatal sepsis (LONS)

and PCT 1 for the diagnosis of EONS and LONS. Acoording to the ROC curves, the sensitivity of this combination was found to be higher than CRP 1 or PCT 1 alone in EONS. In a recently published study, salivary CRP and MPV were investigated for the diagnosis of septic neonates and they found significant difference of CRP levels between septic neonates and controls. At a cut-off of 3.48 ng/L, salivary CRP showed high specifity and sensitivity [21]. In our study, we determined the cut-off of CRP 1 to be 7.0 mg/L for proven sepsis. At this cut-off, the sensitivity, specificity, PPV, and NPV were 76.5, 98.2, 94.9 and 90.5%, respectively. For the diagnosis of clinical sepsis, at the CRP 1 cut-off of 2.6 mg/L, the sensitivity, specificity, PPV and NPV were 73.6, 83.0, 67.2 and 86.9% respectively. For the diagnosis of proven sepsis, we found the cut-off of CRP 2 to be 2.6 mg/L. This second day CRP cut-off was lower than the the cut-off of first day CRP. The specifity, PPV and NPV of this cut-off were also lower than the first day values.

Patrick et al. evaluated 156 newborns and demonstrated that MPV measurements were considerably higher in patients with bacteremia than newborns

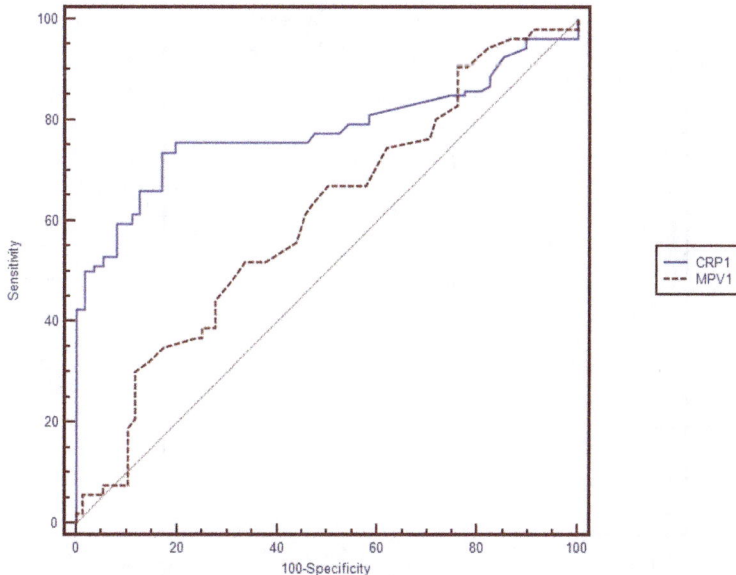

Fig. 3 Pairwise comparison of receiver operating characteristic (ROC) curves of C-reactive protein (CRP 1) and mean platelet volume (MPV 1) level on the first day of sepsis diagnosis in clinical preterm sepsis

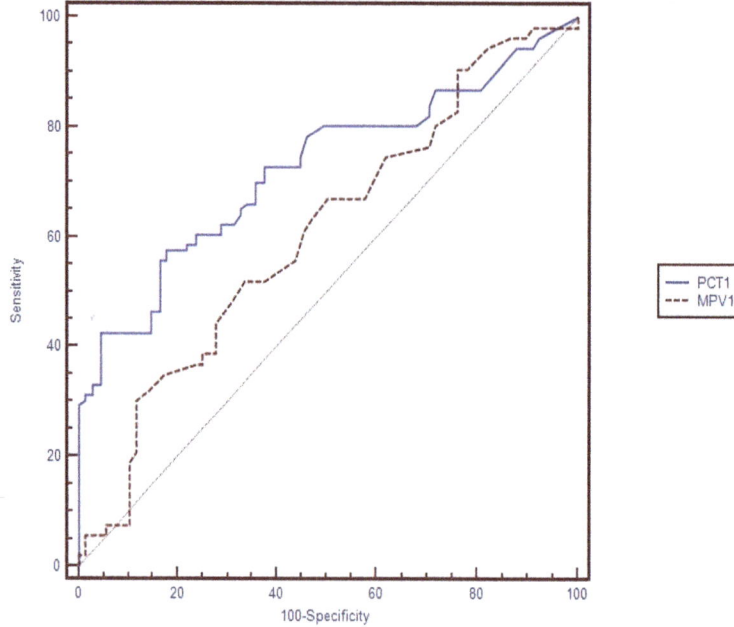

Fig. 4 Pairwise comparison of receiver operating characteristic (ROC) curves of mean platelet volume (MPV 1) and procalcitonin (PCT 1) level on the first day of sepsis diagnosis in clinical preterm sepsis

without infection. The authors reported the sensitivity and specificity of MPV for the diagnosis of sepsis to be 42 and 95%, respectively [22]. Oncel et al. indicated significantly higher MPV and CRP levels in newborns with sepsis than healthy controls [23]. Cekmez et al. investigated the relationship of MPV between the various diseases of newborns other than sepsis. The authors identified high MPV levels within the first hours of these diseases; however, their data showed that higher MPV values were not associated with the development of sepsis [24]. We identified significantly higher MPV levels for the first day of diagnosis in septic premature newborns than non-infectious premature controls. In our study, the median MPV 1 and MPV 2 levels were

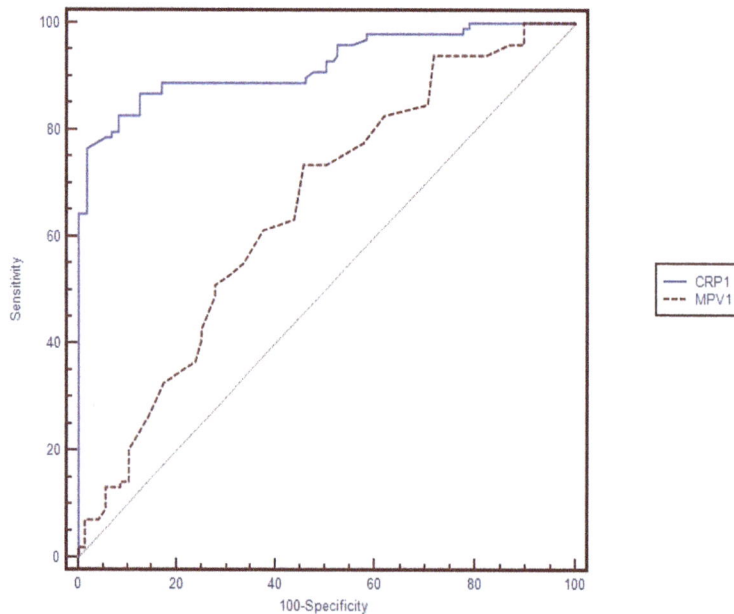

Fig. 5 Pairwise comparison of receiver operating characteristic (ROC) curves of C-reactive protein (CRP 1) and mean platelet volume (MPV 1) level on the first day of sepsis diagnosis in proven sepsis

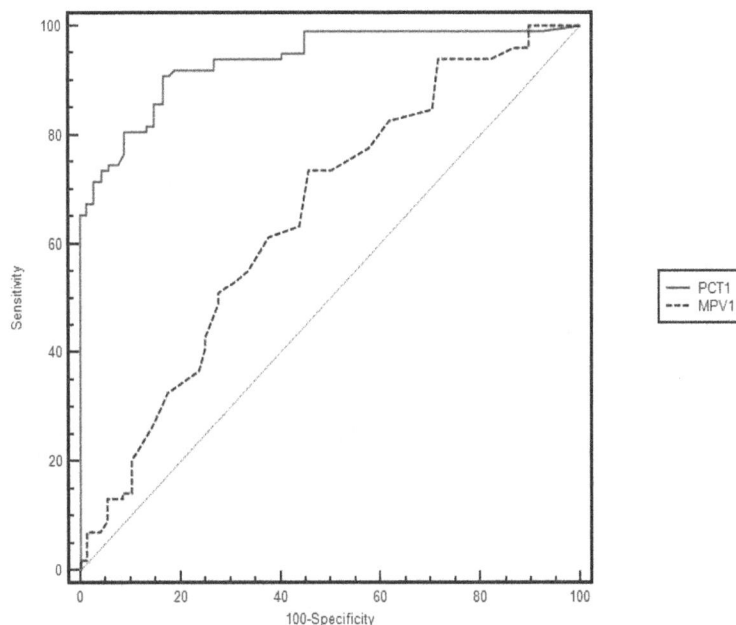

Fig. 6 Pairwise comparison of receiver operating characteristic (ROC) curves of mean platelet volume (MPV 1) and procalcitonin (PCT 1) level on the first day of sepsis diagnosis in proven sepsis

significantly higher in the LONS group than the premature newborns with EONS. We did not find any statistically significant difference in MPV level between patients with proven and clinical sepsis. But in proven sepsis group, we determined significantly higher MPV 2 level than the premature newborns in clinical sepsis group.

Currently, PCT appears to be a specific alternative marker to CRP in the rapid diagnosis of sepsis. The cut-off levels of PCT in newborns with sepsis have been investigated in the literature. Falsely increased PCT concentrations have been reported for hospitalized newborns as a result of non-infectious, critical diseases [25–27]. Moreover, it has been reported that the PCT levels may be normal in severely infected newborns [26–28]. The clinical signs and symptoms of sepsis are silent; low or normal PCT levels may make the diagnosis of sepsis complex. Altunhan et al. compared the PCT levels between septic neonates and non-infectious patients for the diagnosis of EONS. They did not identify a difference between the levels at birth; however, at 24 h of age, the PCT levels were significantly higher in the newborns with suspected sepsis. At 24 h of age, they used a cut-off value of 5.38 ng/mL and determined that the specificity, sensitivity, PPV and NPV were increased when compared with the use of the cut-off value of 0.59 ng/mL at birth [29]. We did not identify a significant difference between the levels of PCT in EONS and LONS. In our study, the median PCT levels at birth and at 24 h of age were significantly higher in patients with proven sepsis. We also determined significant cut-off values for PCT 1

and PCT 2 levels for the diagnosis of proven sepsis. The PCT 1 and PCT 2 cut-off values were found to be 1.4 and 1.1 ng/mL, respectively (sensitivity: 90.8%/75.5%, specificity: 83.4%/81.2%, PPV: 70.6%/63.8% and NPV: 94.4%/88.3%). At a PCT 1 cut-off value of 1.1 ng/mL, the sensitivity, specificity, PPV and NPV were 78.6, 81.2, 64.7 and 89.6% respectively. In a recently published systematic review, it was reported that the evaluation of the clinical usefulness of PCT in ruling in or out neonatal sepsis, in particular EONS, was dependent on the study consistency [25]. In literature we could not find a study included the pairwise comparison of the performance of the parameters of CRP, MPV and PCT in premature neonatal sepsis patients. In this study, the performance of CRP 1 and PCT 1 were found to be significantly higher than the performance of MPV 1 in each sepsis sub-group other than EONS. We did not find a significant cut-off level of birth MPV for the diagnosis of EONS, so pairwise comparisons did not include this parameter. The performances of CRP 1 and PCT 1 did not differ in each sub-group. In the literature, it was reported that serial PCT measurements, not only at the time of clinical suspicion of sepsis but also after 24 h, may be helpful in differentiating between sepsis and noninfectious conditions [28]. In septic neonates who had PCT levels higher than 0.59 ng/mL at birth, the authors determined that these levels subsequently further increased, whereas no significant elevation was identified in the non-infectious group. Although it was reported that increasing PCT levels were valuable for sepsis diagnosis, we did not find a similar elevation in PCT levels [28]. Moreover, we found significantly decrease in PCT levels from the first day values in sepsis groups. In a recently published multicentre study, it was reported that PCT-guided follow up the neonates resulted in a significant reduction in therapy duration. Neonates with EONS were categorized free of PCT values in their study. The normal ranges of PCT were determined according to the birth hours. For the first hours of birth, they accepted the normal ranges of PCT to be 0–0.5 ng/mL. The accepted normal upper range increased to 10 ng/mL in the 36th hours of birth [16].

Our study had some limitations for these measurements. It was not prospective so we could not measure these parameters in the following hours and days of sepsis diagnosis. As we have mentioned in the Methods section, the time interval of blood sampling for these measurements was a part of neonatal sepsis protocol in our hospital. And we could not compare the laboratory parameters between the preterm and full-term neonates, because our study population did not include full-term patients.

In our study, in the proven sepsis group, the isolated pathogens from the blood were approximately equally divided among Gram-negative ($n = 50$, 51%) and Gram-positive ($n = 48$, 49.0%) organisms. The two most common Gram-negative pathogens responsible from sepsis were *Escherichia coli* (22/98, 22.4%), and *Klebsiella pneumoniae* ($n = 20/98$, 20.4%). ESBL production was detected in 13 *E. coli*/*K. pneumoniae* isolates. Methicillin resistance was detected in 82% *S. aureus/epidermidis* isolates. In EONS sepsis, Gram-positive bacteria were more common (27/46, 58.7%), whereas Gram-negative pathogens (30/52, 57.7%) were more commonly isolated from the blood of infants with LONS. Celik et al. determined that Gram-positive bacteria were more common among infants from both EONS and LONS groups [2]. In another published study, it was reported that among the blood culture results of 401 neonatal infants, the most isolated microorganisms were *S. aureus/epidermidis* and Group B Streptococci (GBS) [30]. In our study, GBS did not appear more prominently in the culture positive EONS group. We think it may be due to reduction in GBS infections, owing to the use of intra-partum antibiotic prophylaxis. In literature it was reported that the incidence of EONS due to GBS was decreased because of the same reason [31]. In our control group, no deaths were recorded, whereas 20.6% of premature infants died in the sepsis group. This finding was similar to the literature [28]. *S. epidermidis* was the most commonly isolated Gram-positive pathogen. Although this microorganism in culture may suggest contamination, from the literature it was known that it can be pathogenic in neonates with indwelling vascular catheters or other devices [32]. Our study patients were all preterm and most of them had vascular catheters and other invasive devices.

Conclusions
We determined that the PCT and CRP levels and the MPV measurements are significantly higher in the preterm patients with sepsis. The cut-off levels of CRP and PCT may differ in these subgroups. Furthermore the performances of these tests were found to be different in the diagnosis of premature sepsis subgroups. Although no significantly difference was found between the performances of CRP and PCT measurement in sepsis subgroups, we found that PCT and CRP had higher performances than MPV for the first 24 h of diagnosis of preterm neonatal sepsis.

Abbreviations
AUC: Area under curve; CI: Confidence interval; CLSI: Clinical and laboratory standarts institude; CRP: C-reactive protein; *E. coli*: *Escherichia coli*; ECLIA: Electrochemiluminescence immunoassay; EONS: Early-onset neonatal sepsis; ESBL: Extended-spectrum beta lactamase; *K. pneumonia*: *Klebsiella pneumonia*; LONS: Late-onset neonatal sepsis; MPV: Mean platelet volume; NPV: Negative predictive value; PCT: Procalcitonin; PPV: Positive predictive value; ROC: Receiver operating characteristic; *S. aureus*: *Staphylococcus aureus*; *S. epidermidis*: *Staphylococcus epidermidis*

Authors' contributions
The study was designed by CA. The data was acquired by CA and HA. Drafting of manuscript was made by CA and HA. Analysis and interpretation of data were made by HA and FK. Critical revisions were made by AGM and CK. The major author is CA. All authors read and approved the manuscript.

Competing interests
The authors declare that they have no competing interests.

Author details
[1]Department of Pediatrics, Medical Faculty, Division of Neonatology, Bülent Ecevit University, Zonguldak, Turkey. [2]Department of Infectious Diseases and Clinical Microbiology, Medical Faculty, Bulent Ecevit University, 67600 Zonguldak, Turkey. [3]Department of Biostatistics, Medical Faculty, Bulent Ecevit University, Zonguldak, Turkey. [4]Department of Microbiology, Medical Faculty, Bulent Ecevit University, Zonguldak, Turkey. [5]Department of Biochemistry, Medical Faculty, Bulent Ecevit University, Zonguldak, Turkey.

References
1. Mussap M, Noto A, Cibecchini F, Fanos V. The importance of biomarkers in neonatology. Semin Fetal Neonatal Med. 2013;18:56–64.
2. Celik HT, Portakal O, Yigit S, Hascelik G, Korkmaz A, Yurdakok M. Efficacy of new leukocyte parameters versus serum C-reactive protein, procalcitonin, and interleukin-6 in the diagnosis of neonatal sepsis. Pediatr Int. 2016;58:119–25.
3. Benitz WE. Adjunct laboratory tests in the diagnosis of early-onset neonatal sepsis. Clin Perinatol. 2010;37:421–38.
4. Gerdes JS. Diagnosis and management of bacterial infections in the neonate. Pediatr Clin N Am. 2004;51:939–59.
5. Chiesa C, Natale F, Pascone R, Osborn JF, Pacisico L, Bonci E, et al. C reactive protein and procalcitonin: reference intervals for preterm and term newborns during the early neonatal period. Clin Cim Acta. 2011;412:1053–9.

6.   Turner D, Hammerman C, Rudensky B, Schlesinger Y, Goia C, Schimmel MS. Procalcitonin in preterm infants during the first few days of life: introducing an age related nomogram. Arch Dis Child Fetal Neonatal Ed. 2006;91:F283–6.

7.   Modanlou HD, Ortiz OB. Thrombocytopenia in neonatal infection. Clin Pediatr (Phila). 1982;20:402–7.

8.   Storm W. Use of thrombocytopenia for the early identification of sepsis in critically ill newborns. Acta Paediatr Acad Sci Hung. 1982;23:349–55.

9.   Stephan F, Hollande J, Richard O, Cheffi A, Maier-Redelsperger M, Flahault A. Thrombocytopenia in a surgical ICU. Chest. 1999;115:1363–70.

10. Strauss R, Wehler M, Mehler K, Kreutzer D, Koebnick C, Hahn EG. Thrombocytopenia in patients in the medical intensive care unit: bleeding prevalence, transfusion requirements, and outcome. Crit Care Med. 2002; 30:1765–71.

11. Vanderschueren S, De Weerdt A, Malbrain M, Vankersschaever D, Frans E, Wilmer A, et al. Thrombocytopenia and prognosis in intensive care. Crit Care Med. 2000;28:1871–6.

12. Jackson SR, Carter JM. Platelet volume: laboratory measurement and clinical application. Blood Rev. 1993;7:104–13.

13. Becchi C, Al Malyan M, Fabbri LP, Marsili M, Boddi V, Boncinelli S. Mean platelet volume trend in sepsis: is it a useful parameter? Minerva Anestesiol. 2006;72:749–56.

14. Cohen-Wolkowiez M, Moran C, Benjamin DK, Cotton CM, Clark RH, Benjamin DK Jr, Smith PB. Early and late onset sepsis in late preterm infants. Pediatr Infect Dis J. 2009;28:1052–6.

15. Wheeler DS, Wong HR, Zingarelli B. Pediatric Sepsis - Part I: "Children are not small adults!". Open Inflamm J. 2011;4:4–15.

16. Stocker M, van Herk W, el Helou S, Dutta S, Fontana MS, Schuerman FABA, et al. Procalcitonin-guided decision making for duration of antibiotic therapy in neonates with suspected early-onset sepsis: a multicentre, randomised controlled trial (NeoPIns). Lancet. 2017;390:871–81.

17. Guida JD, Kunig AM, Leef KH, McKenzie SE, Paul DA. Platelet count and sepsis in very low birth weight neonates: is there any organism-spesific response? Pediatrics. 2003;111:1411–5.

18. Hofer N, Zacharias E, Müller W, Resch B. An update on the use of C-reactive protein in early-onset neonatal sepsis: current insights and new tasks. Neonatology. 2012;102:25–36.

19. Ng PC, Lam HS. Diagnostic markers for neonatal sepsis. Curr Opin Pediatr. 2006;18:125–31.

20. Celik IH, Demirel FG, Uras N, Oguz SS, Erdeve O, Biyikli Z, Dilmen U. What are the cut-off levels for IL-6 and CRP in neonatal sepsis? J Clin Lab Anal. 2010;24:407–12.

21. Omran A, Maarof A, Saleh MS, Abdelwahab A. Salivary C-reactive protein, mean platelet volume and neutrophil lymphocyte ratio as diagnostic markers for neonatal sepsis. J Pediatr (Rio J). 2018;94:82–7.

22. Patrick CH, Lazarchick J. The effect of bacteremia on automated platelet measurement in neonates. Am J Clin Pathol. 1990;93:391–4.

23. Oncel MY, Ozdemir R, Yurttutan S, Canpolat FE, Erdeve O, Oguz SS, et al. Mean platelet volume in neonatal sepsis. J Clin Lab Anal. 2012;26:493–6.

24. Cekmez F, Tanju IA, Canpolat FE, Aydinoz S, Aydemir G, Karademir F, et al. Mean platelet volume in very preterm infants: a predictor of morbidities? Eur Rev Med Pharmacol Sci. 2013;17:134–7.

25. Chiesa C, Pacifico L, Osborn JF, Bonci E, Hofer N, Resch B. Early-onset neonatal sepsis: still room for improvement in procalcitonin diagnostic accuracy studies. Medicine (Baltimore). 2015;94:e1230. https://doi.org/10. 1097/MD.0000000000001230.

26. Monneret G, Labaune JM, Isaac C, Bienvenu F, Putet G, Bienvenu J. Procalcitonin and C-reactive protein levels in neonatal infections. Acta Paediatr. 1997;86:209–12.

27. Lapillonne A, Basson E, Monneret G, Bienvenu J, Salle BL. Lack of specificity of procalcitonin for sepsis diagnosis in premature infants. Lancet. 1998;351: 1211–2.

28. Chiesa C, Panero A, Rossi N, Stegagno M. Reliability of procalcitonin concentrations for the diagnosis of sepsis in critically ill neonates. Clin Infect Dis. 1998;26:664–72.

29. Altunhan H, Annagür A, Örs R, Mehmetoğlu I. Procalcitonin measurement at 24 hours of age may be helpful in the prompt diagnosis of early-onset neonatal sepsis. Int J Infect Dis. 2011;15:e854–8. https://doi.org/10.1016/j.ijid. 2011.09.007.

30. Ohlin A, Björkqvist M, Montgomery SC, Schollin J. Clinical signs and CRP values associated with blood culture results in neonates evaluated for suspected sepsis. Acta Pediatr. 2010;99:1635–40.

31. Bauserman MS, Laughon MM, Hornik CP, Smith PB, Benjamin DK Jr, Clark RH, et al. Group B Streptococcus and Escherichia coli infections in the intensive care nursery in the era of intrapartum antibiotic prophylaxis. Pediatr Infect Dis J. 2013;32:208–12.

32. Nizet V, Klein JO. Bacterial sepsis and meningitis. In: Remington JS, et al., editors. Infectious diseases of the fetus and newborn nfant. 8th ed. Philadelphia: Elsevier Saunders; 2016. p. 217.

33. European Medicines Agency (EMA). Report on the Expert Meeting on Neonatal and Pediatric Sepsis, EMA/477725/2010. www.ema.europa.eu/ docs/en_GB/document_library/Report/2010/12/WC500100199.pdf. Accessed 16 Dec 2010.

3

Indirect neonatal hyperbilirubinemia in hospitalized neonates on the Thai-Myanmar border: a review of neonatal medical records from 2009 to 2014

L. Thielemans[1,2]*[iD], M. Trip-Hoving[1], J. Landier[1], C. Turner[3,4,5], T. J. Prins[1], E. M. N. Wouda[1,6], B. Hanboonkunupakarn[7], C. Po[1], C. Beau[1], M. Mu[1], T. Hannay[8], F. Nosten[1,3], B. Van Overmeire[2], R. McGready[1,3] and V. I. Carrara[1]

Abstract

Background: Indirect neonatal hyperbilirubinemia (INH) is a common neonatal disorder worldwide which can remain benign if prompt management is available. However there is a higher morbidity and mortality risk in settings with limited access to diagnosis and care. The manuscript describes the characteristics of neonates with INH, the burden of severe INH and identifies factors associated with severity in a resource-constrained setting.

Methods: We conducted a retrospective evaluation of anonymized records of neonates hospitalized on the Thai-Myanmar border. INH was defined according to the National Institute for Health and Care Excellence guidelines as 'moderate' if at least one serum bilirubin (SBR) value exceeded the phototherapy threshold and as 'severe' if above the exchange transfusion threshold.

Results: Out of 2980 records reviewed, 1580 (53%) had INH within the first 14 days of life. INH was moderate in 87% (1368/1580) and severe in 13% (212/1580). From 2009 to 2011, the proportion of severe INH decreased from 37 to 15% and the mortality dropped from 10% (8/82) to 2% (7/449) coinciding with the implementation of standardized guidelines and light-emitting diode (LED) phototherapy. Severe INH was associated with: prematurity (< 32 weeks, Adjusted Odds Ratio (AOR) 3.3; 95% CI 1.6–6.6 and 32 to 37 weeks, AOR 2.2; 95% CI 1.6–3.1), Glucose-6-phosphate dehydrogenase deficiency (G6PD) (AOR 2.3; 95% CI 1.6–3.3), potential ABO incompatibility (AOR 1.5; 95% CI 1.0–2.2) and late presentation (AOR 1.8; 95% CI 1.3–2.6). The risk of developing severe INH and INH-related mortality significantly increased with each additional risk factor.

Conclusion: INH is an important cause of neonatal hospitalization on the Thai-Myanmar border. Risk factors for severity were similar to previous reports from Asia. Implementing standardized guidelines and appropriate treatment was successful in reducing mortality and severity. Accessing to basic neonatal care including SBR testing, LED phototherapy and G6PD screening can contribute to improve neonatal outcomes.

Keywords: Indirect neonatal hyperbilirubinemia, Jaundice, (LED-) phototherapy, Neonates, Low-resource, Refugee, Migrant, Resource-limited setting, Mortality

* Correspondence: thielemans.laurence@gmail.com
[1]Shoklo Malaria Research Unit, Mahidol-Oxford Tropical Medicine Research Unit, Faculty of Tropical Medicine, Mahidol University, Mae Sot, Thailand
[2]Neonatology-Pediatrics, Cliniques Universitaires de Bruxelles - Hôspital Erasme, Université Libre de Bruxelles, Brussels, Belgium
Full list of author information is available at the end of the article

Background

Jaundice caused by indirect neonatal hyperbilirubinemia (INH) is a common condition and a frequent cause for admission in health care facilities all around the world [1]. Without timely admission and appropriate management, INH can lead to devastating neurologic disorders [1]. Cerebral palsy, auditory disturbances and gaze abnormalities are classical sequelae of INH [2–4]. Worldwide, 80% of severe INH occurs in resource-limited settings with an estimated mortality rate of 25% and with a 13% risk of developing neurological sequelae [1, 5, 6]. In settings with poor access to care, prematurity and Glucose-6-phosphate dehydrogenase (G6PD) deficiency are important causes of INH [1, 7, 8]. Though phototherapy is a proven and cost effective tool to treat INH, it is not accessible to more than 6 million (~ 45%) of at-risk infants worldwide [9]. Unavailable treatment has clinical, public health, and economic impact for both the health care and education systems [5].The 2013 Lancet report on the Global Burden of Disease added INH to the list of estimated causes of death [10] and it was recognized as an important neonatal condition that deserves global health attention in the post-2015 millennium development goal era [5]. Routine reporting of jaundice data at all health care levels has yet to be implemented as most national records report jaundice incidence rate based on tertiary health care studies or registries. In Asia, the latest national incidence estimates vary widely from 7% in Indonesia, 15% in India, 46% in Myanmar and up to 49% in China [5, 6]. In Myanmar jaundice is the most common reason for private and public hospitals admission of neonates [11]. According to the National Hospital Statistic Report, it is the leading cause of morbidity in neonates (37.8%), responsible for 7.4% of the neonatal mortality [12]. In 2008, in Maela, a refugee camp in Thailand for displaced Myanmar people, Shoklo Malaria Research Unit (SMRU) reported an increasing number of neonates admitted for phototherapy in their newly established neonatal unit once recognition of the condition by the local health staff had improved. By 2011, INH became the most common reason for hospitalization in this particular setting [13] but the characteristics of neonates with INH, burden of severe INH and its associated risk factors were not known. We therefore conducted a retrospective analysis of all medical records of neonates admitted at SMRU clinics between 2009 and 2014 with the aim of addressing this knowledge gap. The objective of this manuscript is to describe the characteristics of neonates with INH, estimate the burden of severe INH and identify factors associated with severity; to develop evidence-based recommendations to further reduce INH morbidity and mortality in the area.

Methods

This was an analysis of anonymized medical records of neonates born with a gestational age of 28 weeks or more, admitted either at birth or after discharge from the postnatal ward but within 28 days of life to one of the SMRU Special Care Baby Units between January 1, 2009 and December 31, 2014.

Setting

SMRU is located in Tak province, Northwestern Thailand (Additional file 1). It is an operational field-based research unit combining humanitarian work with research of direct relevance to the local migrant and refugee population. In contrast to refugees, migrants are highly mobile and may have difficulties to access the clinics. SMRU facilities offer basic emergency obstetric and postnatal care; women requiring caesarian section are referred to the nearest Thai hospital within 30–60 min driving time from the clinics. There was no specialized neonatal care facility until 2008 when the first Special Care Baby Unit was established in Maela refugee camp [13], and in 2011, in two additional clinics serving the migrant population. The units provided basic neonatal care including oxygen, intravenous antibiotics, nasogastric feeding and phototherapy. Chest X-ray, assisted ventilation, parenteral feeding and exchange transfusion were not available. Live born neonates with a gestational age below 28 weeks were provided with palliative care [13]. The mortality in this age group approached 100% [14].

Laboratory tests were conducted upon physician request and restricted to blood group testing, hematocrit reading, microscopic examination of urine sediment and cerebrospinal fluid, and serum bilirubin levels (SBR) measurement using a bilirubinometer (Pfaff Medical Bilimeter 2 and 3). Universal G6PD testing of all newborns was not available but the fluorescent spot test [15] was used in cases of INH.

Clinical approach of INH

The decision to use phototherapy was initially based on the Kramer's scale [16]. Once SBR was available at the clinic, SBR gradually replaced Kramer's scale as the primary decision tool for treatment. Records with an SBR level were available from 2009 in the refugee clinic and 2012 in the migrant clinics (Fig. 1). Guidelines to start phototherapy have changed over time (Fig. 1) and since 2011 the British National Institute for Health and Care Excellence (NICE) guidelines have been used [17]. Those guidelines base the need for treatment on thresholds varying by gestational age at birth (https://www.nice.org.uk/guidance/cg98/evidence).

Light intensity was routinely measured with a digital lightmeter (Lightmeter by Medical Technology Transfer

Time line		2008	2009	2010	2011	2012	2013	2014
Setting	*Refugees*	*Special ward dedicated for neonatal care*						
	Migrants	Post-partum ward			Special ward dedicated for neonatal care			
Data management	*Refugees*		*Digitalized data*					
	Migrants				Digitalized data			
Staff	*Refugees*	*Midwives*	*Trained medics, nurses and midwives* *Regular refresher trainings*					
	Migrants	Midwives			Trained medics, nurses and midwives Regular refresher trainings			
Guidelines	*Refugees*	*Local guidelines*			*NICE guidelines*			
	Migrants	Local guidelines				NICE guidelines		
Diagnostic	*Refugees*	*Kramer Zone*	*Serum bilirubin (but systematically used for all jaundice cases from 2011 onwards only)*					
	Migrants	Kramer Zone				Serum bilirubin		
Risk factors assessment		Tested on site: ABO-blood group, CSF-White blood cells count, hematocrit, microscopic urine examination and fluorescent G6PD spot test						
Treatment	*Refugees*	*Sun light*	*Home built phototherapy units with fluorescent light*	*Home built phototherapy units with blue light bulbs (wavelength 315-400nm)*	*LED units*		LED units and possibility to transfer for exchange transfusion to a tertiary Thai hospital	
	Migrants		Sun light				LED units	

Fig. 1 Evolution of care over time. Treatment, diagnostic tools, guidelines and experience of the staff developed over time. Cut off values for phototherapy was based on different guidelines and the type of phototherapy available changed: home built phototherapy units with fluorescent light were available initially and then manufactured bulbs (Philips TL20 W) were used until LED-lights became available. In 2013, collaboration with a tertiary hospital in Thailand was set up to refer neonates who needed exchange transfusion. The condition for referral was a bilirubin more than 550 μmol/L not responding to phototherapy

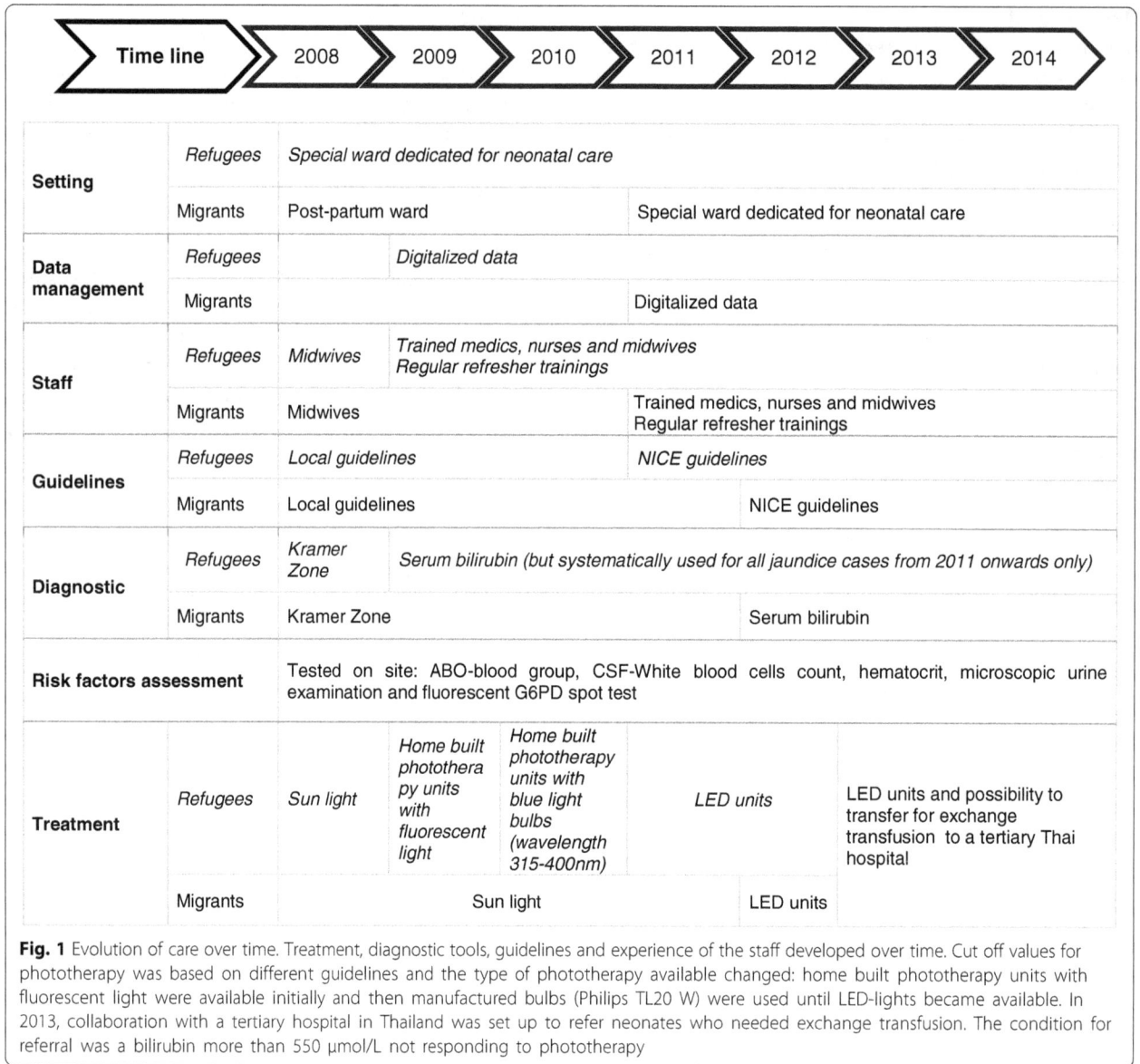

and Services Ltd) prior to starting phototherapy and the conditions were optimized to have the best intensity possible depending on the type of phototherapy available. Data on light intensity or type of phototherapy used per neonate were not available.

Jaundice cases classification
Digital records with a diagnosis of jaundice were classified into three categories: i) clinical jaundice without laboratory confirmation (excluded from the analysis), ii) "moderate" INH if at least one SBR value exceeded the phototherapy threshold of the NICE graphs and iii) "severe" INH if at least one SBR value exceeded the SBR exchange transfusion threshold of the NICE graphs. The NICE guidelines did not provide specific recommendations for the treatment of neonates older than 14 days,

thus neonates with phototherapy started after 2 weeks of life were excluded from the analysis [17].

Variables definitions
Relevant variables used for this analysis were birth history, maternal and newborn characteristics, age and diagnosis on admission; additional diagnosis during hospitalization, laboratory results and outcome at discharge.

Primigravida was defined upon registration to antenatal care as first pregnancy (gravidity 1 parity 0). Maternal literacy was defined on the basis of self-reported ability to read. Gestational age was defined by ultrasound [18] or by Dubowitz score [19] for late presenters to the antenatal consultation (after 24 weeks gestation) and classified as very preterm (28 to < 32 weeks), late preterm (32 to < 37 weeks) and term (≥ 37 weeks) following the recommendations of WHO [20].

Instrumental delivery included both vacuum and forceps delivery. Birthweight was considered valid if measured within the first 72 h of life [21, 22] and small-for-gestational-age (SGA) was a birth weight below the 10th percentile of the normal fetal growth reference curve according to Interbio-21 international standards [23]. Every newborn routinely had a surface examination by a staff who had completed a locally developed training course. A standardized newborn examination sheet was completed and any suspected abnormal findings on surface examination and/or auscultation of the praecordium (heart and lungs) was confirmed by a medical doctor [13].

Reported diagnoses of sepsis, meningitis or pneumonia treated with intravenous antibiotics were regrouped into "severe infection". As laboratory confirmation of these diagnoses was not systematically performed or reported, it was not possible to validate clinically suspected cases. Mild infection was defined as any eye or skin infection treated with oral or topical antibiotics.

Rhesus testing was not available as rhesus incompatibility was deemed very unlikely in this population with very low rates of Rh negative individuals [24]. Coombs test wasn't available either, thus potential ABO incompatibility was considered for newborns of blood groups A or B born to mothers of blood group O. ABO incompatibility was considered unknown if only one of the pair (mother or neonate) had a known blood group [25].

Outcome at discharge was reported as "alive" or "died". The total number of livebirths (from 28 weeks' gestational age) was extracted from SMRU annual reports (http://www.shoklo-unit.com/) and used as denominator for evaluating the changes in proportion of neonates hospitalized with INH.

Statistical analysis

Statistical analysis was performed using SPSS (IBM SPSS Statistics Version 23, IBM Corporation) and Stata (StataCorp 2015, Version 14.1. College Station, Texas, StataCorp LP) softwares. Categorical variables were described using proportions and compared using the Chi-square test, Fisher's exact test or Chi-square test for trends; continuous variables were described by their mean and standard deviation and compared using t-test if normally distributed or by their median and interquartile range (IQR) and compared using Mann-Whitney test if non-normally distributed. Binomial or normal 95% confidence intervals (CI) were calculated for proportions or means as appropriate.

Two main outcomes were considered in the analysis: 1) severe INH and 2) late diagnosis (after 72 h of life). Clinical, demographic characteristics and factors associated with each outcome were identified by logistic regression. Univariate Odds Ratio (OR) and 95% CI were generated excluding missing values for a given variable. For each outcome, variables with p-values lower than 0.25 in univariable analysis, as well as risk-factors for INH described in the literature, were included in a multivariable model. The final model included all remaining variables with p-values below 0.05 and established risk factors for INH described in the literature.

Ethics statement

This retrospective analysis of anonymized data was exempted from formal ethical review (confirmed by Oxford Tropical Research Ethics Committee (OxTREC), UK on February 2017) and discussed with the Tak Province Border Community Ethics Advisory Board (T-CAB-01/FEV/2017).

Results

There were 2980 records of neonates hospitalized between 1st January 2009 and 31st December 2014, representing 23.0% of all live births ($n = 12,948$). Admission within the first 24 h of life contributed to 29.2% ($n = 871$) of hospitalizations. A diagnosis of jaundice was reported in 65.3% (1946/2980) hospitalized neonates of which 87.8% (1708/1946) had at least one SBR value and phototherapy details available. One hundred and twenty records with a maximum SBR level measured below the NICE treatment threshold and eight records with phototherapy started after 14 days of life were excluded. Among the remaining 1580 records, 1368 (86.6%) were classified as moderate INH and 212 (13.4%) as severe INH (Fig. 2). A total of 18,336 SBR measurements in 1580 records were available with a median of 6 SBR measurement [IQR: 3–11] per neonate, ranging from 1 SBR measurement ($n = 7$) to 43 SBR measurement ($n = 1$, recurrent INH). The median SBR value was 249 µmol/l ranging from 24 µmol/l to 1147 µmol/l.

INH trends

Several changes were observed over time (Table 1). Firstly, the proportion of neonates hospitalized with INH in the refugee population changed significantly; between 2009 and 2011 this proportion was low, ranging between 5.4 and 8.8% of all livebirths, but it increased from 2012 onwards to reach 21.8% of all live births ($n = 1102$) in 2014. Proportions observed in the migrant clinics for the period 2012–2014 increased from 10.6% (134/1270) to 14.6% (209/1430). Overall the proportion of INH in 2014 was 17.7% (Table 1). Secondly, the proportion of neonates hospitalized with INH as sole diagnosis increased from 35.4% in 2009 to 66.4% in 2014. Thirdly, INH was diagnosed 1 day

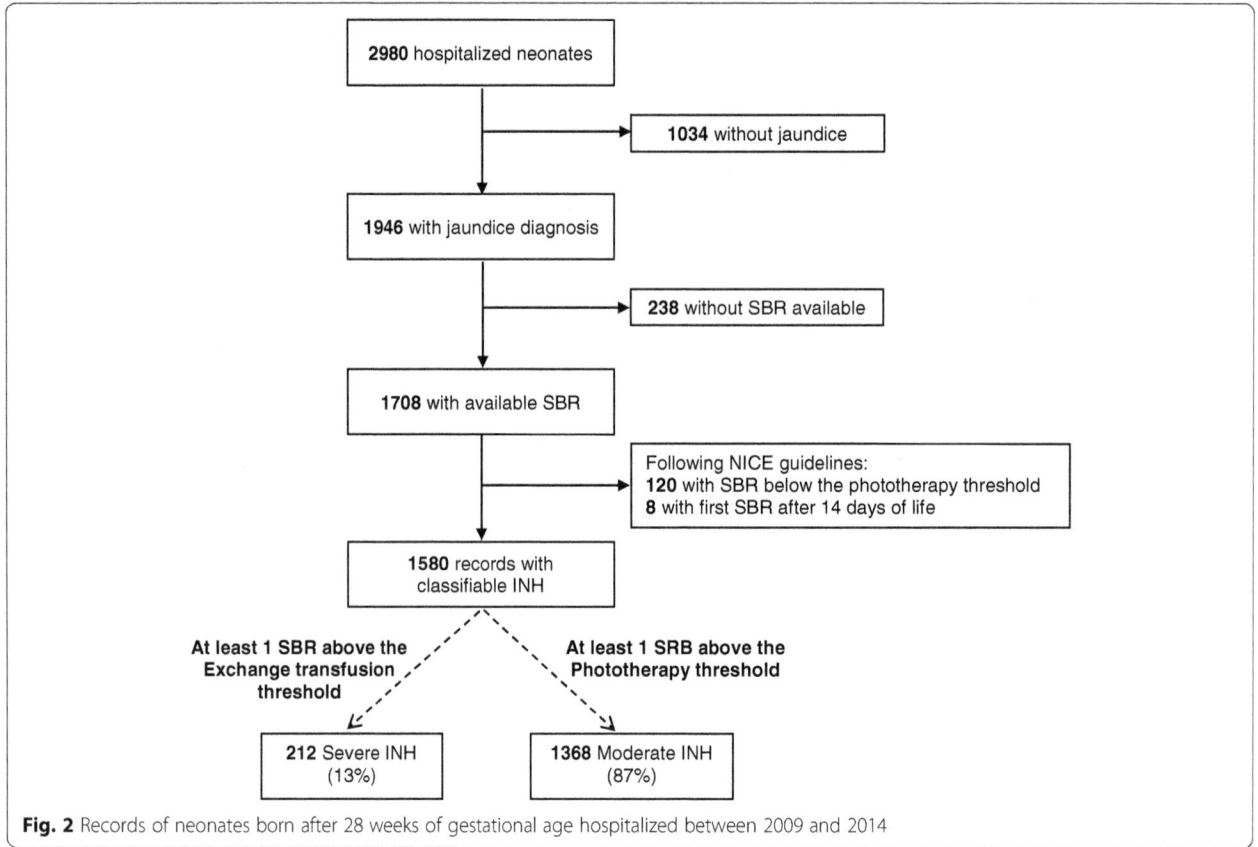

Fig. 2 Records of neonates born after 28 weeks of gestational age hospitalized between 2009 and 2014

Table 1 Changes in proportion of neonates hospitalized for indirect neonatal hyperbilirubinemia (INH), INH as sole clinical diagnosis, postnatal age at diagnosis, severity and mortality rate between 2009 and 2014

Time line	2009	2010	2011	2012	2013	2014
Data available						
Refugee site	✓	✓	✓	✓	✓	✓
Migrants sites				✓	✓	✓
SBR available						
Refugee site	✓	✓	✓	✓	✓	✓
Migrants sites				✓	✓	✓
NICE guidelines and LED phototherapy available [a]			✓	✓	✓	✓
Proportion of NH by total livebirth, n, (%)	82/1520 (5.4)	112/1381 (8.1)	114/1298 (8.8)	364/2573 (14.1)	459/2547 (18.0)	449/2532 (17.7)
NH as sole clinical diagnosis in proportion of total NH [b], n (%)	29/82 (35.4)	48/112 (42.9)	61/114 (53.5)	195/364 (53.6)	280/459 (61.0)	298/449 (66.4)
Postnatal age at diagnosis in hours, median, [IQR]	74.5 [48–106]	73.5 [22–122]	67.5 [47–102]	53.5 [37–91]	52 [33–77]	49 [33–81]
Severe INH in proportion of total INH, n (%)	30/82 (36.6)	39/112 (34.8)	17/114 (14.9)	46/364 (12.6)	43/459 (9.4)	37/449 (8.2)
Mortality rate in neonates with severe INH, n (%)	7/30 (23.3)	4/39 (10.3)	2/17 (11.8)	3/46 (6.5)	1/43 (2.3)	0/37 (0.0)

✓Availability of data, SBR, NICE guidelines and LED phototherapy by sites
[a]NICE guidelines and LED phototherapy became available in 2011 for all sites
[b]Clinical diagnoses do not include prematurity, G6PD deficiency or potential ABO incompatibility

Table 2 Characteristics of 1580 neonates with indirect neonatal hyperbilirubinemia (INH)

Characteristics	Neonates with INH n=1580[a]
Maternal characteristics	
Site, n (%)	
Refugee	1056 (66.8)
Migrant	524 (33.2)
Ethnicity, n (%)	
Karen	1165/1546 (75.4)
Burman	258/1546 (16.7)
Other	123/1546 (8.0)
Age in years, median, (IQR)	24 (20–30) n = 1579
Literacy, n (%)	947/1442 (56.7)
Smoking, n (%)	222/1574 (14.1)
Primigravida, n (%)	763 (48.3)
Multiple pregnancy, n (%)	61 (3.9)
Place of birth, n (%)	
SMRU	1423 (90.1)
Tertiary hospital	68 (4.3)
Home	77 (4.9)
Other	12 (0.8)
Type of delivery	
Normal vaginal delivery, n (%)	1427 (90.3)
Breech and face delivery, n (%)	49 (3.1)
Instrumental vaginal delivery, n (%)	62 (3.9)
Caesarian section, n (%)	42 (2.7)
Newborn characteristics	
Gestational age, n (%)	
< 32 weeks	53/1578 (3.4)
32 < 37 weeks	437/1578 (27.7)
> 37 weeks	1088/1578 (68.9)
Gender (male), n (%)	922 (58.4)
Small for gestational age, n (%)	297/1554 (19.1)
Congenital abnormality, n (%)	44 (2.8)
Hospitalization characteristics	
INH as sole clinical diagnosis[b], n (%)	911 (57.7)
Infection	
Severe infection, n (%)	296 (18.7)
Mild infection, n (%)	206 (13.0)
Age in days at admission, median, (IQR)	2 (1–3)
Age in hours at presentation of INH, median, (IQR)	55 [36–92]
Length of stay in days, median, (IQR)	
1–3 days	588 (37.2)
> 3–5 days	307 (19.4)
> 5–8 days	323 (35.1)

Table 2 Characteristics of 1580 neonates with indirect neonatal hyperbilirubinemia (INH) *(Continued)*

Characteristics	Neonates with INH n=1580[a]
> 8 days	362 (39.3)
Mortality during hospitalization, n (%)	31 (2.0)

[a]Denominator unless stated otherwise
[b]Clinical diagnoses do not include prematurity, G6PD deficiency or potential ABO incompatibility

earlier in 2014 compared to 2009 (Table 1) and it became the most common diagnosis among hospitalized neonates from 2012 onwards.

The proportion of severe INH among confirmed cases which represented over one third of the confirmed INH in 2009–2010 was reduced by half in 2011 and the decreasing trend persisted until 2014, although at a slower pace (Table 1). Overall the proportion of severe INH in 2014 was 1.5% of all livebirths.

Mortality, among neonates with severe INH, initially 23.3% in 2009, significantly decreased over the years to reach zero in 2014 (Table 1). Mortality rate remained constant and low among neonates with moderate INH.

General characteristics of neonates with INH

Maternal, obstetric and neonatal characteristics of neonates hospitalized with INH are shown in Table 2. Half of them (52.8%) had a primiparous mother and one third (31.1%) were born preterm (Table 2). INH was the sole diagnosis reported in 57.7% of the records (Table 2). The three most common factors associated with INH among term neonates were G6PD deficiency (219/1088, 20.1%), potential ABO incompatibility (202/1088, 18.6%) and severe infection (202/1088, 18.6%). Ten neonates (0.6%) with INH were referred to the Thai tertiary hospital for further care of whom 4 received exchange transfusion.

Most INH cases were diagnosed within the first 72 h of life (1009/1580, 63.9%) (Fig. 3). The proportion of neonates with severe INH within the 72 first hours of life was 9.4% (95/1009) and significantly lower ($p < 0.001$) compared to the 20.5% (117/571) of severe INH diagnosed later (> 72 h).

Whilst the proportion of INH cases with G6PD deficiency was equally distributed over the 14 first days of life, there were some striking differences between neonates presenting with an early INH ($\leq$ 72 h of life, $n = 1009$) or late INH (> 72 h of life, $n = 571$) (Additional file 2). After adjustment for other variables, very preterm (< 32 weeks), potential ABO incompatibility and breech or face delivery were independently associated with a diagnosis before 72 h while delivery outside the clinic, severe infection and

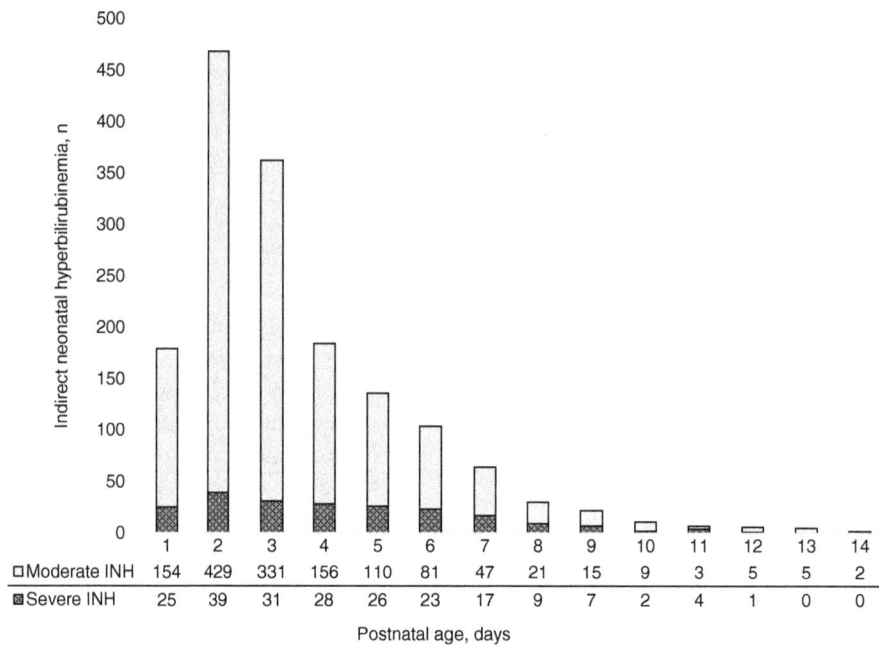

	1	2	3	4	5	6	7	8	9	10	11	12	13	14
☐Moderate INH	154	429	331	156	110	81	47	21	15	9	3	5	5	2
▨Severe INH	25	39	31	28	26	23	17	9	7	2	4	1	0	0

Postnatal age, days

Fig. 3 Timing of first serum bilirubin confirming the degree of severity of INH. Each neonate is represented once, when the SBR measurement reached the moderate threshold (and never passed the severe threshold) or reached the severe threshold for the first time in the first 14 days of life

severe INH were associated with a later diagnosis (Additional file 2).

Characteristics of neonates with severe INH

Seventy-nine of the 212 (37.3%) neonates with severe INH were first treated for moderate INH at a median postnatal age of 48 h IQR [29–88] and later developed severe INH at a median postnatal age of 97 h IQR [64–136] while 133 (62.7%) presented for the first time with a SBR measurement above the severe threshold line at a median postnatal age of 70 h IQR [33–126].

Factors independently associated with severity after adjustment for variables listed in Table 3 were: very premature (Adjusted Odds Ratio (AOR) 3.3; 95% CI 1.6–6.6) and late premature (AOR 2.2; 95% CI 1.6–3.1); or with a congenital abnormality (AOR 2.4; 95% CI 1.1–5.3). Severe infection (AOR 1.8; 95% CI 1.2–2.7), G6PD-deficiency (AOR 2.3; 95% CI 1.6–3.3) and potential ABO incompatibility (AOR 1.5; 95% CI 1.0–2.2) were also associated to severe INH (Table 3).

The risk of death was 8-times higher in severe INH; 17/212, 8.0% vs. moderate INH; 14/1368, 1.0%, $p < 0.001$ (Table 3) and the risk of INH-related death increased by 3.2 fold (95% CI; 2.1–4.8) with each additional risk factors.

Prematurity was the sole factor reported in 20.3% (43/212) of the neonates with severe INH and severe infection was the most commonly additional factor in preterm neonates (31%, 31/100). G6PD deficiency was the

most common factor associated with severe INH among term neonates (32.1%, 36/112), followed by severe infection (22.3%, 25/112) and potential ABO incompatibility (20.5%, 23/112). Overall, the risk to develop severe INH increased significantly with each added risk factor (Table 4).

Discussion

This retrospective analysis confirmed that, with nearly 18% of all livebirths treated for INH, the burden of the disease in this resource-limited area is almost double the worldwide estimates of 10.5% of livebirths that require phototherapy annually [9]. In addition, the high proportion of severe INH and its related mortality contrast with data from high income countries [26] and reinforce the evidence that low-income countries bear the greatest burden of severe INH [1, 26].

The caseload of severe cases was higher in the early years of the Special Baby Care Units while the visual assessment of jaundice was still commonly used. Visual assessment by Kramer zones can be safely used to rule out INH in healthy term neonates if jaundice is limited to the head and torso [27, 28] and might detect severe INH when jaundice has progressed to zones 4 and 5 [29]; however it correlates poorly with measured bilirubin and has limitation for preventing severe INH [28]. The delayed laboratory confirmation likely contributed to the high proportion of severe INH and the higher mortality rate reported during that period.

Table 3 Maternal and newborn characteristics of moderate and severe INH and factors associated with severe INH

Characteristics	Moderate INH, n=1368[a]	Severe INH, n=212[a]	OR [95%CI]	p-value	AOR[b] [95%CI]	p-value
Maternal characteristics						
Site, n (%)						
Migrant	464 (33.9)	60 (28.3)	1	0.107	–	–
Refugee	904 (66.1)	152 (71.7)	1.3 [0.9–1.8]		–	
Ethnicity, n (%)						
Karen	1014/1348 (75.2)	151/198 (76.3)	1	0.434	–	–
Burman	230/1348 (17.1)	28/198 (13.2)	0.8 [0.5–1.2]		–	
Other	104/1348 (7.7)	19/198 (9.0)	1.2 [0.7–2.1]		–	
Age in years, median, (IQR)	24 (20–30)	23 (20–31)	1.0 [0.9–1.0]	0.777	–	–
Literacy, n (%)	846/1280 (66.1)	101/162 (62.3)	0.9 [0.6–1.2]	0.347	–	–
Smoking, n (%)	189/1364 (13.9)	33/210 (15.7)	1.2 [0.8–1.7]	0.477	–	–
Primigravida, n (%)	668 (48.8)	95 (44.8)	0.9 [0.6–1.1]	0.276	–	–
Multiple pregnancy, n (%)	52 (3.8)	9 (4.2)	1.1 [0.5–2.3]	0.758	–	–
Place of birth, n (%)						
SMRU	1241 (90.7)	182 (85.8)	1	0.011	–	–
Tertiary hospital	61 (4.5)	7 (3.3)	0.8 [0.4–1.7]		–	
Home	58 (4.2)	19 (9.0)	2.2 [1.3–3.8]		–	
Other	8 (0.6)	4 (1.9)	3.4 [1.0–11.4]		–	
Breech and face delivery, n (%)	36 (2.6)	13 (6.1)	2.4 [1.3–4.6]	0.008	2.0 [1.0–4.3]	0.056
Instrumental vaginal delivery, n (%)	58 (4.4)	4 (1.9)	0.4 [0.2–1.2]	0.073	–	–
Newborn characteristics						
Gender (male), n (%)	796 (58.2)	126 (59.7)	1.1 [0.8–1.4]	0.731	–	–
Small for gestational age, n (%)	251/1350 (18.6)	46/204 (15.5)	1.3 [0.9–1.8]	0.188	1.3 [0.9–2.0]	0.139
Gestational age, n (%)						
< 32 weeks	38/1367 (2.8)	15/211 (7.1)	3.5 [1.9–6.5]	< 0.001	3.3 [1.6–6.6]	< 0.001
32 < 37 weeks	352/1367 (25.7)	85/211 (40.3)	2.1 [1.6–2.9]		2.2 [1.6–3.1]	
≥ 37 weeks	977/1367 (71.5)	111/211 (52.6)	1		1	
Congenital abnormality, n (%)	34 (2.5)	10 (4.7)	1.9 [1.0–4.0]	0.089	2.4 [1.1–5.3]	0.027
G6PD deficiency, n (%)	213/1364 (15.6)	54 (25.5)	1.9 [1.3–2.6]	< 0.001	2.3 [1.6–3.3]	< 0.001
Potential ABO incompatibility, n (%)	238/1341 (17.7)	45/205 (22.0)	1.3 [0.9–1.9]	0.155	1.5 [1.0–2.2]	0.032
INH as sole clinical diagnosis, n (%)	814 (59.5)	97 (45.8)	1.7 [1.3–2.3]	< 0.001	–	–
Infection, n (%)						
No infection associated	955 (69.8)	123 (58.0)	1	0.003	1	0.006
Associated severe infection	240 (17.5)	56 (26.4)	1.8 [1.3–2.6]		1.8 [1.2–2.7]	
Associated mild infection	173 (12.6)	33 (15.6)	1.5 [0.9–2.3]		1.4 [0.9–2.2]	
Age at presentation, n (%)						
0–24 h	154 (11.3)	37 (17.5)	2.1 [1.4–3.3]	< 0.001	1.5 [0.9–2.4]	0.003
> 24–72 h	160 (55.6)	85 (40.1)	1		1	
> 72 h	454 (33.2)	90 (42.5)	1.8 [1.3–2.4]		1.8 [1.3–2.6]	
Length of phototherapy in hours, median, (IQR)	36 (22–66)	72 (43–133)	–	< 0.001	–	
Mortality during hospitalization, n, (%)	14 (1.0)	17 (8.0)	8.4 [4.1–17.4]	< 0.001	–	–

[a]Denominator unless stated otherwise
[b]Variables included in the final model were: 'Gestational age', 'small for gestational age', 'G6PD deficiency', 'potential ABO incompatibility', infection 'and variables with a p-value < 0.25 in univariable analysis. 'NH as sole clinical diagnosis' (correlated to 'Infection') and 'Place of birth' (correlated to 'Age at presentation') were not included in the final model. Only AOR and [95%CI] of known risk factors and of those remaining significant in the final model are reported in this table

Table 4 Impact of the cumulative number of risk factors on INH severity

Number of risk factors[a]	Moderate INH N = 1368	Severe INH N = 212	Severity OR [95%CI]
No associated factor, n (%)	523 (38.2)	43 (20.3)	1
One associated factor, n (%)	604 (44.2)	95 (44.8)	1.9 [1.3–2.8]
Combination of 2 factors, n (%)	212 (15.5)	54 (25.5)	3.1 [2.0–4.8]
Combination of 3 or 4 factors, n (%)	29 (2.1)	20 (9.4)	8.4 [4.4–16.1]

[a]The considered risk factors were prematurity, G6PD deficiency, potential ABO incompatibility, severe infection and congenital abnormality

After the introduction of the NICE guidelines and of LED-light in 2011, the proportion of severe INH was reduced by half despite the increased number of INH cases diagnosed. This suggests the key-role of increased staff awareness and training in using appropriate guidelines, and the effectiveness of the LED-lights. By providing light at the most effective wavelength ranges close to the infant, LED-lights may keep SBR below the severe threshold [30]. These findings confirm those of the study from Myanmar published in 2015 showing that provision of LED-light and staff's training using standard guidelines reduced severe INH rates drastically [31].

In addition to their impact on the severity of INH these improvements, combined with the possibility to refer for exchange transfusion, had an impact on its mortality which decreased 10-fold between 2009 and 2014.

Apart from prematurity, the three most commonly reported risk factors associated with severe INH in this setting were G6PD deficiency, severe infection and potential ABO incompatibility. They were similar to the risk factors reported previously for low and middle income countries [32].

The prevalence of G6PD deficiency (90% Mahidol variant) in this population is high: 13.7% in adult males [33] and 2–4% in adult females [34]. The increased risk of hyperbilirubinemia in G6PD-deficient neonates might have been further aggravated by an early exposure to naphthalene-containing mothballs used routinely by almost half of the local population [35]. The use of the qualitative fluorescent spot test rather than a quantitative test to diagnose G6PD deficiency in neonates might have underestimated its impact [36]; the G6PD FST has been described not to perform well in neonates possibly due to the higher G6PD activity in neonates then adults [36]. Despite this limitation, G6PD remains significantly associated with severe INH independently of the timing of presentation of INH. Those findings are consistent with those previously described worldwide [17, 37–40].

Potential ABO incompatibility was associated with severity and with an early presentation of INH which is consistent with findings from other studies [32, 41–44]. However, Coombs results were unavailable and the proportion of true ABO alloimmunisation causing INH in this population is still unknown [45, 46].

Nearly a fifth of neonates with INH were treated for a clinically-suspected severe infection. This high proportion of reported infections is consistent with that described in similar low and middle income Asian settings, where 10 to 30% of INH cases are attributed to infections [17, 47]. Its association with the severity of INH might however have been confounded by the similarity of symptoms of a severe infection and of severe INH, and constrained diagnostic laboratory capacity.

Prematurity is an established risk factor for INH [47] but in this particular setting, suboptimal care due to unavailability of parenteral feeding and assisted ventilation, combined with suboptimal visual assessment of jaundice in the preterm neonate [28] might have contributed to the higher rate of severe cases or to the progression from INH to severe INH observed in this setting.

Overall the cumulative effect of risk factors on the risk of severe INH and on the INH-related mortality was significant. This findings support the prediction models based on a combination of risk factors proposed in previous studies [48, 49].

The strength of these results relied on a large dataset of routinely collected clinical and laboratory variables with a low proportion of missing information. The impact of additional factors such as weight loss, bruising or cephalhematoma, having a sibling previously treated for INH, maternal obesity or diabetes, drug-induced labour and rhesus incompatibility were not systematically reported and neither was the intensity or the orientation of the phototherapy lights sources, a limitation of this retrospective design. Those elements should be considered for further evaluation of INH morbidity and mortality in this setting [47, 50].

Conclusion

The implementation of guidelines for the management of INH, early diagnosis by SBR and treatment with LED phototherapy are three simple and relatively inexpensive tools which have the potential to significantly reduce the number of neonates reaching severe levels of INH.

In a setting where G6PD-deficiency is common, this retrospective evaluation supports the implementation of routine neonatal screening for G6PD deficiency and vigilant observation for jaundice, both in hospital and after discharge home to reduce hospitalizations for severe INH [36, 51]. Finally, although controversies remain on the management of prematurity-associated hyperbilirubinemia and its consequences [52], premature neonates are a vulnerable population group for which the use of usual guidelines might be insufficient. In this population, where prematurity increased 2-fold the risk of severity, the use of safe and efficient prophylactic phototherapy as described by the Cochran neonatal group [53] might be indicated. And it would be worth considering applying the same concept for neonates with cumulating risk factors.

Abbreviations
AOR: Adjusted Odds Ratio; CI: Confidence interval; FST: Fluorescent spot test; G6PD: Glucose-6-phosphate dehydrogenase; INH: Indirect Neonatal hyperbilirubinemia; INH: Indirect neonatal hyperbilirubinemia; IQR: Interquartile range; LED: Light-emitting diode; NICE: National Institute for Health and Care Excellence; SBR: Serum bilirubin; SGA: Small-for-gestational-age; SMRU: Shoklo Malaria Research Unit

Acknowledgements
We would like to thank Dr. Cindy Chu and Dr. Jacques Jeugmans for their generous help in revising the manuscript. SMRU is part of the Mahidol Oxford University Research Unit, supported by the Wellcome Trust of Great Britain.

Funding
Funding was obtained from 'The Belgian Kids" Fund for Pediatric Research' which had no role in the design of this manuscript.

Authors' contributions
RM, CT, MHT, VIC, BH conceived and designed the review; VIC and RM obtained the Ethical approvals; CT, MHT, TJP, TH, CB, CP, MM, EMNW made substantial contributions to the acquisition of data. LT, JL, VIC and RM were involved in the analysis and interpretation of data; LT and VIC were involved in drafting the manuscript; CT, RM, FN, and BVO revised the manuscript for important intellectual content. All authors read and contributed to the present manuscript.

Competing interests
All authors declare that they have no competing interests.

Author details
[1]Shoklo Malaria Research Unit, Mahidol-Oxford Tropical Medicine Research Unit, Faculty of Tropical Medicine, Mahidol University, Mae Sot, Thailand. [2]Neonatology-Pediatrics, Cliniques Universitaires de Bruxelles - Hôspital Erasme, Université Libre de Bruxelles, Brussels, Belgium. [3]Centre for Tropical Medicine and Global Health, Nuffield Department of Medicine, University of Oxford, Oxford, UK. [4]Cambodia-Oxford Medical Research Unit, Angkor Hospital for Children, Siem Reap, Cambodia. [5]Angkor Hospital for Children, Siem Reap, Cambodia. [6]University of Groningen, Groningen, The Netherlands. [7]Mahidol-Oxford Tropical Medicine Research Unit (MORU), Faculty of Tropical Medicine, Mahidol University, Salaya, Thailand. [8]University of Glasgow, Glasgow, Scotland, UK.

References
1. Bhutani VK, Zipursky A, Blencowe H, Khanna R, Sgro M, Ebbesen F, et al. Neonatal hyperbilirubinemia and rhesus disease of the newborn: incidence and impairment estimates for 2010 at regional and global levels. Pediatr Res. 2013;74(Suppl 1):86–100.
2. Shapiro SM. Chronic bilirubin encephalopathy: diagnosis and outcome. Semin Fetal Neonatal Med. 2010;15:157–63. Elsevier Ltd
3. Radmacher PG, Groves FD, Owa JA, Ofovwe GE, Amuabunos EA, Olusanya BO, et al. A modified bilirubin-induced neurologic dysfunction (BIND-M) algorithm is useful in evaluating severity of jaundice in a resource-limited setting. BMC Pediatr. 2015;15:1–7.
4. Johnson L, Bhutani VK, Karp K, Sivieri EM, Shapiro SM. Clinical report from the pilot USA kernicterus registry (1992 to 2004). J Perinatol. 2009;29(Suppl 1):S25–45.
5. Lawn JE, Blencowe H, Oza S, You D, Lee ACC, Waiswa P, et al. Every newborn: progress, priorities, and potential beyond survival. Lancet. 2014; 384:189–205.
6. Greco C, Arnolda G, Boo NY, Iskander IF, Okolo AA, Rohsiswatmo R, et al. Neonatal jaundice in low- and middle-income countries: lessons and future directions from the 2015 don Ostrow Trieste yellow retreat. Neonatology. 2016;110:172–80.
7. Blencowe H, Cousens S, Oestergaard MZ, Chou D, Moller AB, Narwal R, et al. National, regional, and worldwide estimates of preterm birth rates in the year 2010 with time trends since 1990 for selected countries: a systematic analysis and implications. Lancet. 2012;379:2162–72.
8. Howes RE, Piel FBFB, Patil AP, Nyangiri OA, Gething PW, Dewi M, et al. G6PD deficiency prevalence and estimates of affected populations in malaria endemic countries: a geostatistical model-based map. PLoS Med. 2012;9(11): e1001339.
9. Bhutani VK. Editorial: building evidence to manage newborn jaundice worldwide. Indian J Pediatr. 2012;79(2):253–5.
10. Naghavi M, Wang H, Lozano R, Davis A, Liang X, Zhou M, et al. Global, regional, and national age-sex specific all-cause and cause-specific mortality for 240 causes of death, 1990-2013: a systematic analysis for the global burden of disease study 2013. Lancet. 2015;385:117–71.
11. Arnolda G, Nwe HM, Trevisanuto D, Thin AA, Thein AA, Defechereux T, et al. Risk factors for acute bilirubin encephalopathy on admission to two Myanmar national paediatric hospitals. Maternal health, neonatology and perinatology. 2015;1:22.
12. Department of Public Health in collaboration with Department of Medical Services. Ministry of Health, Annual Report, 2012–2013: The Republic of the Union of Myanmar; 2013. Available at http://www.mohs.gov.mm/.
13. Turner C, Carrara V, Thein NA, Win NC, Turner P, Bancone G, et al. Neonatal intensive Care in a Karen Refugee Camp: a 4 year descriptive study. PLoS One. 2013;8:1–9.
14. McGready R, Paw MK, Wiladphaingern J, Min AM, Carrara VI, Moore KA, et al. Miscarriage, stillbirth and neonatal mortality in the extreme preterm birth window of gestation in a limited-resource setting on the Thailand-Myanmar border: a population cohort study. Wellcome Open Res. 2016;1:32.
15. Oo NN, Bancone G, Maw LZ, Chowwiwat N, Bansil P, Domingo GJ, et al. Validation of G6PD point-of-care tests among healthy volunteers in Yangon, Myanmar. PLoS One. 2016;11:e0152304.
16. Webster J, Blythe R, Nugent F. An appraisal of the use of the Kramer's scale in predicting hyperbilirubinaemia in healthy full term infants. Birth Issues. 2006;14:83–9.
17. National Institute for Health and Care Excellence (NICE). Neonatal Jaundice, clinical guidelines. http://www.nice.org.uk. 2010;
18. Rijken MJ, Mulder EJH, Papageorghiou AT, Thiptharakun S, Wah N, Paw TK, et al. Quality of ultrasound biometry obtained by local health workers in a refugee camp on the Thai-Burmese border. Ultrasound Obstet Gynecol. 2012;40:151–7.
19. Moore KA, Simpson JA, Thomas KH, Rijken MJ, White LJ, Lu Moo Dwell S, et al. Estimating gestational age in late presenters to antenatal care in a resource-limited setting on the Thai-Myanmar border. PLoS One. 2015; 10:1–17.
20. Howson CP, Kinney MV, Lawn JE, editors. Born too soon: the global action report on preterm birth. Geneva: World Health Organization; 2012. p. 1–26.
21. Turner C, Carrara V, Aye N, Thien M, Moo N, Paw K, et al. Changes in the body weight of term infants, born in the tropics, during the first seven days of life. BMC Pediatr. 2013;13(1):93.
22. Rijken MJ, Rijken JA, Papageorghiou AT, Kennedy SH, Visser GHA, Nosten F, et al. Malaria in pregnancy: the difficulties in measuring birthweight. BJOG Int J Obstet Gynaecol. 2011;118(6):671–8.
23. Villar J, Cheikh Ismail L, Victora CG, Ohuma EO, Bertino E, Altman DG, et al. International standards for newborn weight, length, and head circumference by gestational age and sex: the newborn cross-sectional study of the INTERGROWTH-21st project. The Lancet. 2014;384:857–68.

24. Mya-Tu M, May-May-Yi M, Thin-Thin-Hlaing T. Blood groups of the Burmese population. Hum Hered. 1971;21:420–30.

25. Basu S, Ravneet K, Gagandeep K. Hemolytic disease of the fetus and newborn: current trends and perspectives. Asian J Transfus Sci. 2011;5:3–7.

26. Slusher TM, Zamora TG, Appiah D, Stanke JU, Strand MA, Lee BW, et al. Burden of severe neonatal jaundice: a systematic review and meta-analysis. BMJ Paediatr Open. 2017;1:e000105.

27. Szabo P, Wolf M, Bucher HU, Fauchère JC, Haensse D, Arlettaz R. Detection of hyperbilirubinaemia in jaundiced full-term neonates by eye or by bilirubinometer? Eur J Pediatr. 2004;163:722–7.

28. Keren R, Tremont K, Luan X, Cnaan A. Visual assessment of jaundice in term and late preterm infants. Arch Dis Child Fetal Neonatal Ed. 2009;94:F317–22.

29. Tikmani SS, Warraich HJ, Abbasi F, Rizvi A, Darmstadt GL, Zaidi AKM. Incidence of neonatal hyperbilirubinemia: a population-based prospective study in Pakistan. Trop Med Int Heal. 2010;15:502–7.

30. Sherbiny HS, Youssef DM, Sherbini AS, El-behedy R, Sherief LM. High-intensity light-emitting diode vs fluorescent tubes for intensive phototherapy in neonates. Paediatrics and international child health. 2016; 36(2):127–34.

31. Arnolda G, Thein AA, Trevisanuto D, Aung N, Nwe HM, Thin AA, et al. Evaluation of a simple intervention to reduce exchange transfusion rates among inborn and outborn neonates in Myanmar, comparing pre- and post-intervention rates. BMC Pediatr. 2015;15:216.

32. Olusanya BO, Osibanjo FB, Slusher TM. Risk factors for severe neonatal hyperbilirubinemia in low and middle-income countries: a systematic review and meta-analysis. PLoS One. 2015;10(2):e0117229.

33. Bancone G, Chu CS, Somsakchaicharoen R, Chowwiwat N, Parker DM, Charunwatthana P, et al. Characterization of G6PD genotypes and phenotypes on the northwestern Thailand-Myanmar border. PLoS One. 2014;9:e116063.

34. Bancone G, Gilder ME, Chowwiwat N, Gornsawun G, Win E, Cho WW, et al. Prevalences of inherited red blood cell disorders in pregnant women of different ethnicities living along the Thailand-Myanmar border. Wellcome Open Res. 2017;2:1–17.

35. Prins TJ, Trip-Hoving M, Paw MK, Le Ka M, Win NN, Htoo G, et al. A survey of practice and knowledge of refugee and migrant pregnant mothers surrounding neonatal jaundice on the Thailand-Myanmar border. J Trop Pediatr. 2017;63:50–6. Oxford University Press

36. Thielemans L, Gornsawun G, Hanboonkunupakarn B, Paw MK, Porn P, Moo PK, et al. Diagnostic performances of the fluorescent spot test for G6PD deficiency in newborns along the Thailand-Myanmar border: a cohort study. Wellcome Open Res. 2018;3:1.

37. Kaplan M, Hammerman C. Glucose-6-phosphate dehydrogenase deficiency and severe neonatal hyperbilirubinemia: a complexity of interactions between genes and environment. Semin Fetal Neonatal Med. 2010;15:148–56. Elsevier Ltd

38. Badejoko BO, Owa JA, Oseni SBA, Badejoko O, Fatusi AO, Adejuyigbe EA. Early neonatal bilirubin, hematocrit, and Glucose-6-phosphate dehydrogenase status. Pediatrics. 2014;134:e1082–8.

39. Kaplan M, Herschel M, Hammerman C, Hoyer JD, Stevenson DK. Hyperbilirubinemia among African American, glucose-6-phosphate dehydrogenase-deficient neonates. Pediatrics. 2004;114:e213–9.

40. Watchko JF, Kaplan M, Stark AR, Stevenson DK, Bhutani VK. Should we screen newborns for glucose-6-phosphate dehydrogenase deficiency in the United States? J Perinatol. 2013;33:499–504. Nature Publishing Group

41. Olusanya BO, Osibanjo FB, Mabogunje CA, Slusher TM, Olowe SA. The burden and management of neonatal jaundice in Nigeria: a scoping review of the literature. Niger J Clin Pract. 2016;19(1):1–7.

42. Malla T, Singh S, Poudyal P, Sathian B, Bk G, Malla KKA. Prospective study on exchange transfusion in neonatal unconjugated hyperbilirubinemia–in a tertiary care hospital, Nepal. Kathmandu Univ Med J. 2015;13:102–8.

43. Singla DA, Sharma S, Sharma M, Chaudhary S. Evaluation of risk factors for exchange range hyperbilirubinemia and neurotoxicity in neonates from hilly terrain of India. Int J Appl basic Med Res. 2017;7:228–32. Wolters Kluwer – Medknow Publications

44. Cherepnalkovski AP, Krzelj V, Zafirovska-ivanovska B, Gruev T, Markic J, et al. Evaluation of neonatal laboratory parameters hemolytic Jaundice : clinical and laboratory parameters. OA Maced J Med Sci. 2015;3:694–8.

45. Chen S-H, Lin M, Yang K-L, Lin T-Y, Tsai H-H, Yang S-H, et al. Association of ABO incompatibility with red blood cell indices of cord blood unit. Pediatr Neonatol. 2012;53:138–43.

46. Cherepnalkovski AP, Krzelj V, Zafirovska-ivanovska B, Gruev T, Markic J, Aluloska N, et al. Evaluation of neonatal laboratory parameters hemolytic Jaundice: clinical and laboratory parameters. OA Maced J Med Sci. 2015;3:694–8.

47. Olusanya BO, Slusher TM. Infants at risk of significant hyperbilirubinemia in poorly-resourced countries: evidence from a scoping review. World J Pediatr. 2015;11:293–9.

48. Kaplan M, Herschel M, Hammerman C, Hoyer JD, Heller GZ, Stevenson DK. Neonatal hyperbilirubinemia in African American males: the importance of glucose-6-phosphate dehydrogenase deficiency. J Pediatr. 2006;149: 83–8. Elsevier

49. Norman M, Åberg K, Holmsten K, Weibel V, Ekéus C. Predicting nonhemolytic neonatal hyperbilirubinemia. Am Acad Pediatr. 2015;136: 1087–94.

50. Lee BK, Le Ray I, Sun JY, Wikman A, Reilly M, Johansson S. Haemolytic and nonhaemolytic neonatal jaundice have different risk factor profiles. Acta Paediatr. 2016;105:1444–50.

51. Kaplan M, Hammerman C, Bhutani VK. Parental education and the WHO neonatal G-6-PD screening program: a quarter century later. J Perinatol. 2015;35:779–84. Nature Publishing Group

52. Bhutani VK, Wong RJ, Stevenson DK. Hyperbilirubinemia in Preterm Neonates. Clin Perinatol. 2016;43(2):215–32.

53. Davies MW, Okwundu CI, Okoromah CAN, Shah PS. Cochrane review: prophylactic phototherapy for preventing jaundice in preterm or low birth weight infants. Evidence-Based Child Heal. 2013;8:204–49.

Bacteriological profile and antibiotic susceptibility of neonatal sepsis in neonatal intensive care unit of a tertiary hospital in Nepal

Bhishma Pokhrel[1*] ⓘ, Tapendra Koirala[2], Ganesh Shah[1], Suchita Joshi[1] and Pinky Baral[3]

Abstract

Background: Neonatal sepsis, one of the leading causes of mortality in neonatal intensive care units (NICU) of developing countries like Nepal, is often not extensively studied. In order to decrease the morbidity and mortality associated with neonatal sepsis, neonatologists should have a keen knowledge of the existing bacteriological flora and their antibiotic susceptibility pattern. In this study, we aim to determine the bacteriological profile and antibiotic susceptibility pattern of culture positive neonatal sepsis in the NICU of a tertiary teaching hospital in Nepal.

Methods: This was a retrospective cross-sectional study of all blood culture positive sepsis cases among neonates admitted to the neonatal intensive care unit of Patan Hospital, Nepal between April 15, 2014 and April 15, 2017. All neonates with a clinical suspicion of sepsis with a positive blood culture were identified. Patient demographics, clinical details, maternal risk factors, and laboratory data including bacteriological profiles and antimicrobial susceptibilities were recorded and analyzed.

Results: Of the 336 neonates admitted in the NICU, 69 (20.5%) had culture-positive sepsis. The majority were early-onset sepsis (n = 54, 78.3%) and were among the preterm babies (n = 47, 68.1%). Most bacterial isolates were gram-negative, predominantly the Klebsiella species (n = 23, 33.3%). Klebsiella showed high resistance to commonly used antibiotics such as; Cefotaxime (90.5%), Gentamicin (75%), Ciprofloxacin (76.2%), Ofloxacin (72.2%) and Chloramphenicol (65%). However, they showed good susceptibility to Carbapenems (100%), Colistin (88.8%) and Tigecycline (81.8%). Among cultures with gram-positive species, Coagulase-negative Staphylococci (CONS) (n = 14, 20.3%) predominated. CONS showed high resistance to Oxacillin (80%), Cefotaxime (66.7%) and Meropenem (80%) but good susceptibility (100%) to Vancomycin and Linezolid. Prevalence of multidrug-resistant strain was 73.9%.

Conclusions: Klebsiella species and CONS were the most common causes of neonatal sepsis in our study. A significant proportion of the isolates were multidrug resistant strains, which pose a great threat to neonatal survival, and thereby, warrant modification of existing empirical therapy. Implementation of effective preventive strategies to combat the emergence of antibiotic resistance is urgently needed. We recommend a combination of Piperacillin-Tazobactam and Ofloxacin as the first line therapy and combination of Vancomycin and Meropenem as the second line empirical therapy in our NICU.

Keywords: Antibiotic susceptibility, Klebsiella, Multi-drug resistance, Neonatal sepsis, NICU

* Correspondence: bhishmapokhrel@pahs.edu.np
[1]Department of Pediatrics, Patan Academy of Health Sciences, Lagankhel, PO Box 26500, Lalitpur, Nepal
Full list of author information is available at the end of the article

Background

Sepsis is considered one of the leading causes of neonatal mortality globally, more so in developing countries like Nepal [1]. According to Nepal Demographic and Health Survey 2016, national neonatal mortality rate was 21 per thousand live births. Infections including sepsis contributed to 16% of the neonatal mortality [2]. Emergence of antimicrobial resistance has become a global concern. With a limited reserve of antibiotics, increasing antimicrobial resistance has become a great challenge in the management of neonatal sepsis. Knowledge of prevalent bacterial isolates and their antibiotic susceptibility pattern is crucial when choosing the appropriate empirical therapy in order to decrease morbidity and mortality. There is, however, a paucity of such data in Neonatal Intensive Care Units (NICU) of Nepal. We aim to determine the prevalence of culture-positive neonatal sepsis, its clinico-bacteriological profile and antibiotic susceptibility pattern in the NICU of Patan Hospital, Lalitpur, Nepal.

Methods

This was a retrospective cross-sectional study conducted in the NICU of Patan Hospital. Patan Hospital is the tertiary level teaching hospital of Patan Academy of Health Sciences (PAHS) located in Lalitpur, Nepal. It has a six-bed NICU, caring on average for 120 critically ill neonates annually. Neonates admitted to the NICU between April 15, 2014 and April 15, 2017 with clinical features of sepsis and who had a positive blood culture were included in the study. Blood cultures were sent in neonates with either a clinical suspicion of sepsis or risk factors for it. Sepsis was suspected in the presence of temperature instability, lethargy, feeding intolerance, respiratory distress, hemodynamic instability, convulsion, hypotonia, irritability or bleeding diathesis. Prematurity (< 37 weeks of gestation), low birth weight (< 2500 g), history of resuscitation at birth, rupture of membrane for more than 18 h (PROM), antepartum fever, foul-smelling liquor and repeated (≥3) unclean per vaginal examinations were considered as risk factors for neonatal sepsis.

Patan Hospital follows standard microbiological techniques. Before drawing blood, the skin is disinfected with 10% Povidone-iodine solution for 2 min, followed by 0.5% Chlorhexidine solution for 1 minute. One to three milliliters of blood is taken aseptically from a peripheral vein and injected into the BACTEC PedsPlus™(-Becton Dickinson, Ireland) culture vials. It is then incubated in an automated BACTEC system at 35 ± 2 °C for 5 days as per manufacturer's instructions. Subculture and organism identification is performed as described by Koneman et al. [3]. Antibiotic susceptibility test is done using the Kirby-Bauer disc diffusion method, as per the Clinical and Laboratory Standards Institute (CLSI) guidelines (2014) [4]. After collection of blood for culture, neonates are started on empiric intravenous Ampicillin and Amikacin (first line therapy). If there is no clinical response after 48–72 h, antibiotics are upgraded to intravenous Chloramphenicol and Ofloxacin (second line) or Meropenem and Colistin (third line). These are later modified, based on culture and antibiotic susceptibility results. Coagulase-negative Staphylococcus (CONS) isolated from non-septic neonates, in whom the repeat culture showed no growth, was considered as a contaminant and hence excluded from the study. Early-onset sepsis (EOS) was defined as sepsis occurring within first 72 h of life, that occurring after 72 h of life was defined as late-onset sepsis (LOS) [5]. Multidrug-resistant (MDR) strains were defined as per international standard definitions for acquired resistance and relative to the panel of antibiotics tested for each isolate, as in vitro non-susceptibility to ≥1 agent in ≥3 antimicrobial categories: Penicillins, Cephalosporins, Beta-lactamase inhibitor combinations, Fluoroquinolones, Aminoglycosides, Chloramphenicol, Folate pathway inhibitors, Tetracyclines, Macrolides and Glycopeptides [6].

For data collection, microbiology laboratory blood culture registers were reviewed and all blood culture positive neonates were identified. Their records were subsequently evaluated for clinical evidence of sepsis and enrolled in the study. Data on age at admission, gestational age at birth, birth weight, maternal risk factors, laboratory parameters, blood culture isolates and their susceptibility pattern and clinical outcome were collected. EpiInfo™ for Mobile was used for data entry and Statistical Package for Social Sciences (SPSS) version 21 was used for data analysis. Summary of measures were reported as percentage for categorical variables and as mean with standard deviation for quantitative variables. Fisher's exact test was used to infer any differences between the categorical variables and p-value of less than 0.05 was considered statistically significant. Ethical approval to conduct the study was obtained from the Institutional Review Committee (IRC) of PAHS.

Results

General characteristics and clinical profile

During the study period, 24,516 live births occurred, and 336 neonates were admitted in our NICU of whom 332 had their blood sent for culture. Out of 336 neonates, 69 (20.5%) had culture-positive sepsis. EOS was found in 78.3%. Among neonates with positive cultures, 63.8% had a birth weight less than 2500 g, 68.1% were preterm and 27.5% were delivered by emergency cesarean section (Table 1). Forty-five percent had a maternal history of PROM, which was more common

Bacteriological profile and antibiotic susceptibility of neonatal sepsis in neonatal intensive care unit... 37

Table 1 General characteristics of the enrolled neonates

Variables	EOS group	LOS group	Total	Percent	Fisher's exact test p-value
Neonatal variables					
Gender					
Male	31	6	37	53.6	0.2571
Female	23	9	32	46.4	
Gestational age at birth					
Preterm (< 37 weeks)	42	5	47	68.1	0.0033
Term (> 37 weeks)	12	10	22	31.9	
Birthweight					
< 2500 g	34	10	44	63.8	1.0000
≥ 2500 g	20	5	25	36.2	
Mode of delivery					
Vaginal	35	8	43	62.3	0.5484
Caesarean section	19	7	26	37.7	
APGAR score < 6 at 5 min	5	0	5	7.3	0.6250
Maternal variables					
Maternal fever (within 7 days before delivery)	9	0	9	13.0	0.0039
PROM of > 18 h	29	2	31	44.9	< 0.0001
Foul smelling liquor	2	0	2	2.9	0.5000
Maternal antibiotics (within 7 days before delivery)	19	2	21	30.4	0.0002
Maternal GBS colonization	12	0	12	17.4	0.0004
Neonatal care related variables					
Need for inotropes	39	2	41	59.4	< 0.0001
Need for positive pressure ventilation	54	10	64	92.8	< 0.0001
Central line	47	3	50	72.5	< 0.0001
Mortality	11	0	11	15.9	0.0009

EOS Early onset sepsis, *GBS* Group B Streptococcus, *LOS* Late onset sepsis, *PROM* Prolonged rupture of membrane

among the EOS group (54%). Maternal Group B Streptococcus (GBS) colonization status was unknown in 69.6%.

The common clinical findings observed at admission were respiratory distress (79.7%), tachycardia (60.9%), cyanosis (59.4%) and hypothermia (53.6%). Similarly, low absolute neutrophil count (ANC) ($< 1800/mm^3$), thrombocytopenia ($< 150,000/mm^3$) and raised C-reactive protein (CRP) (> 10 mg/dl) were seen in 20, 75 and 84% respectively. During the course of treatment, feeding intolerance, seizure, and dysglycemia (blood sugar level < 40 mg/dl requiring dextrose bolus or > 250 mg/dl requiring insulin infusion) was observed in 46.4, 31.9 and 27.5% respectively. The mean duration of NICU stay was 16.0 ± 10.7 days and the mortality rate was 15.9%.

Bacteriological profile
The majority of bacterial isolates were gram-negative (77%). Among the total isolates, Klebsiella species, CONS and Enterobacter were the most common (Table 2). Five cases (7.24%) had polymicrobial sepsis of which two had yeast cells along with bacterial growth.

Table 2 Distribution of bacterial isolates with their relative frequency

Bacterial isolate	Number	Percent
Gram-negatives		
Klebsiella species	23	33.3
Enterobacter species	13	18.8
Acinetobacter species	8	11.6
Escherichia coli	3	4.3
Serratia rubidaea	3	4.3
Pseudomonas species	2	2.9
Bacillus species	1	1.4
Gram-positives		
CONS	14	20.3
Staphylococcus aureus	1	1.4
Non-hemolytic streptococcus	1	1.4
Total	69	100.0

CONS Coagulase negative staphylococci

Table 3 Distribution of isolates based on age at admission and gestational age at birth

Bacterial isolate	Age at admission			Gestational age at birth		
	< 72 h (EOS)	> 72 h (LOS)	Fisher's exact test (p-value)	Pre-term	Term	Fisher's exact test (p-value)
Klebsiella	19	4	0.0025	15	8	0.2100
CONS	11	3	0.0573	8	6	0.7905
Enterobacter	9	4	0.2668	10	3	0.0922
Acinetobacter	6	2	0.2890	5	3	0.7265
Serratia rubidaea	3	0	0.2500	2	1	1.0000
Escherichia coli	2	1	1.0000	3	0	0.2500
Pseudomonas	2	0	0.5000	2	0	0.5000
Bacillus	1	0	1.0000	1	0	1.0000
Staphylococcus aureus	1	0	1.0000	1	0	1.0000
Non-hemolytic streptococcus	0	1	1.0000	0	1	1.0000
Total	54	15		47	22	

CONS Coagulase negative staphylococcus, EOS Early onset sepsis, LOS Late onset sepsis

Klebsiella, CONS and Enterobacter species were the most common organisms found in all groups; in both EOS and LOS, term and preterm babies. There was preponderance among EOS and preterm infants (Table 3); however, this observed difference was not statistically significant (p-value> 0.05) except for Klebsiella in EOS group (p-value 0.0025.

Antibiotic susceptibility pattern
Among gram-negative organisms
Within the beta-lactam antibiotics, Klebsiella demonstrated maximum susceptibility to Meropenem (100%), Imipenem (100%) and Piperacillin-Tazobactam (Pip-Taz) (60%) while showing high resistance to Ampicillin-Sulbactam (66.7%) and Cefotaxime (90.5%). Among non-beta-lactam antibiotics, Klebsiella showed maximum susceptibility to Colistin (88.8%) and Tigecycline (81.8%) while showing high resistance to Aminoglycosides and Quinolones.

Enterobacter species demonstrated high susceptibility to Meropenem (80%), Tigecycline (85.7%) and Colistin (87.5%) while demonstrating high resistance to Cefotaxime (83.4%).

Acinetobacter demonstrated good susceptibility to Ciprofloxacin (81.2%), Colistin (80%) and Tigecycline

Table 4 Antibiotics resistance among the major isolates

Antibiotic	Klebsiella (N = 23)		CONS (14)		Enterobacter (N = 13)		Acinetobacter (N = 8)		Escherichia coli (N = 3)		Serratia rubidaea (N = 3)	
	R/(R + S)	R %	R/(R + S)	R %	R/(R + S)	R %	R/(R + S)	R %	R/(R + S)	R %	R/(R + S)	R %
Beta-lactam Antibiotics												
Oxacillin	6/6	100	8/10	80	3/3	100	2/2	100	1/1	100	1/2	50
Cefotaxime	19/21	90.5	4/6	66.7	10/12	83.4	6/7	85.7	3/3	100	1/3	33.3
Meropenem	0/18	0	4/5	80	2/10	20	4/7	57.1	2/3	66.7	0/3	0
Pip-Taz	4/10	40	1/2	50	2/4	50	3/6	50	2/2	100	1/3	33.3
Non-beta-lactam Antibiotics												
Amikacin	12/21	57	5/10	50	0/1	0	7/7	100	3/3	100	1/3	33.3
Gentamicin	15/20	75	7/12	58.3	5/13	38.5	5/7	71.4	2/3	66.7	1/3	33.3
Chloramphenicol	13/20	65	5/11	45.5	8/13	61.5	7/7	100	3/3	100	3/3	100
Ciprofloxacin	16/21	76.2	8/10	80	5/13	38.5	3/16	18.8	3/3	100	1/3	33.3
Ofloxacin	13/18	72.2	8/12	66.7	1/12	8.3	4/6	66.7	3/3	100	1/3	33.3
Linezolid	–	–	0/3	0	–	–	1/1	100	–	–	0/1	0
Vancomycin	1/1	100	0/4	0	1/1	100	–	–	–	–	0/1	0
Tigecycline	2/11	18.2	–	–	1/7	14.3	2/6	33.3	0/2	0	0/1	0
Colistin	2/18	11.2	–	–	1/8	12.5	1/5	20	0/3	0	1/3	33.3

CONS Coagulase negative staphylococci, Pip-Taz Piperacillin-Tazobactam, R Number of resistant isolates, R% Percentage of resistant isolates, S Number of susceptible isolates, [–] Not tested

(66.7%) while it was highly resistant to Amikacin (100%), Chloramphenicol (100%) and Cefotaxime (85.7%).

Escherichia coli demonstrated marked resistance to commonly used antibiotics, showing susceptibility only to reserved antibiotics like Tigecycline and Colistin (Table 4).

Among gram-positive organisms

CONS, Methicillin-resistant *Staphylococcus aureus* (MRSA) and Non-hemolytic Streptococcus were the most common gram-positive organisms associated with neonatal sepsis in our study. The majority of CONS were resistant to commonly used antibiotics (Table 4). A single case of MRSA isolated in our study showed susceptibility to Amikacin, Gentamicin, Ofloxacin, Pip-Taz, and Linezolid. One case of Non-hemolytic Streptococcus isolate showed susceptibility to Amoxicillin, Gentamicin and Chloramphenicol, but surprisingly resistance to Cefotaxime and Ofloxacin.

Status of global antibiotic resistance

Overall resistance to individual antibiotics among gram-positive and gram-negative isolates is summarized in Table 5. It shows alarming rates of resistance to

Table 5 Overall status of antibiotic resistance among the gram-positive and gram-negative isolates

Antibiotics tested	Gram-negative		Gram-positive	
	R	R %	R	R %
Beta-lactam antibiotics				
Amoxicillin	38	100.0	7	87.5
Oxacillin	11	91.7	8	100.0
Cefotaxime	33	80.5	5	62.5
Meropenem	4	11.8	2	40.0
Piperacillin-Tazobactam	9	47.4	1	33.3
Ampicillin-Sulbactam	2	66.7	1	100.0
Imipenem	1	8.3	–	–
Aztreonam	1	50.0		–
Non-beta-lactam antibiotics				
Amikacin	21	50.0	5	45.5
Gentamicin	24	60.0	7	50.0
Tobramycin	1	50.0	1	100.0
Chloramphenicol	29	70.7	6	46.2
Ciprofloxacin	25	62.5	8	61.5
Ofloxacin	18	47.4	9	64.3
Linezolid	–	–	0	0.0
Vancomycin	2	66.7	0	0.0
Tigecycline	3	14.3	–	–
Cotrimoxazole	1	33.3	–	–
Colistin	6	17.6	3	100.0
Teicoplanin	1	50.0	–	87.5

R Number of resistant isolates, *R%* Percentage of resistant isolates

commonly used antibiotics. The resistance to the current first and second line empirical therapy was 72 and 65% respectively.

Discussion

Neonatal sepsis is considered the leading cause of infant mortality and morbidity in the NICU. Two previous studies conducted in neonatal nurseries from Patan Hospital during the period of 2000–2005 and 2006–2007 showed culture positivity of 13.7 and 19.56% respectively [7, 8]. However, our study, which is first of its kind to be conducted in NICU of the same institute, showed culture positivity of neonatal sepsis to be 20.7%. In contrast, studies conducted at KIST Medical College and Manipal College of Medical Sciences, Nepal showed culture positivity to be 48 and 44.9% respectively [9, 10]. Variations in culture positivity rate of neonatal sepsis in different studies seem to arise from differences in culture-techniques and study designs.

The majority of culture positive sepsis was EOS and among preterm and low birth weight neonates, similar to the study findings of Kathmandu University Hospital (KUH), Dhulikhel, Nepal [11].

The most common clinical manifestation of neonatal sepsis in our study was respiratory distress (79%). Similar findings were noted in studies from KIST Medical College, Nepal (54%) and Beni Suef University Hospital, Egypt (36%) [9, 12]. At our center, we take CRP as a biomarker of sepsis and its serial decline is taken as laboratory evidence of improvement. In the initial screening test, the majority had raised CRP (75%) and low platelet count (84%) whereas low ANC was seen only in 20% of the cases.

The majority of the isolates were gram-negative, similar to the findings of Shrestha S et al. and that of investigators of the Delhi Neonatal Infection Study (DeNIS) Collaboration [11, 13]. In contrast, Peterside O et al. in Nigeria and Sharma P et al. in India showed a preponderance of gram-positive organisms of which *Staphylococcus aureus* was the most prevalent [14]. One reason for this variation could be due to the difference in adherence to infection prevention and control measures.

Klebsiella species were the most frequent causative organisms of neonatal sepsis in our study, a similar finding to that of Shrestha S et al. [11]. In contrast, previous studies conducted at the same institute in the neonatal nurseries showed CONS as a major isolate [7, 8]. The variation in the major isolate could be due to differences in study setting, study population and adherence to hand hygiene practices. Similar CONS predominance was reported by Mohamadi P et al. [15]. The same bacterial isolates were attributed to neonatal sepsis among the EOS and LOS groups, in agreement with Shrestha S et al's and Singh HK et al's [11, 16] findings. In contrast, studies by Mahmood A et al. and Ingale HD et al. demonstrated Klebsiella in EOS and Staphylococcus in LOS as common causative organisms [17, 18]. Wu JH et al. in Taiwan, found GBS and Methicillin resistant-CONS to be the most frequent cause among EOS and LOS respectively [19].

Our study shows the majority of causative organisms have developed resistance to these frequently used antibiotics; Amoxicillin, Cefotaxime and Oxacillin from the beta-lactam group. This finding is consistent with studies done in neonatal nurseries of the same institute and NICUs in other parts of Nepal and Pakistan [7, 8, 11, 12, 17]. Both gram-positive and gram-negative organisms showed high susceptibility to Carbapenems, a similar finding to other studies conducted both inside and outside Nepal [11, 12, 17]. Similarly, gram-negative organisms showed high susceptibility to Colistin, which is consistent with the findings of Jessan Bonny et al. [20].

Vancomycin and Linezolid showed high (100%) susceptibility towards gram-positive isolates, similar to the finding's of Mullah SA et al. and Singh HK [16, 21]. Amikacin showed moderate susceptibility against both gram-positive and negatives. Among second-line antibiotics, Chloramphenicol had low susceptibility (29.3%) against gram-negatives compared to gram-positives (53.8%). Whereas Ofloxacin had moderate susceptibility (52.6%) to gram-negatives.

Klebsiella and Enterobacter, the main gram-negative isolates showed maximum susceptibility to Carbapenems, followed by Colistin and Tigecycline respectively. Such high susceptibility toward Carbapenem was also documented by Sheth KV et and Yusuf D et al. [22, 23].

Acinetobacter demonstrated good susceptibility to Ciprofloxacin, Colistin, and Tigecycline. Although our study showed high susceptibility towards Ciprofloxacin various other studies reported low susceptibility [11, 24].

Escherichia coli showed high resistance to the first and second line empirical antibiotics used commonly in our institution, only demonstrating susceptibility towards Colistin and Tigecycline. In contrast to this, Singh HK et al. and Sheth KV et al. showed good susceptibility towards commonly used antibiotics [16, 24]. This indicates the emergence of highly resistant strains of Escherichia coli in our setting.

CONS has been reported in various studies as the most common cause of neonatal sepsis in NICUs [19, 22]. The second commonest cause of neonatal sepsis in our study, CONS showed low susceptibility to Penicillin, third generation Cephalosporin and intermediate to Aminoglycosides and high susceptibility to Linezolid and Vancomycin. Sarangi KK et al.

and Dalal P et al. also demonstrated high Vancomycin susceptibility in their studies [25, 26].

GBS, the most common cause of EOS in high-income countries, has a low reported incidence in low and middle-income countries [27]. Such low incidence of GBS sepsis in EONS is consistent with our findings. Possible reasons for this could include overuse of antibiotics during the antenatal period or substandard culture techniques and microbiological methods [28, 29]. At our institution, intravenous Crystalline Penicillin is given for mothers with PROM and intravenous Metronidazole and Gentamicin along with Crystalline Penicillin for mothers with chorioamnionitis as intrapartum antibiotic prophylaxis. Over diagnosis of PROM and chorioamnionitis and subsequent antibiotic treatment could be the reason for low yield of GBS at our institution.

In our study, the overall mortality rate in culture positive sepsis was 15.94%, which is consistent with the studies from Egypt and India [12, 30, 18]. The highest mortality was seen in the Enterobacter and Klebsiella sepsis group. Though the highest case fatality rate was observed with Pseudomonas sepsis, its limited yield hinders the generalization of this result. A combination of Pip-Taz and Ofloxacin as first line empirical therapy, or Vancomycin and Meropenem as second line would reduce the overall resistance by 22 and 46% respectively. The current first line therapy covers only 28% of the isolates whereas the proposed first line therapy with Pip-taz and Ofloxacin would successfully cover 50% of the isolates.

The emergence of MDR bacteria presents a great challenge to the management of neonatal sepsis, causing significant morbidity and mortality. The prevalence of neonatal sepsis due to MDR strains in our study was 73.91%. MDR among gram-negatives and gram-positives was 80.76 and 52.94% respectively in our study, which is in agreement with the findings of DeNIS Collaboration from India and Labi AK et al. from Ghana [13, 6].

The retrospective design of our study, together with its single centered, small study population and limited yield of some pathogens were all limitations in our study. Hence, large-scale, multi-center prospective studies are needed to validate our findings.

Conclusions

Our study revealed gram-negative isolates as the predominant pathogens in both EOS and LOS groups. Both gram-positive and gram-negative isolates showed high resistance to commonly used antibiotics. Significant proportions of them were MDR strains. Such high antibiotic resistance is associated with significant neonatal morbidity and mortality. Based on our findings, a combination of Pip-Taz and Ofloxacin as first line therapy, or a combination of Vancomycin and Meropenem as second line would be the appropriate empirical therapy. However, the use of the broad-spectrum antibiotics as empirical therapy could be detrimental in the long run and hence they should be used judiciously and modified to narrow spectrum antibiotics, as guided by the culture and susceptibility report at the earliest opportunity. The best prevention of neonatal sepsis comprises of early recognition of high-risk infants and strict infection control practices, such as safe delivery, hand hygiene, avoidance of unnecessary invasive procedures and restricted entry to the NICU. To prevent the emergence of drug resistance, comprehensive approach consisting of evaluation of antibiotic consumption, improvement in laboratory techniques, rational use of empirical therapy and de-escalation/discontinuation of therapy when suitable along with continuous surveillance and monitoring of local epidemiology is needed. Use of synbiotics in a recent trial in India has shown promising results in prevention of neonatal sepsis in developing countries [31]. Use of Matrix assisted laser deserption ionization-time of flight mass spectrometry (MALDI-TOF MS), a nobel technique for the rapid identification of isolates and their antimicrobial susceptibility is yet to be explored in low-income countries like Nepal.

Abbreviations

ANC: Absolute neutrophil count; CONS: Coagulase-negative Staphylococci; CRP: C-reactive protein; EOS: Early-onset sepsis; GBS: Group B Streptococcus; LOS: Late-onset Sepsis; MDR: Multidrug-resistant; MRSA: Methicillin-resistant *Staphylococcus aureus*; NICU: Neonatal intensive care unit; PIP-TAZ: Piperacillin-Tazobactam; PROM: Prolonged rupture of membrane

Acknowledgements

We are grateful to Dr. Katrina Butterworth MD, Professor of General Practice and Dr. Darlene R. House, MD, MS, Assistant Professor of Clinical Emergency Medicine for proofreading our manuscript.

Funding

This work did not receive any funding from any source.

Authors' contributions

BP, TK and PB conceived and designed the study, collected and analyzed the data and drafted the manuscript. SJ and GS revised the manuscript for critically important intellectual content. BP, TK and PB finalized the manuscript. All authors read and approved the final manuscript.

Competing interests

The authors declare they have no competing interests.

Author details

[1]Department of Pediatrics, Patan Academy of Health Sciences, Lagankhel, PO Box 26500, Lalitpur, Nepal. [2]School of Medicine, Patan Academy of Health Sciences, Lagankhel, Lalitpur, Nepal. [3]School of Health and Allied Sciences, Pokhara University, Lekhnath-12, Kaski, Nepal.

References

1. United Nations Inter-agency Group for Child Mortality Estimation (UNIGME). Levels and trends in child mortality report 2017. New York: United Nations Children's Fund; 2017. 36p. Available from: https://www.unicef.org/publications/files/Child_Mortality_Report_2017.pdf. Accessed 1 Dec 2017.

2. Ministry of Health, Nepal; New ERA; ICF. Nepal demographic and health survey 2016. Kathmandu, Nepal: Ministry of Health, Nepal; 2017 Nov. 411p. Available from: https://www.dhsprogram.com/pubs/pdf/FR336/FR336.pdf. Accessed 1 Dec 2017.

3. Winn WC, Allen SD, Janda WN, Koneman E, Procop G, Schreckenberger P, Woods G. Koneman's color atlas and textbook of diagnostic microbiology. 6th ed. Philadelphia: Lippincott; 2006.

4. Clinical and Laboratory Standards Institute (CLSI). Performance standards for antimicrobial susceptibility testing; twenty-fourth informational supplement. Wayne (PA): Clinical and Laboratory Standard Institute; 2014 Jan. Report No.: CLSI document M 100-S24.

5. National Neonatology Forum NNPD Network, India. National neonatal-perinatal database report 2002–2003. New Delhi: National Neonatology Forum NNPD Network, India; 2005 Jan. 70p. Available from: http://www.newbornwhocc.org/pdf/nnpd_report_2002-03.PDF. Accessed 4 Dec 2017.

6. Labi AK, Obeng-Nkrumah N, Bjerrum S, Enweronu-Laryea C, Newman MJ. Neonatal bloodstream infections in a Ghanaian tertiary hospital: are the current antibiotic recommendations adequate? BMC Infect Dis. 2016 16:598. Available from: https://doi.org/10.1186/s12879-016-1913-4. Accessed 4 Dec 2017.

7. Shrestha S; Adhikari N; Shakya D; Manandhar L, Chand A. Bacteriological profile of neonatal blood cultures at Patan hospital. J Nepal Paediatr Soc. 2007 26(1):1–4. Available from: https://www.popline.org/node/198598. Accessed 5 Dec 2017.

8. Shrestha S, Adhikari N, Rai BK, Shreepaili A. Antibiotic resistance pattern of bacterial isolates in neonatal care unit. J Nepal Med Assoc. 2010 49 (180): 277–281. Available from: http://www.jnma.com.np/jnma/index.php/jnma/article/view/54/416. Accessed 5 Dec 2017.

9. Lakhey A, Shakya H. Role of sepsis screening in early diagnosis of neonatal sepsis. J Pathol Nepal. 2017;7(1):1103–1110. Available from: https://doi.org/10.3126/jpn.v7i1.16944. Accessed 6 Dec 2017.

10. Shrestha NJ, Subedi KU, Rai GK. Bacteriological profile of neonatal sepsis: a hospital based study. J Nepal Paediatr Soc. 2011;31 (1):1–5. Available from: https://doi.org/10.3126/jnps.v31i1.4158. Accessed 9 Dec 2017.

11. Shrestha S, Shrestha NC, Dongol Singh S, Shrestha RPB, Kayestha S, Shrestha M. Bacterial isolates and its antibiotic susceptibility pattern in NICU. Kathmandu Univ Med J. 2013;41(1):66–70. Available from: http://www.kumj.com.np/issue/41/66-70.pdf. Accessed 9 Dec 2017.

12. Fahmey SS. Early-onset sepsis in a neonatal intensive care unit in Beni Suef, Egypt: bacterial isolates and antibiotic resistance pattern. Kor J Pediatr 2013; 56(8):332–337. Available from: https://doi.org/10.3345/kjp.2013.56.8.332. Accessed 12 Dec 2017.

13. Investigators of the Delhi Neonatal Infection Study (DeNIS) collaboration. Characterisation and antimicrobial resistance of sepsis pathogens in neonates born in tertiary care centres in Delhi, India: a cohort study. Lancet Glob Health. 2016; e752–e760. Available from: https://doi.org/10.1016/S2214-109X(16)30148-6. Accessed 16 Feb 2018.

14. Sharma P, Kaur P, Aggarwal A. Staphylococcus aureus- the predominant pathogen in the neonatal ICU of a tertiary care hospital in Amritsar, India. J Clin Diagn Res. 2013;7(1): 66–69. Available from: https://doi.org/10.7860/JCDR/2012/4913.2672. Accessed 14 Dec 2017.

15. Mohammadi P, Kalantar E, Bahmani N, Fatemi A, Naseri N, Ghotbi N, Naseri MH. Neonatal bacteriemia isolates and their antibiotic resistance pattern in neonatal intensive care unit (NICU) at Beasat hospital, Sanandaj, Iran. Acta Medica Iranica. 2014 52(5):337–40. Available from: http://acta.tums.ac.ir/index.php/acta/article/download/4624/4414 Accessed 14 Dec 2017.

16. Singh HK, Sharja P, Onkar K. Bacteriological profile of neonatal sepsis in neonatal intensive care unit (NICU) in a tertiary care hospital: prevalent bugs and their susceptibility patterns. Eur J Pharmaceutical Med Res 2016; 3(3):241–245. Available from: http://www.ejpmr.com/admin/assets/article_issue/1457056566.pdf . Accessed 14 Dec 2017.

17. Mahmood A, Karamat KA, Butt T. Neonatal sepsis: high antibiotic resistance of the bacterial pathogen in a neonatal intensive care unit in Karachi. J Pak Med Assoc.200252(8):348–350. Available from: http://www.jpma.org.pk/full_article_text.php?article_id=2358. Accessed 15 Dec 2017.

18. Ingale HD, Kongre VA, Bharadwaj RS. A study of infections in neonatal intensive care unit at a tertiary care hospital. Int J Contemp Pediatr. 20174(4):1349–1356. Available from: https://doi.org/10.18203/2349-3291.ijcp20172664. Accessed 16 Dec 2017.

19. Wu JH, Chen CY, Tsao PN, Hsieh WS, Chou HC. Neonatal sepsis: a 6-year analysis in a neonatal care unit in Taiwan. Pediatr Neonatol. 200950(3):88–95. Available from: https://doi.org/10.1016/S1875-9572(09)60042-5. Accessed 16 Dec 2017.

20. Jasani B, Kannan S, Nanavati R, Gogtay NJ, Thatte U. An audit of colistin use in neonatal sepsis from a tertiary care centre of a resource-limited country. Indian J Med Res. 2016144(3):433–439. Available from: https://doi.org/10.4103/0971-5916.198682. Accessed 18 Dec 2017.

21. Mulla SA, Revdiwala SB. Neonatal High antibiotic resistance of the bacterial pathogens in a neonatal intensive care unit of a tertiary Care hospital. J Clin Neonatol. 2012;1(2):72–75. Available from: https://doi.org/10.4103/2249-4847.96753. Accessed 18 Dec 2017.

22. Sheth KV, Patel TK, Tripathi CB. Antibiotic sensitivity pattern in neonatal intensive care unit of a tertiary care hospital of India. Asian J Pharm Clin Res. 2012 5(3):46–50. Available from: http://www.ajpcr.com/Vol5Issue3/965.pdf. Accessed 18 Dec 2017.

23. Yusef D, Shalakhti T, Awad S, Algharaibeh H, Khasawneh W. Clinical characteristics and epidemiology of sepsis in the neonatal intensive care unit in the era of multi-drug resistant organisms: a retrospective review. Pediatr Neonatol. 2017 June;59(1):35-41. Available from: https://doi.org/10.1016/j.pedneo.2017.06.001. Accessed 18 Dec 2017.

24. Shaw CK, Shaw P, Thapalial A. Neonatal sepsis bacterial isolates and antibiotic susceptibility patterns at a NICU in a tertiary care hospital in western Nepal: A retrospective analysis. Kathmandu Univ Med J. 2007;5(18):153–160. Available from: http://www.kumj.com.np/issue/18/153-160.pdf. Accessed 20 Dec 2017.

25. Sarangi KK, Pattnaik D, Mishra SN, Nayak MK, Jena J. Bacteriological profile and antibiogram of blood culture isolates done by automated culture and sensitivity method in a neonatal intensive care unit in a tertiary care hospital in Odisha, India: Int J. Adv Med. 2015;2(4):387–92. Available from: https://doi.org/10.18203/2349-3933.ijam20151015. Accessed 20 Dec 2017

26. Dalal P, Gathwala G, Gupta M, Singh J. Bacteriological profile and antimicrobial sensitivity pattern in neonatal sepsis: a study from North India. Int J Res Med Sci. 2017:5(4):1541–1545. Available from: https://doi.org/10.18203/2320-6012.ijrms20171261. Accessed 20 Dec 2017.

27. Fuchs A, Bielici J, Mathur S, Sharland M, van den Anker JN. Antibiotic use for sepsis in neonates and children: 2016 evidence update. WHO-Reviews; 2016. 25 p. Available from: http://www.who.int/selection_medicines/committees/expert/21/applications/s6_paed_antibiotics_appendix4_sepsis.pdf. Accessed 21 Dec 2017.

28. Moore MR, Schrag SJ, Schuchat A. Effects of intrapartum antimicrobial prophylaxis for prevention of group B streptococcal disease on the incidence and ecology of early-onset neonatal sepsis. Lancet Infect Dis. 20033(4):201–13. Available from: http:// doi.org/10.1016/S1473-3099(03)00577-2. Accessed 21 Dec 2017.

29. Stoll BJ, Schuchat A. Maternal carriage of group B streptococci in developing countries. Pediatr Infect Dis J. 1998;17:499–503. Available from: http://journals.lww.com/pidj/Abstract/1998/06000/Maternal__carriage_of_group_B_streptococci_in.13.aspx. Accessed 22 Dec 2017.

30. Mohsen L, Ramy N, Saied D, Akmal D, Salama N, Abdel Haleim MM, Aly H. Emerging antimicrobial resistance in early and late-onset neonatal sepsis. Antimicrob Resist Infect Control. 2017;6(63):1–9. Available from: http:// doi.org/10.1186/s13756-017-0225-9. Accessed 22 Dec 2017.

31. Panigrahi P, Parida S, Nanda NC, Satpathy R, Pradhan L, Chandel DS, Baccaglini L, Mohapatra A, Mohapatra SS, Misra PR, Chaudhry R, Chen HH, Johnson JA, Morris JG, Paneth N, Gewolb IH. A randomized synbiotic trial to prevent sepsis among infants in rural India. Nature 2017;548(7668):407–412. Available from: https://doi.org/10.1038/nature23480. Accessed 2018 Feb 15.

Prevalence and seasonality of common viral respiratory pathogens, including Cytomegalovirus in children, between 0–5 years of age in KwaZulu-Natal, an HIV endemic province in South Africa

Temitayo Famoroti[1]* (ID), Wilbert Sibanda[2] and Thumbi Ndung'u[3]

Abstract

Background: Acute respiratory tract infections contribute significantly to morbidity and mortality among young children in resource-poor countries. However, studies on the viral aetiology of acute respiratory infections, seasonality and the relative contributions of comorbidities such as immune deficiency states to viral respiratory tract infections in children in these countries are limited.

Methods: A retrospective analysis of laboratory test results of upper or lower respiratory specimens of children between 0 and 5 years of age collected between 1st January 2011 and 31st July 2015 from hospitals in KwaZulu-Natal, South Africa. Respiratory specimens were tested for viral respiratory pathogens using multiplex polymerase chain reaction (PCR), HIV testing was performed either by serological or PCR methods. Cytomegalovirus (CMV) respiratory infection was determined using the CMV R-gene PCR kit.

Results: In total 2172 specimens were analysed, of which 1175 (54.1%) were from males. The median age was 3.0 months (interquartile range [IQR] 1–7). Samples from the lower respiratory tract accounted for 1949 (89.7%) of all specimens. Respiratory multiplex PCR results were positive in 834 (45.7%) specimens. Respiratory syncytial virus (RSV) was the most commonly detected virus in 316 (32.1%) patients, followed by adenovirus (ADV) in 215 (21.8%), human rhinovirus (Hrhino) in 152 (15.4%) and influenza A (FluA) in 50 (5.1%). A seasonal time series pattern was observed for ADV (winter peak), enterovirus (EV) (autumn), human bocavirus (HBoV) (summer), and parainfluenza viruses 1 and 3 (PIV1 and 3) (spring). Stationary or untrended seasonal variation was observed for FluA (winter peak) and RSV (summer). HIV results were available for 1475 (67.9%) specimens; of these 348 (23.6%) were positive. CMV results were available for 714 (32.9%) specimens, of which 416 (58.3%) were positive. There was a statistically significant association between the coinfection of HIV and CMV with ADV.

Conclusions: In this study, we identified the most common respiratory viral pathogens detected among hospitalized children in KwaZulu-Natal. The coinfection between HIV and CMV was found to be associated with an increased risk of only adenovirus infection. Most viral pathogens showed a seasonal trend of occurrence. Our data has implications for the rational design of public health programmes.

Keywords: Children, Respiratory virus, Seasonality, South Africa

---

* Correspondence: famoroti@ukzn.ac.za; teeboy555@yahoo.co.uk
[1]Department of Virology, National Health Laboratory Service, Nelson R Mandela School of Medicine, University of KwaZulu-Natal, Durban, KwaZulu-Natal, South Africa
Full list of author information is available at the end of the article

Background

Respiratory tract infections are common in children and account for significant cases of absenteeism from school, hospitalization and sometimes death [1]. Viruses are a leading cause of these infections in children under 5 years of age and are associated with significant morbidity and mortality [2, 3]. Among children aged 1–59 months acute respiratory infection, diarrhoea, and malaria are the leading cause of death with over 15% caused by acute respiratory tract infection (ARTI) [4]. It is estimated that up to 53% of infants will have a viral respiratory tract infection in the first year of life and about 3% of children less than 1 year of age may require hospitalization with moderate or severe respiratory infections [5].

Costs attributable to viral respiratory tract infections in both outpatient and inpatient settings are an important burden on national healthcare budgets [5]. Children from poor socio-economic backgrounds are more susceptible to viral respiratory tract infection, as are malnourished children [6]. Overcrowding, especially among children attending day care centres, lack of breastfeeding, poor weaning methods, and exposure of children to passive smoking by their parents are other factors associated with viral respiratory infection [6]. Other important factors are the immunization status of the children as well as the human immunodeficiency virus (HIV) infection status [6, 7].

Respiratory viruses are generally transmitted through inhalation of aerosols or direct contact with respiratory secretions. Transmission is often associated with climatic factors such as low temperatures, low ultraviolet radiation and low humidity which prolong the survival of respiratory viruses in the environment [8]. The seasonality of respiratory viral infections in temperate countries is associated with temperature changes [8]. This can be partly explained by behavioural changes whereby individuals seek shelter and tend to congregate together due to reduced environmental temperature associated with seasonal changes [2]. Viral respiratory infection has also been linked to an increase in susceptibility to bacterial infections by altering physical and immune system barriers leading to increased bacterial super infection [6, 9].

In tropical and subtropical countries, correlation of respiratory viral infections with climatic factors is not well defined, a situation exacerbated by lack of adequate diagnostic facilities [2, 10, 11]. The province of KwaZulu-Natal, in the eastern region of South Africa is defined as having a sub-tropical climate [12] and it is also the epicentre of the HIV epidemic in the country [13]. The aim of this study was to determine the most common viral pathogens associated with ARTI among children between 0 and 5 years of age in KwaZulu-Natal, to describe seasonal patterns for identified viral pathogens, to assess the effect of HIV status on viral respiratory disease pattern, and the impact HIV status has on respiratory cytomegalovirus (CMV) infection.

We also investigated the association of CMV and HIV co-infection on viral respiratory infection. A detailed understanding of the prevalence, seasonality and interactions between viral respiratory pathogens would form the basis for the development of public health interventions to prevent associated morbidity and mortality.

Methods

Study design

This study involved retrospective data mining of a laboratory information database system. The study population consisted of patients between 0 and 5 years of age whose lower or upper respiratory tract specimens were sent to the National Health Laboratory Services (NHLS) at Inkosi Albert Luthuli Central Hospital (IALCH) in Durban, KwaZulu-Natal, South Africa.

Specimen types and test methods

Upper respiratory tract samples were either nasopharyngeal swabs or aspirates while lower tract specimens were bronchoalveolar lavages, tracheal aspirates, or endotracheal aspirates. Respiratory specimens were used for both respiratory multiplex and CMV respiratory tests. The samples were collected between 1st January 2011 and 31st July 2015. Laboratory analysis for the respiratory specimens was performed using the multiplex Fast Track Diagnosis (FTD) respiratory pathogens 21 polymerase chain reaction (PCR) test kit (Fast Track Diagnostics, Luxembourg City, Luxembourg). At the IALCH virology laboratory, this kit has been validated for the detection of adenovirus (ADV), enterovirus (EV), influenza A (FluA), influenza B (FluB), human bocavirus (HBoV), human metapneumovirus (HMPV), parainfluenza viruses 1–4 (PIV 1–4), human rhinovirus (Hrhino) and respiratory syncytial virus (RSV) only and therefore these were the pathogens evaluated in this study.

CMV was tested for using the CMV R-gene PCR kit (Biomerieux SA Marcy-l'Étoile, France) while blood specimens were used for HIV testing either by Abbott Architect i4000 ELISA (Abbott, IL, USA) or *Cobas AmpliPrep/ Cobas TaqMan* HIV-1 Test (*CAP/CTM*) (Roche Diagnostics) for screening. In children less than 18 months HIV confirmatory testing was conducted using *Cobas AmpliPrep/Cobas TaqMan* HIV-1 Test (*CAP/CTM*) (Roche Diagnostics) and for children older than 18 months of age, Roche Cobas 6000 (Roche diagnostics) was used if the previous HIV test result was positive. Non-viral pathogens (e.g bacteria and fungi) were detected using appropriate culture media.

In this study, NHLS data was collected retrospectively by retrieving test results from the corporate data warehouse (CDW). Information retrieved included demographic and clinical data such as age, sex, specimen type, date of specimen collection, unique hospital number, location of patient in the health facility, respiratory multiplex, HIV, CMV and non-viral isolate test results.

Statistical analysis

The data retrieved was cleaned by discarding duplicated viral pathogen test results for the same patient within a two-week period only using the first positive results and removing the second duplicated positive results. Laboratory results with the following missing data were excluded: date of birth, specimen type, date of specimen collection and test set requested. Continuous variables such as age were summarised using mean ± standard deviation or median (IQR) and categorical variables such as sex, age groups, facility types, respiratory multiplex and CMV results were summarized using proportions and percentages. We carried out sub-group analysis to determine the between groups p value and on the basis of the between groups p value, we conducted pair wise comparisons for all the sub-group pairs while adjusting the alpha level using a Bonferroni correction. The effect of HIV and CMV on viral respiratory infection was investigated by comparing the proportion of respiratory specimens with HIV and CMV coinfection compared with specimens that were HIV and CMV negative using a z test. Categorical variables were compared using Pearson's chi-squared test or Fisher's exact test, as appropriate. All analysis was conducted using IBM SPSS version 25 (IBM Corp. Released 2018. IBM SPSS Statistics for Windows, Version 25.0. Armonk, NY: IBM Corp). The level of significance was set at $p < 0.05$.

An objective of the study was to identify and describe seasonal patterns of respiratory viruses using the Autoregressive Integrated Moving Averages (ARIMA) model. ARIMA models are generalisations of Autoregressive Moving Averages and these models are fitted to time series data to understand the data and predict future points in the series [14]. In this study, ARIMA models were used to isolate the seasonal component by removing the underlying trend [15]. The trend was estimated by means of a centred 12 point moving averages. The resulting values were averaged for each month over the duration of the study and expressed as percentages. The 12 percentages were taken as representing the seasonal profile of each respiratory virus. Autocorrelation Function (ACF) and Partial Correlation Function (PACF) plots were used to identify the number of autoregressive and moving average terms, thereby assisting in determining the stationarity and seasonality of the time series. Seasonal indices were calculated as a measure of how the prevalence of the respiratory viruses changed during a given season compared with the season's average. A seasonal index is a measure of how the prevalence of a respiratory virus compares with the season's average.

Ethical considerations

The protocol for the study was approved by the University of KwaZulu-Natal Biomedical Research Ethics Committee (BREC-BCA 143/09), while approval was obtained from the National Health Laboratory Services (NHLS) for the use of the data.

Results

Demographic distribution and specimen characteristics

Out of 2172 respiratory specimens during the period under review, 932 (42.9%) came from females and 1175 (54.1%) from males and the remaining 65 (3.0%) specimens did not indicate gender from which they came. The age range of patients studied, were from 0 to 60 months. The median age was 3.0 months, with an interquartile range (IQR) of 1–7 months, with the majority of patients 1599 (73.6%) aged 0 to 6 months.

One thousand nine hundred and forty-nine (89.7%) specimens were from the lower respiratory tract, with 223 (10.3%) upper respiratory specimens. One thousand eight hundred and twenty-three (83.9%) had results available for the multiplex viral respiratory pathogens PCR, with 834 (45.7%) positive and 989 (54.3%) negative (Table 1). The majority of the specimens, 1678 (77.3%) were from patients admitted to the intensive care unit (ICU), 454 (20.9%) specimens were from general hospital ward patients, 38 (1.7%) were from nursery and 2 (0.1%) were from the out-patient department (OPD) (Table 1).

A total of 984 viral pathogens were isolated from 834 positive specimens analysed for respiratory pathogens, out of which 715 (85.7%) had only one viral isolate, 92 (11.0%) had two isolates, 23 (2.8%) had three isolates and 4 (0.5%) possessed four different isolated viruses (Fig. 1). RSV was the most frequently detected virus pathogen in 316 (32.1%) isolates, followed by ADV in 215 (21.8%), Hrhino viruses in 152 (15.4%), PIV3 virus in 90 (9.1%), FluA in 50 (5.1%), FluB in 33 (3.4%) and PIV2 was the least common of the viruses detected, found in only 5 (0.5%) of isolates (Fig. 2).

Out of the total 2172 specimens, 814 (37.5%) had non-viral isolates, in which *Klebsiella pneumoniae was* the most common isolated non-viral isolate detected in 190 (23.3%), followed by *Staphylococcus aureus* in 108 (13.3%), *Acinetobacter baumannii* in 104 (12.8%), *Candida albicans* in 45 (5.5%), *Pseudomonas aeruginosa* in 56 (6.9%) and *Streptococcus pneumoniae* in 29 (3.6%).

Out of 984 viral pathogens, 579 (58.8%) were from HIV negative individuals, 142 (14.4%) were from HIV positive individuals, while the rest 263 (26.7%) were of unknown HIV status. Five hundred and ninety-nine (60.9%) out of the total 984 viral pathogens were from patients between the ages of 0–6 months, 326 (54.4%) were males and 261 (43.6%) were females and the remaining 12 (2.0%) were of unknown gender (Table 2).

Table 1 Demographic distribution and specimen characteristics

Variables	N	%
Male	1175	54.1
Female	932	42.9
Gender not stated	65	3.0
Total	2172	100
Age (months)		
0–6	1599	73.6
7–12	232	10.7
13–24	204	9.4
25–60	137	6.3
Total	2172	100
Facility type[a]		
District	245	11.3
Tertiary	374	17.2
Specialised	1553	71.5
Total	2172	100
Respiratory multiplex results		
Positive	834	45.7
Negative	989	54.3
Total	1823	100
CMV results		
Positive	416	58.3
Negative	298	41.7
Total	714	100

[a]In South Africa health facilities are categorised into district, tertiary and specialised according to the level of care

HIV results were available for 1475 (67.9%) specimens with 348 (23.6%) positive and 1127 (76.4%) negative, with the remaining 697 (32.1%) of unknown HIV result. There were only 714 specimens with CMV data available of which 416 (58.3%) were positive. Out of 1475 specimens with HIV results 536 (36.3%) had both CMV and HIV results available, of these 161 (84.7%) were both CMV positive and HIV positive. One hundred and sixty eight (48.6%) were CMV positive and HIV negative, 178 (51.4%) were both CMV negative and HIV negative and 29 (15.3%) were CMV negative and HIV positive. Using a chi-square test a statistically significant association was found between CMV and HIV infection ($p = 0.0001$). This indicates that HIV positive results are more likely to be associated with CMV positive results.

An investigation into the relationship between the presence of respiratory viruses, age, sex, HIV and CMV results using a one-way analysis-of-variance (ANOVA), revealed that there was a statistically significant difference between the four age groups (0–6, 7–12, 13–24 and 25–60 months) with respect to the frequency of respiratory viruses ($p < 0.0001$). There was a statistically higher proportion of ADV results that were coinfected with CMV and HIV than specimens that were not coinfected with CMV and HIV, 5.1 and 0.5% respectively ($p = 0.004$) suggesting an association between ADV and coinfection with CMV and HIV. However, a different picture was observed for RSV, where CMV and HIV negative associated results had higher proportion of RSV compared to coinfected CMV and HIV results (10.4 and 1.9% respectively, $p = 0.001$). In the case of FluA and Hrhino there was no statistically significant difference in the proportion found between CMV and HIV coinfection with p values of 0.91 and 0.93 respectively.

The youngest group aged between 0 and 6 months demonstrated the highest number of viral isolates detected at

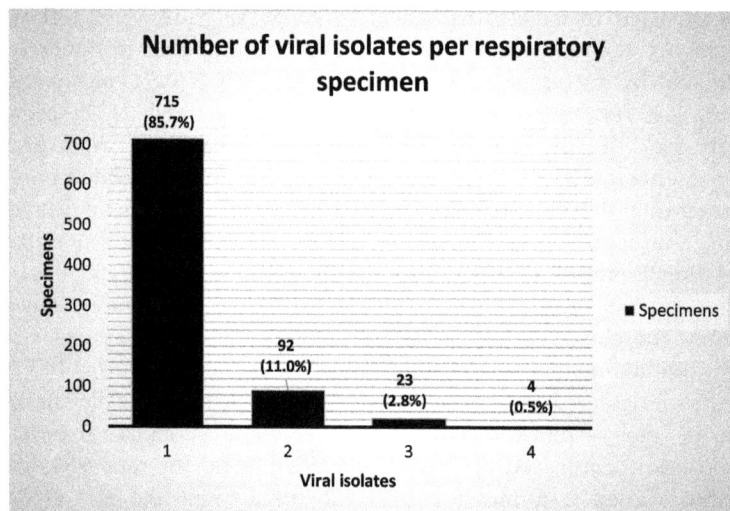

Fig. 1 Number of viral isolates

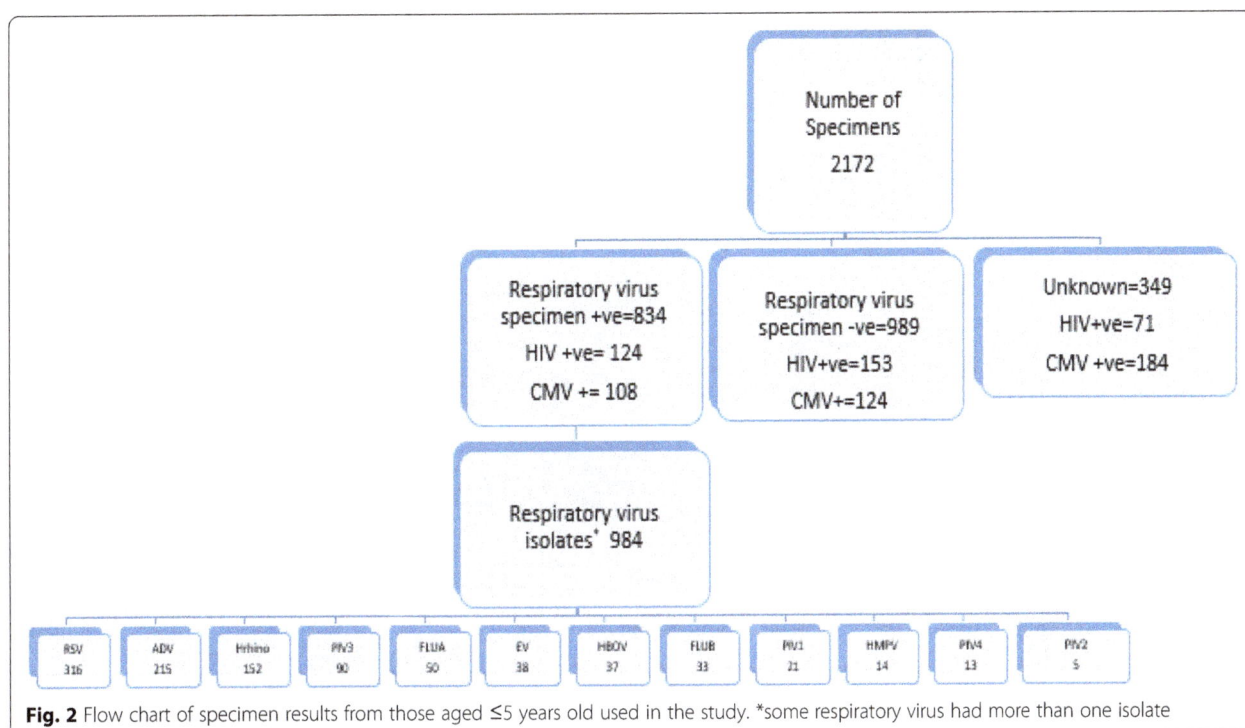

Fig. 2 Flow chart of specimen results from those aged ≤5 years old used in the study. *some respiratory virus had more than one isolate

599 (60.9%), out of the total number of 984 specimens with at least one isolate detected. There was no statistically significant difference in frequency of respiratory viruses between males and females comparing all the age groups ($p = 0.08$).

Seasonality

South Africa has 4 annual seasons, namely autumn, winter, spring and summer [16]. Figure 3 shows the pattern of viral respiratory pathogen isolated during the study period between 1st January 2011 and 31st July 2015. A seasonal time series pattern was observed for ADV (winter peak in August), EV (autumn peak in May), HBoV (summer peak in February), PIV1 (spring peak in November) and PIV3 (spring peak in November). Stationary or untrended seasonal variation was observed for FluA (winter peak in August) and RSV (summer peak in February). Irregular cyclical time series trends were observed for HMPV, PIV2 and Hrhino, where the trends exhibited rises and falls that were not of fixed period. A seasonal time series pattern is characterised by a regular and predictable change that occurs every calendar year, while stationary or untrended seasonal variation is characterised by a constant seasonal variation that neither increases or decreases over time.

Seasonal indices are shown in Table 3. A seasonal index is a measure of how the prevalence of a respiratory virus compares with the season's average. It shows that in autumn and winter, ADV was detected 1.287 and 1.340 times more than the average. An autumn seasonal index

of 2.353 for PIV4, indicates that in autumn more than twice the average prevalence of PIV4 was observed. Based on seasonal indices, all the viruses demonstrated a seasonal spread, with some viruses detected two seasons per year (a biannual pattern), such as ADV (autumn and winter), FluA (autumn and winter), HMPV (summer and spring), PIV3 (summer and spring) and RSV (summer and autumn).

Discussion

Viral agents play an important role in respiratory infections associated with disease in young children but their prevalence, seasonality and predisposing factors are not well understood in resource-poor countries. The results in this study show that RSV was the most commonly detected viral pathogen in the respiratory specimens, consistent with the view that RSV is a leading cause of respiratory tract infection in infants and young children worldwide [10] causing an estimated 66,000 to 199,000 deaths per year globally in children less than 5 years of age [17]. The overall prevalence of RSV (32.1%) is comparable to previous studies done in other developing countries with tropical and sub-tropical climates such as Ghana [10] and Malaysia [8] though in a South African study conducted in Pretoria [18], RSV was more common in HIV-uninfected children than in HIV-infected children which was consistent with our study.

ADV was the second most commonly detected virus (21.8%) in this study, similar to a Ghanaian study although the prevalence was lower at 10.2% [10]. A Malaysian study

Table 2 Classification of respiratory viruses according to age, sex, HIV and CMV results

Virus	RSV n (%)	ADV n (%)	Hrhino n (%)	PIV3 n (%)	FluA n (%)	EV n (%)	HBoV n (%)	FluB n (%)	PIV1 n (%)	HMPV n (%)	PIV4 n (%)	PIV2 n (%)	Total	P Value
Age														
0–6	250 (79.1)	102 (47.4)	91 (59.9)	59 (65.6)	27 (54)	22 (57.9)	9 (24.3)	15 (45.5)	12 (57.1)	3 (21.4)	6 (46.2)	3 (60)	599 (60.9)	< 0.0001
7–12	10 (3.2)	25 (11.6)	11 (7.2)	9 (10)	3 (6)	4 (10.5)	8 (21.6)	2 (6.1)	4 (19)	3 (21.4)	2 (15.4)	0 (0)	81 (8.2)	
13–24	49 (15.5)	72 (33.5)	40 (26.3)	16 (17.8)	17 (34.0)	6 (23.7)	18 (48.6)	14 (42.4)	4 (19.0)	7 (50.0)	5 (38.5)	2 (40.0)	253 (25.7)	
25–60	7 (2.2)	16 (7.4)	10 (6.6)	6 (6.7)	3 (6)	3 (7.9)	2 (5.4)	2 (6.1)	1 (4.8)	1 (7.1)	0 (0)	0 (0)	51 (5.2)	
Total	316	215	152	90	50	38	37	33	21	14	13	5	984	
Sex														
Male	181 (58.6)	128 (60.7)	75 (50.7)	39 (43.8)	27 (55.1)	26 (70.3)	20 (54.1)	19 (57.6)	10 (50.0)	5 (35.7)	5 (41.7)	2 (40)	537 (55.7)	0.08
Female	128 (41.4)	83 (39.3)	73 (49.3)	50 (56.2)	22 (44.9)	11 (29.7)	17 (45.9)	14 (42.4)	10 (50.0)	9 (64.3)	7 (58.3)	3 (60)	427 (44.3)	
Total	309	211	148	89	49	37	37	33	20	14	12	5	964	
Facility type														
District	30 (9.5)	24 (11.1)	19 (12.5)	14 (15.6)	7 (14.0)	2 (5.3)	4 (10.8)	5 (15.2)	0 (0.0)	1 (7.1)	0 (0.0)	2 (40.0)	108 (11.0)	0.84
Tertiary	54 (17.1)	33 (15.3)	25 (16.4)	17 (18.9)	10 (20.0)	8 (21.1)	3 (8.1)	3 (9.1)	8 (38.1)	3 (21.4)	8 (61.5)	1 (20.0)	173 (17.6)	
Specialised	232 (73.5)	158 (73.5)	108 (71.1)	59 (65.6)	33 (66.0)	28 (73.7)	30 (81.1)	25 (75.8)	13 (61.9)	10 (71.4)	5 (38.5)	2 (40.0)	703 (71.4)	
Total	316	215	152	90	50	38	37	33	21	14	13	5	984	
HIV Positive	27 (11.6)	33 (21.0)	29 (25.2)	20 (29.0)	4 (12.1)	4 (17.4)	7 (24.1)	8 (30.8)	6 (40.0)	2 (16.7)	2 (25.0)	0 (0.0)	142 (19.7)	0.006
HIV negative	205 (88.4)	124 (79.0)	86 (74.8)	49 (71.0)	29 (87.9)	19 (82.6)	22 (75.9)	18 (69.2)	9 (60.0)	10 (83.3)	6 (75.0)	2 (100.0)	579 (80.3)	
Total	232	157	115	69	33	23	29	26	15	12	8	2	721	
CMV Positive	28 (41.8)	29 (74.4)	21 (58.3)	14 (70.0)	9 (50.0)	5 (71.4)	9 (81.8)	5 (62.5)	4 (80.0)	2 (66.7)	7 (100.0)	1 (100.0)	134 (60.4)	0.042
CMV negative	39 (58.2)	10 (25.6)	15 (41.7)	6 (30.0)	9 (50.0)	2 (28.6)	2 (18.2)	3 (37.5)	1 (20.0)	1 (33.3)	0 (0.0)	0 (0.0)	88 (39.6)	
Total	67	39	36	20	18	7	11	8	5	3	7	1	222	

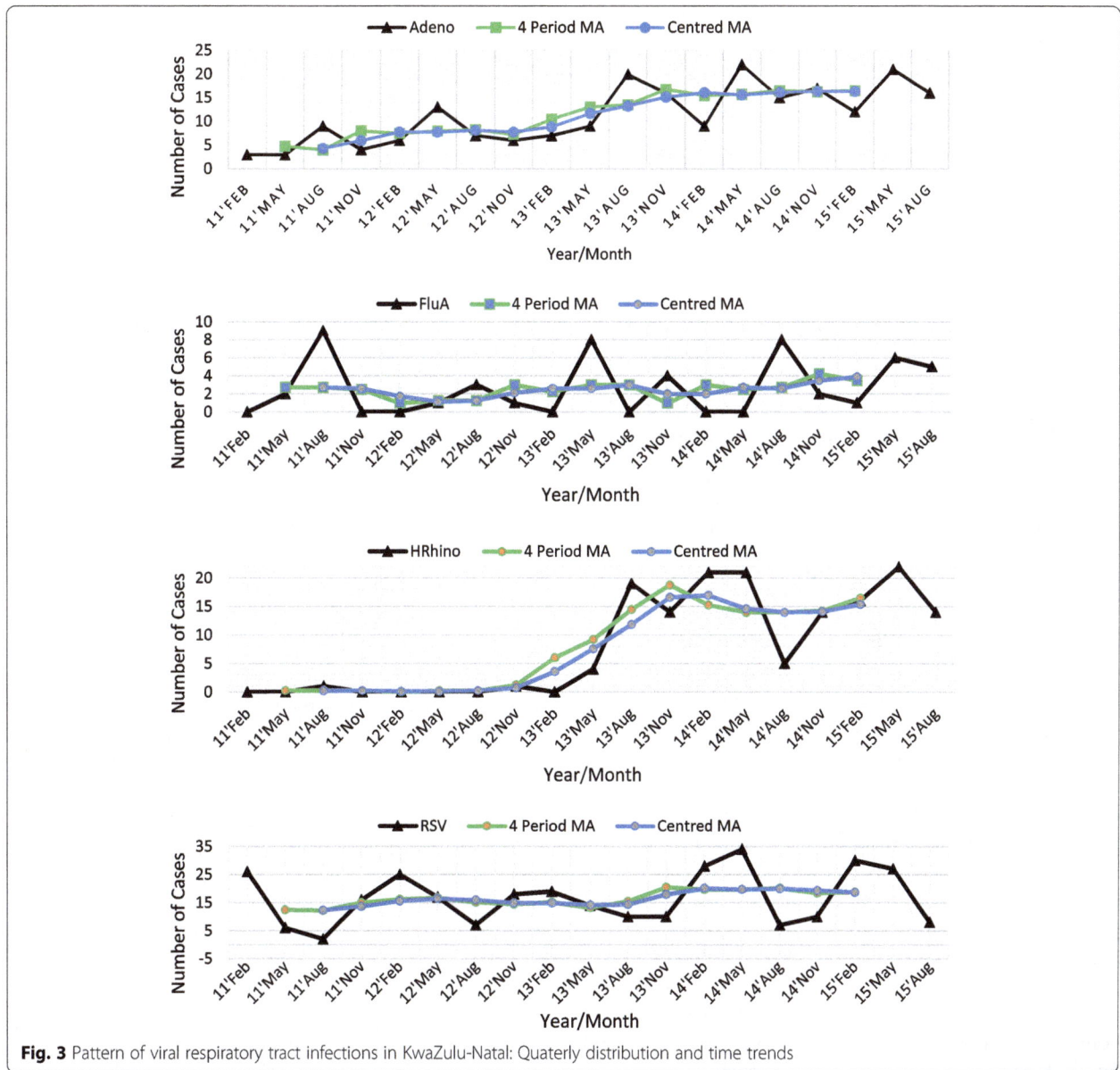

Fig. 3 Pattern of viral respiratory tract infections in KwaZulu-Natal: Quaterly distribution and time trends

also found ADV to be one of the most common respiratory viral isolates, although it ranked fourth in that study [8]. In another South African study done in Cape Town [19], ADV respiratory infections was isolated in 10.9% of all respiratory tract samples tested and it was linked to severe morbidity with 36.9% needing ICU admission and 14.1% developing persistent lung disease. The latter study is comparable to our study where 66.0% of the specimens were from the ICU which is an indirect indicator of disease severity.

Table 3 Seasonal indices

Season	Seasonal Indices											
	ADV	EV	FluA	FluB	HBOV	HMPV	PIV1	PIV2	PIV3	PIV4	Hrhino	RSV
Summer	0.713	1.011[a]	0	0	2.471[a]	1.714[a]	0.686	0.667	1.112[a]	0.571	0.569	1.450[a]
Autumn	1.287[a]	1.449[a]	1.312[a]	0	1.000	0	1.067[a]	0	0.480	2.353[a]	0.653	1.450[a]
Winter	1.340[a]	0.458	2.180[a]	0.841	0	0.533	0.741	0	0.875	0.308	1.489[a]	0.412
Spring	0.885	0.695	0.761	1.844[a]	0.242	1.949[a]	2.115[a]	0.889	1.650[a]	0.308	0.792	0.864

[a]Boldface indicates Seasonal indices above 1 means that prevalence of a respiratory virus is above average

Hrhino virus was the third most commonly isolated pathogen in this study, in contrast to studies by Pretorius et al. (2012) and Annamalay et al. (2016) in which it was commonest [11, 18]. Both studies highlight that Hrhino virus is an important viral pathogen in children in the South African setting. In the Annamalay et al. (2016) study Hrhino virus detection was highest in the 18–24 months age group [18] compared to our study where it was commonest in the age group 0–6 months. In a study by Abadom et al. (2016) in South Africa, HIV was more prevalent among cases of influenza associated with severe acute respiratory infection [20]. However, this is different in our study, where most of the specimens with a positive influenza result were linked to an HIV negative result 29 (87.9%) compared to an HIV positive result 4 (12.1%).

Out of all the detected viral pathogens 599 (60.9%) were isolated from the age group 0–6 months, emphasizing the high infection burden in this group and likely associated morbidity and mortality, similar to a study by Khor et al. (2012, Malaysia) where 76.2% of the positive cases were isolated from children less than 1 year old [8]. Cytomegalovirus has been implicated as a cause of increased morbidity and mortality and associated with respiratory disease, especially in immunocompromised individuals such as those infected with HIV, transplant patients and patients on therapy for autoimmune diseases [21–23]. In this current study, there was significant association between coinfected HIV and CMV results which is similar to a study conducted by Zampoli et al. (2011) in Cape Town where CMV associated respiratory disease was more common in HIV infected than uninfected children [21].

An important finding from our study is that most viral pathogens detected displayed seasonal prevalence trends, with most having peak periods between autumn and winter, suggestive of increased susceptibility to respiratory viral infections during the colder months. Overall, these results are consistent with other studies from Malaysia, Brazil and South Africa that all indicate that seasonality is a common feature of viral respiratory infections [2, 8, 11]. However, there are some contrasting findings between our study and other studies, such as a study conducted in Malaysia were no seasonal trend was observed for ADV [8]. Some studies have also documented that ADV is normally isolated all year round with no distinct seasonal trends [24].

Hrhino virus was isolated all year round with the trends exhibiting rises and falls that were not of fixed period in our study which is different from a study by Gardinassi et al. (2012), that was conducted in Brazil where outbreaks were observed in spring, autumn and winter [2]. In our study a seasonality pattern was noted for FluA from 2011 to 2015, with first yearly isolations in autumn and a peak in winter, which is similar to previous surveillance reports where the virus was first isolated in autumn, peaked in winter and tapered off in late winter [25–29]. However, in 2015, more Flu B than Flu A was detected in our study, which is similar to the influenza-like illness (ILI) surveillance report by NICD [29] and this could be an emerging trend in the prevalence of Flu B.

The limitations of our study could be due to the fact that it was retrospective in nature and therefore it was not possible to differentiate between community acquired and nosocomial infections. Emerging respiratory viruses were not tested for in this study, which can also pose a significant public health risk especially in children with immature immune systems. In the same vein, inferring whether a pathogen was a bystander or contributing to disease was a challenge in our study due to the probability of patients having other co-morbidities and therefore more detailed epidemiological and clinical studies are required to evaluate the relative importance of respiratory viral pathogens in this setting. The diagnostic kit used for detection of viral infections was also not exhaustive, and therefore important viral infections that may contribute to morbidity and mortality in children may have been missed.

Conclusions

Viruses play an important role in respiratory diseases in young children and this report shows the high burden of infection in children especially the younger age group of 0 to 6 months. The association between HIV infected children and CMV respiratory infection highlights the importance of investigating CMV in sick young children.

The data on seasonality shows that most viral respiratory pathogens showed seasonal patterns with slight differences from other studies with pathogens such as ADV previously thought to show no seasonal pattern showing regular predictable peaks and trends in this study. Our study highlights the need for more comprehensive studies on viral associated respiratory tract infections with the goal of developing more effective interventional strategies to prevent and treat these infections that impose a huge public health and socio-economic burden in resource-limited countries. Overall, more comprehensive studies are needed to identify prevalence and seasonal trends of respiratory viral agents relevant to developing countries.

Abbreviations

ADV: Adenovirus; ARTI: Acute respiratory tract infection; CDW: Corporate data warehouse; CMV: Cytomegalovirus; EV: Enterovirus; FluA: Influenza A; FluB: Influenza B; HBoV: Human boca virus; HIV: Human immunodeficiency virus; HMPV: Human metapneumovirus; Hrhino: Human Rhino virus; ICU: Intensive care unit; IFA: Immunofluorescence assay; NHLS: National Health Laboratory Services; PCR: Polymerase chain reaction; PIV1: Parainfluenza virus 1; PIV2: Parainfluenza virus 2; PIV3: Parainfluenza virus 3; PIV4: Parainfluenza virus 4; RSV: Respiratory syncytial virus

Acknowledgements

We wish to thank the National Health Laboratory Services (NHLS) for the data and staff of the Department of Virology, Inkosi Albert Luthuli Central Hospital. Open access publication of this article has been made possible through support from the Victor Daitz Information Gateway, an initiative of the Victor Daitz Foundation and the University of KwaZulu-Natal.

Authors' contributions

Research idea and study design: TF and TN; Data acquisition: TF and TN; Data analysis and Interpretation: TF, WS and TN; Statistical analysis: WS; Supervision and Mentoring: TN. Each author contributed important intellectual content during manuscript drafting or revision and accepts accountability for the overall work by ensuring that questions pertaining to the accuracy or integrity of any portion of the work are appropriately investigated and resolved. All authors read and approved the final manuscript.

Competing interests

The authors declare that they have no competing interests.

Author details

[1]Department of Virology, National Health Laboratory Service, Nelson R Mandela School of Medicine, University of KwaZulu-Natal, Durban, KwaZulu-Natal, South Africa. [2]Biostatistics Unit, School of Nursing and Public Health, College of Health Sciences, University of KwaZulu-Natal, Durban, KwaZulu-Natal, South Africa. [3]HIV Pathogenesis Programme, Doris Duke Medical Research Institute, Nelson R Mandela School of Medicine, University of KwaZulu-Natal, Durban, KwaZulu-Natal, South Africa.

References

1. McLean HQ, Peterson SH, King JP, Meece JK, Belongia EA. School absenteeism among school-aged children with medically attended acute viral respiratory illness during three influenza seasons, 2012-2013 through 2014-2015. Influenza Other Respir Viruses. 2017;11(3):220–9. https://www.ncbi.nlm.nih.gov/pmc/articles/PMC5410714/pdf/IRV-11-220. pdf. Accessed 21 May 2018

2. Gardinassi LG, Simas PV, Salomão JB, Durigon EL, Trevisan DM, Cordeiro JA, Lacerda MN, Rahal P, Souza FP. Seasonality of viral respiratory infections in southeast of Brazil: the influence of temperature and air humidity. Braz J Microbiol. 2012;43(1):98–108.

3. Wong-Chew RM, Espinoza MA, Taboada B, Aponte FE, Arias-Ortiz MA, Monge-Martínez J, Rodríguez-Vázquez R, Díaz-Hernández F, Zárate-Vidal F, Santos-Preciado JI, López S. Prevalence of respiratory virus in symptomatic children in private physician office settings in five communities of the state of Veracruz, Mexico. BMC research notes. 2015;8(1):261.

4. World Health Organization. World Health Statistics 2018: Monitoring health for the sustainable development goals. http://apps.who.int/iris/bitstream/ handle/10665/272596/9789241565585-eng.pdf?ua=1. Accessed 9 June 2018.

5. Van Woensel JB, Van Aalderen WM, Kimpen JL. Viral lower respiratory tract infection in infants and young children. BMJ: British Medical Journal. 2003;327(7405):36.

6. Ujunwa FA, Ezeonu CT. Risk factors for acute respiratory tract infections in under-five children in Enugu Southeast Nigeria. Annals of medical and health sciences research. 2014;4(1):95–9.

7. Lonngren C, Morrow BM, Haynes S, Yusri T, Vyas H, Argent AC. North–south divide: distribution and outcome of respiratory viral infections in paediatric intensive care units in Cape Town (South Africa) and Nottingham (United Kingdom). J Paediatr Child Health. 2014;50(3):208–15.

8. Khor CS, Sam IC, Hooi PS, Quek KF, Chan YF. Epidemiology and seasonality of respiratory viral infections in hospitalized children in Kuala Lumpur, Malaysia: a retrospective study of 27 years. BMC pediatrics. 2012;12(1):32.

9. Tregoning JS, Schwarze J. Respiratory viral infections in infants: causes, clinical symptoms, virology, and immunology. Clin Microbiol Rev. 2010;23(1):74–98.

10. Kwofie TB, Anane YA, Nkrumah B, Annan A, Nguah SB, Owusu M. Respiratory viruses in children hospitalized for acute lower respiratory tract infection in Ghana. Virol J. 2012;9(1):78.

11. Pretorius MA, Madhi SA, Cohen C, Naidoo D, Groome M, Moyes J, Buys A, Walaza S, Dawood H, Chhagan M, Haffjee S. Respiratory viral coinfections identified by a 10-plex real-time reverse-transcription polymerase chain reaction assay in patients hospitalized with severe acute respiratory illness—South Africa, 2009–2010. J Infect Dis. 2012;206(suppl_1):S159–65.

12. Medical education partner initiative (MEPI), University of KwaZulu-Natal. Geography-South Africa: http://mepi.ukzn.ac.za/OtherInfo/Geographyaspx. Accessed 15 July 2017.

13. KwaZulu-Natal, Department of health. HIV counselling and testing campaign (HCT) in KwaZulu-Natal. 2010. http://www.kznhealth.gov.za/ simama/hct.htm. Accessed 16 June 2017.

14. Helfenstein U. Box-Jenkins modelling of some viral infectious diseases. Stat Med. 1986;5(1):37–47.

15. Chadsuthi S, Iamsirithaworn S, Triampo W, Modchang C. Modeling seasonal influenza transmission and its association with climate factors in Thailand using time-series and ARIMAX analyses. Computational and mathematical methods in medicine. 2015;2015

16. Department of Environmental Affairs. South African weather services (SAWS). http://www.weathersa.co.za/learning/weather-questions/82-how-are-the-dates-of-the-four-seasons-worked-out. Accessed 18 July 2017.

17. Mazur NI, Bont L, Cohen AL, Cohen C, Von Gottberg A, Groome MJ, Hellferscee O, Klipstein-Grobusch K, Mekgoe O, Naby F, Moyes J. Severity of respiratory syncytial virus lower respiratory tract infection with viral coinfection in HIV-uninfected children. Clin Infect Dis. 2016; 64(4):443–50.

18. Annamalay AA, Abbott S, Sikazwe C, Khoo SK, Bizzintino J, Zhang G, Laing I, Chidlow GR, Smith DW, Gern J, Goldblatt J. Respiratory viruses in young south African children with acute lower respiratory infections and interactions with HIV. J Clin Virol. 2016;81:58–63.

19. Zampoli M, Mukuddem-Sablay Z. Adenovirus-associated pneumonia in south African children: presentation, clinical course and outcome. SAMJ: South African Medical Journal. 2017;107(2):123–6.

20. Abadom TR, Smith AD, Tempia S, Madhi SA, Cohen C, Cohen AL. Risk factors associated with hospitalisation for influenza-associated severe acute respiratory illness in South Africa: a case-population study. Vaccine. 2016; 34(46):5649–55.

21. Zampoli M, Morrow B, Hsiao NY, Whitelaw A, Zar HJ. Prevalence and outcome of cytomegalovirus-associated pneumonia in relation to human immunodeficiency virus infection. Pediatr Infect Dis J. 2011;30(5): 413–7.

22. Govender K, Jeena P, Parboosing R. Clinical utility of bronchoalveolar lavage cytomegalovirus viral loads in the diagnosis of cytomegalovirus pneumonitis in infants. J Med Virol. 2017;89(6):1080–7.

23. Adland E, Klenerman P, Goulder P, Matthews P. Ongoing burden of disease and mortality from HIV/CMV coinfection in Africa in the antiretroviral therapy era. Front Microbiol. 2015;6:1016.

24. Richman DD, Whitley RJ, Hayden FG. Clinical virology 4th edition ed. Washington DC: ASM press; 2017. Pg 9.

25. National Health Laboratory Services (NHLS), Communicable diseases surveillance bulletin. National institute for communicable diseases (NICD). 2011. http:// www.nicd.ac.za/assets/files/CommDisBull%2010(2)-May%20final2012.pdf. Accessed 17 Feb 2016.

26. National Health Laboratory Services (NHLS), Communicable diseases surveillance bulletin. National institute for communicable diseases 2012 http://www.nicd.ac. za/assets/files/Communicable%20Diseases%20Surveillance%20Bulletin%20April %202013.pdf. Accessed 17 Feb 2016.

27. National Health Laboratory Services (NHLS), Communicable diseases surveillance bulletin. National institute for communicable diseases 2013 http://www.nicd.ac.za/assets/files/CommDisBull%2012(1)-April%202014_Fin. pdf. Accessed 17 Feb 2016.

28. National Health Laboratory Services (NHLS), Communicable diseases surveillance bulletin. National institute for communicable diseases 2014 http://www.nicd.ac.za/assets/files/CommDisBull%2013(1)-April%202015.pdf. Accessed 17 Feb 2016.

29. National Health Laboratory Services (NHLS), Communicable diseases surveillance bulletin. National institute for communicable diseases 2015 http://www.nicd.ac.za/assets/files/CommDisBull%2014(1)-Mar2016(1).pdf. Accessed 17 Feb 2016.

6

Effect of increased enteral protein intake on plasma and urinary urea concentrations in preterm infants born at < 32 weeks gestation and < 1500 g birth weight enrolled in a randomized controlled trial –a secondary analysis

Michaela Mathes[1]* , Christoph Maas[1], Christine Bleeker[1], Julia Vek[1], Wolfgang Bernhard[1], Andreas Peter[3,4,5], Christian F. Poets[1] and Axel R. Franz[1,2]

Abstract

Background: Feeding breast milk is associated with reduced morbidity and mortality, as well as improved neurodevelopmental outcome but does not meet the high nutritional requirements of preterm infants. Both plasma and urinary urea concentrations represent amino acid oxidation and low concentrations may indicate insufficient protein supply.

This study assesses the effect of different levels of enteral protein on plasma and urinary urea concentrations and determines if the urinary urea-creatinine ratio provides reliable information about the protein status of preterm infants.

Methods: Sixty preterm infants (birthweight < 1500 g; gestational age < 32 weeks) were enrolled in a randomized controlled trial and assigned to either a lower-protein group (median protein intake 3.7 g/kg/d) or a higher-protein group (median protein intake 4,3 g/kg/d). Half the patients in the higher-protein group received standardized supplementation with a supplement adding 1.8 g protein/100 ml milk, the other half received individual supplementation depending on the respective mother's milk macronutrient content. Plasma urea concentration was determined in two scheduled blood samples (BS1; BS2); urinary urea and creatinine concentrations in weekly spot urine samples.

Results: The higher-protein group showed higher plasma urea concentrations in both BS1 and BS2 and a higher urinary urea-creatinine-ratio in week 3 and 5–7 compared to the lower-protein group. In addition, a highly positive correlation between plasma urea concentrations and the urinary urea-creatinine-ratio ($p < 0.0001$) and between actual protein intake and plasma urea concentrations and the urinary urea-creatinine-ratio (both $p < 0.0001$) was shown.

Conclusions: The urinary urea-creatinine-ratio, just like plasma urea concentrations, may help to estimate actual protein supply, absorption and oxidation in preterm infants and, additionally, can be determined non-invasively. Further investigations are needed to determine reliable cut-off values of urinary urea concentrations to ensure appropriate protein intake.

(Continued on next page)

* Correspondence: michaela.mathes@med.uni-tuebingen.de
[1]Department of Neonatology, University Children's Hospital, Tübingen
University Hospital, Calwerstr. 7, Tübingen, Germany
Full list of author information is available at the end of the article

(Continued from previous page)

Keywords: Infant, premature, Very low birth weight infant, Infant, newborn, Enteral feeding, Nutrition, Protein supply, Milk, human, Supplementation, Targeted fortification, Urea concentration

Background

Feeding human milk has a lot of beneficial effects on preterm and term newborn infants. It contains immunoglobulins and cytokines and therefore offers protection against infections [1–3]. Besides, the ingestion of maternal milk reduces the incidence of necrotizing enterocolitis [4, 5], retinopathy of prematurity [5] and diabetes type 1 and 2, as well as obesity in later life [6, 7]. Furthermore, it is associated with improved neurocognitive and psychomotor development [8]. Therefore, mother's milk is considered the optimal nutritional source for preterm infants [9]. However, human milk does not meet the high nutrient needs of preterm infants, hence requires supplementation with multicomponent fortifiers [10]. Nevertheless, many preterm infants show early postnatal growth retardation despite having been fed fortified human milk [11].

In general, an average composition of breast milk is assumed and fortifiers are added in a standardized manner, but this assumption is rarely appropriate [12], because human milk is a biological product with considerable intra- and inter-individual variation of its macro- and micronutrient content, particularly protein [13].

To ensure an optimal supplementation with protein in the daily neonatal intensive care unit (NICU) routine, it is necessary to establish a feasible method to assess the individual protein supply and, ideally, protein availability for growth in very preterm infants.

Frequent measurements of the individual breast milk macronutrient content using a milk analyzer (mid-infrared spectroscopy) is an easy and valid method to assess macronutrient supply [14]. Nevertheless, due to the immaturity of the gastrointestinal system of a preterm infant and the individual intestinal microbiome the calculation of actual macronutrient supply might not reflect the effectively absorbed amount of protein, fat and energy ('actual intake'). Our concept of the interaction of actual protein intake and growth on plasma (PUC) and urinary urea concentrations (UUC) is illustrated in Fig. 1.

The PUC represents amino acid oxidation and therefore offers information about availability of protein after absorption and incorporation for growth, provided that fluid intake, kidney function and quality of the nutritional protein remain unchanged. However, associated blood samples are painful, contribute to blood loss and carry the risk for additional complications. In contrast, urine can be collected non-invasively and painlessly, and is frequently collected to guide calcium and phosphate supplementation in preterm infants [15]. Because the UUC may be confounded by fluid homeostasis, normalization of urinary urea for the creatinine excretion as the urinary-urea-creatinine-ratio (UUCR) may be appropriate.

The aim of this study was to determine 1) the impact of increased enteral protein intake on PUC and UUCR in very preterm infants and 2) if the UUCR

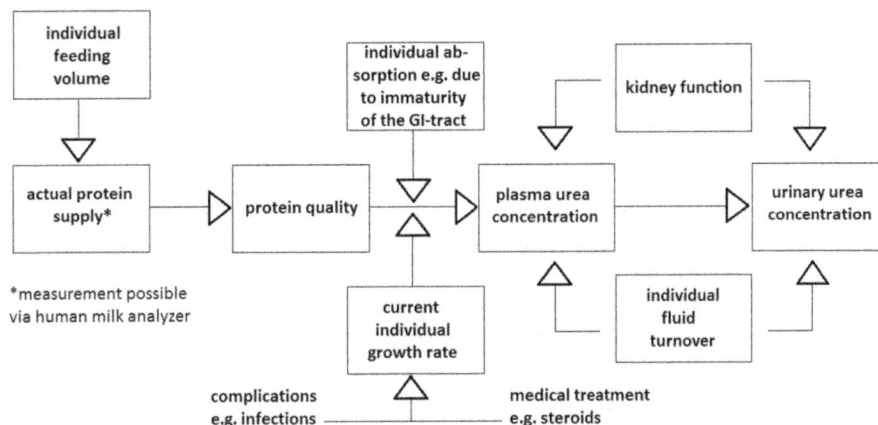

Fig. 1 Concept of the interaction of actual protein intake and growth on plasma and urinary urea concentrations

represent PUCs and actual enteral protein supply in this population.

Methods

Detailed information on the underlying randomized controlled trial has been previously reported [16]; in short:

From October 2012 to October 2014, this partially blinded randomized controlled trial was conducted at the department of neonatology at Tübingen university children's hospital, Germany. The Institutional Review Board approved the protocol and written informed parental consent was obtained. The trial was registered with Clinicaltrials.gov as NCT01773902.

The primary objective of the randomized controlled trial was to evaluate the effects of different target levels of enteral protein supplementation on growth in predominantly human milk fed very preterm infants [16], where no significant difference regarding the growth velocity (g/kg/d) from birth to end of intervention was shown. Both groups achieved near-fetal growth-rates. Secondary objectives of this trial were analysis of UUCR and PUC.

Participants

Sixty preterm infants born at our hospital within the above time frame, and with gestational age < 32 weeks at birth and weight < 1500 g were included. Main exclusion criteria were major congenital or chromosomal abnormalities.

Intervention

Infants were randomly assigned in proportions of 2/1/1 to one of three parallel treatment groups (after reaching 100 ml/kg enteral nutrition per day and informed consent was given) including:

1) a lower-protein group (LPG) (standardized fortification adding 5 g/100 ml of the commercially available multicomponent fortifier FM 85* (Nestlé Nutrition, Frankfurt, Germany; the standard fortifier in our unit, ingredients shown in Table 1) resulting in supplementation of 1 g protein/100 ml);

2) a higher-protein group (HPG) which comprised subgroups:

2a) with standardized higher protein supplementation using 5 g/100 ml of an investigational multicomponent fortifier. The study fortifier administered to group 2a) contained 1.8 g protein/5 g fortifier (10.01.DE.INF, Nestlé Nutrition, Frankfurt, Germany, ingredients shown in Table 1).

2b) individually adjusted fortification based on the individual human milk macronutrient content on top of standardized fortification as in group 1.

Table 1 Ingredients of the multicomponent fortifiers

	5 g BEBA FM 85	5 g Study fortifier 10.01.DE.INF
	74 kJ / 18 kcal	90 kJ / 22 kcal
Protein	1,0 g	1,8 g
Total carbohydrates (including:)	3,3 g	1,8 g
lactose	0 g	0 g
maltodextrin	3,2 g	1,8 g
Other carbohydrates	0,1 g	0 g
Total lipids (incuding:)	0,02 g	0,87 g
docosahexaenic acid (DHA)		0,0075 g
arachidonic acid (AA)		0,0006 g
Sodium	20 mg	33 mg
Potassium	42 mg	83 mg
Chloride	17 mg	29 mg
Calcium	75 mg	94 mg
Phosphor	45 mg	56 mg
Magnesium	2 mg	5 mg
Iron	1,3 mg	0,94 mg
Copper	0,04 mg	0 mg
Zinc	0,8 mg	0 mg
Iodine	15 µg	19 µg
Selenium	1,5 µg	4,25 µg
Vitamin A	0,15 mg	0,5 mg
Vitamin D	2,5 µg	5 µg
Vitamin E	2,0 mg	5 mg
Vitamin K	4,0 µg	10 µg
Vitamin C	10 mg	25 mg
Vitamin B1	0,05 mg	0,19 mg
Vitamin B2	0,10 mg	0,25 mg
Vitamin B6	0,05 mg	0,16 mg
Folic Acid	40 µg	50 µg
Vitamin B5	0,4 mg	0,88 mg
Vitamin B12	0,1 µg	0,25 µg
Biotin	3 µg	4 µg

In all three study groups, multicomponent fortifier was added at a fixed dose of 2.5 g/100 ml breast milk at enteral intakes between 100 and 149 ml/kg/d and at 5 g/100 ml breast milk once ≥150 ml/kg/d of enteral feeds had been reached and always thereafter.

In infants randomized to individual fortification (group 2b), the protein dosage was adjusted according to breast milk content aiming for 4.5 g/kg/d of enteral protein if the weight was < 1500 g or 4.0 g/kg/d of enteral protein if the weight was > 1500 g according to recommendations of the European Society of Paediatric Gastroenterology, Hepatology and Nutrition

Table 2 Comparison of the comorbidities of LPG and HPG

	LPG	HPG	p-value
NEC (≥ Bell stage 2A)	0(0)	0(0)	1
PDA therapy (indomethacin or ibuprofen)	4(13)	3(10)	1
BPD (physiological definition[a])	0(0)	2(7)	0,49
ROP[b/c]	0(0)	1(3)	1
IVH[d]	3(10)	0(0)	0,24
PVL / intra-parenchymal bleeding	0(0) / 0(0)	0(0) / 0(0)	1 / 1
Corticosteroid administration inhaled / systemic[e]	0(0) / 1(3)	5(17) / 1(3)	0,05 / 1

[a]moderate or severe BPD indicated by need for positive pressure respiratory support or supplemental oxygen at a postmenstrual age of 36 weeks to maintain an SpO2 > 90%, verified by a room air test where indicated
[b]no ophthalmologic examination in 6 patients
[c]max. Stage of ROP in all participants: stage I
[d]max. Grade of IVH in all participants: grade I
[e]budesonide inhalation, systemic supply of hydrocortisone (no patient received dexamethasone)

[17]. Moreover, fat was supplemented to ensure a cumulative fat intake > 4.8 g/kg/d. Aptamil Eiweiß+°, (Milupa, Friedrichsdorf, Germany) was used as an additional protein source in individually supplemented infants and a generic medium-chain triglyceride oil (Oleum neutrale) was used as an additional source of enteral fat. In the following, group 2a (mean protein intake 4,38 g/kg/d) and 2b (mean protein intake 4,12 g/kg/d) were combined (HPG; mean protein intake 4,30 g/kg/d) for further investigations.

Measurement of serum and urine urea
According to the study protocol, venous blood samples to measure PUC were scheduled on day 14 (±2) and day 28 (±4) after randomization, but had to be re-scheduled until clinical indication arose to avoid study-driven needle-sticks, which resulted in an earlier collection of BS 1. BS 1 was taken on day 9 (7–

10) after randomization, BS 2 on day 27 (24–32). Since UUCs were measured weekly, the closest urine sample (BS max. + / - 3 days) was matched to each blood sample. For BS1 sample size was 54; for BS2 sample size was 41 (available serum-urine-urea-pair).

To take the individual fluid turnover of the preterm infants into account UUCs are shown as urinary urea to urinary creatinine ratio (urea concentration (mg/dl) /creatinine concentration (mg/dl) of the same urine sample) (UUCR).

Every week the urinary urea and creatinine concentrations were measured from clinically indicated spot urine samples used for guidance of calcium and phosphorus supplementation as described in [15]. Urine was collected non-invasively with an absorbent fleece placed in the diaper.

Biochemical analyses
Determination of PUC and UUC was performed on the ADVIA XPT clinical chemistry analyzer (Siemens Healtheneers, Eschborn, Germany). Internal and external quality controls were always within the allowed ranges. The inter assay coefficient of variation was < 2.5% for plasma and < 4% for urine.

Actual daily protein supply
The median actual daily protein supply (based on mother's milk protein content (measured twice a week with a human milk analyzer (Miris, Uppsala, Sweden; infrared spectroscopy; calibration was carried out once a day as recommended by the manufacturer using a check solution); formula's protein content, protein content of the fortifier and parenteral amino acid supply) was calculated for the 5 days prior to the respective blood sample to ensure that variations due to clinical nutrition restriction/ lack of mother's milk were taken into account.

Table 3 Patient details lower-protein group vs. higher-protein group, data shown as number n (%), respectively median (p25-p75), or *mean (±SD)

	Lower-protein group	Higher-protein group	p-value
Sex female	19(63)	14(47)	0,3
Gestational age in weeks	30,0(29,0–31,1)	29,7(27,9–31,0)	0,2
Birth weight in g	1215(1065–1393)	1193(984–1326)	0,61
Day of randomisation in days after birth	7(6–7)	7(6–8)	0,75
Length of hospital stay	52(42–65)	52(37–70)	0,6
Mean protein supply in g/kg/d (birth to end of intervention)	3,82(3,59–3,93)	4,30(4,11–4,43)	< 0,0001
Mean energy supply in kcal/kg/d (birth to end of intervention)	136(133–143)	137(135–147)	0,62
Weight gain in g/kg/d (birth to end of intervention, primary outcome of the underlying study)*	16,25 (±2,22)*	16,02 (±2,48)*	0,71

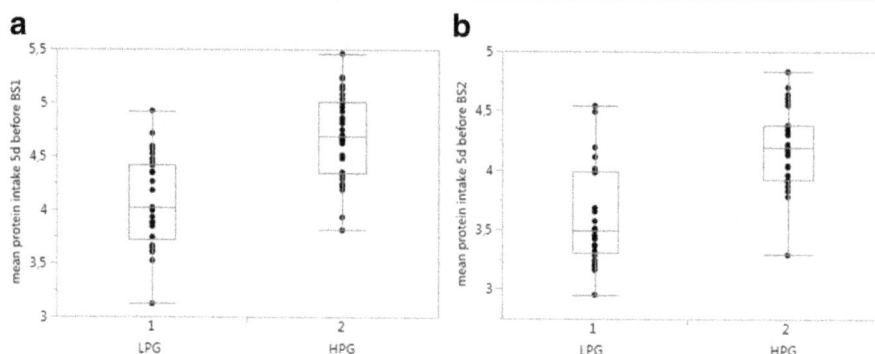

Fig. 2 Protein intake 5 days before blood samples (BS) were taken **a** BS1: lower-protein group (4.02 (3.72–4.42)) vs. higher-protein group (4.69 (4.34–5.01)) $p < 0.001$; **b** BS2 - lower protein group (3.49 (3.30–3.99)) vs. higher-protein group (4.19 (3.92–4.38)) $p < 0.0001$

Single samples of breast milk were used to measure macronutrient content as the mean of three individual measurements.

Statistical analyses

Statistical analyses were performed using Microsoft Excel and the statistic software JMP. Data was tested with non-parametric Wilcoxon-Test and Spearman's rank correlation coefficient (rho) was used for analysis of correlation, since not all data showed normal distribution. Results are shown as median and p25-p75.

Results

There were no differences in birth weight, gestational age at birth, gender or length of hospital stay between the LPG and the HPG [16], no statistic differences regarding the comorbidities due to early preterm birth between the two groups were shown (Table 2). The HPG had a significant higher protein supply while no difference in median energy supply was shown considering the time from birth to end of intervention and no difference in weight gain was shown (Table 3).

In comparison to the LPG, the HPG had also a significantly higher mean actual daily protein supply 5 days before blood sampling (Fig. 2); accordingly, in both samples higher PUC in the HPG were detected (Fig. 3).

The UUCR in the whole cohort ranged from 3.7 to 87.1 (median: 30.0) with a 2.5 Percentile of 9.3.

The UUCRs in both groups were similar in week 2 of life, but significantly higher in the HPG in week 3, as well as in weeks 5 through 7, with a trend to higher UUCRs in the HPG in week 4 ($p = 0.08$) (Table 4).

UUCRs and PUCs showed a highly significant positive correlation when all samples were compared ($p < 0.0001$), with $\rho = 0.72$ (Fig. 4).

In addition, median actual daily protein intake in the last 5 days before BS was calculated and PUC as well as the matched UUCR samples showed a highly significant positive correlation (Fig. 5).

No correlation of median daily growth rate during 5 days prior to BS was observed with PUC ($p = 0.7$; $\rho = -0.03$) and UCC ($p = 0.56$; $\rho = -0.04$) in this generally well-thriving cohort (Difference of weight-SDS between end of intervention and birth were LPG: 0.26 (-0.18–0.60) and HPG: 0.13 (-0.11–0.60), respectively).

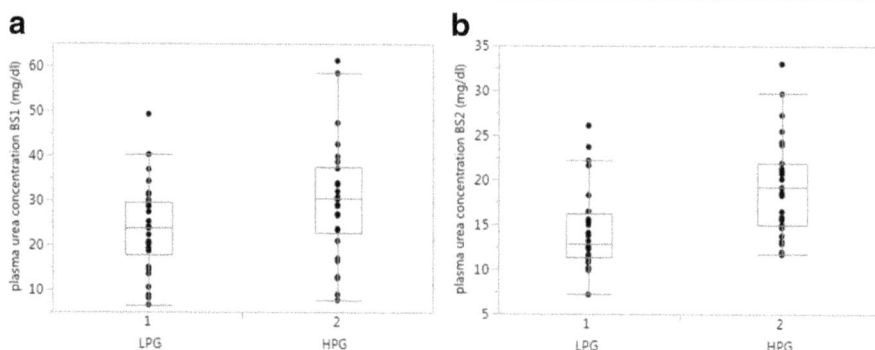

Fig. 3 Plasma urea (PU) concentrations (mg/dl) – **a** Blood sample (BS) 1 lower-protein group 23.9 (17.7–29.6)) vs. higher-protein group 30.6 (22.8–37.6) $p = 0.03$; **b** BS2 lower-protein group 12.9 (11.4–16.3) vs. higher-protein group 19.2 (15.0–21.9) $p = 0.0008$

Table 4 Urinary urea-creatinine-ratio in the lower protein group versus high protein group in week two to seven after birth, showing significant difference in week 3 and from week 5 to week 7

Weeks	Lower-protein group urinary urea-creatinine-ratio	Higher-protein group urinary urea-creatinine-ratio	p-value
2	38,0 (24,1–52,7)	43,3 (30,2–49,5)	0.77
3	25,8 (16,9–41,1)	39,9 (33,5–51,0)	0.0019
4	26,2 (20,7–31,3)	30,9 (24,4–46,5)	0.086
5	21,0 (14,9–26,0)	30,7 (26,2–38,5)	0.0024
6	25,3 (17,4–29,6)	33,7 (25,1–42,2)	0.029
7	16,3 (12,1–30,8)	34,0 (27,8–52,0)	0.0083

Discussion

Inadequate postnatal enteral protein supply (and absorption, hence intake) may contribute to early postnatal growth failure of preterm infants [18], which may be associated with poor neurocognitive outcome in later life [19]. In cases of intrauterine growth retardation, reduced plasma amino acid concentrations were observed in cord blood samples during the third trimester [20–22].

At the contrary, an excess in protein supply may no longer improve growth [16, 23] and may theoretically also have adverse effects and should therefore be avoided.

Beyond defining the actual protein supply to a preterm infant, the immaturity of the gastrointestinal tract (as well as the individual microbiome) may impair individual absorption of administered protein. Therefore, further information is required to estimate whether the actual protein intake is adequate, i.e. to determine whether additional protein supply may help to optimize growth or is inadequate because the infant already oxidizes excessively administered protein.

High enteral protein intake results in higher blood urea nitrogen levels in preterm infants, which can be used as a guidance to estimate optimal protein supply in enterally fed preterm infants. In addition, an excess of protein leads to higher PUCs and therefore high PUCs might identify a surplus of protein [16, 23].

Our investigations show a highly significant correlation between PUCs and UUCRs and in addition a highly significant positive correlation between UUCRs and PUCs and actual protein intake in fairly stable fully enterally fed very preterm infants.

Measuring UUCs and its normalization for creatinine excretion as UUCRs, as indicator (surrogate parameter) of amino acid oxidation, would be an easy, non-invasive way to estimate oxidation of surplus protein (as result of enteral protein supply and absorption and growth) in preterm infants. Measuring UUCs is already used in older children and adults to evaluate protein turn-over and intake, e.g. in the context of renal failure. In the late 1960's, a decrease in UUCs during periods of prolonged starvation was detected in adults [24], and therefore UUCR could become a marker for protein malnutrition in preterm infants, too. Polberger et al. showed in 1990 that low protein intakes result in low serum and urinary urea concentrations, and vice versa [25]. Despite a lack of good correlation between parenteral supply of protein and blood urea nitrogen levels in unstable preterm infants during the first days of life [26], Roggero et al. identified blood urea nitrogen as a potential marker of protein intake in low-birth-weight preterm infants on full enteral feeds [27]. The major advantage of assessing UUCRs is that urine is regularly disposed with the diapers; non-invasive collection of urine is painless and does not bear any risk for the infant. In our institution, urine collection is performed every week to assess calcium and phosphate metabolism in very low birth weight infants [15], so routine measurements of UUCR can be easily established. Considering that preterm infants continuously receive enteral nutrition every 2–3 h, spot urine sampling is considered to be sufficiently precise regarding the mineral homeostasis in a stable preterm infant [28] and may be sufficient to assess UUCRs as well.

Patients from this study with an actual protein supply of 4.0–4.5 g/kg/d during the 5 days prior to BS,

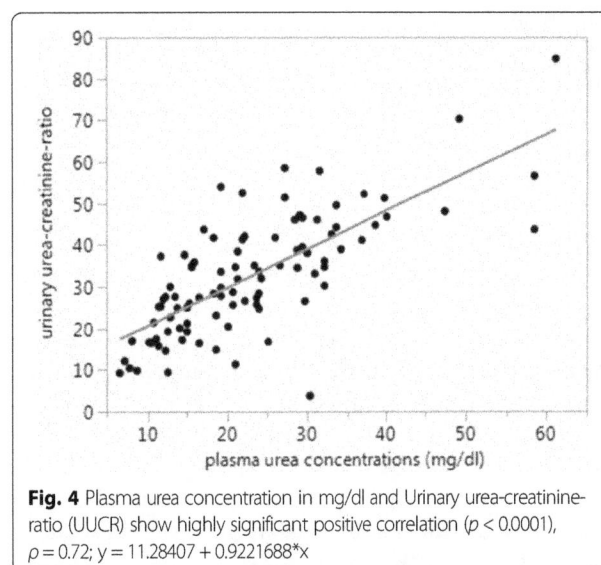

Fig. 4 Plasma urea concentration in mg/dl and Urinary urea-creatinine-ratio (UUCR) show highly significant positive correlation (p < 0.0001), $\rho = 0.72$; y = 11.28407 + 0.9221688*x

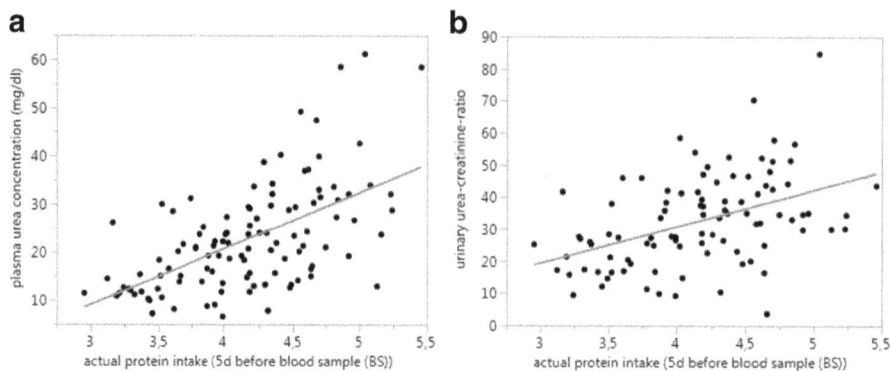

Fig. 5 Actual protein intake (5d before blood sample (BS)) and **a** Plasma urea concentration ($p < 0.0001$; $\rho = 0.59$); $y = -25.8499 + 11.644884 \cdot x$ and **b** Urinary urea-creatinine ratio (UUCR) ($p < 0.0001$; $\rho = 0.47$) showed highly significant positive correlation; $y = -14.80586 + 11.401612 \cdot x$

standardized feeding regimens and near-optimal growth along their intrauterine birth trajectories [16], had UUCRs ranging from 3.7 to 84.7 (min; max); median: 36.1. This wide range indicates that variability of protein oxidation and urea elimination is high, even if protein supply is adequate, probably due to variability in protein absorption, growth rate, need for protein oxidation for gluconeogenesis and energy metabolism, as well as kidney function. Consequently, confounding factors as well as mediators and modifiers need to be considered when interpreting UUCRs (Fig. 1).

In this well thriving cohort (SDS-difference for weight between birth and end of intervention 0.18 (- 0.165–0. 59)) [16] with adequate actual protein supply 4.0 (3.8–4. 3) g/kg/d the 2.5 percentile of UUCR was 9.3. Lower UUCRs (< 9 mg/mg) may indicate a low protein availability. Hence in preterm infants with inadequate weight gain and UUCRs < 9 insufficient protein availability should be considered as cause for growth failure.

Nevertheless, further investigations addressing the before mentioned confounding factors and mediators in a larger population are needed to determine reliable cutoff values and to establish an algorithm based on UUCR and confounding factors to indicate adequacy of protein intake in clinical routine.

Limitations and strengths of the study
In this randomized controlled study, the primary goal was to determine the effect of two levels of protein supply on weight gain. Nitrogen intake and balance weren't measured directly and the study population lacks infants with clearly insufficient protein intake. At the contrary, actual protein intakes, weight gain and longitudinal growth, PUCs and UCCs (and respectively UUCRs) were assessed prospectively, and the whole cohort showed near-intrauterine weight gain throughout the study.

Conclusion
In very preterm infants, determination of urinary urea/ urinary creatinine ratios (UUCR) is a promising approach to estimate adequacy of protein supply noninvasively, since urinary urea/urinary creatinine ratios show highly positive correlation with plasma urea concentrations and actual protein supply.

Abbreviations
BS: Blood sample; PUC: Plasma urea concentration; UUC: Urinary urea concentration; UUCR: Urinary urea-creatinine-ratio; LPG: Lower-protein group; HPG: Higher-protein group; Fig.: Figure; SDS: Standard deviation score; NEC: Necrotizing enterocolitis; PDA: Patent ductus arteriosus; BPD: Bronchopulmonary dysplasia; ROP: Retinopathy of prematurity; IVH: Intraventricular hemorrhage

Funding
The study fortifier administered to group 2a) (10.01.DE.INF) was provided by Nestlé Nutrition, Frankfurt, Germany. In addition the University of Tuebingen offered a scholarship for one of the contributory doctoral candidates (M.M.). We acknowledge support by Deutsche Forschungsgemeinschaft and Open Access Publishing Fund of University of Tuebingen.

Authors' contributions
Conception/Design of the work: AF; CM. Data collection: AF,CM,CB, JV,MM, AP. Data analysis: CM, MM. Drafting the article: MM. Critical revision of the article: AF, CM, CB, WB, JV, CP, MM, AP. Final approval of the version to be published; AF, CM, CB, WB, JV, CP, MM, AP.

Competing interests
The authors declare that they have no competing interests.

Author details
[1]Department of Neonatology, University Children's Hospital, Tübingen University Hospital, Calwerstr. 7, Tübingen, Germany. [2]Center for Pediatric Clinical Studies, University Children's Hospital, Tübingen University Hospital, Tübingen, Germany. [3]Department of Internal Medicine IV, Division of Endocrinology, Diabetology, Vascular Medicine, Nephrology and Clinical Chemistry and Pathobiochemistry, University of Tuebingen, Tübingen, Germany. [4]Institute of Diabetes Research and Metabolic Diseases (IDM) of the Helmholtz Center Munich at the University of Tuebingen, Tübingen, Germany. [5]German Center for Diabetes Research (DZD), Muenchen-Neuherberg, Germany.

References

1. Narayanan I, Prakash K, Bala S, Verma RK, Gujral VV. Partial supplementation with expressed breast-milk for prevention of infection in low-birth-weight infants. Lancet. 1980;2(8194):561–3.

2. Duijts L, Jaddoe VW, Hofman A, Moll HA. Prolonged and exclusive breastfeeding reduces the risk of infectious diseases in infancy. Pediatrics. 2010;126(1):e18–25.

3. Patel AL, Johnson TJ, Engstrom JL, Fogg LF, Jegier BJ, Bigger HR, Meier PP. Impact of early human milk on sepsis and health-care costs in very low birth weight infants. J Perinatol. 2013;33(7):514–9.

4. Sisk PM, Lovelady CA, Dillard RG, Gruber KJ, O'Shea TM. Early human milk feeding is associated with a lower risk of necrotizing enterocolitis in very low birth weight infants. J Perinatol. 2007;27(7):428–33.

5. Maayan-Metzger A, Avivi S, Schushan-Eisen I, Kuint J. Human milk versus formula feeding among preterm infants: short-term outcomes. Am J Perinatol. 2012;29(2):121–6.

6. Hoddinott P, Tappin D, Wright C. Breast feeding. BMJ. 2008;336(7649):881–7.

7. Ip S, Chung M, Raman G, Chew P, Magula N, DeVine D, Trikalinos T, Lau J. Breastfeeding and maternal and infant health outcomes in developed countries. Evid Rep Technol Assess. 2007;153:1–186.

8. Vohr BR, Poindexter BB, Dusick AM, McKinley LT, Higgins RD, Langer JC, Poole WK. Persistent beneficial effects of breast milk ingested in the neonatal intensive care unit on outcomes of extremely low birth weight infants at 30 months of age. Pediatrics. 2007;120(4):e953–9.

9. Victora CG, Bahl R, Barros AJ, Franca GV, Horton S, Krasevec J, Murch S, Sankar MJ, Walker N, Rollins NC. Breastfeeding in the 21st century: epidemiology, mechanisms, and lifelong effect. Lancet. 2016;387(10017):475–90.

10. Ziegler EE. Breast-milk fortification. Acta Paediatr. 2001;90(7):720–3.

11. Clark RH, Thomas P, Peabody J. Extrauterine growth restriction remains a serious problem in prematurely born neonates. Pediatrics. 2003;111(5 Pt 1):986–90.

12. Arslanoglu S, Moro GE, Ziegler EE. Preterm infants fed fortified human milk receive less protein than they need. J Perinatol. 2009;29(7):489–92.

13. Weber A, Loui A, Jochum F, Buhrer C, Obladen M. Breast milk from mothers of very low birthweight infants: variability in fat and protein content. Acta Paediatr. 2001;90(7):772–5.

14. Menjo A, Mizuno K, Murase M, Nishida Y, Taki M, Itabashi K, Shimono T, Namba K. Bedside analysis of human milk for adjustable nutrition strategy. Acta Paediatr. 2009;98(2):380–4.

15. Maas C, Pohlandt F, Mihatsch WA, Franz AR. Prevention of bone mineral deficiency in premature infants: review of the literature with focus on monitoring of urinary calcium and phosphate. Klinische Padiatrie. 2012;224(2):80–7.

16. Maas C, Mathes M, Bleeker C, Vek J, Bernhard W, Wiechers C, Peter A, Poets CF, Franz AR. Effect of increased enteral protein intake on growth in human milk-fed preterm infants: a randomized clinical trial. JAMA Pediatr. 2017;171(1):16–22.

17. Agostoni C, Buonocore G, Carnielli VP, De Curtis M, Darmaun D, Decsi T, Domellof M, Embleton ND, Fusch C, Genzel-Boroviczeny O, et al. Enteral nutrient supply for preterm infants: commentary from the European Society of Paediatric Gastroenterology, hepatology and nutrition committee on nutrition. J Pediatr Gastroenterol Nutr. 2010;50(1):85–91.

18. Arslanoglu S, Moro GE, Ziegler EE. Adjustable fortification of human milk fed to preterm infants: does it make a difference? J Perinatol. 2006;26(10):614–21.

19. Franz AR, Pohlandt F, Bode H, Mihatsch WA, Sander S, Kron M, Steinmacher J. Intrauterine, early neonatal, and postdischarge growth and neurodevelopmental outcome at 5.4 years in extremely preterm infants after intensive neonatal nutritional support. Pediatrics. 2009;123(1):e101–9.

20. Cetin I, Corbetta C, Sereni LP, Marconi AM, Bozzetti P, Pardi G, Battaglia FC. Umbilical amino acid concentrations in normal and growth-retarded fetuses sampled in utero by cordocentesis. Am J Obstet Gynecol. 1990;162(1):253–61.

21. Cetin I, Marconi AM, Bozzetti P, Sereni LP, Corbetta C, Pardi G, Battaglia FC. Umbilical amino acid concentrations in appropriate and small for gestational age infants: a biochemical difference present in utero. Am J Obstet Gynecol. 1988;158(1):120–6.

22. de Boo HA, Harding JE. Protein metabolism in preterm infants with particular reference to intrauterine growth restriction. Arch Dis Child Fetal Neonatal Ed. 2007;92(4):F315–9.

23. Bellagamba MP, Carmenati E, D'Ascenzo R, Malatesta M, Spagnoli C, Biagetti C, Burattini I, Carnielli VP. One extra gram of protein to preterm infants from birth to 1800 g: a single-blinded randomized clinical trial. J Pediatr Gastroenterol Nutr. 2016;62(6):879–84.

24. Owen OE, Felig P, Morgan AP, Wahren J, Cahill GF Jr. Liver and kidney metabolism during prolonged starvation. J Clin Invest. 1969;48(3):574–83.

25. Polberger SK, Axelsson IE, Raiha NC. Urinary and serum urea as indicators of protein metabolism in very low birthweight infants fed varying human milk protein intakes. Acta Paediatr Scand. 1990;79(8–9):737–42.

26. Ridout E, Melara D, Rottinghaus S, Thureen PJ. Blood urea nitrogen concentration as a marker of amino-acid intolerance in neonates with birthweight less than 1250 g. J Perinatol. 2005;25(2):130–3.

27. Roggero P, Gianni ML, Morlacchi L, Piemontese P, Liotto N, Taroni F, Mosca F. Blood urea nitrogen concentrations in low-birth-weight preterm infants during parenteral and enteral nutrition. J Pediatr Gastroenterol Nutr. 2010;51(2):213–5.

28. Mihatsch W, Trotter A, Pohlandt F. Calcium and phosphor intake in preterm infants: sensitivity and specifity of 6-hour urine samples to detect deficiency. Klinische Padiatrie. 2012;224(2):61–5.

7

Neonatal hypothermia and associated factors among neonates admitted to neonatal intensive care unit of public hospitals in Addis Ababa, Ethiopia

Birhanu Wondimeneh Demissie[1]* (iD), Balcha Berhanu Abera[2], Tesfaye Yitna Chichiabellu[1] and Feleke Hailemichael Astawesegn[3]

Abstract

Background: Neonatal hypothermia is a worldwide problem and an important contributing factor for Neonatal morbidity and mortality especially in developing countries. High prevalence of hypothermia has been reported from countries with the highest burden of Neonatal mortality. So the aim of this study was to assess the prevalence of Neonatal hypothermia and associated factors among newborn admitted to Neonatal Intensive Care Unit of Public Hospitals in Addis Ababa.

Methods: An institutional based cross-sectional study was conducted from March 30 to April 30, 2016, in Public Hospitals in Addis Ababa and based on admission rate a total of 356 Neonates with their mother paired were enrolled for the study. Axillary temperate of the newborn was measured by a digital thermometer at the point of admission. Multivariate binary logistic regression, with 95% confidence interval and a p-value < 0.05 was used to identify variables which had a significant association.

Results: The prevalence of Neonatal hypothermia in the study area was 64%. Preterm delivery (AOR = 4.81, 95% CI: 2.67, 8.64), age of Neonate ≤24 h old (AOR = 2.26, 95% CI: 1.27, 4.03), no skin to skin contact with their mother immediately after delivery (AOR = 4.39, 95% CI: 2.38, 8.11), delayed initiation of breastfeeding (AOR = 3.72, 95% CI: 2.07, 6.65) and resuscitation at birth (AOR = 3.65, 95%CI: 1.52, 8.78) were significantly associated with hypothermia.

Conclusions: The prevalence of Neonatal hypothermia in the study area was high. Preterm delivery, age ≤ 24 h old, no skin to skin contact immediately after delivery, delayed initiation of breastfeeding and resuscitation at birth were independent predictors of Neonatal hypothermia. Therefore attention is needed for thermal care of preterm newborn and use of low-cost thermal protection principles of warm chain especially on early initiation of breastfeeding, skin to skin contact immediately after delivery and warm resuscitation.

Keywords: Hypothermia, Newborn, NICU, Addis Ababa

* Correspondence: birhanuwondimeneh@gmail.com
[1]Department of Nursing, College of Health Sciences and Medicine, Wolaita Sodo University, Sodo, Ethiopia
Full list of author information is available at the end of the article

Background

World Health Organization (WHO) defined Neonatal hypothermia as an axillary temperature less than 36.5 °c. Reduction of thermal stability has a long-term physiologic effect that leads to, death due to hypoxia, and hypotension [1]. Globally an estimated of four million newborns die within the first four weeks of life, which accounts 2/3rd of all deaths in the first year of life and 40% of under five deaths. Most Neonatal deaths (99%) arise in low and middle-income countries [2, 3]. In Ethiopia also there is high Neonatal mortality, 37 deaths per 1000 live birth [4].

Hypothermia is one of the important causes for Neonatal death and morbidity in developing countries, which increases mortality by five times, and recent studies showed that every 1 °c decrement of body temperature increases mortality by 80% [2, 5, 6]. The prevalence is high among countries with the highest burden of Neonatal mortality [7]. It is a problem of both home delivered (32 - 85%) and institutional delivery (11 to 90%) [8]. A study in Bangladesh reported 34% of Neonates had hypothermia out of NICU admission [9]. Reports in developing country show that greater than 90% of Neonates were hypothermic (temperature less than 36.5 °C) and 10.7% of the newborn were at less than 35.0 °C [10, 11]. In West African sub-region, a prevalence rate of 62% at the point of admission was reported [12]. In Ethiopia also there was a prevalence of hypothermia ranging from 53 to 69.8% [8, 13].

Prematurity is one of the risk factors for Neonatal hypothermia and it is the leading cause of Neonatal mortality which accounts 37% of Neonatal death in Ethiopia [4]. And the prevalence of preterm birth ranges from 10 - 25.9% [14, 15]. Both physical characteristics and environmental factors predispose the preterm infant to hypothermia [16].

In Ethiopia lack of adequate perinatal care is one of the factors for onset of hypothermia, there is a high prevalence of home delivery which accounts 73% and Institutional deliveries accounts only 26% [17]. Low socio-economic status, poor kangaroo mother care practice, low birth weight, bathing of a newborn within 24 h, delayed initiation of breastfeeding, a traditional practice of oil massage of Neonates and inadequate knowledge of thermal care among health workers are determinant factors for hypothermia [2, 18, 19].

Although hypothermia is rarely a direct cause of death, it contributes to Neonatal mortality as a comorbidity of severe Neonatal infections, preterm birth, and asphyxia [8]. Mortality rate was significantly higher among hypothermic babies (RR = 2.26, CI = 1.14–4.48).

Even though predisposing factors for hypothermia are easily preventable the problem of hypothermia remains an unanswered question and it is highly prevalent in developing nations including sub-Sahara Africa [2].

Ethiopia applies thermal care principle which is one of the components of essential newborn care (ENBC) recommended by WHO. Despite this intervention, the problem of hypothermia remains a challenge in Ethiopia [1, 20]. And the achievement of sustainable development goal (SDG) 3 of ensuring healthy lives and promote well-being for all at all age requires a remarkable reduction of Neonatal death. Even though reduction of Neonatal hypothermia contributes to the achievement of SDG 3, it sustains as a challenge [21].

Providing ENBC including thermal care or prevention of Neonatal hypothermia is one part of nursing care, but the problem of Neonatal hypothermia remains a worldwide problem, especially in sub-Saharan Africa. Therefore, the purpose of this study was to determine the prevalence of Neonatal hypothermia and associated factors among Neonates admitted to NICU of Public Hospitals in Addis Ababa. So, this study will provide baseline data on the prevalence of Neonatal hypothermia and identification of possible factors for the onset of Neonatal hypothermia in the area will have greater input to program managers and policy makers for designing, proper implementation and evaluation programs on reduction of Neonatal mortality and improvement of newborn care to achieve SDG 3. In addition, the study will help to improve quality of newborn care in the nursing profession, specifically thermal protection, by low - tech preventive measures and early detection and referral of hypothermia.

Methods

Study design and period

An institutional based cross -sectional study design was conducted from March 30 to April 30, 2016, to determine the prevalence of Neonatal hypothermia and associated factors among Neonates admitted to Neonatal Intensive Care Unit of Public Hospitals in Addis Ababa.

Study setting

The study was conducted in six Public Hospitals in Addis Ababa, Ethiopia, that have their own NICU; namely; Tikur Anbessa Specialized Teaching Hospital that has its own Neonatal Intensive Care Unit (NICU) with an average NICU admission of 240 Neonates per month, St. Paul's Hospital Millennium Medical College with an average NICU admission of 210 Neonates per month, Yekatit 12 Hospital Medical College with an average NICU admission of 170 Neonates per month, Gandhi Memorial Specialized Hospital with an average NICU admission of 192 Neonates per month, Zewditu Memorial Hospital with an average NICU admission of 110 Neonates per month and Tirunesh Beijing General Hospital with an average NICU admission of 60 Neonates per month. The study was conducted in all Public Hospitals in Addis Ababa that has their own NICU, because the level of perinatal care given, standards of NICU, and accessibility of thermal prevention materials are somewhat different in each Hospital.

Population
Source population
The source populations were all Neonates who were admitted to NICU of public Hospitals in Addis Ababa.

Study population
Randomly Selected Neonates admitted to NICU of public Hospitals in Addis Ababa from March 30 to April 30, 2016, were the study population.

Eligibility criteria
Inclusion criteria
All Neonates with their mother admitted to NICU of Public Hospitals in Addis Ababa during the study period were included in the study.

Sample size determination
Sample size was calculated by using single population proportion formula:

$$n = \frac{(za/2)2^* \; pq}{d2}$$

By considering 10% none response rate of participants, the final sample size was **356**.

Where n = the required sample size.

$d = m$ arg*in of error between the sample and population* $= 5\% = 0.05$
$Z = s$ tan*dard normal distribution value at* 95%*confidence level*
$Z\,\alpha/2 = 1.96$ *for* 95%*confidence* interval
$p = $ Prevalence of Neonatal hypothermia (69.8%)

from the previous study conducted in Gondar University Teaching and Referral Hospital, Northwest Ethiopia [13].

Sampling technique and procedure
There were a total of six Public Hospitals in Addis Ababa that have their own organized NICU and they have a total average number of 982 admissions to NICU per month and a total sample size of 356 Neonates were selected from the six Hospitals. Then participants was selected by using systematic random sampling technique, that is every three admission until the required sample size was obtained (K = 2.75, approximately every 3 admissions was taken). The number of Neonates surveyed from each Hospital was allocated proportionally to the total average number of admission per month from all Hospitals.

Method of data collection
The instrument for data collection was semi-structured pre-tested questionnaire which was adopted and modified

from a study conducted in Ethiopia, Gondar University Hospital, Nigeria and Uganda [12, 13, 19]. The questionnaire contains items to assess the temperature of the newborn during admission to NICU and associated factors for the onset of hypothermia (Additional file 1).

Axillary temperate of the newborn was measured for three minute by using digital thermometer (model of MT-101 MT-111) which can measure from 32.0 °C to 42.9 °C (89.6 °F to 109.9 °F) that had measurement accuracy of ±0.1 °C for the temperature range of (35.5 °C – 42.0 °C) and ± 0.2 °C for the temperature range of (32.0 °C - 35.5 °C or above 42.0 °C) at point of admission. The thermometer was disinfected by using 70% ethyl alcohol disinfectant with a damp cloth after every measure of axillary temperature of the newborn to prevent infection transmission.

And other data such as; medical diagnosis, and CPR history was collected from the chart of the newborn and socio-demographic data and obstetric history was collected from their mother by using semi-structured pre-tested questionnaire. Infrared thermometer (model of Kintrex IRT0421) with a measurement range of (– 60 °C to 50 °C) and measurement accuracy of ±2 °C was used to measure the room temperature of the NICU. And data collection was done carefully by six BSc nurses.

Study variables
Dependent variable

- Neonatal hypothermia

Independent variables

1. Socio-demographic characteristics of the mother
   Maternal age, parity, residence, ethnicity, educational status, occupation and income.

2. Neonatal, obstetric and environmental factors of the neonate:

Age of newborn in hour, sex of newborn, low birth weight, mode of delivery, pregnancy type (single / multiple), prematurity, skin to skin contact with mother immediately after delivery, bathing before age of 24 h, CPR, delayed initiation of breastfeeding, room temperature of NICU, place of delivery, application of oil massage, obstetric complication during pregnancy and Medical diagnosis during admission.

Operational definitions

- **Hypothermia**: an axillary temperature of less than 36.5 °c

- **Cold stress(mild hypothermia)**: an axillary temperature of 36.0 to 36.4 °C
- **Moderate hypothermia**: an axillary temperature of 32.0 to 35.9 °C
- **Severe hypothermia:** an axillary temperature of < 32.0 °C
- **Normothermic:** an axillary temperature of 36.5 to 37.5 °C
- **Hyperthermia:** an axillary temperature of > 37.5 °C
- **Admission temperature**: The first temperature obtained from neonates at admission to NICU
- **Inborn**: a new born that was delivered from the study Hospital
- **Out born:** a new born that was deliver other than the study Hospital

Data quality and control

The questionnaire was prepared in English and translated to Amharic, and back-translated into English by two language experts to check for consistency of the questionnaire. The data was collected by six BSc. nurse experts. Thermometer calibration was done for the reliability of the thermometer before using the instrument for data collection. Three day training and clear orientation were provided on the process of data collection for data collectors. A pretest was done by 5% of the study population in another Hospital three weeks before the actual data collection to evaluate the clarity of questions and validity of the instrument and reaction of respondents to the questions. Data collectors were closely monitored and guided by two MSc. nurse supervisors during data collection.

Data entry and analysis

The data was cleaned manually, coded and entered into Epi info version 3.5 and exported to SPSS version 20 software for further analysis. After coding, and entering the data to the software descriptive statistics were used to calculate the result in proportion, frequencies, cross tabulation, and measure of central tendency. Tables and graphs were used to present the result. A bivariate binary logistic regression was used to identify candidate variables for the final model (multivariate binary logistic regressions) at p - value < 0.20. Finally the independent predictors or variables which had significant association were identified by using multivariate binary logistic regressions. The cut point to declare the presence of an association between the dependent and independent variable was p - value < 0.05 or AOR, 95% CI.

Results

Socio - demographic characteristics

A total of 356 mothers with their neonates were included in the study with 100% response rate. The mean age of mothers was 28 years (SD = 5.6) and more than half of the mothers were in the age group between 20 and 29 (51.1%) years of age. One hundred twenty seven (35.7%) were Oromo in ethnicity and majority of the mothers 206 (57.9%) were Orthodox followers. Two hundred seventy six (77.5%) were urban residents. Eighty respondents (22.2%) were unable to read and write and 144 (40.4%) of respondents were housewife. The mean monthly income of the family was 54 US dollar (SD = 11US dollar) and 117 (32.9%) had a monthly income of below average. And 191 respondents (53.7%) were primiparous (Table 1).

Table 1 Socio-demographic characteristics of mothers of neonates admitted to Neonatal Intensive Care Unit of Public Hospitals in Addis Ababa, Ethiopia, 2016 [$n = 356$]

Variables	Categories	Frequency	Percentage (%)
Age of mother (years)	15–19	17	4.8
	20–29	182	51.1
	30–39	145	40.7
	40–49	12	3.4
Ethnicity	Amhara	121	34.0
	Tigre	55	15.4
	Oromo	127	35.7
	Gurage	37	10.4
	Other	16	4.5
Religion	Orthodox	206	57.9
	Protestant	59	16.6
	Muslim	88	24.7
	Other	3	0.8
Residence	Urban	276	77.5
	Rural	80	22.5
Educational status	Unable to read and write	80	22.5
	Primary school	77	21.6
	Secondary school	102	28.7
	Diploma and above	97	27.2
Occupation	House wife	144	40.4
	Government employ	79	22.2
	Private business	92	25.8
	Student	27	7.6
	Farmer	14	3.9
Monthly income of the family	Below average	117	32.9
	Average (43–65 US dollar)	129	36.2
	Above average	110	30.9
Parity	Primiparous	191	53.7
	Multiparous	165	46.3

Neonatal factors

Majority of Neonates were males 204 (57.3%) and the median age of the newborn was 3 h. And most of the neonates 233 (65.4%) were in the age group of ≤24 h. The mean birth weight was 2440 g (SD 721 g). More than half 183 (51.4%) of the Neonates had birth weight ≥ 2500 g. The mean gestational age (GA) was 36 weeks ±2.8 weeks, most of them, 202 (56.7%) were with GA < 37 weeks. Only 126 (35.4%) of Neonates had early initiation of breastfeeding within one hour after birth. Eighty four (23.6%) had received resuscitation (CPR) during birth (Table 2).

Obstetric and environmental factors

Most of the pregnancies 311 (87.4%) were single and the majority of Neonates 286 (80.3%) were born without any obstetric complication. More than half 213 (59.8%) were delivered through SVD. Sixty five (18.3%) of the newborn were bathed before 24 h old and more than half of Neonates 188 (52.8%) had no skin to skin contact immediately after birth. And 41 (11.5%) had Oil massage of the skin after birth. One hundred seventy (47.8%) were out born neonates and of them, nine (2.5%) delivered at home. More than half 190 (53.4%) deliver during day time. Majority of Neonates 329 (92.4%) were admitted to NICU at room Temperature ≥ 25 °C (Table 3).

Table 2 Neonatal characteristics of respondents among Neonates admitted to Neonatal Intensive Care Unit of Public Hospitals in Addis Ababa, Ethiopia, 2016 [n = 356]

Variables	Categories	Frequency	Percentage (%)
Age of Newborn (hour)	≤24	233	65.4
	24–72	60	16.9
	> 72	63	17.7
Sex of new born	Male	204	57.3
	Female	152	42.7
Birth weight(grams)	< 1000	10	2.8
	1000–1499	32	9.0
	1500–2499	131	36.8
	2500–4000	179	50.3
	> 4000	4	1.1
Gestational age (weeks)	< 28 weeks	2	0.6
	28- < 32 weeks	25	7.0
	32- < 37 weeks	175	49.2
	37-42 weeks	152	42.7
	> 42 weeks	2	.6
Started breast feeding within one hour after birth	Yes	126	35.4
	No	230	64.6
Received CPR during birth	Yes	84	23.6
	No	272	76.4

Table 3 Obstetric and Environmental characteristics of respondents among Neonates admitted to Neonatal Intensive Care Unit of Public Hospitals in Addis Ababa, Ethiopia, 2016 [n = 356]

Variables	Categories	Frequency	Percentage (%)
Obstetric complication during pregnancy	Yes	70	19.7
	No	286	80.3
pregnancy type	Single	311	87.4
	Twine	41	11.5
	Triple	4	1.1
Mode of delivery	SVD	213	59.8
	Instrumental	32	9.0
	C/S	111	31.2
skin to skin contact immediately after delivery	Yes	168	47.2
	No	188	52.8
Place of delivery	Inborn	186	52.2
	Out born	170	47.8
setting for out born delivery	Missing (Inborn)	186	52.2
	Other Hospital	69	19.4
	Health Centre	76	21.3
	Private health facility	13	3.7
	Traditional birth center	3	0.8
	Homes	9	2.5
Oil massage of the skin immediately after birth	Yes	41	11.5
	No	315	88.5
Bathed the new born before 24 h old	Yes	65	18.3
	No	291	81.7
Time of delivery	Day time	190	53.4
	Night time	166	46.6
Room Temperature of NICU	< 25 °C	27	7.6

Medical diagnosis of the neonate

Medical diagnoses during admission were reviewed from medical record of the newborn and 116 (32.6%) were admitted for the reason of respiratory distress, 173 (48.6%) diagnosed as low birth weight and 202 (56.7%) were diagnosed as preterm, and 84 (23.6%) diagnoses as perinatal asphyxia (Table 4).

The prevalence of neonatal hypothermia

The prevalence of neonatal hypothermia among Neonates admitted to Neonatal Intensive Care Unit of Public Hospitals in Addis Ababa was 228 (64%). Among them, more than half 184 (80.7%) were moderate hypothermic and the remaining 44 (19.3%) were mild hypothermic babies (Fig. 1).

Table 4 Medical diagnoses of neonates during admission among Neonates admitted to Neonatal Intensive Care Unit of Public Hospitals in Addis Ababa, Ethiopia, 2016 [n = 356]

Variable	Categories	Frequency	Percentage (%)
Diagnosis during Admission	Respiratory distress	116	32.6
	Preterm	202	56.7
	Jaundice	55	15.4
	Sepsis	83	23.3
	LBW	173	48.6
	Perinatal asphyxia	84	23.6
	Congenital anomaly	35	9.8
	Meconium aspiration syndrome	22	6.2
	Small for gestational age	15	4.2
	hypoglycemia	15	4.2
	Other	16	4.5

The total cumulative frequency for diagnosis is greater than 100% because the Neonate may have more than one clinical diagnosis during admission.

And the prevalence of hypothermia was high among preterm 155 (76.7%), low birth weight 127 (73.4%), age ≤ 24 h 171 (73.4%), and among out born delivery 112 (65.9%) (Fig. 2).

Factors associated with neonatal hypothermia

In bivariate logistic regression analysis the following factors were significantly associated with hypothermia; age of newborn ≤24 h old, low birth weight, preterm delivery, no skin to skin contact to their mother immediately after delivery, no early initiation of breastfeeding within one hour, resuscitation at birth (CPR), obstetric complication during pregnancy, multiple Pregnancy and night-time delivery. Then those variables which are significant on bivariate analysis were entered to multiple logistic regressions to see independent predictors.

Accordingly, Neonates with the age of ≤24 h old were 2 times more likely to have hypothermia when compared to age greater than 24 h (AOR = 2.26, 95% CI: 1.27, 4.03).

Preterm Neonates were 4.8 times more likely to have hypothermia when compared to term delivery (AOR = 4.81, 95% CI: 2.67, 8.64). And newborn who had no skin to skin contact to their mother immediately after delivery were 4.3 times more likely to be hypothermic when compared to those who have skin to skin contact (AOR = 4.39, 95% CI: 2.38, 8.11). Those Neonates who had no early initiation of breastfeeding within one hour after birth were 3.7 times more likely to develop hypothermia when compared to those who have started within one hour after birth (AOR = 3.72, 95% CI: 2.07, 6.65). And Neonates who had resuscitation at birth (CPR) were 3.6 times more likely to be hypothermic when compared to those who had no resuscitation (AOR = 3.65, 95% CI: 1.52, 8.78) (Table 5).

Discussion

The prevalence of Neonatal hypothermia among newborn in this study was 64%. This was almost similar with a study conducted in Nigeria (62%) [12], in Bahir Dar, Ethiopia (67%) [22] and Gondar, Northwest Ethiopia (69.8%) [13]. And it was lower than a study conducted in Nepal (92.3%) [10], Zimbabwe (85%) [8] and Uganda (83%) [19]. But it was higher than a study conducted in South Africa (21%) [23], Bangladesh (34%) [9] and Pakistan (49.5%) [24]. This variation might be due to the difference in temperature measurement site,

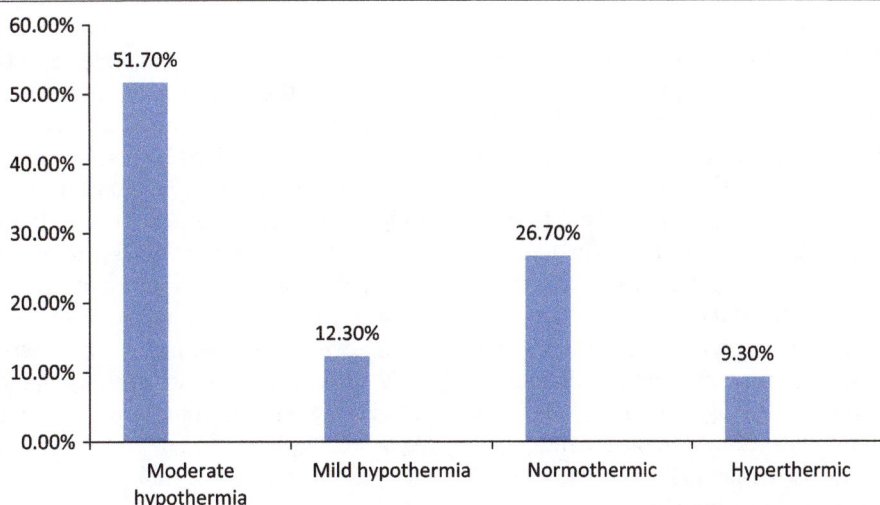

Fig. 1 Classification of temperature among Neonates admitted to Neonatal Intensive Care Unit of Public Hospitals in Addis Ababa, Ethiopia, 2016 [n = 356]

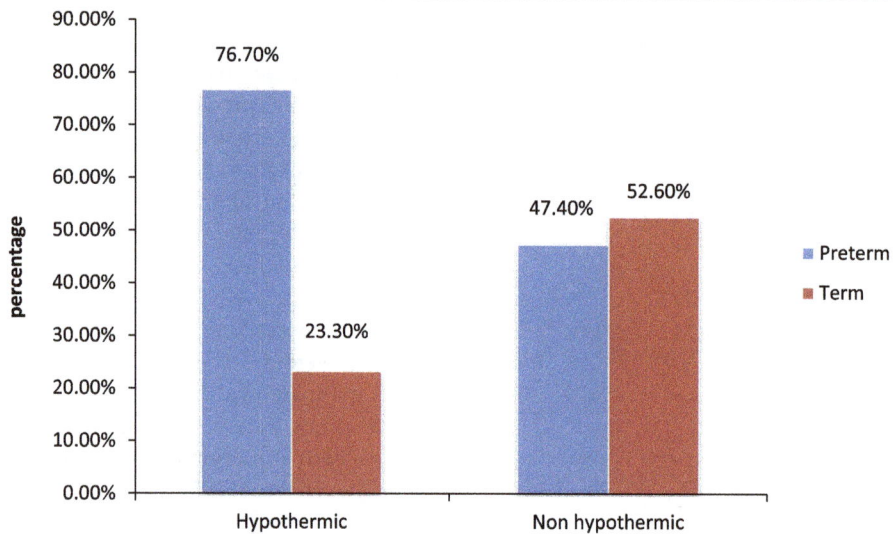

Fig. 2 Comparison of Hypothermia with gestational age among Neonates admitted to Neonatal Intensive Care Unit of Public Hospitals in Addis Ababa, Ethiopia, 2016 [n = 356]

ecological, economic and cultural difference between the study areas.

There was high prevalence of hypothermia among out born delivery (65.9%); this might be due to lack of proper thermal care practice during inter-facility transportation. Neonates are transported from ward to ward or to other Hospital without proper wrapping. This finding was higher than a study done in Bangladesh which was 43% for out born and 22% for inborn but lower than Nigeria which was 90.9% for out born and 61.1% for inborn [9, 12, 23]. This might be due to the difference in inter-Hospital transport thermal care services, distance traveled to the hospital and economical difference.

This study revealed that Neonates with the age of 24 h old or less were 2 times more likely to have hypothermia than age greater than 24 h (AOR = 2.26, 95%CI: 1.27, 4.03). This could be due to the fact that newborns have no adequate adipose brown tissue and had no shivering thermogenesis so they are not capable for thermoregulation. This is similar to a study conducted in Bangladesh, (AOR = 2.23 95% CI: 1.22, 4.0) [9].

Preterm Neonates were 4.8 times more likely to have hypothermia when compared to term Neonates (AOR = 4.81, 95% CI: 2.67, 8.64). The possible reason might be preterm Neonates have immature and thin skin that increase heat loss through radiation, underdeveloped hypothalamic control, they lack efficient neural mechanisms for temperature control by shivering, have decreased glycogen stores, have decreased fat for insulation and have less brown adipose tissue, so they have decreased ability to regulate their body temperature, by producing heat through non - shivering thermogenesis [2, 25, 26]. This is almost similar to a study done in Pakistan in which

preterm Neonates were 4 times more likely to develop hypothermia when compared to term newborn [24]. But it is higher than a study conducted in Iran in which preterm Neonates were 1.73 times more likely to be hypothermic than term one [27]. This variation might be due to the difference in the thermal care of preterm newborn, standard of delivery room and NICU.

Neonates who had no skin to skin contact with their mother immediately after delivery were 4.3 times more likely to develop hypothermia when compared with those who have skin to skin contact immediately after delivery (AOR = 4.39, 95% CI: 2.38, 8.11). The possible reason could be in the utero body temperature of the fetus is consistent with maternal temperature; Neonates who had skin to skin contact immediately after delivery with their mother gain heat through conduction which is consistent with their temperature in the womb during exposure of the newborn to extra uterine environment [28]. This finding is almost similar with a study conducted in Gondar, North west Ethiopia in which those who had no skin to skin contact were 3 times more likely to develop hypothermia [13]. Putting newborn together with the mother or kangaroo mother care is an important means of prevention of hypothermia [29].

Those Neonates who had no early initiation of breastfeeding within one hour after birth were 3.7 times more likely to be hypothermic when compared to those who had started breastfeeding within one hour after birth (AOR = 3.72, 95% CI: 2.07, 6.65). This might be due to the reason that breast milk is the source of energy or calories to produce heat for thermoregulation and they have no adequate adipose tissue for glucose breakdown which results in hypothermia [25]. And it is consistent

Table 5 Bivariate and multivariate logistic regression analysis of associated factors among Neonates admitted to Neonatal Intensive Care Unit of Governmental Hospitals in Addis Ababa, Ethiopia, 2016 [$n = 356$]

Variables	Hypothermic (228)	Non Hypothermic (128)	COR (95% CI)	AOR (95% CI)	P - value
	N (%)	N (%)			
Age of Neonate (hour)					
≤ 24	171(73.4)	62(26.6)	3.19(2.02,5.05)	2.26(1.27, 4.03)	.005*
> 24	57(46.3)	66(53.7)	1.0	1.0	
Birth weight (grams)					
< 2500	127(73.4)	46(26.6)	2.24(1.44,3.5)	1.33(0.75,2.36)	0.331
≥ 2500	101(55.2)	82(44.8)	1.0	1.0	
Gestational age (weeks)					
< 37	155(76.7)	47(23.3)	3.66(2.32,5.76)	4.81(2.67, 8.64)	0.001*
≥ 37	73(47.4)	81(52.6)	1.0	1.0	
skin to skin contact					
Yes	71(42.3)	97(57.7)	1.0	1.0	0.001*
No	157(83.5)	31(16.5)	6.92(4.23,11.32)	4.39(2.38, 8.11)	
Early initiation of breast feeding					
Yes	45(35.7)	81(64.3)	1.0	1.0	0.001*
No	183(79.6)	47(20.4)	7.0(4.32,11.38)	3.72(2.07, 6.65)	
CPR received					
Yes	76(90.5)	8(9.5)	7.5(3.48, 16.15)	3.65(1.52, 8.78)	0.004*
No	152(55.9)	120(44.1)	1.0	1.0	
Obstetric complication during pregnancy					
Yes	62(88.6)	8(11.4)	5.6(2.59, 12.13)	1.43(0.57, 3.56)	0.440
No	166(58)	120(42)	1.0	1.0	
Pregnancy type					
Single	190(61.1)	121(38.9)	1.0	1.0	0.145
Multiple	38(84.4)	7(15.6)	3.46(1.45,7.99)	2.14(0.77, 5.97)	
Time of delivery					
Day time	108(56.8)	82(43.2)	1.0	1.0	0.352
Night time	120(72.3)	46(27.7)	1.98(1.26, 3.09)	1.32(0.73, 2.37)	

* Significant at p-value ≤ 0.05

with a study done in Nigeria but lower than a study done in Gondar, North west Ethiopia in which those who were delayed in initiation of breast feeding were 7.5 times more likely to be hypothermic [13, 18]. This difference in magnitude might be due to difference in study setup, knowledge of mothers on good positioning and attachment of breast feeding and difference in place of delivery.

Neonates who had resuscitation at birth were 3.6 times more likely to be hypothermic when compared to those who had no resuscitation (AOR = 3.65, 95% CI: 1.52, 8.78). This is due to the fact that Neonates who need resuscitation are those who had birth asphyxia; there is no enough oxygen which is needed for mitochondrial oxidation in the brown adipose tissue, for heat production. And during resuscitation at birth temperature control

may not be properly taken care of; during emergency condition resuscitation may be done without wrapping the baby and in cold table. This finding is higher than study done in Bangladesh in which Neonates that had resuscitation were 2 times more likely to be hypothermic(AOR = 2.15, 95% CI:1.4–3.32) [9] and a study done in Iran in which those who had resuscitation at birth were almost 2 times more likely to be hypothermic (AOR =1.91, p value = 0.001) [27]. This variation may be due to the difference in thermal care practice during resuscitation, warm resuscitation or not and difference in time of resuscitation.

In bivariate analysis, low birth weight was statistically significant with the onset of hypothermia but in multiple logistic regression analysis it was not significant but there was a high prevalence of hypothermia among low birth weight neonates 127 (73.4%) compared with 101 (55.2%) normal birth weight. This is consistent with a study done in Pakistan 58.1%, Nigeria 89.1% and Gondar, Northwest Ethiopia 58 (89.2%) [13, 18, 24].

Limitation of the study

Even though the study was conducted in multiple Hospitals, it was done with small sample size and it was conducted with short period of time or in one season so factors like climatic changes or seasonal variations were not addressed.

Conclusions

The prevalence of Neonatal hypothermia among Neonates admitted to Neonatal Intensive Care Unit of Public hospitals in Addis Ababa was high 228 (64%). Preterm delivery, age of newborn ≤24 h, and absence of skin to skin contact with their mother immediately after delivery, delayed in early initiation of breastfeeding within one hour after birth and resuscitation at birth were factors that had significant association with Neonatal hypothermia. Therefore attention is needed for thermal care of preterm newborn and on the principle of WHO warm chain especially on early initiation of breast feeding, skin to skin contact and warm resuscitation. It is better to increase the practice of skin to skin contact immediately after delivery which is the effective warm chain principle especially in developing countries in which advanced warming instruments and incubators are not present.

Abbreviations
^{0}c: Degree centigrade; °F: Degree farhanite; AOR: Adjusted odds ratio; CI: Confidence interval; CPR: Cardio pulmonary resuscitation; ENBC: Essential newborn care; GA: Gestational age; MDG: Millennium development goal; NICU: Neonatal Intensive Care Unit; RR: Relative risk; SDG: Sustainable development goal; SPSS: Statistical Package for Social Sciences; WHO: World Health Organization

Acknowledgements
The authors would like to thank Addis Ababa University for funding this study. Our thanks also goes to for all study participants, supervisors and data collectors for their unreserved efforts and willingness to take part in this study.

Funding
Addis Ababa University had covered all the costs for data collection instruments, data collection, data entry and payments for supervisors and advisors.

Authors' contributions
BW was involved in the conception, design, analysis, interpretation, report and manuscript writing; BB and TY were participated in the design, analysis,

interpretation and report writing. FH was involved in designing the study, analysis, report and manuscript writing. And all authors have read and approved the final manuscript.

Competing interests
The authors declare that they have no competing interests.

Author details
^{1}Department of Nursing, College of Health Sciences and Medicine, Wolaita Sodo University, Sodo, Ethiopia. ^{2}School of Nursing and Midwifery, College of Health Science, Addis Ababa University, Addis Ababa, Ethiopia. ^{3}School of Public Health, College of Medicine and Health Sciences, Hawassa University, Hawassa, Ethiopia.

References
1. World Health Organization. Thermal Protection of the Newborn: a practical guide. Maternal and Safe Motherhood unit. Geneva: World Health Organization; 2006.
2. Onalo R. Neonatal hypothermia in sub-Saharan Africa : A review. Niger J Clin Pract. 2013;16(2):129–38.
3. United Nations (UN). The Millennium Development Goals Report 2014. New York: United Nations; 2014.
4. Central Statistical Agency [Ethiopia] and ICF International. Ethiopia Demographic and Health Survey 2011. Addis Ababa, Ethiopia and Calverton, Maryland: Central Statistical Agency and ICF International; 2012. p. 1–452.
5. Sodemann M, Nielsen J, Veirum J, Jakobsen MS, Biai S, Aaby P. Hypothermia of newborns is associated with excess mortality in the first 2 months of life in Guinea- Bissau, West Africa. Trop Med Int Heal. 2008;13(8):980–6.
6. Mullany LC, Katz J, Khatry SK, LeClerq SC, Darmstadt GL, Tielsch JM. Risk of mortality associated with neonatal hypothermia in southern Nepal. Arch Pediatr Adolesc Med. 2010;164(7):650–6.
7. Kumar V, Shearer JC, Kumar A, Darmstadt GL. STATE-OF-THE-ART neonatal hypothermia in low resource settings : a review. J Perinatol. Nature Publishing Group. 2009;29(6):401–12.
8. Lunze K, Bloom DE, Jamison DT, Hamer DH. The global burden of neonatal hypothermia: systematic review of a major challenge for newborn survival. BMC Med. 2013;11(1):24.
9. Akter S, Parvin R, Yasmeen BHN. Admission hypothermia among neonates presented to neonatal intensive care unit. J Nepal Paediatr Soc. 2013;33(3):166–71.
10. Mullany LC, Katz J, Khatry SK, LeClerq SC, Darmstadt GL, Tielsch JM. Incidence and seasonality of hypothermia among newborns in southern Nepal Luke. Arch Pediatr Adolesc Med. 2010;164(1):71–7.
11. Zayeri F, Kazemnejad A, Ganjali M, Babaei G, Nayeri F. Incidence and risk factors of neonatal hypothermia at referral hospitals in Tehran, Islamic Republic of Iran. East Mediterr Heal J. 2007;13(6):1308–18.
12. Ogunlesi TA, Ogunfowora OB, Adekanmbi FA, Fetuga BM, Olanrewaju DM. Point-of-admission hypothermia among high-risk Nigerian newborns. BMC Pediatr. 2008;8:40.
13. Seyum T, Ebrahim E. Proportion of neonatal hypothermia and associated factors among newborns at Gondar University teaching and Refferal hospital, Northwest Ethiopia: a hospital based cross sectional study. Gen Med. 2015;03(04):1–7.
14. Bekele, et al. Prevalence of Preterm Birth and its Associated Factors among Mothers Delivered in Jimma University Specialized Teaching and Referral Hospital, Jimma Zone, Oromia Regional State, South West Ethiopia. J Women's Health Care. 2017;6(1)
15. UNICEF Ethiopia. Preterm babies may be saved with simple inexpensive measures [Internet]. Addis Ababa: UNICEF Ethiopia; 2013. Available from: https://unicefethiopia.org/2013/11/16/preterm-babies-may-be-saved-with-simple-inexpensive-measures/.
16. Manani M, Jegatheesan P, DeSandre G, Song D, Showalter L, Govindaswami B. Elimination of admission hypothermia in preterm very low-birth-weight infants by standardization of delivery room management. Perm J. 2013;17(3):8–13.
17. Central Statistical Agency (CSA) [Ethiopia] and ICF. Ethiopia Demographic and Health Survey 2016. Addis Ababa, Ethiopia, and Rockville, Maryland: CSA and ICF; 2016.
18. Ogunlesi TA, Ogunfowora OB, Ogundeyi MM. Prevalence and risk factors for hypothermia on admission in Nigerian babies < 72 h of age. J Perinat Med. 2009;37(2):180–4.
19. Byaruhanga R, Bergstrom A, Okong P. Neonatal hypothermia in Uganda: prevalence and risk factors. J Trop Pediatr. 2005;51(4):212–5.
20. World Health Orgnatization. Pocket book of Hospital care for children: Guidlines for the mannagment of common childhood illness. 2nd ed; 2013. p. 49 51.
21. Osborn D, Cutter A and Ullah F. Universal sustainable Development goals. Understanding the Transformational Challenge for Developed Countries; report of a study by stakeholder forum. 2015;
22. Fulton C. Improving neonatal mortality in an Ethiopian referral hospital. BMJ Qual Improv Reports. 2013:1–4.

23. Thwala MD. The quality of neonatal inter-facility transport systems within the Johannesburg metropolitan region; 2009. p. 1–75. Available from: Http:/handle/10539/11031

24. Ali R, Mirza R, Qadir M, Ahmed S, Bhatti Z, Dema S. Neonatal hypothermia among hospitalized high risk newborns in a developing country. Pak J Med Sci January. 2012;28(1):49–53.

25. Knobel RB. Fetal and neonatal thermal physiology. Newborn Infant Nurs Rev. 2014;14(2):45–9.

26. Lunze K, Hamer DH. Thermal protection of the newborn in resource-limited environments. J Perinatol Nature Publishing Group. 2012;32(5):317–24.

27. Zayeri F, Kazemenejad A, Ganjali M, Babaei G, Nayeri F. Incidence and risk factors of neonatal hypothermia at referal hospitals in tehran, islamic republic of Iran. East Mediterr Heal J. 2007;13(6):1308–18.

28. Waldron S, Mackinnon R. Neonatal thermoregulation. Journal of Infant. 2007; 3(3):101–6

29. Lawn JE, et al. Kangaroo mother care to prevent neonatal deaths due to preterm birth complications. Int J Epidemiol. 2010;3(1):144–54.

8

Effectiveness of early intervention programs for parents of preterm infants: a meta-review of systematic reviews

Shuby Puthussery[1]* (iD), Muhammad Chutiyami[1], Pei-Ching Tseng[1], Lesley Kilby[2] and Jogesh Kapadia[2]

Abstract

Background: Various intervention programs exist for parents of preterm babies and some systematic reviews (SRs) have synthesised the evidence of their effectiveness. These reviews are, however, limited to specific interventions, components, or outcomes, and a comprehensive evidence base is lacking. The aim of this meta-review was to appraise and meta-synthesise the evidence from existing SRs to provide a comprehensive evidence base on the effectiveness of interventions for parents of preterm infants on parental and infant outcomes.

Methods: We conducted a comprehensive search of the following databases to identify relevant SRs: Cochrane library, Web of science, EMBASE, CINAHL, British Nursing Index, PsycINFO, Medline, ScienceDirect, Scopus, IBSS, DOAJ, ERIC, EPPI-Centre, PROSPERO, WHO Library. Additional searches were conducted using authors' institutional libraries, Google Scholar, and the reference lists of identified reviews. Identified articles were screened in two stages against an inclusion criteria with titles and abstracts screened first followed by full-text screening. Selected SRs were appraised using the AMSTAR tool. Extracted data using a predesigned tool were synthesised narratively examining the direction of impact on outcomes.

Results: We found 11 SRs eligible for inclusion that synthesised a total of 343 quantitative primary studies. The average quality of the SRs was 'medium'. Thirty four interventions were reported across the SRs with considerable heterogeneity in the structural framework and the targeted outcomes that included maternal-infant dyadic, maternal/parental, and infant outcomes. Among all interventions, Kangaroo Care (KC) showed the most frequent positive impact across outcomes ($n = 19$) followed by Mother Infant Transaction Program (MITP) ($n = 14$). Other interventions with most consistent positive impact on infant outcomes were Modified-Mother Infant Transaction Program (M-MITP) ($n = 6$), Infant Health and Development Program (IHDP) ($n = 5$) and Creating Opportunities for Parent Empowerment (COPE) ($n = 5$). Overall, interventions with both home and facility based components showed the most frequent positive impact across outcomes.

Conclusions: Neonatal care policy and planning for preterm babies should consider the implementation of interventions with most positive impact on outcomes. The heterogeneity in interventions and outcomes calls for the development and implementation of an integrated program for parents of preterm infants with a clearly defined global set of parental and infant outcomes.

Keywords: Preterm infants, Early intervention programs, Parents, Meta-review, Neonatal health

* Correspondence: shuby.puthussery@beds.ac.uk
[1]Maternal and Child Health Research Centre, Institute for Health Research, University of Bedfordshire, Putteridge Bury, Hitchin Road, Luton, Bedfordshire LU2 8LE, UK
Full list of author information is available at the end of the article

Background

Preterm birth, defined as birth at less than 37 completed weeks of gestation, remains a significant cause of infant mortality and morbidity worldwide. Preterm births are on the increase globally with about 15 million babies born preterm annually [1]. Compared to babies born at term, preterm babies carry a higher risk of developmental delays and learning disabilities and are increasingly vulnerable to conditions such as cerebral palsy, respiratory illnesses, feeding difficulties, and vision problems [1–6].

Caring for a preterm baby can be challenging and stressful to parents. Studies have consistently documented higher levels of stress and parenting difficulties among parents of preterm babies compared to those of babies born at term [7–15]. Parents are central to children's health and development and successful parenting is a key element in promoting overall parental wellbeing as well as children's physical and psychosocial development. The importance of supporting parents in the early years of their children's lives is reflected in a range of parenting programs developed over the years [16]. There is good quality evidence to demonstrate the effectiveness of early interventions in facilitating effective parenting and thereby promoting children's health and psychosocial development [17–20].

Various early intervention programs have been developed and delivered for parents of preterm babies and some systematic reviews (SRs) have synthesised the evidence on the effectiveness of these programmes [21–24]. While individual reviews have been successful in identifying the components and assessing the effectiveness of certain interventions on parental and infant outcomes, they often focus on specific interventions [21], components [25], or outcomes [26], which limit their ability to provide a comprehensive picture of the effectiveness of early intervention programs for the parents of preterm babies.

The aim of this review of SRs, referred to as meta-review, was to appraise and meta-synthesise the evidence from SRs to provide a comprehensive evidence base on the effectiveness of interventions for parents of preterm infants on various parental and infant outcomes.

Methods

We followed the Preferred Reporting Items for Systematic Reviews and Meta Analyses (PRISMA) guidelines [27] for this meta-review. The review question was framed using Population, Intervention, Comparator, Outcome and Study design (PICOS) framework. The population comprised of parents of preterm babies. The interventions comprised of interventions aimed at supporting parents of preterm babies. The outcome measures were indicators of health and/or psycho social wellbeing of parents and infants. SRs were included if they met the following criteria: searched at least two electronic databases; included a method of describing how the studies were included and/or excluded; synthesised findings from individual primary studies on the effectiveness of interventions for parents of preterm babies; and have drawn conclusions on at least one parental or infant outcome. No restrictions on language or the year of publication was applied as part of the inclusion criteria. The protocol was reviewed and agreed by the members of the team.

We conducted a comprehensive systematic search of the following databases to identify all existing SRs: Cochrane library, Web of science, EMBASE, CINAHL, British Nursing Index, PsycINFO, PubMed/Medline, ScienceDirect, Scopus, IBSS, DOAJ, ERIC, EPPI centre, PROSPERO, and the electronic libraries of the authors' institutions. Additional sources searched included Google Scholar, WHO Library, and the reference list of identified reviews. The key search terms used included [parent* OR famil* OR mother* OR father* OR preterm OR prematur* OR preterm birth OR preterm infant* OR premature infant*] AND [Intervention* OR initiative* OR process* OR program* OR effect* OR implication* OR scheme* OR strategy* OR outcome* OR educat* OR impact OR evaluat* OR support* OR delivery* OR implement*] AND ["systematic review" OR "SLR" OR "SR" OR meta-analysis* OR meta-review* OR meta-regression* OR meta-synthesis* OR "realistic review" OR "descriptive review" OR "research review" OR "thematic review" OR "explanatory review" OR "narrative review" OR "integrative review" OR "mixed method review" OR "qualitative review" OR "quantitative review" OR "research synthesis" OR "evaluation review" OR "evidence mapping" OR "evidence map review" OR "impact review" OR overview OR "evidence synthesis" OR "narrative synthesis"]. The main search was conducted between 1 February – 31 March 2016 and a subsequent updated search was conducted in August 2017. We registered ourselves on key databases such as PUBMED, Cochrane library and CINAHL to receive alerts on the publication of new articles. Identified SRs were screened by two researchers (SP and MC) using a two stage process. The first stage involved screening of all titles and abstracts based on the inclusion and exclusion criteria. Full text articles of all the included SRs in stage 1 were retrieved and screened for eligibility in stage 2.

Methodological quality assessment and data analysis

All the included SRs were assessed for methodological quality using the Assessing the Methodological Quality of Systematic Reviews (AMSTAR) tool [28]. Both the second (MC) and third (PcT) authors independently rated the methodological quality of all the SRs. Any discrepancies in scores were examined by the first author (SP) to make the final decision. SRs were assessed on eleven items on AMSTAR with the scores for individual items summed up. A total score of 11 represented an SR of the highest quality. The scores were grouped into three equal categories by the review team: score of 8–11 represented 'high' quality; score of 4–7 represented 'medium' quality; and a score of 0–3 represented 'low' quality.

The data from individual SRs were extracted using a predesigned review specific tool. The tool included details on the population and interventions (components, mode & place of delivery, duration); the numerical or narrative summary findings on outcomes; and the recommendations and implications for policy and practice outlined in the SRs. Author statements about the quality of the included studies to draw conclusions, their concerns, whether they agreed with the findings, and the recommendations were also recorded.

The extracted data were synthesised narratively in line with the review objective. This involved a detailed examination of the numerical and narrative summary findings and conclusions with respect to the effectiveness on outcomes and the categorisation of effectiveness as 'positive impact', 'no impact' and 'inconclusive' taking into account, wherever possible, the statistical significance, and the design and quality of the included studies as reported in the SR. Meta-analysis was deemed inappropriate for this review as this was a review of SRs and meta-analysis was already conducted in some of the included SRs [29]. The outcomes were classified into three categories: mother-infant dyadic outcomes; maternal/parental outcomes; and infant outcomes.

Results
Study selection
The results of the search and SR selection are shown in Fig. 1. The initial keyword search and updates from registered databases produced a total of 2171 titles and abstracts, of which 2038 were excluded due to either discordance with the inclusion criteria or duplication from multiple databases. Full texts of the remaining 133 articles were retrieved. Four more full text articles were retrieved following reference list searches. Altogether 137 full text articles were screened against the inclusion criteria. Following full text screening, 126 articles were further excluded due to discordance with the inclusion criteria resulting in 11 SRs eligible for inclusion in the meta-review (Table 1).

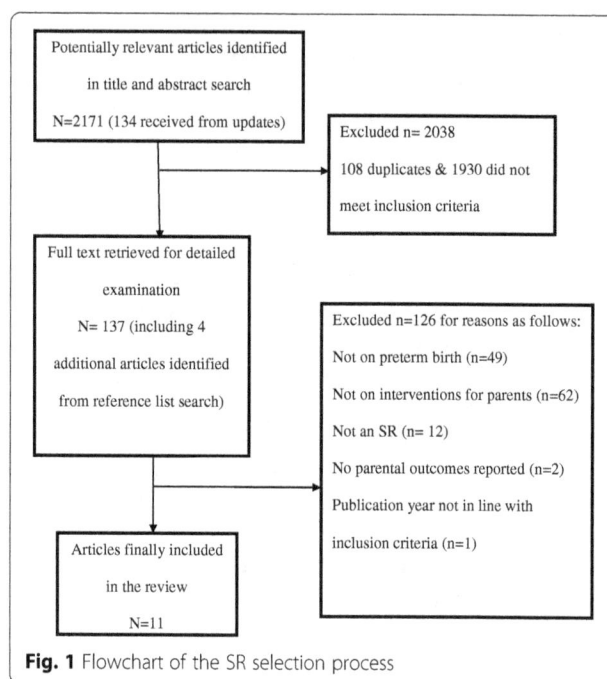

Fig. 1 Flowchart of the SR selection process

Characteristics of the included systematic reviews
A total of 343 quantitative primary studies were synthesised in the 11 SRs, of which 179 were Randomised Controlled Trials (RCTs). Meta-analysis was conducted in eight SRs [21, 23, 26, 30–34] and the remaining ones reported narrative syntheses. Four SRs included RCTs only [23, 24, 30, 32], while the rest included studies irrespective of the design. All except one SR [33] included primary studies without restriction to any specific geographical area although the reported interventions were mainly developed in countries such as the USA, UK, Australia, Germany, Japan, Italy, Netherlands, Norway and Columbia. One SR [33] was specifically focused on studies conducted in the US and Canada. All the included studies in another SR [31] were from low and middle income countries including Colombia, Ethiopia, Ecuador, Ethiopia, Indonesia, Bangladesh, India, Mexico and South Africa.

All the included SRs were critically appraised for methodological quality using AMSTAR tool. The result of the quality appraisal is presented in Table 2. The methodological quality assessment showed one SR with 'high' (score 8 to 11) quality, eight SRs with 'medium' (score 4 to 7) quality and two SRs with 'low' (0–3) quality. The included SRs had a mean AMSTAR score of 4.90. All the reviews met the AMSTAR criteria 3 and 6 (comprehensive literature search conducted and characteristics of included studies provided). The least met AMSTAR criteria among the reviews included criterion 1 (priori design provided), criterion 5 (list of included and excluded studies provided) and criterion 8 (use of scientific quality of the studies in formulating

Table 1 Characteristics of the included reviews

Authors and year of publication	Title of the study	Aim	Study designs	Included databases	Number of studies included
Evans et al., 2014 [26]	Are parenting interventions effective in improving the relationship between mothers and their preterm infants?	To systematically review the efficacy of parenting interventions in improving the quality of the relationship between mothers and preterm infants	RCTs and quasi-experimental designs	The Cochrane Library, PubMed, CINAHL, PsycINFO and Web of Science	17
Benzies et al., 2013 [30]	Key components of early intervention programs for preterm infants and their parents: a systematic review and meta-analysis	To categorise the key components of early intervention programs and determine the direct effects of components on parents, as well as their preterm infants	RCTs	MEDLINE, EMBASE, CINAHL, ERIC, and Cochrane Database of Systematic Reviews	18
Brett et al., 2011 [25]	A systematic mapping review of effective interventions for communicating with, supporting and providing information to parents of preterm infants	To identify and map out effective interventions for communication with, supporting and providing information for parents of preterm infants.	RCTs, quasi-experimental and non-intervention studies	Medline, Embase, PsychINFO, the Cochrane library, CINAHL, Midwives Information and Resource Service, Health Management Information Consortium, Health Management and Information Service	72
Herd, et al., 2014 [32]	Efficacy of preventative parenting interventions for parents of preterm infants on later child behaviour: a systematic review and meta-analysis	To determine the efficacy of parenting interventions for parents of preterm infants to improve child behaviour	RCTs	PubMed, CINAHL, Scopus, PsychINFO, web of science, Cochrane library	12
Goyal et al., 2013 [33]	Home Visiting and Outcomes of Preterm Infants: A Systematic Review	To review evidence regarding home visiting and outcomes of preterm infants	RCTs and Cohort studies	Medline, CINAHL, Cochrane library, PsycINFO, EMBASE	17
Vanderveen et al., 2009 [23]	Early interventions involving parents to improve neurodevelopmental outcomes of premature infants a meta-analysis	To determine whether interventions for infant development that involve parents, improve neurodevelopment at 12 months corrected age or older	RCTs	MEDLINE, CINAHL, PsychINFO, Cochrane library	25
Spittle al., 2015 [34]	Early developmental intervention programmes provided post hospital discharge to prevent motor and cognitive impairment in preterm infants	To compare the effectiveness of early developmental intervention programmes provided post hospital discharge to prevent motor or cognitive impairment in preterm (< 37 weeks) infants versus standard medical follow-up of preterm infants at infancy (zero to < three years), preschool age (three to < five years), school age (five to < 18 years) and adulthood (≥ 18 years)	RCTs and Quasi- RCTs	Cochrane Central Register of Controlled Trials, MEDLINE, CINAHL, PsycINFO, Embase	25
Boundy et al., 2016 [21]	Kangaroo Mother Care and Neonatal Outcomes: A Meta-analysis	To conduct a systematic review and meta-analysis estimating the association between KMC and neonatal outcomes	RCTs and observational studies	PubMed, Embase, Web of Science, Scopus, African Index Medicus (AIM), Latin American and Caribbean Health Sciences Information System (LILACS), Index Medicus for the Eastern Mediterranean Region (IMEMR), Index Medicus for the South-East Asian Region	124

Table 1 Characteristics of the included reviews (Continued)

Authors and year of publication	Title of the study	Aim	Study designs	Included databases	Number. of studies included
				(IMSEAR), and Western Pacific Region Index Medicus (WPRIM).	
Lawn et al., 2010 [31]	Kangaroo mother care' to prevent neonatal deaths due to preterm birth complications	To review the evidence, and estimate the effect of KMC on neonatal mortality due to complications of preterm birth.	RCTs and observational studies	Cochrane Libraries, PubMed, LILACS, African Medicus, EMRO and all World Health Organization Regional Databases	15
McGregor et al., 2012 [35]	Enhancing parent-infant bonding using kangaroo care: a structured review	To review the literature on the effectiveness of kangaroo care with premature infants for enhancing bonding.	RCTs and observational studies	Medline, CINAHL, OTDBASE, PsycINFO, Applied Social Sciences Index and Abstracts (ASSIA), Allied and Complimentary Medicine Database (AMED), and British Nursing Index (BNI)	6
Zhang et al., 2014 [24]	Early Intervention for preterm infants and their mothers	To evaluate the efficacy of early interventions on maternal emotions, mother-infant interaction and infant development outcomes	RCTs	PubMed, CINAHL, EMBASE, PsychINFO, Cochrane library	12

Table 2 Quality assessment of the reviews using AMSTAR

Study	1	2	3	4	5	6	7	8	9	10	11	Total
Benzies et al., 2013 [30]	0	0	1	0	0	1	1	1	1	1	0	6
Boundy et al., 2016 [21]	0	1	1	1	0	1	0	0	1	1	1	7
Brett et al., 2011 [25]	0	1	1	1	0	1	0	0	0	0	1	5
Evans et al., 2014 [26]	0	0	1	0	0	1	1	0	1	0	0	4
Goyal et al., 2013 [33]	0	0	1	0	0	1	1	0	1	0	0	4
Herd, et al., 2014 [32]	0	0	1	0	0	1	1	0	1	0	1	5
Lawn et al., 2010 [31]	0	0	1	0	0	1	1	0	1	0	1	5
McGregor and Casey, 2012 [35]	0	0	1	0	0	1	0	0	0	0	0	2
Spittle et al., 2015 [34]	1	1	1	0	1	1	1	0	1	1	1	9
Vanderveen et al., 2009 [23]	0	0	1	0	0	1	0	0	1	0	0	3
Zhang et al., 2014 [24]	0	1	1	0	0	1	1	0	0	0	0	4

AMSTAR TOOL Key: 1 = Yes, 0 = No/Unclear/Not applicable. Areas assessed are numbered 1 to 11 on horizontal axis; 1-Priori design provided, 2-Duplicate selection/extraction, 3-Comprehensive literature search conducted, 4-Status of publication (i.e, grey literature) used as an inclusion criterion, 5-List of included & excluded studies provided, 6-Characteristics of included studies provided, 7-Quality of included studies assessed and documented, 8-Use of the scientific quality of the studies in formulating conclusions, 9-Use of appropriate methods to combine the findings of studies, 10-Assessment of publication bias, 11- Conflict of interest included

conclusions). The highest quality SR [34] was a Cochrane Collaboration review conducted using set guidelines.

Participants
Consistent with the focus of this meta-review, the participants were parents of preterm infants with or without their infants. The parents included mothers [21, 23, 26, 30, 31, 34, 35], fathers [30] or both parents [25, 32, 33], although the distinction was not clearly explicit in some SRs. One SR was focused on interventions targeted at black teenage mothers and mothers of lower socioeconomic status [23]. The participants in another SR were mainly first-time mothers [24] whereas two other SRs [26, 30] included only parents of first born infants who were preterm. Three SRs [21, 31, 33] included interventions for both preterm and low birth weight infants. The number of participants included in the SRs ranged from 1940 [26] to 5556 [32] although this information was not reported in two SRs [25, 35]. Participants identified in the reviews were broadly from low, middle, and high income countries, including USA, UK, Australia, Germany, Japan, Italy, Netherlands, Norway, Colombia, Ethiopia, Ecuador, Ethiopia, Indonesia, Bangladesh, India, Mexico, Sweden, Israel, South Africa, Zimbabwe and Mozambique.

Interventions
A total of 34 parenting interventions were reported in the included reviews (Table 3). Most of the SRs reported the components of the interventions and the mode of delivery although none of the SRs included complete details of the interventions to enable replication. The intervention components were broadly classified into three categories: parent education consisting of aspects such as teaching, sensitisation, training or awareness creation; parent support consisting of guidance, encouragement or other forms of support; and infant support/therapy consisting of infant care or therapy elements. Parent support and parent education was reported as a component in 23 and 21 interventions respectively whereas infant support/therapy was included as a component in 15 interventions.

The most frequently reported interventions were Kangaroo Care (KC) ($n = 8$) followed by Mother Infant Transaction Programme (MITP) ($n = 7$) and Infant Health and Development Program (IHDP) ($n = 5$). Fourteen interventions including Avon Premature Infant Project (APIP), Demonstration and interaction Group (DIG), Education group (EG), Home Based intervention programme (HBIP), Infant Behavioural Assessment and Intervention Program (IBAIP), Interaction Coaching (IC), Individualized family-based intervention (IFBI), Japanese Infant Mental Health Programme (JIMHP), Kinesthetic stimulation (KS), Nursing Systems Towards Effective Parenting-Preterm (NSTEP-P), Physiotherapy Intervention (PI), Support Group (SG), Supporting Play Exploration and Early Development Intervention (SPEEDI), Victorian Infant Brain Studies (VIBeS Plus) were home based. Facility based interventions included Clinic-Based Intervention programme (CBIP), Hospital to Home (H-HOPE), Individualised Developmental Plan (IDP), Newborn Individualised Developmental & Assessment Programme (NIDCAP), and Standardised Individualised Intervention (SII). Interventions with both home and facility based components included KC, MITP, IHDP, Creating Opportunities for Parent Empowerment (COPE), Cues programme (CP), Early intervention (EI),

Table 3 Characteristics of the interventions

Name of the intervention programme	Reviews reporting the intervention		Intervention components			Intervention focus		Mode of delivery		Place of delivery		Frequency/Duration	Additional details of the intervention
	Total number	Details provided	Parent education	Parent support	Infant support/therapy	Mother/Parent	Child	Individual	Group	Hospital	Community/Home		
APIP	N=4	N=2	N=2	N=1	–	√	–	√	–	–	√	Weekly session for 2 years	Initiated from discharge
CAMS	N=1	N=1	N=1	–	N=1	√	√	NR	NR	NR	NR	Not Reported (NR)	Information was reported only on the intervention component
CBIP	N=1	N=1	N=1	–	N=1	√	√	√	–	√	–	5 inpatient sessions	–
COPE	N=4	N=3	N=3	–	–	√	–	√	–	√	√	1–8 sessions before discharge (BD) and 1 week session after discharge (AD)	–
CP	N=1	N=1	N=1	N=1	–	√	–	√	–	√	√	5 sessions in the Neonatal Intensive Care Unit,1 home visit	Home visit within 4 weeks AD
DIG	N=1	N=1	N=1	–	–	√	–	–	√	–	√	Once a day for period of 1 week	Initiated immediately AD
EG	N=1	N=1	N=1	–	–	√	–	–	√	–	√	Once a day for period of 1 week	Initiated immediately AD
EI	N=1	N=1	N=1	–	–	√	–	√	–	√	√	1NICU session, 1 home visit session	Home visit is done within first 60 weeks of adjusted infant age
GP	N=2	N=1	N=1	N=1	–	√	–	–	√	√	√	6 session	–
HBIP	N=1	N=1	–	N=1	N=1	√	√	–	–	–	√	8 neonatal clinic visits	Neonatal visit is initiated AD from hospital
H-HOPE	N=1	N=1	N=1	–	N=1	√	√	√	–	√	–	4 sessions at NICU	Sessions within 1 month adjusted infant age
IBAIP	N=3	N=3	N=2	–	N=3	√	√	√	–	–	√	6 to 8 home visits	Within 6 months AD
IC	N=1	N=1	–	N=1	N=1	√	√	√	–	–	√	8 sessions AD	Within 12-15 weeks
IDP	N=1	N=1	–	N=1	N=1	√	√	√	–	√	–	3-4weekly session in the hospital	Initiated AD
IFBI	N=1	N=1	N=1	N=1	N=1	√	√	√	–	–	√	3-17 sessions	Within 8 weeks AD
IHDP	N=5	N=5	N=1	N=2	N=5	√	√	√	–	√	√	Weekly home visits for a year, then 1 visit/2 weeks for next 2 years	Sessions from discharge to 3 years of infant age
JIMHP	N=1	N=1	–	N=1	–	√	–	√	–	–	√	5 sessions AD	Sessions at 1,3,5 and 12 months
KC	N=8	N=6	–	N=5	N=3	√	√	√	–	√	√	Up to 10 sessions AD	Frequency of hospital sessions not reported
KS	N=1	N=1	N=1	N=1	–	√	–	NR	NR	–	√	4 times per day for 1 month	Start from term
MITP	N=7	N=5	N=3	N=3	–	√	√	√	–	√	√	1 session BD and 4 sessions AD	AD sessions within first 3 months
M-MITP	N=3	N=3	N=3	N=3	–	√	–	√	–	√	√	1 session BD and 4 sessions AD	AD sessions within first 3 months

Table 3 Characteristics of the interventions (Continued)

Name of the intervention programme	Reviews reporting the intervention		Intervention components			Intervention focus		Mode of delivery		Place of delivery		Frequency/Duration	Additional details of the intervention
	Total number	Details provided	Parent education	Parent support	Infant support/therapy	Mother/Parent	Child	Individual	Group	Hospital	Community/Home		
NBAS	N=1	N=1	N=1	–	–	✓	–	NR	NR	NR	NR	NR	–
NCATS	N=4	N=1	N=1	–	–	✓	–	✓	–	NR	NR	NR	–
NIDCAP	N=2	N=1	–	N=1	N=1	✓	✓	✓	–	✓	–	NR	–
NSTEP-P	N=2	N=2	N=2	N=2	–	✓	–	✓	–	–	✓	9 home visits	Within 5 months AD
PBIP	N=4	N=2	N=1	–	–	✓	–	✓	–	✓	✓	Weekly session BD and 6 sessions AD	Session before discharge starts at birth
PPI	N=1	N=1	N=1	N=1	–	✓	–	✓	✓	✓	✓	5 sessions BD and 1 session AD	Sessions at home within 1-12 weeks AD
PI	N=1	N=1	–	N=1	–	✓	–	NR	NR	–	✓	Once a month session for 12 months	Home or out-patient department
SG	N=1	N=1	N=1	N=1	–	✓	–	–	✓	–	✓	Weekly sessions for 0-3 months, 2 sessions per month 3–9 months 1session per month 9-12 months	Start from term
SII	N=1	N=1	–	N=1	N=1	✓	✓	✓	–	✓	–	3 sessions BD	Last session on discharge day
SM	N=1	N=1	–	N=1	N=1	✓	✓	✓	–	✓	✓	1 session BD or AD	–
SPEEDI	N=1	N=1	N=1	–	N=1	✓	✓	✓	–	–	✓	20 min sessions 5 times/week	Each family received at least 10 visits
TH	N=1	N=1	–	N=1	N=1	✓	✓	✓	–	✓	✓	1 h blanket holding daily	Frequency not specified
VIBeS Plus	N=2	N=2	N=2	N=2	–	✓	–	✓	–	✓	✓	9 sessions in 12 months	Initiated from discharge

Key: *AD* After discharge, *BD* Before discharge, *NR* Not Reported. Interventions: *APIP* Avon Premature Infant Project, *CBIP* Clinic-Based Intervention programme, *COPE* Creating Opportunities for Parent Empowerment, *CP* Cues programme, *CAMS* Curriculum and Monitoring System, *DIG* Demonstration and interaction Group, *EI* Early intervention, *EG* Education group, *GP* Guided participation, *HBIP* Home Based intervention programme, *H-HOPE* Hospital to Home, *IDP* Individualised developmental plan, *IFBI* Individualized family-based intervention, *IBAIP* Infant Behavioural Assessment and Intervention Program, *IHDP* Infant Health and Development Program, *IC* Interaction Coaching, *JIMHP* Japanese Infant Mental Health Programme, *KC* Kangaroo Care, *KS* Kinesthetic stimulation, *M-MITP* Modified Mother Infant transaction programme, *MITP* Mother–Infant Transaction Program, *NBAS* Neonatal Behavioural Assessment Scale, *NIDCAP* Newborn Individualised Developmental & Assessment Programme, *NCATS* Nursing Child Assessment Teaching scale, *NSTEP-P* Nursing Systems Towards Effective Parenting-Preterm, *PBIP* Parent-Baby Interaction Programme, *PPI* Preventative Psychotherapy Intervention, *PI* Physiotherapy Intervention, *SII* Standardised Individualised Intervention, *SM* State Modulation, *SG* Support Group, *SPEEDI* Supporting Play Exploration and Early Development Intervention, *TH* Traditional Holding, *VIBeS Plus* Victorian Infant Brain Studies

Guided participation (GP), Modified-Mother Infant trans-action programme (M-MITP), Parent-Baby Interaction Programme (PBIP), Preventative Psychotherapy Interven-tion (PPI), State Modulation (SM), Traditional Holding (TH) had both home and facility based components. All of the interventions were focused on mothers/parents although programs such as CAMS, CBIP, HBIP, H-HOPE, IDP, IHDP, IFPI, IC, KC, NIDCAP, SM, SII, SPEEDI, TH, and IBAIP had components for the parents and their babies.

Most of the interventions were provided on an individ-ual basis ($n = 27$) and were administered by a range of pro-fessionals including nurses, psychologists sociologists, community health workers, physiotherapists, educationists and graduate students. Half of the interventions ($n = 17$) were initiated soon after birth in the Neonatal Intensive Care Unit (NICU) whereas the others had components delivered before and after discharge from the hospital. The control groups reported in the SRs consisted of par-ents and babies who received the usual care for preterm infants or those who received conventional/standard information given to parents following the birth of a pre-term baby. Two SRs reported follow up measurements for infant outcomes up to 18 years of the infant's age [32, 34].

Effectiveness of interventions on outcomes
Mother-infant dyadic outcomes
As presented in Table 4, the effectiveness of various interventions on mother-infant dyadic outcomes were reported in five SRs [24, 26, 30, 33, 35], with three reporting findings from meta-analyses [26, 30, 33]. All of these SRs reported improvements with respect to different mother-infant dyadic outcomes. In their meta-analysis, Evans et al., [26] found statistically signifi-cant improvements in the quality of the maternal-infant relationship for the intervention groups with effect sizes ranging from small, 0.38 to large, 2.81 from SM, NSTEP-P, KC, TH, and MITP. The same review [26] also found positive impact with large effect sizes for KC on the outcomes of symmetrical co-regulation (2.72) and asymmetrical co-regulation (– 2.81) and for mutual attention from MITP (1.95).

Positive impact on maternal sensitivity and responsive-ness while interacting with the infant was reported from five interventions including H-HOPE, MITP, COPE, and EI [24] although the effect size was not available. In their meta-analysis, Benezies et al., [30] found limited impact of early intervention programs including PBIB, COPE, MITP, M-MITP, NSTEP-P on maternal sensitivity and responsiveness. The authors, however, stated that two of the included studies showed a positive impact of MITP and M-MITP [30]. McGregor et al., [35] reported signifi-cant improvements in mother-infant attachment follow-ing KC based on findings from five of the six studies

included in their review. Overall improvements in mother-infant interaction were reported from MITP, M-MITP, COPE, H-HOPE, EI [24] and KC [35] and from home based interventions with active parental involvement [33].

Overall, KC and MITP showed most consistent positive impact on mother–infant dyadic outcomes. KC had positive impact on the quality of the mother-infant relationship, symmetrical co-regulation, asymmetrical co-regulation [26], mother-infant attachment [35], and mother-infant interaction [35]. MITP showed positive impact on the quality of the mother-infant relationship, mutual attention [26], maternal sensitivity and/or re-sponsiveness [24, 30] and mother-infant interaction [24]. Most of the interventions (KC, MITP, TH, COPE, EI) with positive impact on various mother-infant dyadic outcomes had both home and facility based components [24, 26, 35]. Among interventions that are exclusively home based, NSTEP-P improved mother infant relationship (effect size 0.38) [26] but had no effect on sensitivity/responsiveness [30]. Among facility based interventions, H-HOPE showed positive impact on sensitivity/responsiveness although no effect size was indicated [24].

Maternal/ parental outcomes
The effectiveness of the interventions on a range of maternal/ parental outcomes was reported across the SRs as shown in Table 5. Improvement in the quality of the mother–infant relationship for mothers was reported in two of the SRs [25, 26]. In their meta-analysis of RCTs, Evans et al., [26] found significant improvements in mother – infant relationship for the mothers who took part in GP and for mothers with low education in State Modulation-Nursing System Towards Effective Parenting-Preterm (SM-NSTEP-P) based on self-report questionnaires from the mother's perspective [26]. Par-ent led peer support groups in the NICU also improved mother – infant relationship for mothers of critically ill preterm babies although the reported evidence was based on a non- RCT study [25].

Reduction in maternal and/or overall parenting stress was reported in three SRs from the following interven-tions: M-MITP, COPE, MITP [24], COPE, MITP, NID-CAP [25] and KC [35]. Brett et al.'s [25] findings relating to MITP, COPE and NIDCAP were based on well conducted RCTs. Brett et al., [25] also indicated a recent RCT suggesting no significant reduction in parental stress from NIDCAP at 1–2 weeks after the baby was born. McGregor et al., [35] reported significant reduction in maternal stress from KC, while Zhang et al., [24] reported MITP to be effective in alleviating maternal stress up to 12 months. In their meta-analysis, Benzies et al., [30] reported inconclusive evidence on the impact of

Table 4 Effectiveness on mother - infant dyadic outcomes

Mother- infant dyadic outcomes	Review	Intervention	Effectiveness on the outcome			Additional information on impact
			Positive impact	No impact	Inconclusive	
Quality of the mother–infant relationship	Evans et al., 2014 [26]	SM, NSTEP-P, KC, TH, MITP	√	–	–	Effect sizes ranged from small, 0.38 to large, 2.81
Symmetrical co-regulation		KC	√	–	–	large effect size 2.72
Asymmetrical co-regulation		KC	√	–	–	large effect size −2.81
Mutual attention		MITP	√	–	–	large effect size 1.95
Maternal sensitivity and/or responsiveness in interactions with the infant	Benzies et al., 2013 [30]	PBIP, COPE, MITP, M-MITP, NSTEP-P	–	–	√	Overall effect was not significant. Pooled effect Z = 1.84 (P = 0.07). Included studies showed positive effect of MITP and M-MITP
	Zhang et al., 2014 [24]	H-HOPE, MITP, COPE, EI	√			No effect size reported
Mother –infant attachment	McGregor et al., 2012 [35]	KC	√	–	–	Five of the six studies reported significant improvements
Mother-infant interaction	Goyal et al., 2013 [33]	Home based interventions (unspecified)	√	–	–	No effect size reported. 13 of the 14 studies reported positive intervention effect on any parent-infant interaction measures
	McGregor et al., 2012 [35]	KC	√	–	–	At 6 months, mother-infant interactions were significantly more optimal for the KC group (p < 0.05).
	Zhang et al., 2014 [24]	MITP, M-MITP, COPE, H-HOPE, EI	√	–	–	No effect size reported

Interventions: *COPE* Creating Opportunities for Parent Empowerment, *EI* Early intervention, *H-HOPE* Hospital to Home, *KC* Kangaroo Care, *M-MITP* Modified Mother Infant Transaction Programme, *MITP* Mother–Infant Transaction Program, *NSTEP-P* Nursing Systems Towards Effective Parenting-Preterm, *PBIP* Parent-Baby Interaction Programme, *SM* State Modulation, *TH* Traditional Holding

M-MITP, Neonatal Behavioural Assessment Scale (NBAS), COPE, PBIP, IBAIP on stress (z = 0.40 p = 0.69).

Three SRs [24, 25, 30] reported changes in maternal/parental anxiety, with one [30] reporting strong effect from COPE, NBAS and VIBeS Plus on maternal anxiety reduction based on a meta-analysis (z = 2.54 p = 0.01) and another [25] reporting positive effect on maternal anxiety reduction from KC. The third SR [24] found no statistically significant effect on parental anxiety reduction from early interventions in general although the interventions were not specified. One SR [30] reported reduction in maternal depressive symptoms from COPE, VIBeS Plus, and M-MITP with strong statistical effect (z = 4.04 P < 0.0001). Although two SRs reported impact of MITP, COPE [24] and KC [25] on reduction in maternal depressive symptoms, the statistical significance was not reported.

Benzies et al., [30] found improvements in maternal self-efficacy from NBAS with strong statistical effect [z = 2.05 (P = 0.04)]. Home visiting interventions in general were found to significantly improve mother's confidence and satisfaction at 6 months postnatally [33]. MITP, KC, breast feeding support [25] and home visiting programmes [33] showed positive impact on maternal confidence and competence. NIDCAP had no significant impact on parental confidence at 1–

2 weeks [25]. Discharge planning programs, home support programs and KC appeared to improve maternal/parental interaction with infants [25]. Zhang et al., [24] reported significant improvements in mother's coping skills from COPE.

Overall, the interventions with positive impact on most parental/maternal outcomes were KC (n = 5), MITP (n = 3) and COPE (n = 3). KC had positive impact on stress alleviation [35], reduction in maternal anxiety [25], reduction in depressive symptoms [25], parental confidence/competence/satisfaction [25] and parent's interaction with infants [25]. MITP had positive impact on stress alleviation, parental confidence/competence/satisfaction [25], and reduction in depressive symptoms [24]. COPE had positive impact on stress alleviation [24, 25], reduction in anxiety [30] and reduction in depressive symptoms [30]. Most of the interventions (KC, MITP, COPE, GP, SM-NSTEP-P, COPE, M-MITP), with positive impact on maternal/parental outcomes had both home and facility based components [24–26, 30, 35]. Few home-based interventions (NSTEP-P, SG, VIBeS Plus) showed positive impact on mother's quality of relationship, parental confidence and reduction in anxiety/depressive symptoms [25, 26, 30, 33]. It would appear interventions that were exclusively facility-based had little impact on maternal/parental outcomes.

Table 5 Effectiveness on maternal/parental outcomes

Maternal/parental outcomes	Review	Intervention	Effectiveness of the intervention on outcome			Additional information on impact
			Positive impact	No impact	Inconclusive	
Quality of mother–infant relationship for mothers	Evans et al., 2014 [26]	GP	√	–	–	Large effect sizes using observation measure (2.09) and interview measure (1.20)
		SM-NSTEP-P	√	–	–	Positive impact for mothers with low education, with effect size 0.86
	Brett et al., 2011 [25][a]	Parent support groups/parent led peer support	√	–	–	Evidence reported from a non-RCT study for mothers of critically ill preterm babies
Maternal/parental stress alleviation	Benzies et al. 2013 [30]	M-MITP, NBAS, COPE, PBIP, IBAIP	–	–	√	Pooled effect $z = 0.40$ ($p = 0.69$)
	Brett et al., 2011 [25][a]	COPE, MITP, NIDCAP	√	–	–	Evidence reported from four high quality and well conducted RCTs. No significant reduction in parental stress from NIDCAP at 1–2 weeks after the baby was born
		Home support programmes where parents are visited regularly for the first year and for upto three years afterwards	√	–	–	Based on RCT evidence with high risk of bias. Specific details of the intervention unclear
	McGregor et al., 2012 [35]	KC	√	–	–	Reduction in stressful situations (32%), heart rate (7%) and Pain Visual Analogue Scale score (89%)
	Zhang et al., 2014 [24]	M-MITP, COPE, MITP	√	–	–	Impact until the baby is 12 months old with MITP
Reduction in maternal/parental anxiety	Benzies et al. 2013 [30]	COPE, VIBeS Plus, NBAS	√	–	–	Positive pooled effect $z = 2.54$ ($P = 0.01$)
	Zhang et al., 2014 [24]	Not specified	–	√	–	Used State Trait Anxiety Inventory scale to measure anxiety
	Brett et al., 2011 [25][a]	KC	√	–	–	Significant reduction in maternal anxiety around her infant. RCT evidence showing music during KC resulted in significantly lower maternal anxiety
Reduction in maternal depressive symptoms	Benzies et al. 2013 [30]	COPE, VIBeS Plus, M-MITP,	√	–	–	Positive pooled effect $z = 4.04$ ($P < 0.0001$)
	Zhang et al., 2014 [24]	MITP, COPE	√	–	–	Positive impact on depressive symptoms after the infant was discharged home. Statistical significance not reported
	Brett et al., 2011 [25][a]	KC	√	–	–	Significantly less postnatal depression compared with the controls at 37 weeks
Maternal self-efficacy	Benzies et al. 2013 [30]	NBAS	√	–	–	Pooled effect $z = 2.05$ ($P = 0.04$)
Parental confidence/ competence/ satisfaction	Goyal et al., 2013 [33]	Home visiting programmes	√	–	–	Name of the interventions not specified
	Brett et al., 2011 [25][a]	MITP, KC	√	–	–	MITP significantly improved maternal satisfaction and maternal self-confidence. KC provided the mother with a significantly greater sense of competence with their infant

Table 5 Effectiveness on maternal/parental outcomes (Continued)

Maternal/parental outcomes	Review	Intervention	Effectiveness of the intervention on outcome			Additional information on impact
			Positive impact	No impact	Inconclusive	
		Breast feeding support programmes	√	–	–	Improved the confidence of mothers in breastfeeding
		NIDCAP	–	√	–	RCT evidence showing no impact at 1–2 weeks after birth
Mother's/Parents' interaction with infants	Brett et al., 2011 [25][a]	Discharge planning programmes	√	–	–	Based on RCT evidence with high risk of bias. Specific details of the intervention unclear
		Home support programmes	√	–	–	Based on RCT evidence with high risk of bias. Specific details of the intervention unclear
		KC	√	–	–	Significantly greater sensitivity towards her infant. Effect size not reported. Better infant interaction, more touch, better adaptation to infant cues and better perception of their infant at all time periods.
Mother's coping skills	Zhang et al., 2014 [24]	COPE	–	–	√	Both positive and no impact reported.
Preparing parents to see infant for first time	Brett et al., 2011 [25][a]	Use of photograph	√	–	–	Reported positive effect based on a well conducted RCT
Parents' emotional and practical guidance	Brett et al., 2011 [25][a]	Home based support programmes	√	–	–	[a]RCT (1-), interventions unclear

[a]Brett et al., [25] used evidence from RCTs with the strength of evidence reported using Scottish Intercollegiate Grading Network guideline
Interventions: COPE Creating Opportunities for Parent Empowerment, G? Guided participation, IBAIP Infant Behavioural Assessment and Intervention Program, KC Kangaroo Care, M-MITP Modified Mother Infant transaction programme, MITP Mother–Infant Transaction Program, NBAS Neonatal Behavioural Assessment Scale, NIDCAP Newborn Individualised Developmental & Assessment Programme, NSTEP-P Nursing Systems Towards Effective Parenting-Preterm, PBIP Parent-Baby Interaction Progamme, SM State Modulation, VIBeS Plus Victorian Infant Brain Studies

Infant outcomes

The effectiveness of interventions on a range of infant outcomes was reported across the reviews as shown in Table 6. The impact was measured using a range of tools at various ages; examples included Bayley Scales of Infant Development [23, 33, 34]; Griffiths Mental Development Scale, McCarthy Scales of Children's Abilities, Stanford-Binet Intelligence Scale, Wechsler Preschool and Primary Scale of Intelligence [23, 34]; Differential Abilities Scale Edition II, Wechsler Intelligence Scale for Children - Full Scale IQ, Kaufman Assessment Battery for Children, British Abilities Scale, Wechsler Abbreviated Scale of Intelligence [34]; and Behaviour Assessment System for Children-Preschool version [32].

Improvement in the quality of the mother–infant relationship for infants was reported from KC, TH, SM, NSTEP– P with effect sizes ranging from small, 0.35 to large, – 1.60 [26]. Small, but significant, improvements were reported in child's general behaviour at different ages from M-MITP (at 5 years), VIBeS Plus (at 4 years) and IHDP (at 3 years) [32]. Similarly, MITP and COPE were found to be effective towards improving symbolic behaviour of infants with respect to understanding spoken language/object use during play [24]. Benzies et al., [30] and Zhang et al., [24] found positive effect of M-MITP [24, 30] and COPE [24] on child temperament although the strength of the effect was not reported.

The impact of IHDP on physical growth and nutritional status was inconclusive [33] while KC had no clear positive impact on weight gain or body length growth [21]. Kangaroo Care had positive impact on exclusive breast feeding KC [21] while MITP and COPE resulted in improvements in general breast feeding [24]. KC was also beneficial in improving head circumference [21, 35] and height [35]. The impact of KC in reducing infant heart rate and pain was inconsistent with one SR reporting no impact [21] and another SR reporting positive impact [35].

Morbidity related outcomes were reported in three SRs [21, 31, 33]. Goyal et al., [33] found mixed impact of IHDP on reduction of morbidities with small, statistically significant increase in maternally reported minor illnesses at 3 years of age, but only for infants weighing 1500 g, and no effect on serious health conditions or on rates of hospitalization or acute care visits. KC significantly reduced relative risk (RR) of morbidities generally [21, 31], especially neonatal sepsis, hypothermia, hypoglycaemia and hospital readmission [21]. The significant protective effect of KC on infant mortality was reported in two of the SRs [21, 23] based on evidence from RCTs exclusively in one [21] and a combination of RCTs and non-RCTs in the other [31].

Positive impact of various interventions on a number of child developmental outcomes from both RCT and non-RCT studies were reported in five SRs [23, 24, 30, 33, 34]. Vanderveen et al., [23] examined child mental development outcomes including the level of cognitive, language and personal-social development at ages of 6 months, 12 months, 24 months, 36 months and 5 years, and found statistically significant impact at different ages with the impact peaking at 36 months. The impact decreased thereafter, eventually becoming insignificant at 5 years [23]. Zhang et al., [24] found MITP and COPE to be effective in promoting symbolic behaviour including understanding of spoken language and object use in play and communication. Similarly, Spittle et al., [34] examined the impact of early developmental interventions in general on cognitive and motor outcomes and found strong positive effect on cognitive development from 0 to 5 years. The effect on cognitive development was not maintained after 5 years. The same SR also found that the effect on motor development remained positive with small effect size for 0 to 2 years, but became insignificant thereafter [34]. Based on evidence from RCTs, Benzies et al., [30] found positive impact of M-MITP (3–6 months) and NBAS (4 months) on early cognitive development. Vanderveen et al., [23] found positive impact of early interventions including IHDP and NIDCAP on psychomotor development. Zhang et al., [24], Benzies et al., [30] and Goyal et al., [33] reported positive impact of MITP, M-MITP and COPE up to 12 months of infant age [24], VIBeS Plus upto 24 months [30], and home visiting interventions (age unspecified) [33] on general infant development.

Overall, KC had the most frequent positive impact on infant outcomes (*n* = 9) followed by MITP (*n* = 7), COPE (*n* = 5), M-MITP (n = 5) and IHDP (n = 5). KC had positive impact on infant's quality of relationship with mother [26], breast feeding [21, 24], height [35], height and head circumference [21, 35], decrease in infant heart rate and pain [35], reduction in morbidity [21, 31], reduction in hospital readmission [21], lower mortality [21, 31], early mental development/ neurodevelopment [23]. Most of the interventions (KC, MITP, COPE, M-MITP, IHDP, TH, SM) that showed positive impact on various infant outcomes (infant's quality of relationship, infant's behaviour, breast feeding, head circumference, infant's height, mental development, psychomotor development, early motor development, early cognitive development, general development at infancy, temperament and reduced hospital readmission/mortality had both home and facility based components [21, 23, 24, 26, 30, 32, 34, 35]. Interventions that were exclusively home based (NSTEP-P, VIBeS Plus, IBAIP, HBIP, SPEEDI) improved infant's quality of relationship, behaviour, cognitive development, early motor development and overall development in

Table 6 Effectiveness on infant outcomes

Infant outcomes	Review	Intervention	Effectiveness of the intervention on the outcome			Additional information on impact
			Positive impact	No impact	Inconclusive	
Infant's quality of relationship with mother	Evans et al. 2014 [26]	KC, TH, SM NSTEP-P	✓	–	–	Effect sizes ranged from small, 0.35 to large, −1.60. Large effect size observed with KC (1.60) and TH (−0.87)
Behaviour improvement	Herd et al. 2014 [32]	IHDP, M-MITP, VIBeS Plus	✓	–	–	Small, but significant, effect on behaviour outcomes. IHDP improved behaviour up to 3 years of age, the VIBeS Plus program up to 4 years and the M-MITP up to 5 years
	Zhang et al., 2014 [24]	APIP	–	✓	–	No improvement in child behaviour
	Zhang et al., 2014 [24]	MITP, COPE	✓	–	–	Symbolic behaviour (understanding spoken language /object use in play)
Temperament	Benzies et al. 2013 [30]	M-MITP	✓	–	–	Positive effect at 3 and 6 months. Effect size not reported
	Zhang et al., 2014 [24]	MITP, COPE	✓	–	–	Statistical significance not reported
Nutrition and growth	Goyal et al. 2013 [33]	IHDP, others not specified	–	–	✓	Mixed findings with one study demonstrating a significant intervention effect on weight and length during infancy (at 4 and 12 months)
	Boundy et al., 2016 [21]	KC	–	✓	–	No improvements in weight gain or body length growth
Breast feeding	Boundy et al., 2016 [21]	KC	✓	–	–	Improvements in exclusive breast feeding
	Zhang et al., 2014 [24]	MITP, COPE	✓	–	–	Improvements in general breast feeding
Height and head circumference	McGregor et al., 2012 [35]	KC	✓	–	–	Improvements in height & head circumference reported by one study
Head circumference	Boundy et al., 2016 [21]	KC	✓	–	–	Improvements in head circumference
Decrease in infant heart rate and pain	Boundy et al., 2016 [21]	KC	–	✓	–	Ineffective with respect to heart rate, respiration, and pain experience
	McGregor et al., 2012 [35]	KC	✓	–	–	Infant's heart rates and pain scores significantly decreased during intervention ($p = .007$ and $p = .005$, respectively) and post-intervention ($p = .03$ and $p = .04$, respectively), although there was no significant differences in infants' stress levels
Reduction in morbidity and health service utilisation	Goyal et al., 2013 [33]	IHDP	–	–	✓	Mixed findings. Small, statistically significant increase in maternally reported minor illnesses at 3 years of age, but only for infants weighing 1500 g, and no effect on serious health conditions. No significant effects on rates of hospitalization or acute care visits
	Boundy et al., 2016 [21]	KC	✓	–	–	RR = 0.53 (Neonatal sepsis), RR = 0.22 (Hypothermia), RR = 0.12 (Hypoglycemia)
	Lawn et al., 2010 [31]	KC	✓	–	–	RR = 0.34 (RCT evidence)

Table 6 Effectiveness on infant outcomes (Continued)

Infant outcomes	Review	Intervention	Effectiveness of the intervention on the outcome			Additional information on impact
			Positive impact	No impact	Inconclusive	
Reduction in hospital readmission	Boundy et al., 2016 [21]	KC	√	–	–	Reduced hospital readmission by 58%
Lower mortality	Boundy et al., 2016 [21]	KC	√	–	–	Significant protective effect on mortality. Mortality 36% lower among low birth weight new borns.
	Lawn et al., 2010 [31]	KC	√	–	–	Large effect size, RR = 0.49 (RCT evidence) and RR = 0.68 (non-RCT evidence)
Early mental development/ neurodevelopment	Vanderveen et al., 2009 [23]	APIP, KC, COPE, IHDP, NIDCAP, others not specified	√	–	–	Large effect size at 6 months Weighted Mean Difference (WMD) = 3.55, p = 0.05), 12 months (WMD = 5.57, p = 0.0009), 24 months (WMD = 7.59, p = 0.0003) and 36 months (WMD = 9.66, p < 0.0001)
	Zhang et al., 2014 [24]	MITP, COPE	√	–	–	Statistical significance not reported
Long term mental development (at 5 years)	Vanderveen et al., 20,092 [23]	APIP, IHDP, others not specified	–	√	–	WMD = −1.36, (P = 0.24)
Early cognitive development (infancy & preschool age)	Spittle et al., 2015 [34]	Early interventions including MITP, IHDP, M-MITP, IBAIP, CBIP, HBIP, SPEEDI, others not specified	√	–	–	Infancy -developmental quotient (DQ): standardised mean difference (SMD) 0.32 [0.16, 0.47]; P < 0.001; 16 studies; 2372 participants. Preschool age -intelligence quotient (IIQ): SMD 0.43 [0.32–0.54]; P < 0.001; eight studies; 1436 participants.
	Benzies et al. 2013 [30]	M-MITP, NBAS	√	–	–	Effective at 4 months (NBAS) and 3 and 6 months (M-MITP)
Long term cognitive development	Spittle et al., 2015 [34]	MITP, IHDP, APIP	–	√	–	School age – IQ: SMD 0.18 [−0.08, 0.43]; P = 0.17; five studies; 1372 participants
Early motor development	Spittle et al., 2015 [34]	Early interventions including MITP, IHDP, M-MITP, IBAIP, CBIP, HBIP, SPEEDI, others not specified	√	–	–	Small significant effect in motor development in infancy. Motor scale DQ: SMD 0.10 [0.10, 0.19]
Long term motor development	Spittle et al., 2015 [34]		–	√	–	SMD −0.18, 95% CI −0.47 to 0.11; P = 0.22. Only five included studies reported outcomes at preschool age (n = 3) or at school age (n = 2).
Early psychomotor development	Vanderveen et al., 2009 [23]	IHDP, NIDCAP, others not specified	√	–	–	6 months WMD = 3.47 (3.92, 10.86) P = 0.36, 12 months WMD = 5.10 (1.44, 8.75) P = 0.006, 24 months WMD = 2.47 (2.01, 6.94) P = 0.28)
General child development	Benzies et al. 2013 [30]	VIBeS Plus	√	–	–	Short term 0–24 months
	Goyal et al., 2013 [33]	Home visiting interventions	√	–	–	Overall effect at infancy, z = 6.98 (p < 0.001)
	Zhang et al., 2014 [24]	M-MITP, COPE, MITP	√	–	–	Overall development up to 12 months

Interventions: *APIP* Avon Premature Infant Project, *CBIP* Clinic-Based Intervention programme, *COPE* Creating Opportunities for Parent Empowerment, *HBIP* Home Based intervention programme, *IBAIP* Infant Behavioural Assessment and Intervention Program, *IHDP* Infant Health and Development Program, *KC* Kangaroo Care, *M-MITP* Modified Mother Infant transaction programme, *MITP* Mother–Infant Transaction Program, *NBAS* Neonatal Behavioral Assessment Scale, *NIDCAP* Newborn Individualised Developmental & Assessment Programme, *NSTEP-P* Nursing Systems Towards Effective Parenting–Preterm, *SM* State Modulation, *SPEEDI* Supporting Play Exploration and Early Development Intervention, *TH* Traditional Holding, *VIBeS Plus* Victorian Infant Brain Studies

infancy [26, 32–34]. Two facility-based interventions (CBIP, NIDCAP) were found to improve cognitive development, psychomotor development and motor development in infancy, although the effect did not sustain in later ages [23, 34].

Discussion

This meta-review appraised and synthesised the evidence from 11 SRs on the effectiveness of early interventions on mother-infant dyadic, maternal/parental, and infant outcomes. To our knowledge, this is the first meta-review that was conducted with a specific focus on the effectiveness of interventions for parents of preterm infants on both parental and infant outcomes. Majority of the SRs were rated as of high or medium methodological quality. We found 34 interventions reported in the included SRs with differing components delivered by various professionals in the health facility and/or home settings. All the identified interventions started after the baby was born, either at the health facility or at home after discharge. Great majority of the interventions were focused on mothers whereas interventions specifically focusing on fathers or both the parents were relatively few. Although some SRs focused on interventions targeted at specific groups such as black teenage mothers and mothers of lower socioeconomic status [23], first-time mothers [24] and parents of first born infants who were preterm, we could not find any reviews specific to groups at higher risk of preterm birth, or reviews exclusively based on studies from low and middle income countries for interventions other than KC.

The most frequently reported interventions in our meta-review included the well-established programs: KC, MITP and IHDP. While KC has been defined with four key components - early, continuous, and prolonged skin-to-skin contact between the new-born and mother; exclusive breastfeeding; early discharge from the health facility; and close follow-up at home [36], there were variations in their implementation across the SRs. The theoretical foundations of MITP and IHDP have been highlighted by some SRs to demonstrate their positive impact. MITP is rooted in the transactional theory of development [37] arguing that children's developmental outcomes are shaped by the dynamic interplay between the child's behaviour, the caregiver's response, and the contextual factors that may influence both the child's behaviour and the caregiver response [38]. This framework emphasised children's active role in a reciprocal interaction that influences their own development [37]. MITP helps to enable the parents to appreciate their infant's unique characteristics, temperament and developmental potential, gradually sensitizing parents to infant cues, thereby improving the interaction between the parents and the infants [25]. The modified version,

M-MITP was designed to support mothers of preterm infants up to 5 years of age based on the premise that mothers' experiences of the preterm infant will transform over time and improve connection between the mother and the infant [32, 37]. The programme also encouraged engagement from both fathers and mothers, which eventually appeared to enhance their commitment to the programme. IHDP is underpinned by the wider bio-psychosocial model of early development which views the child's social and cognitive development as influenced by the extent of parent support, cultural environment, health status and genetics [39]. The programme included both home and facility based approaches designed to enhance the cognitive, behavioural, and health status of the infant, with the parent considered as an essential participant.

The interventions with most frequent positive impact across all the outcomes were KC and MITP, with KC standing out as the programme with the most positive impact on mother–infant dyadic, maternal/parental and infant outcomes. COPE also showed effectiveness on maternal/parental and infant outcomes. COPE provided an educational programme for parents at the neonatal unit including aspects such as the appearance and behavioural characteristics of preterm infants, how parents can participate in their infant's care, and how parents can make more positive interactions with their infant [25]. Other programs that showed consistent positive impact on infant outcomes were M-MITP and IHDP. Several outcomes such as mother-infant interaction; maternal/parental stress alleviation; reduction in maternal anxiety; depressive symptom reduction; reduction in infant morbidity and health service utilisation were reported in at least three reviews. However, the outcomes that were reported with consistent positive impact in at least three reviews were maternal/parental stress alleviation; depressive symptom reduction; and general child development.

Our meta-review provided a comprehensive evidence base on the range of interventions to support parents of preterm babies and their effectiveness on parents and preterm infants. The rigorous methodological approach based on a focused research question with a comprehensive search strategy, clear inclusion and exclusion criteria, and structured data extraction and quality assessment using standardised techniques make our findings robust and reliable. However, our findings are limited to SRs that either involve parents or reported parent outcomes and some of the inconsistent findings with respect to the effectiveness on the outcomes may be attributed to methodological factors including the variability in the definitions and measurement approaches of individual outcomes, variability in the intervention components and their delivery, and the quality of the individual studies included in the SRs. While all the reviews provided some description of the intervention components, none of the reviews reported complete details of all the interventions to enable replication. There was considerable heterogeneity in the structural framework of the interventions and the outcomes with a range of mother-infant dyadic, parental (mainly maternal), and infant outcomes making it challenging to compare and contrast the effectiveness of different interventions. There were also inconsistencies in the way individual outcomes were measured and reported both within and across the SRs. These are significant limitations of the existing SRs.

As a meta-review of SRs, our findings are limited to the direction of the association, with indications of significance wherever possible, rather than providing the magnitude of the association itself [29]. We were able to neither assess results separately by study designs nor account for any overlapping effects that might have existed due to the studies being included in more than one SR [40]. We were also unable to assess any moderating effects of the operational or contextual factors that could have impacted the effectiveness of the interventions. Although we did not restrict language of publication, we could only identify SRs published in English which might have led to the inadvertent exclusion of relevant papers published in other languages although this is likely to be minimum.

Conclusion

Our findings offer relevant insights and directions towards planning and implementing early intervention programs for parents to improve both parental and infant wellbeing following preterm birth. While we found a large number of interventions with considerable heterogeneity in structural framework and the outcomes, some interventions were more successful than others in achieving the intended outcomes. Neonatal care policy and planning for preterm babies should consider interventions with the most positive impact on parental and infant outcomes. The heterogeneity in interventions and outcomes calls for the development and implementation of an integrated intervention program for parents of preterm infants with a clearly defined standardised set of parental and infant outcomes.

Future meta-reviews should focus on the variations in contextual and implementation factors that can moderate the effectiveness on interventions, and on summarising the evidence by study design. Individual SRs should be conducted on the impact of interventions on groups potentially at higher risk of preterm birth such as parents from ethnic minority groups and those from low socio-economic status; and on interventions exclusively from low and middle income countries.

Abbreviations
AMSTAR: Assessing the Methodological Quality of Systematic Reviews; APIP: Avon Premature Infant Project; CBIP: Clinic Based Intervention Programme; COPE: Creating Opportunities for Parent Empowerment; EI: Early Intervention; HBIP: Home Based Intervention Programme; H-HOME: Hospital to Home; IBAIP: Infant Behavioural Assessment and Intervention Program; IHDP: Infant Health and Development Program; KC: Kangaroo Care; MITP: Mother Infant Transaction Programme; M-MITP: Modified mother infant transaction programme; NBAS: Neonatal Behavioral Assessment Scale; NICU: Neonatal Intensive Care Unit; NIDCAP: Newborn Individualised Developmental & Assessment Programme; NSTEP-P: Nursing Systems Towards Effective Parenting-Preterm; PBIP: Parent-Baby Interaction Programme; PI: Physiotherapy Intervention; PICOS: Population, Intervention, Comparator, Outcome, Study design; PRISMA: Preferred Reporting Items for Systematic Reviews and Meta Analyses; RCTs: Randomised Controlled Trials; RR: Relative Risk; SM: State Modulation; SM-NSTEP-P: State Modulation-Nursing System Towards Effective Parenting – Preterm; SPEEDI: Support Play Exploration and Early Development Intervention; SRs: Systematic Reviews; TH: Traditional Holding; VIBeS PLUS: Victorian Infant Brain Studies Program

Acknowledgements
We thank the subject librarian at the University of Bedfordshire, Janine Bhandol, for her assistance in conducting the searches.

Funding
No external funding received for this manuscript.

Authors' contributions
SP conceptualised and designed the study; coordinated and supervised the searches, SR selection, quality appraisal, data extraction and synthesis; and drafted the manuscript. MC conducted the searches, SR selection, quality appraisal, data extraction and synthesis. PcT contributed to the literature review, the searches, SR selection, quality appraisal, data extraction and synthesis. LK contributed to the literature review and reviewed the manuscript for important intellectual content. JK contributed to the literature review and reviewed the manuscript for important intellectual content. All authors approved the final manuscript as submitted and agree to be accountable for all aspects of the work.

Competing interests
The authors declare that they have no competing interests.

Author details
Maternal and Child Health Research Centre, Institute for Health Research, University of Bedfordshire, Putteridge Bury, Hitchin Road, Luton, Bedfordshire LU2 8LE, UK. [2]Neonatal Unit, Luton and Dunstable Hospital, Lewsey Rd, Luton LU4 0DZ, UK.

References
1. World Health Organization. Preterm Birth. 2015. http://www.who.int/mediacentre/factsheets/fs363/en/. Accessed 17 April 2016.
2. Petrou S, Mehta Z, Hockley C, Cook-Mozaffari P, Henderson J, Goldacre M. The impact of preterm birth on hospital inpatient admissions and costs during the first 5 years of life. Pediatrics. 2003;112
3. Feinberg ME, Roettger ME, Jones DE, Paul IM, Kan ML. Effects of a psychosocial couple-based prevention program on adverse birth outcomes. Matern Child Health J. 2015;19(1):102–11.
4. Centres for Disease Control. Preterm Birth. 2015. http://www.cdc.gov/reproductivehealth/MaternalInfantHealth/PretermBirth.htm. Accessed 28 March 2016.
5. Boyle EM, Poulsen G, Field DJ, Kurinczuk JJ, Wolke D, Alfirevic Z, et al. Effects of gestational age at birth on health outcomes at 3 and 5 years of age: population based cohort study. BMJ. 2012;344:1–14.
6. Kerstjens JM, de Winter AF, Bocca-Tjeertes IF, ten Vergert EM, Reijneveld SA, Bos AF. Developmental delay in moderately preterm-born children at school entry. J Pediatr. 2011;159(1):92–8.

7. Miles MS, Funk SG, Kasper MA. The stress response of mothers and fathers of preterm infants. Res Nurs Health. 1992;15(4):261–9.

8. Forcada-Guex M, Pierrehumbert B, Borghini A, Moessinger A, Muller-Nix C. Early dyadic patterns of mother-infant interactions and outcomes of prematurity at 18 months. Pediatrics. 2006;118(1):e107–14.

9. Kaaresen PI, Rønning JA, Ulvund SE, Dahl LB. A randomized, controlled trial of the effectiveness of an early-intervention program in reducing parenting stress after preterm birth. Pediatrics. 2006;118(1):9–19.

10. Talmi A, Harmon RJ. Relationships between preterm infants and their parents: disruption and development. Zero to Three (J). 2003;24(2):13–20.

11. Raju TN, Higgins RD, Stark AR, Leveno KJ. Optimizing care and outcome for late-preterm (near-term) infants: a summary of the workshop sponsored by the national institute of child health and human development. Pediatrics. 2006;118(3):1207–14.

12. Blencowe H, Cousens S, Chou D, Oestergaard M, Say L, Moller AB, et al. Born too soon: the global epidemiology of 15 million preterm births. Reprod Health. 2013;10(1):1–14.

13. Wang ML, Dorer DJ, Fleming MP, Catlin EA. Clinical outcomes of near-term infants. Pediatrics. 2004;114(2):372–6.

14. Smith V, Devane D, Begley CM, Clarke M, Higgins S. A systematic review and quality assessment of systematic reviews of randomised trials of interventions for preventing and treating preterm birth. Eur J Obstet Gynecol Reprod Biol. 2009;142(1):3–11.

15. Ravn IH, Lindemann R, Smeby NA, Bunch EH, Sandvik L, Smith L. Stress in fathers of moderately and late preterm infants: a randomised controlled trial. Early Child Dev Care. 2012;182(5):537–52.

16. The United Nations Office on Drugs and Crime's (UNODC): Compilation of Evidence-Based Family Skills Training Programmes. https://www.issup.net/knowledge-share/publications/2017-08/compilation-evidence-based-family-skills-training-programmes. Accessed 1 Oct 2017.

17. Day C, Michelson D, Thomson S, Penney C, Draper L. Evaluation of a peer led parenting intervention for disruptive behaviour problems in children: community based randomised controlled trial. BMJ. 2012;344:e1107.

18. Petrie J, Bunn F, Byrne G. Parenting programmes for preventing tobacco, alcohol or drugs misuse in children< 18: a systematic review. Health Educ Res. 2006;22(2):177–91.

19. Ferrari AJ, Whittingham K, Boyd R, Sanders M, Colditz P. Prem baby triple P a new parenting intervention for parents of infants born very preterm: acceptability and barriers. Infant Behav Dev. 2011;34(4):602–9.

20. Landsem IP, Handegård BH, Ulvund SE, Kaaresen PI, Rønning JA. Early intervention influences positively quality of life as reported by prematurely born children at age nine and their parents; a randomized clinical trial. Health Qual Life Outcomes. 2015;13(1):1–11.

21. Boundy EO, Dastjerdi R, Spiegelman D, Fawzi WW, Missmer SA, Lieberman E, et al. Kangaroo mother care and neonatal outcomes: a meta-analysis. Pediatrics. 2016;137(1):2015–238.

22. Orton J, Spittle A, Doyle L, Anderson P, Boyd R. Do early intervention programmes improve cognitive and motor outcomes for preterm infants after discharge? A systematic review. Dev Med Child Neurol. 2009;51(11):851–9.

23. Vanderveen J, Bassler D, Robertson C, Kirpalani H. Early interventions involving parents to improve neurodevelopmental outcomes of premature infants: a meta-analysis. J Perinatol. 2009;29(5):343–51.

24. Zhang X, Kurtz M, Lee SY, Liu H. Early intervention for preterm infants and their mothers: a systematic review. J Perinat Neonatal Nurs. 2014;18(11):1–14.

25. Brett J, Staniszewska S, Newburn M, Jones N, Taylor L. A systematic mapping review of effective interventions for communicating with, supporting and providing information to parents of preterm infants. BMJ Open. 2011;1(1):1–13.

26. Evans T, Whittingham K, Sanders M, Colditz P, Boyd RN. Are parenting interventions effective in improving the relationship between mothers and their preterm infants? Infant Behav Dev. 2014;37(2):131–54.

27. Moher D, Liberati A, Tetzlaff J, Altman DG; The PRISMA Group. Preferred Reporting Items for Systematic Reviews and Meta-Analyses: The PRISMA Statement. PLoS Med. 2009;6(7):e1000097. https://doi.org/10.1371/journal.pmed.1000097.

28. Shea BJ, Hamel C, Wells GA, et al. AMSTAR is a reliable and valid measurement tool to assess the methodological quality of systematic reviews. J Clin Epidemiol. 2009;62(10):1013–20.

29. Smith V, Devane D, Begley CM, Clarke M. Methodology in conducting a systematic review of systematic reviews of healthcare interventions. BMC Med Res Methodol. 2011;11(1):15.

30. Benzies KM, Magill-Evans JE, Hayden KA, Ballantyne M. Key components of early intervention programs for preterm infants and their parents: a systematic review and meta-analysis. BMC Pregnancy Childbirth. 2013;13(S1):S10.

31. Lawn JE, Mwansa-Kambafwile J, Horta BL, Barros FC, Cousens S. 'Kangaroo mother care' to prevent neonatal deaths due to preterm birth complications. Int J Epidemiol. 2010;39(1):144–54.

32. Herd M, Whittingham K, Sanders M, Colditz P, Boyd RN. Efficacy of preventative parenting interventions for parents of preterm infants on later child behavior: a systematic review and meta-analysis. Infant Ment Health J. 2014;35(6):630–41.

33. Goyal NK, Teeters A, Ammerman RT. Home visiting and outcomes of preterm infants: a systematic review. Pediatrics. 2013;132(3):502–16.

34. Spittle A, Orton J, Anderson PJ, Boyd R, Doyle LW. Early developmental intervention programmes provided post hospital discharge to prevent motor and cognitive impairment in preterm infants. Cochrane Database Syst Rev. 2015;11:1–74.

35. McGregor J, Casey J. Enhancing parent-infant bonding using kangaroo care: a structured review. Evidence Based Midwifery. 2012;10(2):50–6.

36. World Health Organization. Reproductive Health. Kangaroo Mother Care: A Practical Guide. http://www.who.int/maternal_child_adolescent/documents/9241590351/en/. Accessed 1 May 2017.

37. McDonald Culp A. The transactional model of development: How children and contexts shape each other. Edited by Arnold Sameroff. American Psychological Association, Washington, DC, 2009;115–117.

38. Sameroff AJ, MacKenzie MJ. A quarter-century of the transactional model: how have things changed? Zero to Three (J). 2003;24(1):14–22.

39. Borrell-Carrio F, Suchman AL, Epstein RM. The biopsychosocial model 25 years later: principles, practice, and scientific inquiry. Ann Fam Med. 2004;2(6):576–82.

40. Hartling L, Vandermeer B, Fernandes RM. Systematic reviews, overviews of reviews and comparative effectiveness reviews: a discussion of approaches to knowledge synthesis. Evid Based Child Health. 2014;9(2):486–94.

9

Review of guidelines on expression, storage and transport of breast milk for infants in hospital, to guide formulation of such recommendations in Sri Lanka

Ranmali Rodrigo[1,2]* (iD), Lisa H. Amir[2] and Della A. Forster[2,3]

Abstract

Background: Sick newborns in neonatal units who are unable to breastfeed are fed expressed breast milk. In Sri Lanka, most mothers stay in hospital throughout baby's stay to provide this milk freshly. In other countries mothers go home, express breast milk at home and bring it to hospital. There are concerns about the safety of transported expressed milk if used in a tropical middle-income country. The aim of this paper is to compare and contrast advice offered by different hospitals and organizations on how to express, store and transport breast milk safely.

Methods: We assessed guidelines used by hospital staff of the four Level 3 neonatal units in Melbourne, Australia, National Health Service UK, guidelines and training manuals of the Human Milk Banking Association of North America, the World Health Organization and an information leaflet from Family Health Bureau, Sri Lanka. Information on breast milk expression, storage and transport provided by the guidelines were tabulated under seven topics: general information; container for milk collection; hand expression; using a pump for expression; storage; thawing / warming; and transport of expressed breast milk. The AGREE II tool was used to assess the guidelines written for hospital staff.

Results: There was considerable agreement on most recommendations provided by these sources, but no single source covered all topics in full. Most recommend hand expression as the initial method for expressing of breast milk, followed by breast pump use, except the Sri Lankan recommendations which strongly discourages the use of breast pumps. Durations of storage under various conditions are generally similar in the different recommendations. Most guidelines recommend a 'cool box' or container with ice or freezer packs for transportation of milk.

Conclusion: A single document containing recommendations on all aspects of expressing, storing and transporting breast milk should be available for each unit, with the same basic information for mothers and the healthcare staff and further technical details for staff if required. The Sri Lankan recommendations need to be updated based on current worldwide practices and further studies are needed to establish a safe method of transport of expressed breast milk in Sri Lanka.

Keywords: Expressed breast milk, Storage, Transport, Preterm infant

* Correspondence: ranmali_waduge@yahoo.com
[1]Department of Paediatrics, University of Kelaniya, 6 Thalagolla Road, Ragama 11010, Sri Lanka
[2]Judith Lumley Centre, La Trobe University, 215 Franklin Street, Melbourne, VIC 3000, Australia
Full list of author information is available at the end of the article

Background

Breastfeeding has numerous advantages to the baby and mother including reduced infections and higher intelligence in the breastfed children and reduced breast cancer with lower risk of diabetes for the mothers [1]. Showing all mothers how to '.. . maintain lactation even if they should be separated from their infants' is one of the ten steps to successful breastfeeding, identified under the Baby Friendly Hospital Initiative (BFHI) [2].

A considerable number of babies who are in neonatal units either due to prematurity or other illness are unable to breastfeed directly as they are receiving invasive ventilatory support or are too premature to have coordinated, safe, sucking and swallowing reflexes [3]. These babies need to be provided with expressed breast milk, which can be given to the baby via several different methods including nasogastric or orogastric tubes, cup feeds, and syringe or dropper feeds [4]. The numbers of babies using these different methods have not been published in Sri Lanka or elsewhere. The monthly statistics of the unit that the first author is attached to, reveal that there were 3382 births in 2017, with 744 admissions to the neonatal unit including 61 babies born in other hospitals. This unit is a referral centre for fetal medicine. The number of babies less than 36 weeks gestation who were admitted to the neonatal unit, who would certainly have been given expressed breast milk at some point, was 272, that is 36% of the admitted babies. Some of the other babies more than 36 weeks who were on the ventilator or double phototherapy would also have received expressed breast milk.

In most developed countries like Australia, the United Kingdom and the United States of America, mothers are discharged from hospital even if their infants remain in the neonatal unit. Therefore, if they are providing breast milk for their babies they have to express breast milk at home and bring it to the hospital. In Sri Lanka, most mothers spend the entire time their baby is in the neonatal unit in hospital, and they provide fresh expressed breast milk for each feed. However, with increasingly lower gestation babies surviving in the neonatal units in Sri Lanka, mothers have to spend many weeks in the hospital, which becomes difficult in practice for some mothers. Mothers whose babies are in the neonatal unit do not even get a bed of their own at times due to overcrowding in the postnatal ward; there are situations where several mothers whose babies are in the neonatal unit have had to share a single bed. Meals are provided by the hospital, but most mothers wish to have their meals brought from home by relatives in the belief that lactating mothers should be provided with special home-made meals. A restricted number of relatives are allowed to visit the mother during the three visiting hours per day, but children are not allowed to come to the postnatal ward.

As there are concerns about the safety of using breast milk expressed at home and brought into hospital, this is currently not encouraged, especially from long distances; a safe method of expressing, storing and transporting breast milk for sick newborns in Sri Lanka therefore needs to be established. Currently there is no written feeding guideline for the unit at which the principal author works in Sri Lanka, but the hospital strives to adhere to the 10 steps of BFHI [2] in taking decisions regarding the feeding plan for individual babies. The different modes of feeding have not been formally evaluated or described in a study yet, in Sri Lanka.

A written guidance is used in the unit in assessing fitness for discharge, with the minimum criterion being that the baby is fully breast milk fed, using a combination of breastfeeding and cup-feeding (without use of bottles and teats) and being 1.2 kg by weight (around 34 weeks). The mothers receive intensive support in lactation management during hospital stay and the babies are closely followed-up for weight gain after discharge.

Having access to a refrigerator is essential for breast milk storage if it is to be expressed at home, stored and transported to the hospital later. National Sri Lankan data from 2009/10 which is the latest available, show that 60% of urban households and 38% of rural households have a refrigerator [5]. This number is certainly higher now although no more recent data are available, either for the country or for any particular hospital.

The bacteriological contamination of stored human milk and fresh milk has shown varied results in studies conducted under different conditions leading to differences in recommendations made by different institutes [6–10]. Studies have also examined the biochemical properties of stored milk [11, 12]. As there is currently no gold standard in best practice for expressing, storing and transporting human milk from home to hospital specifically for sick and preterm infants, we set out to review recommendations from a number of sources.

Methods

In order to establish safe standards for transporting expressed breast milk in Sri Lanka we initially identified information sources from Melbourne, Australia, where the researchers had access to the detailed protocols and guidelines of the Level 3 neonatal units, and other countries where transportation of expressed breast milk is common practice. The information sources we used are given in Table 1. The resources written for hospital staff were evaluated using the Appraisal of Guidelines for Research & Evaluation – II (AGREE-II) instrument [13] to assess the quality of guidelines. The information sources for which the AGREE II instrument was used has been indicated in Table 1. Guidance given by the Level 3 neonatal units in Melbourne, Australia and recognized

Table 1 List of information sources reviewed

Institute	Year	Names of guidelines / protocols / webpage titles / fact sheets	Audience	AGREE II Instrument [13]
MHW	2013	1. Breastfeeding guide [17]	Mothers	Not used
	2012	2. Breast Milk Expression Procedure [18]	Staff	Used
	2014	3. Breast Milk Expressing Equipment Management Procedure [19]	Staff	Used
	2015	4. Expressed Breast Milk (EBM): Storage and Management in Neonatal Services Procedure [20]	Staff	Used
	2014	5. Expressing breast milk [34]	Mothers	Not used
		6. Cleaning your breast pump equipment [36]	Mothers	Not used
RWH	2015	1. Expressing breast milk for sick or preterm babies [21]	Mothers	Not used
	2013	2. Expressing breast milk [22]	Mothers	Not used
	2011	3. Infant Feeding: Expressed Breast Milk: Management in Newborn Services [37]	Staff	Used
	2008	4. Using a breast pump [35]	Mothers	Not used
Monash	2014	1. Expressed breast milk (EBM) safe management and storage [23]	Mothers	Not used
	2011	2. Expressing breast milk [24]	Mothers	Not used
RCH	2013	1. Breastfeeding a baby in hospital [25]	Mothers	Not used
	2013	2. Breastfeeding at The Royal Children's Hospital [26]	Mothers	Not used
NHS (UK)	2016	1. Expressing and storing breast milk [27]	Mothers	Not used
	2014	2.Breastfeeding your premature baby [28]	Mothers	Not used
HMBANA	2011	1. Best Practice for Expressing, Storing and Handling Human Milk in Hospitals, Homes, and Child Care Settings.© HMBANA. 3rd Edition [30]	Staff	Used
WHO/UNICEF/ Wellstart	2009	1. Baby-Friendly Hospital Initiative - revised, updated and expanded for integrated care. Section "Results" Breastfeeding Promotion and Support in a Baby-Friendly Hospital. A 20-h course for maternity staff [31]	Staff	Used
SL		How to express breast milk [32]	Mothers	Not used

MHW Mercy Hospital for Women, Melbourne, Australia, *RWH* Royal Women's Hospital, Melbourne, Australia, *Monash* Monash Melbourne, Australia, *RCH* Royal Children's Hospital, Melbourne, Australia, *NHS* National Health Service, UK webpages, *HMBANA* Human Milk Banking Association of North America, *WHO/UNICEF* World Health Organization / United Nations Children's Emergency Fund, *SL* Sri Lanka

health authorities in UK, USA, and Sri Lanka as well as the World Health Organization (WHO) recommendations were used. The documents from Australia, UK and USA are meant for neonatal intensive care unit hospital staff and mothers. The Sri Lankan fact sheet is mostly used in the community, but is given to some mothers with babies in the neonatal unit as a written guidance to the method of expressing breast milk by hand. The WHO recommendations, which are meant for global usage including resource limited settings, are used by the Family Health Bureau of the Ministry of Health, Sri Lanka, for training of all health care personnel in the country on breastfeeding issues.

The guidelines of the National Health and Medical Research Council, Australia and the Academy of Breastfeeding Medicine, USA protocol were not used as these guidelines focus on expressing and storing human milk for healthy term babies when mothers are separated from this infants, e.g. for paid employment [14, 15]. A recent review by Peters et al. provides one of the most comprehensive systematic literature reviews on the safe management of expressed breast milk [16]. However that review did not make a clear distinction between expressing milk for sick preterm babies in hospital and healthy term infants at home [16].

The guidelines for hospital staff and fact sheets for parents provided to mothers from the four hospitals in Melbourne, Australia which have level 3 neonatal units, namely Mercy Hospital for Women (MHW) [17–20], the Royal Women's Hospital (RWH) [21, 22], Monash Health (MH) [23, 24] and the Royal Children's Hospital (RCH) [25, 26]; the National Health Service (NHS) website from the United Kingdom [27, 28]; the guideline of the Human Milk Banking Association of North America [29, 30]; information provided in the World Health Organization training course for maternity staff on breastfeeding promotion and support in a baby friendly hospital [31]; and the fact sheet for mothers on breast milk expression published by the Ministry of Health, Sri Lanka [32] were used to identify the recommendations made regarding storage and transport of expressed breast milk for sick babies in hospital. If these information sources provided advice separately for both categories of babies – those in neonatal units and those at home, only those relevant to the hospitalized infants was used. Two of the institutes whose recommendations were reviewed (Mercy Hospital for Women, Melbourne and HMBANA) also provided advice regarding milk being brought in for human milk banking and milk donation, but this information was not considered in the review.

The RCH and RWH recommendations are available online for access by the general public, while the MHW and Monash guidelines are available only on the intranet of each hospital for internal use only. The NHS, UK has a web page accessible by the general public with useful attractive illustrations regarding expression of breast milk, and advises to contact hospital staff regarding storage of milk for sick newborns.

Guideline quality assessment by the AGREE II instrument

The guidelines written for hospital staff were appraised by two assessors using the AGREE-II instrument. The assessment is done based on 23 items classified into six domains – namely scope and purpose, stakeholder involvement, rigor of development, clarity of presentation, applicability and editorial independence [13]. Each item is scored on a 7-point scale. The scores given by the assessors are presented as percentages based on the maximum possible score for each domain. The maximum possible score depends on the number of assessors and number of items in a particular domain that were assessed. In our assessments all 23 items were scored and none were left out. In some of the documents from Mercy Hospital for Women, stakeholder involvement was unclear and clarifications were made by contacting the staff of the Department of Paediatrics and Human Milk Bank at the hospital.

Review of the recommendations provided by the information sources

The recommendations provided by the chosen information sources were categorized under the following topics and tabulated.

1. General information on expression of breast milk and preparation for expression (Additional file 1: Table S1)
2. Container for collection and storage of expressed breast milk (Additional file 2: Table S2)
3. Hand expression of breast milk (Additional file 3: Table S3)
4. Using a pump for expression of breast milk (Additional file 4: Table S4)
5. Storage of expressed breast milk (Additional file 5: Table S5)
6. Thawing and warming of stored expressed breast milk (Additional file 6: Table S6)
7. Transport of expressed breast milk (Additional file 7: Table S7)

A detailed section on developing the healthcare workers' communication skills to counsel and build the self-confidence of mothers is available only in the WHO guidance [31].

Results

Assessment of guideline quality using the AGREE II instrument

The percentages obtained for each domain by the six guidelines appraised using the AGREE II instrument are given in Table 2. All six guidelines scored well in the two categories of scope and purpose, and clarity of presentation, but poorly in the category of rigor of

Table 2 Assessment of guideline quality by AGREE II tool

	MHW 2 (%)	MHW 3 (%)	MHW 4 (%)	RWH 3 (%)	HMBANA (%)	WHO (%)
Scope and purpose	97	94	94	89	78	94
Stakeholder involvement	42	61	50	25	22	100
Rigor of development	16	13	13	9	44	56
Clarity and presentation	92	89	89	92	94	100
Applicability	25	58	38	40	29	96
Editorial independence	13	25	25	13	50	100

MHW 2 Breast milk Expression Procedure (2012) from Mercy Hospital for Women [18], MHW 3 Breast Milk Expressing Equipment Management Procedure (2014) from Mercy, Hospital for Women [19], MHW 4 Expressed Breast Milk (EBM): Storage and Management in Neonatal Services, Procedure from Mercy Hospital for Women [20], RWH 3 Infant Feeding: Expressed Breast Milk: Management in Newborn Services from, Royal Women's Hospital [37], HMBANA Best Practice for Expressing, Storing and Handling Human Milk in Hospitals, Homes, and Child Care Settings.© HMBANA. 3rd Edition from Human Milk Banking Association of North America [30], WHO Baby-Friendly Hospital Initiative - revised, updated and expanded for integrated care, Section 3 - Breastfeeding Promotion and Support in a Baby-Friendly Hospital. A 20-hour course for maternity staff from the World Health Organization, UNICEF and Wellstart [31]

development. Editorial independence was also a weak point in most except for the WHO guideline [31]. Applicability of most guidelines, except the WHO guidelines had room for improvement. Overall, the WHO guideline was of the highest quality according to the AGREE II assessment, however the most amount of evidence based information was available in the HMBANA guideline [30].

Review of information provided by the information sources

General information on expression of breast milk and preparing for expression

The Melbourne hospitals with maternity units, HMBANA and WHO all mentioned the need to commence expression of breast milk as soon as possible after birth with the latter two mentioning that it should ideally be within 6 h of delivery [18, 21, 22, 24, 30, 31]. The Sri Lankan fact sheet and the NHS website did not comment on the timing of commencement of breast milk expression. All guidelines / institutes which provided recommendations on how to initiate breast milk expression suggested hand expression as the initial method. Subsequently they all recommended the pump as the preferred method with the exception of the Sri Lankan fact sheet [32].

The need for regular expression of breast milk – 3 to 4 hourly – along with the need for night time expression was stressed by all guidelines [18, 21, 22, 24, 25, 27, 30–33].

All guidelines advised women to wash their hands before expression, with the NHS, HMBANA and Sri Lankan recommendations being specific about mentioning that soap and water should be used for washing [27, 30, 32]. HMBANA guidelines also advise women to clip nails, remove rings and nail polish and recommended single-use towels for drying the hands after washing [30].

In order to encourage the mother's let-down reflex and maximize milk output, most of the guidelines advise mothers to be seated, relaxed and observe a photograph of their baby if the expression is being done away from the bedside of the baby [21, 25, 30, 31, 34]. The Sri Lankan fact sheet does not mention these, although use of warm compresses and gentle massage are advised [32].

Container for collection and storage of expressed breast milk

There is a mix of recommendations about containers to collect and store milk in, with some recommending only 'clean' containers [30–32] while others recommend 'sterile' containers [20, 21, 23, 25, 27] . In the first few days after giving birth a mother may have only small amounts of colostrum available. It is easier to collect this small quantity in a syringe. Sterile syringes for colostrum are specifically mentioned by MHW and RWH [20, 21]. Single use sealable plastic containers are mentioned by the

RWH and MHW whereas the Sri Lankan fact sheet recommends wide-mouthed containers which should be washed, boiled and reused. As there is no storage involved at present in Sri Lanka; the same container is usually used for cup-feeding the baby [20, 21, 32]. The filling of the container by expressed milk was most often recommended to be restricted to three quarters, by institutes where milk is stored by freezing [20, 21, 30]. MHW, RWH and RCH guidelines refer to the number of expressions that can be included in one container, with a range from two to several within 1 day [20, 21, 25] being recommended. RWH specifies that the fresh milk should be chilled before adding to the already frozen milk in the storage container [21].

The need for clear labelling of expressed milk was mentioned by most guidelines. Most hospitals provide the mother with printed labels which have the baby's identification details, and also request the mother to write the date and time of expression, with some having labels on which date and time of thawing and additive use can also be mentioned [20, 21, 23].

Hand expression of breast milk

The placement of the fingers on the breast for hand expression was explained in slightly different ways. In essence, all the recommendations advise placing the fingers at the edge of the areola / several centimeters back from the nipple with thumb opposite the forefinger / other four fingers to hold the areola in between. The WHO description is complicated as it makes statements like 'compress the breast over the *ducts*' and '*try* pressing your thumb and fingers back towards your chest' [31] p.164, rather than providing simple, directed, stepwise statements.

The need to press backwards towards the chest wall prior to compression is mentioned by most. Compression is very basically described as 'press thumb and 1st finger together' in the Sri Lankan pamphlet, while the WHO and NHS stress the importance of avoiding sliding or rubbing along the breast to avoid damage to the skin [27, 31, 32]. Most advise to move around areola to express from all ducts. The fact that hand expression of breast milk should not be painful if done correctly is mentioned clearly.

Most information sources advised to express from one breast until the flow slows down and then to switch over to the other breast. The Sri Lankan fact sheet advises to express for 20–25 min, while the MHW guideline says to switch over to the other breast or different site on the same breast when milk flow slows, with no specific duration being given [18, 32]. The RWH guideline mentions clearly that in the first few days the volume would only be a few drops [22].

The Sri Lankan fact sheet explicitly states that pressing or pulling on the nipple or massaging the breast does not result in expression of breast milk [32].

Using a pump for expression of breast milk

As mentioned earlier the Sri Lankan fact sheet strongly discourages use of pumps for expression of breast milk [32]. Personal experience has found the reason given for this is the idea, especially among midwives and nurses, that pumps are painful and ineffective as staff have not had much exposure to technologically advanced equipment in this field. There are also concerns regarding hygiene: pumps are thought to be a potential source of harmful bacteria [32]. The MHW guideline advises to hand express prior to use of a pump to stimulate the let-down reflex [18]. Only the MHW and RWH guidelines provided details on how to use an electric breast pump [34, 35]. They advise to place the breast shield centrally over the nipple and to initially use low suction with high speeds and vice versa as the milk starts flowing. Mothers are advised to use single breast pumps for 20–30 min and a double for 10–15 min each time [34]. The RCH guideline advises to seek the assistance of the nursing staff [25].

Clear cleaning instructions are given by the MHW and RWH [35, 36]. HMBANA states that majority of hospitals give each mother a sterile kit but only advises cleaning between use [30]. The MHW advises the same for reusable pump kits, except when the baby is preterm or sick when daily sterilisation is recommended [19]. The NHS advises to sterilise before and after each use [27, 28].

Storage of expressed breast milk

Expressed breast milk can be stored under different conditions. The recommended safe time period given by the different guidelines for keeping in room temperature ranges from 4 to 8 h. The ambient room temperature is not mentioned. If fresh milk is to be chilled / frozen RWH mentions that it should be done within 1 h of being expressed, while the MHW states that excess fresh milk placed in the refrigerator for < 48 h can be frozen [18, 20, 37].

The recommended duration of safe storage in a refrigerator for a baby in the hospital ranged from 24 h in the Sri Lankan pamphlet to 2–4 days by HMBANA [30, 32]. The MHW and RWH guidelines recommend 48 h while the RCH requests mothers to bring in the expressed milk, which has been kept in the refrigerator, to the hospital within 24 h of expression, for freezing [20, 21, 25]. The recommendation by the WHO and the Sri Lanka pamphlet for all babies in general, and by MHW specifically for babies in hospital, is that milk should be stored for ≤3 months in the freezer [20, 31, 32]. The RWH guidelines recommend safe frozen storage times of a) 2 weeks or b) 3 months c) 6 months respectively for milk stored in

a freezer that is a a) compartment within the refrigerator or b) the freezer has a separate door from that of the refrigerator or c) if the freezer is completely separate without being part of a refrigerator [21]. The RCH guideline does not clearly state the maximum duration that milk for a sick baby can be stored in hospital [25]. The Monash guideline recommends the safe duration of refrigeration for freshly expressed breast milk as being up to 72 h, but does not specify a safe time period for frozen milk [23].

Thawing and warming of stored expressed breast milk

The sources mention a wide range of methods to thaw frozen milk and safe usage times following thawing. If thawed in room temperature, the MHW guideline states that it should be used within 12 h or maximum 24 h if placed in the refrigerator immediately after thawing outside the refrigerator [20]. The HMBANA guideline however recommends only a 4 h safety period (until next feed) for the latter method [30]. Others do not mention this method of thawing.

If the expressed breast milk is thawed by placing in the refrigerator (one of the two commonly recommended methods) the WHO guideline recommends 12 h and the RWH guideline recommends 48 h, while the guidelines of MHW [20, 23, 30, 31, 37], Monash and HMBANA recommend 24 h as the safe period for usage. The HMBANA guideline additionally mentions that it should be used within 4 h once placed in room temperature [30].

Thawing by rapid warming using luke warm water was the other method mentioned by the guidelines from MHW, RWH, HMBANA, WHO, and it was the only method mentioned by the RCH guidelines [20, 25, 30, 31, 37]. Of these, the RWH and Monash guidelines said to use within 4 h, while MHW and HMBANA recommended to keep outside the refrigerator only until the end of the feed and mentioned that reusing any remainder that has been separated before the feed commenced is possible within 4 h if placed in refrigerator until then [20, 23, 30, 37]. The WHO recommendation was to use within 1 h [31].

All guidelines stated that there should be no refreezing after thawing. All sources also stated that a microwave should not be used for thawing.

The Sri Lankan fact sheet did not provide any information on methods of thawing or safe usage durations following thawing [32]. This guideline mentioned that refrigerated milk needs to warmed by placing in luke warm water, but advised not to boil or reheat. The latter advice was given by the WHO guideline as well [31]. Refraining from boiling was not mentioned by any other sources, while avoidance of reheating was specifically not mentioned by the MHW, RWH, RCH or HMBANA guidelines [20, 21, 25, 30, 37].

Transport of expressed breast milk

The RCH guideline advised not to bring frozen milk in to the hospital and Monash mentioned that frozen milk should be maintained in frozen state for transport while refrigerated should be maintained between 1 and 4 °C [23, 25].

An insulated food container or cool-box was recommended by all the Melbourne hospitals for transport of expressed breast milk. The RWH, Monash and RCH guidelines requested transportation with ice or freezing blocks [21, 23, 25]. The MHW guideline showed preference for gel or cold packs over ice for transport [20]. If the amount of thawed milk was < 25% the MHW guideline advised to place the milk in the freezer while it was to be placed in the refrigerator if the amount thawed was more extensive [20]. The RCH guideline did not encourage mothers to bring in frozen milk and advised mothers to bring in refrigerated milk less than 24 h old to hospital [25]. The RWH guideline recommended refrigerating the expressed breast milk within 1 h of expression, and freezing within 24 h if it was not possible to bring in the milk within 48 h to hospital [37]. The Monash guideline also recommended to freeze the expressed breast milk if it will not be transported within 24 h [24]. Similar to MHW, the RWH guideline recommended frozen milk that was partially thawed on arrival to be thawed completely in the refrigerator and be used within 24 h [20, 37].

There were no Sri Lankan recommendations on transportation of expressed breast milk.

Other information

The Sri Lankan pamphlet mentioned that there is no difference in the taste or goodness of expressed breast milk (which is used fresh in Sri Lanka) versus milk obtained by direct breastfeeding [32]. This pamphlet also mentioned not to use bottles with teats for feeding the milk and to use a cup or spoon instead.

Discussion

The purpose of this paper was to review selected guidelines and factsheets on expression and storage of breast milk, both at home and in the neonatal unit, and on transport of expressed breast milk from home to hospital, in order to assist in establishing safe standards for transporting expressed breast milk in Sri Lanka from home to neonatal units in the hospital for mothers who are unable to stay in hospital with their sick newborns. In reviewing the selected guidelines and fact sheets we noted that most recommendations on general aspects of breast milk expression, how to hand-express and freezer storage guidelines were similar in the different guidelines. However, when taking each information source individually there were gaps, wide variations and unclear areas with regard to the method of transport. There is

therefore a need for a written single guideline, for each unit which contains recommendations on all aspects of expressing, storing and transporting breast milk which has the same basic information for mothers and the healthcare staff and further technical details for staff if required. The Sri Lankan fact sheet strongly discourages the use of pumps, even going to the extent of stating that it is more painful. Concerns about cleanliness have also contributed to the discouragement [32]. In Sri Lanka – especially for hospital based use, only fresh expressed breast milk is generally used. Therefore, currently there is no necessity for expressing large volumes for storage in Sri Lanka. This may be the reason for discouragement of pump use along with concerns about the cost of pumps as well – although hand pumps are now available for very reasonable prices. The available guidelines have been written nearly a decade ago and neonatal care, especially in terms of survival of preterm infants has improved greatly since then. Therefore, the Sri Lankan information sheet needs to be updated with more evidence-based recommendations that are relevant to the current situation of sick newborns in the country. There is an urgent need to identify safe modes of storage and transport of expressed breast milk in Sri Lanka, taking into consideration available modes of storage and transport along with weather conditions. Sri Lanka is an island situated within the tropics where the mean annual temperature varies between 27 °C in the coastal lowlands to 16 °C in the central highlands. Even in the highlands the maximum daytime temperatures are more than 18.5 °C [38]. The average relative humidity is > 65% in all parts of the country and above 75%, up to 95%, in the wet zone [39].

The Sri Lankan fact sheet does not mention the use of photographs of the baby to stimulate hormonal responses in the mother because it is currently not relevant as mothers will be doing most of the expression of breast milk in the neonatal unit itself [32]. However, it would be very useful for the mothers who are unwell in intensive care unit themselves and therefore may not even have seen the baby yet. There are hospital regulations in Sri Lanka which prohibit photography of patients which would need to be addressed. Other methods of stimulating a hormonal response which enhance milk secretion, that could be mentioned in a guideline or fact sheet for mothers include kangaroo mother care and back massage for the mothers [31].

With regard to containers, the Sri Lankan recommendation is the use of wide-mouthed containers as they can then be used directly for cup-feeding of the baby. In Sri Lanka, in keeping with the ten steps of the Baby Friendly Hospital Initiative, the recommended method of feeding expressed breast milk even at home is by cup or rarely spoon; mothers are advised to avoid teats and bottles for feeding the expressed breast milk; it is always cups or spoons that are used for feeding of supplementary expressed breast milk even after the babies are discharged home. This recommendation should be considered by other institutes worldwide as well, if they are hoping to achieve baby-friendly hospital status.

This paper is the first component of a series of studies to establish the necessity and safety of an economical method of expressing, storing and transporting breast milk in Sri Lanka from home to hospital, for mothers who are unable to stay in hospital for a prolonged period with their sick newborns. A Hazard Analysis and Critical Control Points is a system designed to ensure food safety by preventing hazards due to microbiological contamination, biochemical and physical changes that occur in food items from the stage of raw material to the finished product that would be consumed and a previous study in Belgium has studied this in 2011 for expressed breast milk on a neonatal unit [8]. When the final version of the recommendations for Sri Lanka are prepared, the points that need to be addressed e.g. method of hand expression including cleaning of hands before expression of milk, type of container used for storage, cleansing of the container for storage, methods of storage and transportation of the expressed breast milk that will maintain desired temperatures and acceptable microbiological status, will be identified using the guidelines and protocols that have been studied in this paper, taking economical and sociocultural aspects of Sri Lanka into consideration. The availability of a refrigerator or freezer at home and transport modes that will be used by mothers or the person bringing in milk from home to hospital will be studied prior to making any recommendations. The guideline we prepare will include a section on breastfeeding counselling and supporting a mother to build her self-confidence.

Conclusion

A single document containing recommendations on all aspects of expressing, storing and transporting breast milk should be available for each unit, with the same basic information for mothers and the healthcare staff and further technical details for staff if required. The Sri Lankan recommendations need to be updated based on current worldwide practices and further studies are needed to establish a safe method of transport of expressed breast milk in Sri Lanka.

Abbreviations

AGREE-II: Appraisal of Guidelines for Research & Evaluation – II; HMBANA: Human Milk Banking Association of North America; MHW: Mercy Hospital for Women, Melbourne, Australia; Monash: Monash Melbourne, Australia; NHS: National Health Service, UK webpages; RCH: Royal Children's Hospital, Melbourne, Australia; RWH: Royal Women's Hospital, Melbourne, Australia; SL: Sri Lanka; WHO/UNICEF: World Health Organization / United Nations Children's Emergency Fund

Authors' contributions

RR gathered and tabulated the information from the different sources under the guidance and supervision of LHA and DAF. All authors contributed to the writing of the manuscript and approved the final manuscript.

Competing interests

The authors declare that they have no competing interests.

Author details

Department of Paediatrics, University of Kelaniya, 6 Thalagolla Road, Ragama 11010, Sri Lanka. [2]Judith Lumley Centre, La Trobe University, 215 Franklin Street, Melbourne, VIC 3000, Australia. [3]Royal Women's Hospital, Locked Bag 300, Parkville, VIC 3052, Australia.

References

1. Victora CG, Bahl R, Barros AJ, Franca GV, Horton S, Krasevec J, Murch S, Sankar MJ, Walker N, Rollins NC, et al. Breastfeeding in the 21st century: epidemiology, mechanisms, and lifelong effect. Lancet. 2016;387(10017): 475–90.
2. World Health Organization, UNICEF, Wellstart International. Baby-friendly hospital initiative : revised, updated and expanded for integrated care. Section 1 - Background and implementation. Geneva: World Health Organisation and UNICEF; 2009.
3. Lau C. Development of suck and swallow mechanisms in infants. Ann Nutr Metab. 2015;66(Suppl 5):7–14.
4. Maggio L, Costa S, Zecca C, Giordano L. Methods of enteral feeding in preterm infants. Early Hum Dev. 2012;88(Suppl 2):S31–3.
5. Department of Census and Statistics, Ministry of Finance and Planning Sri Lanka. Household Income and Expenditure Survey 2009/10. Colombo: Department of census and statistics; 2011.
6. Ogundele MO. Techniques for the storage of human breast milk: implications for anti-microbial functions and safety of stored milk. Eur J Pediatr. 2000;159(11):793–7.
7. Igumbor EO, Mukura RD, Makandiramba B, Chihota V. Storage of breast milk: effect of temperature and storage duration on microbial growth. Cent Afr J Med. 2000;46(9):247–51.
8. Cossey V, Jeurissen A, Thelissen MJ, Vanhole C, Schuermans A. Expressed breast milk on a neonatal unit: a hazard analysis and critical control points approach. Am J Infect Control. 2011;39(10):832–8.
9. Hososaka Y, Nukita H, Ishii Y, Onishi A, Isonishi S, Ito F. Bacteriological safety of human milk storage. Jikeikai Med J. 2013;60:17–22.
10. Ukegbu PO, Uwaegbute AC, Ijeh II, Ukegbu AU. Bacterial load in expressed and stored breast milk of lactating mothers in Abia state, Nigeria. Afr J Food Agric Nutr Dev. 2013;13(4):8139–54.
11. Hamosh M, Ellis LA, Pollock DR, Henderson TR, Hamosh P. Breastfeeding and the working mother: effect of time and temperature of short-term storage on proteolysis, lipolysis, and bacterial growth in milk. Pediatrics. 1996;97(4):492–8.
12. Ghoshal B, Lahiri S, Kar K, Sarkar N. Changes in biochemical contents of expressed breast milk on refrigerator storage. Indian Pediatr. 2012;49(10):836–7.
13. Brouwers MC, Kho ME, Browman GP, Burgers JS, Cluzeau F, Feder G, Fervers B, Graham ID, Grimshaw J, Hanna SE, et al. AGREE II: advancing guideline development, reporting and evaluation in health care. CMAJ. 2010;182(18):E839–42.
14. National Health and Medical Research Council. Infant Feeding Guidelines: Information for Health Workers. Canberra: National Health and Medical Research Council; 2012.
15. Academy of Breastfeeding Medicine Protocol Committee. ABM clinical protocol #8: human milk storage information for home use for full-term infants (original protocol march 2004; revision #1 march 2010). Breastfeed Med. 2010;5(3):127–30.
16. Peters MD, McArthur A, Munn Z. Safe management of expressed breast milk: a systematic review. Women Birth. 2016;29(6):473–81.
17. Inc MPH. Breastfeeding guide. Melbourne: Mercy Public Hospitals Inc; 2013.

18. Mercy Hospital for Women. Breast Milk Expression Procedure. Melbourne: Mercy Hospital for Women; 2012.

19. Mercy Hospital for Women. Breast Milk Expressing Equipment Management Procedure. Melbourne: Mercy Hospital for Women; 2014.

20. Mercy Hospital for Women. Expressed Breast Milk (EBM): Storage and Management in Neonatal Services Procedure. Melbourne: Mercy Hospital for Women; 2015.

21. Expressing breast milk for sick and preterm babies [file:///C:/Users/Admin/Downloads/Breastfeeding-Expressing-breast-milk-for-sick-preterm-babies2%20(2).pdf].

22. Expressing breast milk [https://thewomens.r.worldssl.net/images/uploads/fact-sheets/Breastfeeding-Expressing-breast-milk.pdf].

23. Health M. Expressed breast milk (EBM) safe management and storage. Melbourne: Monash Health; 2014.

24. Monash Children's Hospital. Expressing breast milk. Melbourne: Monash Children's Hospital; 2011.

25. Breastfeeding a baby in hospital [http://www.rch.org.au/kidsinfo/fact_sheets/Breastfeeding_a_baby_in_hospital/].

26. Breastfeeding at The Royal Children's Hospital [http://www.rch.org.au/kidsinfo/fact_sheets/Breastfeeding_at_The_Royal_Children_s_Hospital/].

27. Expressing and storing breast milk [http://www.nhs.uk/Conditions/pregnancy-and-baby/pages/expressing-storing-breast-milk.aspx].

28. Breastfeeding your premature baby [http://www.nhs.uk/Conditions/pregnancy-and-baby/Pages/breastfeeding-premature-baby.aspx].

29. Human Milk Banking Association fo North America (HMBANA). Guidelines for the Establishment and Operation of Donor Human Milk Bank. Texas: HMBANA; 2015.

30. Jones F. Best practice for expressing, storing and handling human milk in hospitals, homes, and child care settings. 3rd ed. Texas: Human milk banking Association of North America; 2011.

31. World Health Organization, UNICEF, Wellstart International. Baby-friendly hospital initiative : revised, updated and expanded for integrated care. Section 3 - Breastfeeding promotion and support in a baby-friendly hospital: a 20-hour course for maternity staff. Geneva: World Health Organization and UNICEF; 2009.

32. Ministry of Health. How to express breast milk? Colombo: Family Health Bureau, Ministry of Health; 2000.

33. Mercy Public Hospitals Inc: Breastfeeding guide. In. Edited by Inc MPH; 2015.

34. Mercy Hospital for Women. Expressing breast milk. Melbourne: Mercy Hospital for Women; 2014.

35. The Royal Women's Hospital. Using a breast pump. Melbourne: Royal Women's Hospital; 2008.

36. Mercy Hospital for Women. Cleaning your breast pump equipment. Melbourne: Mercy Hospital for Women; 2014.

37. The Royal Women's Hospital. Infant feeding: expressed breast milk: Management in Newborn Services. Melbourne: The Royal Women's Hospital; 2011.

38. Climate of Sri Lanka [http://www.meteo.gov.lk/index.php?option=com_content&view=article&id=94&Itemid=310&lang=en].

39. Annual and monthly average relative humidity , 2008–2013 [http://www.statistics.gov.lk/Abstract2014/CHAP1/1.5.pdf].

10

Sex-specific effects of perinatal dioxin exposure on eating behavior in 3-year-old Vietnamese children

Anh Thi Nguyet Nguyen[1], Muneko Nishijo[1*], Tai The Pham[2], Nghi Ngoc Tran[1], Anh Hai Tran[2], Luong Van Hoang[2], Hitomi Boda[3], Yuko Morikawa[3], Yoshikazu Nishino[1] and Hisao Nishijo[4]

Abstract

Background: We previously reported that perinatal dioxin exposure increased autistic traits in children living in dioxin-contaminated areas of Vietnam. In the present study, we investigated the impact of dioxin exposure on children's eating behavior, which is often altered in those with developmental disorders.

Methods: A total of 185 mother-and-child pairs previously enrolled in a birth cohort in dioxin-contaminated areas participated in this survey, conducted when the children reached 3 years of age. Perinatal dioxin exposure levels in the children were estimated using dioxin levels in maternal breast milk after birth. Mothers were interviewed using the Children's Eating Behaviour Questionnaire (CEBQ). A multiple linear regression model was used to analyze the association between dioxin exposure and CEBQ scores, after controlling for covariates such as location, parity, maternal age, maternal education, maternal body mass index, family income, children's gestational age at delivery, and children's age at the time of the survey. A general linear model was used to analyze the effects of sex and dioxin exposure on CEBQ scores.

Results: There was no significant association between most dioxin congeners or toxic equivalencies of polychlorinated dibenzo-*p*-dioxins/furans (TEQ-PCDDs/Fs) and CEBQ scores in boys, although significant associations between some eating behavior sub-scores and 1,2,3,4,6,7,8,9-octachlorodibenzofuran were observed. In girls, there was a significant inverse association between levels of TEQ-PCDFs and enjoyment of food scores and between levels of TEQ-PCDFs and TEQ-PCDDs/Fs and desire to drink scores. Two pentachlorodibenzofuran congeners and 1,2,3,6,7,8-hexachlorodibenzofuran were associated with a decreased enjoyment of food score, and seven PCDF congeners were associated with a decreased desire to drink score. The adjusted mean enjoyment of food score was significantly lower in children of both sexes exposed to high levels of TEQ-PCDFs. There was, however, a significant interaction between sex and TEQ-PCDF exposure in their effect on desire to drink scores, especially in girls.

Conclusions: Perinatal exposure to dioxin can influence eating behavior in children and particularly in girls. A longer follow-up study would be required to assess whether emotional development that affects eating styles and behaviors is related to dioxin exposure.

Keywords: Dioxin, Breast milk, Perinatal exposure, Children, Eating behavior, Vietnam

* Correspondence: ni-koei@kanazawa-med.ac.jp
[1]Department of Public Health and Epidemiology, Kanazawa Medical University, 1-1, Daigaku, Uchinada, Ishikawa 920-0293, Japan
Full list of author information is available at the end of the article

Background

Dioxin contamination in Vietnam has had a long-term impact on the environment and human health, particularly in hotspots of high contamination [1–4]. This has mainly been related to the use of herbicides, especially Agent Orange, which contains 2,3,7,8-tetrachlorodibenzo-*p*-dioxin (TCDD) during the Vietnam War. We found that dioxin levels in maternal breast milk in contamination hotspots in southern Vietnam were 3–4 times the levels in unsprayed areas of northern Vietnam, even though four decades had passed [5]. As breast milk reflects the maternal body burden of dioxin, we carried out various studies on the health effects of dioxin exposure in infants using dioxin levels in maternal breast milk as a marker of perinatal exposure. We found that perinatal dioxin exposure was associated with reduced growth during the first 4 months of life, particularly in boys [6], lower cognitive and fine motor skill scores in infants aged 4 months [7], and lower social emotional scores in toddlers aged 1 year [8].

When our cohort reached 3 years of age, we performed a health impact survey to determine whether there was an association between perinatal dioxin exposure and autistic traits measured using the Autism Spectrum Rating Scales (ASRS), and found that perinatal TCDD exposure increased social emotional difficulties in these children [9]. We also investigated the longitudinal effects of perinatal dioxin exposure on growth and neurodevelopment in the children during the first 3 years of life, and reported that increased dioxin exposure was associated with sex-specific effects on growth and neurodevelopment. We found that exposure decreased various body measurements in boys, increased head and abdominal circumferences in girls, and decreased neurodevelopmental motor and expressive language scores in boys [10]. These findings highlight the need to investigate sex-specific effects of perinatal dioxin exposure on children's eating behavior, which may lead to differences in size, particularly in children with poor neurodevelopment. In clinical studies, eating behavior has been linked to problems in social behavior in children with neurodevelopmental disorders such as autism spectrum disorder [11, 12], which are more prevalent in boys.

Animal studies have reported that dioxin exposure affected brain regions in the limbic system such as the hypothalamus, nucleus accumbens, amygdala, and orbitofrontal cortex [13–16] that are involved in controlling appetite and food rewards [17, 18], and altered taste preference in female rats exposed to dioxin perinatally [19]. Based on these findings, we hypothesized that dioxin may alter eating behaviors in children perinatally exposed to dioxin by affecting these brain regions. In the present study, we investigated whether dioxin exposure affected the eating behaviors of Vietnamese children, and whether such an effect was sex-specific.

Methods

Study subjects

The study was conducted in the Thanh Khe and Son Tra districts of Da Nang City near Da Nang airbase, where extremely high dioxin levels have been recorded in soil and sediment samples collected in 2006 (858–361,000 pg/g dry weight of TCDD in soil and 674–8580 pg/g dry weight in sediment from a nearby lake and from the airbase's drainage system) [4]. The Vietnamese and US governments have been carrying out soil remediation activities at the Da Nang airbase since 2012 [20], but environmental contamination remains high.

In 2008–9, a total of 241 mother-and-newborn pairs (159 pairs in Thanh Khe and 82 in Son Tra) were recruited in district hospitals. These pairs were selected based on the following criteria: i) Mothers resided in Thanh Khe or Son Tra at least during their pregnancy; ii) babies were born at term; iii) mothers had no birth complications. Breast milk samples (20 mL) were collected from these mothers 1 month postpartum with the assistance of midwives and were stored in sterile polyethylene containers at $-4\,°C$ at local health centers.

A total of 198 mother-child pairs (82.2%) participated in the survey when the children reached 3 years of age. Forty-one other pairs were lost to follow-up owing to relocation or failure to appear at the examination; two infants died in their first postnatal month. There were no significant differences in the characteristics of mothers and children or dioxin levels in breast milk between study participants and the 43 pairs lost to follow-up. Some demographic information was missing for 13 of the mothers, so the final sample for analysis included 185 mother-child pairs, representing 76.8% of the original sample.

At the follow-up surveys at 4 months, 1 year, and 3 years of age, neurodevelopmental measurements were obtained using the Bayley Scales of Infant and Toddler Development, Third Edition (NCS Pearson, Inc., Bloomington, MN, USA) to assess infant development in the areas of cognition, language, and motor functions. The findings were reported in our previous studies [6–9]. At the 3-year survey, full-length parent rating forms of the Autism Spectrum Rating Scales (ASRS; MHS, Inc., North Tonawanda, NY, USA) and the Children's Eating Behaviour Questionnaire (CEBQ) [21] were used to measure behaviors associated with autism spectrum disorder and eating behavior, respectively. We previously reported an association between dioxin exposure and ASRS [9].

Dioxin measurement in breast milk samples

Breast milk samples were frozen after collection and transported to the High Technology Center, Kanazawa Medical University, Japan to analyze concentrations of 17 2,3,7,8-substituted dioxin congeners. After extracting fat from 10 mL of sample and a series of purifying operations, measurement was performed using a gas chromatograph (HP-6980; Hewlett-Packard, Palo Alto, CA, USA) equipped with a high-resolution mass spectrometer (MStation-700, JEOL, Tokyo, Japan). The established analytical method has been described in detail previously [5]. Concentrations of the 17 congeners of polychlorinated dibenzo-p-dioxins/furans (PCDDs/Fs) were lipid-base calculated. Toxic equivalency factors (TEFs) for each congener were referenced from the World Health Organization 2005-TEF list [22]. Toxic equivalencies (TEQs) of polychlorinated dibenzo-p-dioxins (PCDDs), polychlorinated dibenzofurans (PCDFs), and PCDDs/Fs were calculated by multiplying each congener concentration by its TEF and summing the values. The values of the concentrations that were below the limit of detection were set to equal half of the limit of detection for the analysis. Table 1 lists the concentrations of each congener in breast milk samples, stratified by the sex of the child.

Lower TEQ levels of dioxin-like polychlorinated biphenyls (dl-PCBs) measured in the present study were compared with levels in samples collected in unsprayed areas in northern Vietnam, although dl-PCB levels were measured in only four samples [6]. Those findings suggested that TEQ-PCDDs/Fs can be used as an indicator of dioxin toxicity in the Da Nang sampling area because of the lower contribution of dl-PCBs to the total TEQ.

Questionnaire survey

Structured questionnaires were used to obtain information related to childbirth and the growth and neurodevelopment of children (gestational weeks at birth and birth weight) and to maternal demographics at the 4-month survey. Maternal height and weight were obtained from medical records in the hospitals' obstetrics departments. Table 2 lists the characteristics of the participants, stratified by the sex of the child. All children were born at full term, and breast milk served as the only or main food supply of all

Table 1 Dioxin concentrations in maternal breast milk stratified by child's sex

	LOD (ppt)	Samples with below LOD N (%)	Boys (N = 106) Median	GM	GSD	Girls (N = 79) Median	GM	GSD
PCDD congeners (pg/g lipid)								
2,3,7,8-TetraCDD	0.004	11 (5.9)	1.5	1.3	2.1	1.7	1.4	2.6
1,2,3,7,8-PentaCDD	0.011	0	4.2	4.3	1.6	4.5	4.1	1.7
1,2,3,4,7,8-HexaCDD	0.004	0	2.2	2.3	1.6	2.4	2.3	1.7
1,2,3,6,7,8-HexaCDD	0.01	0	8.3	8.2	1.6	8.4	8.2	1.8
1,2,3,7,8,9-HexaCDD	0.008	0	2.5	2.6	1.6	2.7	2.7	1.7
1,2,3,4,6,7,8-HeptaCDD	0.008	0	12.1	12.0	1.5	11.4	12.1	1.6
OctaCDD	0.008	0	63.9	67.7	1.5	68.1	67.7	1.6
PCDF congeners (pg/g lipid)								
2,3,7,8-TetraCDF	0.005	13 (7.0)	0.5	0.5	2.0	0.6	0.5	2.2
1,2,3,7,8-PentaCDF	0.006	0	1.2	1.2	1.7	1.3	1.2	2.1
2,3,4,7,8-PentaCDF	0.01	0	7.2	7.1	1.5	8.1	7.2	1.7
1,2,3,4,7,8-HexaCDF	0.008	0	16.5	16.7	1.6	19.9	18.0	1.9
1,2,3,6,7,8-HexaCDF	0.003	0	10.8	10.2	1.6	12.0	11.1	1.9
1,2,3,7,8,9-HexaCDF	0.004	12 (13.5)	0.2	0.2	2.2	0.3	0.3	2.7
2,3,4,6,7,8-HexaCDF	0.006	0	1.3	1.2	1.5	1.5	1.4	1.9
1,2,3,4,6,7,8-HeptaCDF	0.01	0	10.8	11.6	1.6	13.5	12.9	2.0
1,2,3,4,7,8,9-HeptaCDF	0.004	3 (1.6)	1.2	1.1	1.9	1.6	1.2	2.7
OctaCDF	0.013	47 (25.4)	0.5	0.6	2.4	0.5	0.6	2.6
TEQs (pg-TEQ/g lipid)								
TEQ-PCDDs			7.4	7.3	1.6	8.0	7.3	1.8
TEQ-PCDFs			5.2	5.3	1.5	5.7	5.6	1.8
TEQ-PCDDs/Fs			12.5	12.6	1.5	14.2	13.0	1.7

CDD chlorinated dibenzo-p-dioxin, *CDF* chlorinated dibenzofuran, *GM* geometrical mean, *GSD* geometrical standard deviation, *LOD* limit of detection, *PCDD* polychlorinated dibenzo-p-dioxin, *PCDF* polychlorinated dibenzofuran, *ppt* parts per trillion, *TEQ* toxic equivalency

Table 2 Characteristics of study participants and Children's Eating Behaviour Questionnaire (CEBQ) scores stratified by sex

	Characteristics, CEBQ scores	Boys (N = 106)		Girls (N = 79)	
		Mean, N (%)	SD	Mean, N (%)	SD
Mothers	Age (years)	27.9	5.7	28.4	6.6
	Primiparae (%)	30 (28.3)		25 (32.9)	
	Weight during pregnancy (kg)	58.4	6.3	56.7	7.1
	Height (cm)	154.4	4.9	154.0	5.3
	BMI	24.5	2.6	23.9	2.5
	Family income (VND)	2986	1489	3012	1717
Children	Age at the survey (months)	36.3	1.5	36.8	1.6
	Birth weight (g)	3280	384	3187	352
	Gestational weeks at birth	39.6	0.8	39.5	0.8
	Weight at the survey (kg)	14.1	1.9	13.4	1.9
	Height at the survey (cm)	93.2	3.2	91.9	3.6
	BMI at the survey	16.2	1.5	15.8	1.6
	CEBQ scores				
	Satiety Responsiveness (SR)	2.3	0.7	2.5	0.7
	Slowness in Eating (SE)	2.7	0.8	3.0	0.9
	Fussiness (FU)	3.1	0.4	3.2	0.4
	Food Responsiveness (FR)	2.6	1.0	2.9	1.0
	Enjoyment of Food (EF)	4.1	0.8	4.0	0.8
	Desire to Drink (DD)	3.3	1.3	3.4	1.2
	Emotional of Undereating (EU)	3.2	0.9	3.5	0.9
	Emotional of Overeating (EO)	2.0	0.6	2.3	0.8
	Food Approach (FAPP)	3.0	0.7	3.1	0.6
	Food Advoident (FAVD)	2.8	0.4	3.1	0.4

The food approach score was calculated from the food responsiveness, enjoyment of food, desire to drink, and emotional over-eating scores
The food avoidance score was calculated from the satiety responsiveness, slowness in eating, fussiness, and emotional under-eating scores
N number of subjects, *SD* standard deviation, *BMI* body mass index, *VND* Vietnam Dong

infants for the first 4 months. The children's age at the time of the present survey was 34–40 months.

Mothers were asked about the children's eating behavior in face-to-face interviews using the CEBQ, a multi-dimensional, parent-reported questionnaire [21]. This scale was applied after it had been translated from the original English into Vietnamese and then back-translated into English for validation. The CEBQ comprises 35 questions, scored on a 1–4 scale. The questions are divided into eight subscales, as follows, and the mean of each subscale was calculated: Satiety responsiveness, slowness in eating, fussiness, food responsiveness, enjoyment of food, desire to drink, emotional under-eating, and emotional over-eating. We summed the food responsiveness, enjoyment of food, desire to drink, and emotional over-eating scores to calculate the food approach (FAPP) score, and summed the satiety responsiveness, slowness in eating, fussiness, and emotional under-eating scores to calculate the food

avoidance (FAVD) score. Significant correlations were observed between each of the subscales and the score under which it was categorized, suggesting internal CEBQ consistency among the present subjects. Table 2 lists the means and standard deviation of the eight subscales and the FAPP and FAVD scores, stratified by sex. In general, the CEBQ scores in the present study were higher than those reported in two European studies [23, 24]. Because of different distributions, we transformed the scores into standardized z-scores prior to analysis, which allowed calculation of the probability of a score occurring within our normal distribution.

Informed consent to participate in the present study was obtained from all mothers. The Institutional Ethics Boards of Medical and Epidemiological Studies at Kanazawa Medical University and Vietnam Military Medical University approved the study design. The Department of Health and Prevention of Diseases of Da Nang City government reviewed and approved the informed consent process.

Statistical analysis

Statistical analysis was performed using SPSS ver. 11.0 for Windows (IBM SPSS, Armonk, NY, USA). Concentrations of PCDDs and PCDFs congeners and TEQ levels of PCDDs, PCDFs, and PCDDs/Fs in breast milk were used for analysis after base-10 logarithmical transformation to improve normality. A linear regression model was used to analyze the association between each CEBQ score (a response variable) and congener concentration and TEQ in breast milk (a predictor variable) after adjusting for the following covariates: Location (Thanh Khe or Son Tra), maternal age, parity, body mass index (BMI) during pregnancy, maternal education, family income, gestational weeks to delivery, and children's age at the time of the survey. Regression analysis was stratified by sex because we previously found that the effects of dioxin exposure on growth and neurodevelopment differed between boys and girls in this cohort [5–10]. Next, a general linear model was used to analyze the effects of sex and dioxin levels on CEBQ scores by two-way ANCOVA after adjusting for the same covariates.

Results

Tables 3 and 4 list the values calculated for the association between dioxin congener levels in breast milk and CEBQ scores in boys and girls aged 3 years, respectively. In boys, no significant association was found for TCDD or TEQ-PCDDs/Fs, although there were significant inverse associations of food responsiveness, enjoyment of food, and FAPP with 1,2,3,4,6,7,8,9-octachlorodibenzofuran, a PCDF isomer whose levels in breast milk were low (25.4% of samples were below the limit of detection; Table 1). Levels of 1,2,3,7,8,9-hexachlorodibenzofuran and 1,2,3,4,7,8,9-heptachlorodibenzofuran were also associated with enjoyment of food scores in boys (Table 3). Levels of 1,2,3,4,6,7,8,9-octachlorodibenzo-p-dioxin in boys were inversely associated with the fussiness score ($\beta = -0.225$, $p = 0.044$), suggesting a connection between this dioxin congener and decreased food avoidance behavior.

In girls, we found significant inverse associations between levels of TEQ-PCDFs and enjoyment of food scores, and between levels of TEQ-PCDFs and TEQ-PCDDs/Fs and desire to drink scores. Among PCDF isomers, two pentachlorodibenzofuran isomers with high TEFs and 1,2,3,6,7,8-hexachlorodibenzofuran were associated with lower enjoyment of food scores, and seven PCDF isomers were associated with lower desire to drink scores in girls (Table 4). In addition, four PCDD isomers had an inverse association with desire to drink scores, contributing to an association between TEQ-PCDDs/Fs and decreased desire to drink scores (Table 4). FAPP was not significantly associated with any dioxin TEQs or isomers in girls. No significant association was found between dioxins and scores of food-avoidance behaviors such as satiety responsiveness,

slowness in eating, fussiness, emotional under-eating, or FAVD in girls.

The findings suggested significant associations between exposure to dioxin, as indicated by TEQ-PCDF and/or TEQ-PCDD/F values, and enjoyment of food and desire to drink scores, with sex-specific differences. We therefore analyzed the effects of the two main factors, sex and dioxin type (low- and high-exposure groups; < and ≥ 75th percentile of TEQ-PCDF and TEQ-PCDD/F levels, respectively) on enjoyment of food and desire to drink scores using the general linear model after adjusting for covariates (Table 5). We found no significant effects of sex or TEQ-PCDD/F levels on enjoyment of food or desire to drink scores. TEQ-PCDF levels, however, were significantly associated with enjoyment of food scores (F[1173] = 6.983, $p = 0.009$), without a significant effect by sex. The adjusted mean enjoyment of food score was 3.8, significantly lower in the high-exposure TEQ-PCDF group than in the low-exposure group (4.1). The effect of TEQ-PCDFs on the desire to drink score was borderline significant (F[1173] = 2.927, $p = 0.089$), but interaction between sex and TEQ-PCDF levels was significant (F[1173] = 4.897, $P = 0.028$), with a lower adjusted mean in the high-exposure TEQ-PCDF group (2.8) than in the low-exposure group (3.5) in girls.

Discussion

Dioxin exposure and eating behavior in children aged 3 years

In the present study, high levels of TEQ-PCDFs and TEQ-PCDDs/Fs were associated with reduced food approach, but no association was found between eating behavior scores and levels of TCDD, the main congener in Agent Orange. In girls, high- and low-level exposures to TEQ-PCDDs/Fs were not associated with height, weight, or BMI (data not shown). BMI was not associated with CEBQ scores, and a decrease in positive eating score was not related to emaciation. In boys, while dioxin exposure was not related to eating behavior, BMI was positively associated with enjoyment of food scores and inversely correlated with satiety responsiveness scores, suggesting that eating behavior affects BMI.

In our previous study performed in the same cohort, we reported that perinatal exposure to TCDD was associated with an increase in autistic traits, particularly in boys [9]. Children with autism are known to eat a significantly narrower range of foods [11] and are more likely to exhibit fussy eating behavior [12] than typically developed children. The present findings suggest a possible alteration in eating behavior in boys with autistic traits exposed to high levels of TCDD, but we did not find an association between TCDD and CEBQ scores, although there were significant associations between the ASRS and slowness in eating and emotional under-eating scores. These unexpected findings

Table 3 Associations between dioxin levels and Children's Eating Behaviour Questionnaire scores in boys aged 3 years

	FR		EF		DD		EO		FAPP	
	Beta	(95% CI)	Beta	(95% CI)	Beta	(95% CI)	Beta	(95% CI)	Beta	(95% CI)
2,3,7,8-TetraCDD	0.063	(− 0.167, 0.292)	0.080	(− 0.154, 0.315)	0.047	(− 0.172, 0.266)	0.101	(− 0.126, 0.328)	0.101	(−0.125, 0.326)
1,2,3,7,8-PentaCDD	0.012	(− 0.204, 0.228)	− 0.156	(− 0.374, 0.063)	0.119	(− 0.085, 0.323)	0.061	(− 0.152, 0.274)	− 0.039	(− 0.250, 0.173)
1,2,3,4,7,8-HexaCDD	− 0.059	(− 0.288, 0.171)	− 0.186	(− 0.417, 0.046)	−0.006	(− 0.224, 0.213)	−0.002	(− 0.229, 0.225)	− 0.110	(− 0.335, 0.114)
1,2,3,6,7,8-HexaCDD	0.031	(− 0.183, 0.246)	−0.121	(− 0.339, 0.098)	0.012	(− 0.192, 0.217)	− 0.033	(− 0.179, 0.246)	− 0.023	(− 0.234, 0.189)
1,2,3,7,8,9-HexaCDD	0.011	(− 0.194, 0.217)	− 0.159	(− 0.366, 0.048)	0.092	(− 0.103, 0.287)	− 0.023	(− 0.226, 0.181)	− 0.068	(− 0.269, 0.134)
1,2,3,4,6,7,8-HeptaCDD	0.024	(−0.247, 0.199)	− 0.049	(− 0.277, 0.180)	−0.006	(− 0.219, 0.207)	− 0.151	(− 0.370, 0.068)	− 0.082	(− 0.301, 0.137)
OctaCDD	0.036	(−0.178, 0.250)	−0.003	(− 0.221, 0.216)	−0.029	(− 0.233, 0.174)	−0.080	(− 0.291, 0.131)	− 0.007	(− 0.217, 0.203)
2,3,7,8-TetraCDF	0.084	(−0.115, 0.283)	0.028	(−0.176, 0.231)	0.013	(−0.177, 0.203)	−0.044	(− 0.241, 0.153)	0.043	(− 0.152, 0.239)
1,2,3,7,8-PentaCDF	−0.008	(− 0.204, 0.189)	−0.118	(− 0.317, 0.081)	−0.003	(− 0.190, 0.184)	−0.124	(− 0.317, 0.069)	0.094	(− 0.286, 0.098)
2,3,4,7,8-PentaCDF	−0.030	(− 0.248, 0.189)	−0.152	(− 0.373, 0.069)	0.048	(− 0.159, 0.256)	0.028	(− 0.188, 0.244)	−0.071	(− 0.285, 0.143)
1,2,3,4,7,8-HexaCDF	−0.064	(− 0.263, 0.135)	−0.162	(− 0.363, 0.039)	− 0.007	(− 0.197, 0.182)	0.001	(− 0.198, 0.197)	− 0.103	(− 0.298, 0.091)
1,2,3,6,7,8-HexaCDF	− 0.067	(− 0.236, 0.163)	−0.158	(− 0.359, 0.043)	0.014	(− 0.176, 0.204)	0.018	(− 0.180, 0.215)	−0.081	(− 0.276, 0.115)
1,2,3,7,8,9-HexaCDF	0.053	(− 0.161, 0.266)	− 0.216	(− 0.431, − 0.002)*	0.015	(− 0.098, 0.308)	− 0.165	(− 0.374, 0.044)	− 0.115	(− 0.324, 0.094)
2,3,4,6,7,8-HexaCDF	− 0.158	(− 0.363, 0.048)	− 0.121	(− 0.332, 0.090)	− 0.013	(− 0.211, 0.185)	− 0.042	(− 0.248, 0.164)	− 0.151	(− 0.353, 0.051)
1,2,3,4,6,7,8-HeptaCDF	−0.079	(− 0.275, 0.118)	−0.180	(− 0.378, 0.018)	−0.040	(− 0.228, 0.147)	−0.044	(− 0.239, 0.150)	− 0.133	(− 0.325, 0.059)
1,2,3,4,7,8,9-HeptaCDF	−0.090	(− 0.281, 0.100)	− 0.204	(− 0.395, − 0.010)*	−0.044	(− 0.226, 0.138)	− 0.081	(− 0.270, 0.108)	− 0.161	(− 0.346, 0.024)
OctaCDF	− 0.250	(− 0.434, − 0.066)**	− 0.263	(− 0.451, − 0.080)**	−0.003	(− 0.185, 0.179)	− 0.151	(− 0.338, 0.035)	− 0.296	(− 0.474, − 0.120)**
TEQ-PCDDs	0.029	(− 0.197, 0.255)	− 0.126	(− 0.356, 0.104)	0.096	(− 0.118, 0.311)	0.067	(− 0.156, 0.291)	− 0.015	(− 0.237, 0.207)
TEQ-PCDFs	− 0.045	(− 0.252, 0.161)	− 0.166	(− 0.375, 0.043)	0.017	(− 0.180, 0.214)	0.012	(− 0.193, 0.217)	− 0.091	(− 0.293, 0.112)
TEQ-PCDDs/Fs	− 0.010	(− 0.232, 0.212)	− 0.159	(− 0.384, 0.066)	0.063	(− 0.148, 0.274)	0.040	(− 0.179, 0.260)	−0.059	(− 0.277, 0.159)

Beta: Standardized regression coefficient controlling the following covariates: Location, maternal age, parity, maternal body mass index, maternal education, family income, gestational weeks at birth, and children's age at the time of the survey
CDD chlorinated dibenzo-p-dioxin, CDF chlorinated dibenzofuran, CI confidence interval, DD desire to drink, EF enjoyment of food, EO emotional over-eating, FAPP food approach, FR food responsiveness, PCDD polychlorinated dibenzo-p-dioxin, PCDF polychlorinated dibenzofuran, TEQ toxic equivalency
The FAPP was calculated as FR + EF + DD + EO
*$p < 0.05$; **$p < 0.01$

may be explained by the report of Nadon and colleagues that children with autistic traits have fewer sensory processing problems than are frequently observed in autism spectrum disorder children with eating problems [25].

In the present study, TEQ-PCDFs of congeners with comparatively lower TEFs than PCDDs were associated with decreased CEBQ scores. Some high-chlorinated PCDD isomers with lower TEF values, such as hepta-chlorodibenzo-p-dioxin and octachlorodibenzo-p-dioxin, were associated with eating behaviors; this suggests that the mechanism altering eating behavior in these children may not be the toxicity of TCDD-like aryl hydrocarbon receptor agonists. A similar study in areas contaminated by PCDFs and high-chlorinated PCDD isomers in other countries than Vietnam would be required to validate the effects on eating behavior in young children.

Neurotoxic effects of dioxin exposure on appetite and taste preference in animals

We conducted the present study to assess whether dioxin exposure might alter eating behaviors in children. Animal studies have linked perinatal dioxin exposure with poor neurodevelopment. Pretreatment with TCDD was reported to completely block the effects of lesions in the ventromedial hypothalamus of the rat brain, leading to hypophagia and weight loss, suggesting that TCDD exposure affects neurological control of appetite [13]. Food intake has been reported to be regulated by a neuronal network in the limbic system of the rat brain, and involvement of GABAergic neurons in this network has been suggested to control feeding responses, both excitation and suppression, via bidirectional interactions [26]. Because low doses of TCDD have been shown to influence development of GABAergic neurons in the rat brain [27], perinatal dioxin exposure may affect GABAergic neurons in the brain network that control food intake and appetite in humans as well.

Previous studies have suggested that perinatal dioxin exposure affects taste preference in rats, particular in females. Perinatal TCDD and dioxin-like PCB exposure altered the expression of saccharin preference behavior in adult female rats [28]. Nishijo and colleagues reported that female pups exposed to TCDD during the perinatal period preferred the bitter taste of histidine and lysine solutions using a choice paradigm of six amino acid solutions [19].

Table 4 Associations between dioxin levels and Children's Eating Behaviour Questionnaire scores in girls aged 3 years

	FR		EF		DD		EO		FAPP	
	Beta	(95% CI)	Beta	(95% CI)	Beta	(95% CI)	Beta	(95% CI)	Beta	(95% CI)
2,3,7,8-TetraCDD	−0.220	(−0.458, 0.017)	−0.079	(−0.327, 0.168)	−0.012	(−0.249, 0.224)	0.016	(−0.230, 0.262)	−0.156	(−0.394, 0.082)
1,2,3,7,8-PentaCDD	−0.131	(−0.399, 0.138)	−0.219	(−0.490, 0.052)	−0.325	(−0.576, −0.074)*	−0.169	(−0.439, 0.101)	−0.251	(−0.512, 0.009)
1,2,3,4,7,8-HexaCDD	−0.002	(−0.268, 0.263)	−0.272	(−0.535, −0.010)*	−0.291	(−0.539, −0.043)*	−0.086	(−0.353, 0.181)	−0.166	(−0.426, 0.093)
1,2,3,6,7,8-HexaCDD	0.011	(−0.255, 0.277)	−0.246	(−0.510, 0.019)	−0.239	(−0.491, 0.013)	−0.085	(−0.353, 0.183)	−0.146	(−0.407, 0.115)
1,2,3,7,8,9-HexaCDD	−0.036	(−0.281, 0.210)	−0.293	(−0.533, −0.053)*	−0.311	(−0.537, −0.085)**	−0.078	(−0.325, 0.170)	−0.192	(−0.430, 0.047)
1,2,3,4,6,7,8-HeptaCDD	0.032	(−0.225, 0.289)	−0.274	(−0.528, −0.021)*	−0.316	(−0.554, −0.079)*	−0.052	(−0.312, 0.207)	−0.133	(−0.385, 0.119)
OctaCDD	0.053	(−0.189, 0.295)	−0.074	(−0.320, 0.172)	−0.188	(−0.419, 0.043)	−0.025	(−0.368, 0.118)	−0.059	(−0.298, 0.180)
2,3,7,8-TetraCDF	−0.097	(−0.351, 0.157)	−0.226	(−0.480, 0.028)	−0.186	(−0.429, 0.057)	0.178	(−0.076, 0.432)	−0.083	(−0.334, 0.169)
1,2,3,7,8-PentaCDF	0.170	(−0.064, 0.403)	−0.270	(−0.503, −0.037)*	−0.298	(−0.517, −0.080)*	0.190	(−0.045, 0.425)	0.055	(−0.179, 0.289)
2,3,4,7,8-PentaCDF	−0.059	(−0.327, 0.210)	−0.276	(−0.542, −0.01)*	−0.280	(−0.533, −0.028)*	−0.084	(−0.355, 0.187)	−0.200	(−0.462, 0.061)
1,2,3,4,7,8-HexaCDF	0.011	(−0.245, 0.267)	−0.248	(−0.502, 0.006)	−0.357	(−0.590, −0.124)**	−0.076	(−0.334, 0.181)	−0.143	(−0.394, 0.107)
1,2,3,6,7,8-HexaCDF	−0.007	(−0.261, 0.246)	−0.280	(−0.529, −0.031)*	−0.331	(−0.563, −0.098)**	−0.107	(−0.362, 0.148)	−0.182	(−0.429, 0.064)
1,2,3,7,8,9-HexaCDF	0.012	(−0.238, 0.263)	−0.224	(−0.474, 0.226)	−0.213	(−0.441, 0.036)	−0.011	(−0.264, 0.243)	−0.102	(−0.349, 0.144)
2,3,4,6,7,8-HexaCDF	0.029	(−0.228, 0.286)	−0.192	(−0.450, 0.066)	−0.276	(−0.516, −0.035)*	−0.127	(−0.385, 0.131)	−0.129	(−0.381, 0.123)
1,2,3,4,6,7,8-HeptaCDF	0.069	(−0.177, 0.314)	−0.223	(−0.468, 0.022)	−0.352	(−0.575, −0.128)**	−0.013	(−0.262, 0.236)	−0.071	(−0.314, 0.172)
1,2,3,4,7,8,9-HeptaCDF	0.076	(−0.175, 0.328)	−0.098	(−0.354, 0.158)	−0.292	(−0.527, −0.058)*	0.039	(−0.216, 0.293)	0.015	(−0.235, 0.264)
OctaCDF	0.005	(−0.215, 0.224)	0.016	(−0.208, 0.240)	−0.204	(−0.411, 0.004)	0.189	(−0.028, 0.406)	0.094	(−0.122, 0.309)
TEQ-PCDDs	−0.138	(−0.402, 0.126)	−0.182	(−0.450, 0.085)	−0.220	(−0.473, 0.032)	−0.109	(−0.376, 0.158)	−0.212	(−0.470, 0.046)
TEQ-PCDFs	−0.012	(−0.274, 0.249)	−0.276	(−0.533, −0.018)*	−0.331	(−0.572, −0.090)*	−0.080	(−0.343, 0.183)	−0.171	(−0.426, 0.084)
TEQ-PCDDs/Fs	−0.086	(−0.351, 0.179)	−0.237	(−0.502, 0.028)	−0.279	(−0.528, −0.030)*	−0.101	(−0.368, 0.167)	−0.204	(−0.463, 0.054)

Beta: Standardized regression coefficient controlling the following covariates: Location, maternal age, parity, maternal body mass index, maternal education, family income, gestational weeks at birth, and children's age at the time of the survey

CDD chlorinated dibenzo-p-dioxin, CDF chlorinated dibenzofuran, CI confidence interval, DD desire to drink, EF enjoyment of food, EO emotional over-eating, FAPP food approach, FR food responsiveness, PCDD polychlorinated dibenzo-p-dioxin, PCDF polychlorinated dibenzofuran, TEQ toxic equivalency

The FAPP was calculated as FR + EF + DD + EO

*$p < 0.05$; **$p < 0.01$

Sex-specific effects in humans

Growth restriction has been reported in infants with Yusho disease whose mothers ingested rice oil contaminated with PCDDs/Fs and PCBs during pregnancy, and particularly in boys [29]. In our previous follow-up studies of the same birth cohort [6–10], we also found adverse health effects of perinatal dioxin exposure on weight, and height, and head and abdominal circumferences, and neurodevelopment that were more pronounced in boys. A study in Dutch children aged 6–8 reported endocrine-disrupting effects of perinatal exposure to PCDDs/Fs and PCBs manifesting as more feminized play behavior in boys [30], suggesting a greater susceptibility to dioxin in males. In the present study of eating behaviors, however, a significant influence of perinatal dioxin exposure was found in girls.

In children, eating behaviors have been targeted in preventing obesity and over-eating. One study reported that boys were more inclined to have a post-meal snack than girls, a habit leading to weight gain [31]. A study of elementary school children in Japan found that boys were more interested in food and preferred fatty foods, and that food interest scores were associated with energy density, fat energy content, and saturated fatty acid scores [32]. A cohort study of 2-year-old children born at preterm found

that being female was associated with eating difficulties [33], while a study in 5-year-old American children concluded that parental pressure on girls to eat more was associated with the emergence of dietary restraint and emotional disinhibition, as well as with decreased responsiveness to internal hunger and satiety cues [34]. In addition, Nordin and colleagues found that in young Swedish adults, food rejection and aversion were more common in women [35]. These studies indicate that females are more inclined than males to develop aversion to foods, and further suggest that the 3-year-old girls in the present study may be susceptible to dioxin-induced effects on emotion-related food aversion. Longer follow-up periods would be required to elucidate the sex-specific effects of dioxin exposure on emotion-related eating and food preferences in this cohort.

Sources of dioxin contamination and prevention of health effects

We found that TEQ-PCDFs contributed more to increased FAPP scores in girls than TEQ-PCDDs, including TCDD. Our previous study of dioxin exposure sources indicated that PCDF levels may increase with increased intake of marine food sources such as shrimp and with longer

Table 5 Effects of sex and dioxin type on Children's Eating Behaviour Questionnaire (CEBQ) scores

CEBQ	Main effects and interaction	df	Mean SS	F-value	P-value
EF	Sex (Girls/Boys)	1	0.292	0.312	0.577
	TEQ-PCDDs/Fs (High/Low)	1	2.649	2.832	0.094
	Sex * TEQ-PCDDs/Fs	1	0.163	0.175	0.676
	Sex (Girls/Boys)	1	0.056	0.061	0.806
	TEQ-PCDFs (High/Low)	1	6.388	6.983	0.009
	Sex * TEQ-PCDFs	1	0.007	0.007	0.932
DD	Sex (Girls/Boys)	1	1.397	1.664	0.199
	TEQ-PCDDs/Fs (High/Low)	1	2.047	2.438	0.120
	Sex * TEQ-PCDDs/Fs	1	2.047	2.438	0.120
	Sex (Girls/Boys)	1	1.917	2.325	0.129
	TEQ-PCDFs (High/Low)	1	2.413	2.927	0.089
	Sex * TEQ-PCDFs	1	4.037	4.897	0.028

The general linear model was adjusted for the following covariates: Location, maternal age, parity, maternal body mass index, maternal education, family income, gestational weeks at birth, and children's age at the time of the survey
DD desire to drink, *df* degrees of freedom, *EF* enjoyment of food, *PCDD* polychlorinated dibenzo-*p*-dioxin, *PCDF* polychlorinated dibenzofuran, *SS* sum of squares, *TEQ* toxic equivalency
The cutoff value of TEQ-PCDFs for high- and low-exposure groups was 7.6 pg-TEQ/g lipid (75th percentile)
The cutoff value of TEQ-PCDDs/Fs for high- and low-exposure groups was 17.8 pg-TEQ/g lipid (75th percentile)

residency in contaminated areas [36]. Ongoing remediation of dioxin contamination in the former US airbases should be completed to decrease maternal dioxin body burdens leading to perinatal exposure.

Conclusion

Perinatal exposure to dioxin affected eating behavior in 3-year-old children and particularly in girls. Future research should clarify the effects of dioxins on emotional development that affects eating styles and behaviors, leading to health problems such as emaciation or obesity in later life.

Abbreviations
ASRS: Autism Spectrum Rating Scales; CEBQ: Children's Eating Behaviour Questionnaire; dl-PCBs: Dioxin-like polychlorinated biphenyls; FAPP: Food approach; FAVD: Food avoidance; PCDDs: Polychlorinated dibenzo-p-dioxins; PCDFs: Polychlorinated dibenzofurans; TCDD: 2,3,7,8-tetrachlorodibenzo-p-dioxin; TEF: Toxic equivalency factor; TEQ: Toxic equivalency

Acknowledgments
We thank all mother-and-child pairs for participating in this study. We are grateful to the doctors and nurses in the Health Department of Da Nang City government, Thanh Khe and Son Tra District Hospitals, and Commune Health Centers in the Thanh Khe and Son Tra districts, Da Nang City, for their collaboration. We also thank Dean Meyer, PhD, ELS from Edanz Group (https://www.edanzediting.co.jp/) for editing a draft of this manuscript.

Funding
Sources of funding for the research were Project Research from the JSPS Asian Core Program, the Japan Society for the promotion of science (Grant-in-Aid for Scientific Research (B), numbers 25305024 and 25290005), and a grant for collaboration research from Kanazawa Medical University (C-2014-2). The authors declare that these funding bodies had no role in the design of the study, collection, analysis, and interpretation of the data, or in writing the manuscript.

Authors' contributions
MN, THA and HN participated in the design and coordination of the study. NTNA, PTT, TNN, and HVL carried out the survey and collected the data. YM and HB performed the statistical analysis. NTNA, MN, and YN prepared the manuscript. All authors read and approved the final manuscript.

Consent for publication
The manuscript contains no individual person's information in any form.

Competing interests
The authors declare that they have no competing interests.

Author details
[1]Department of Public Health and Epidemiology, Kanazawa Medical University, 1-1, Daigaku, Uchinada, Ishikawa 920-0293, Japan. [2]Biomedical and Pharmaceutical Research Center, Vietnam Military Medical University, Ha Noi, Vietnam. [3]School of Nursing, Kanazawa Medical University, 1-1 Daigaku, Uchinada, Ishikawa 920-0293, Japan. [4]System Emotional Science, Graduate School of Medicine and Pharmaceutical Sciences, University of Toyama, 2630 Sugitani, Toyama 930-0194, Japan.

References
1. Dwernychunk LW. Dioxin hot spots in Vietnam. Chemosphere. 2005;60:998–9.
2. Schecter A, Hoang TQ, Päpke O, Tung KC, Constable JD. Agent Orange, dioxins, and other chemicals of concern in Vietnam: update 2006. J Occup Environ Med. 2006;48:408–13.
3. Mai TA, Doan TV, Tarradellas J, Felippe de Alencastro L, Grandjean D. Dioxin contamination in soils of southern Vietnam. Chemosphere. 2007;67:1802–7.
4. Hatfield Consultants and the Office of National Steering Committee 33. Comprehensive assessment of dioxin contamination in Da Nang airport, Vietnam: Environmental levels, human exposure and options for mitigating impacts, Final report. November 2009. http://www.hatfieldgroup.com/wpcontent/uploads/AgentOrangeReports/DANDI-II1450/Da%20Nang%202009%20Report.pdf
5. Tai PT, Nishijo M, Kido T, Nakagawa H, Maruzeni S, Anh NTN, et al. Dioxin concentrations in breast milk of Vietnamese nursing mothers: a survey four decades after the herbicide spraying. Environ Sci Technol. 2011;45:6625–32.
6. Nishijo M, Tai PT, Nakagawa H, Maruzeni S, Anh NTN, Luong HV, et al. Impact of perinatal dioxin exposure on infant growth: a cross-sectional and longitudinal studies in dioxin-contaminated areas in Vietnam. PLoS One. 2012;7:e4027.
7. Pham TT, Nishijo M, Nguyen TNA, Maruzeni S, Nakagawa H, Luong HV, et al. Dioxin exposure in breast milk and infant neurodevelopment in Vietnam. Occup Environ Med. 2013;70:656–62.
8. Pham TT, Nishijo M, Nguyen AT, Tran NN, Hoang VL, Tran AH, et al. Perinatal dioxin exposure and the neurodevelopment of Vietnamese toddlers at 1 year of age. Sci Total Environ. 2015;536:575–81.
9. Nishijo M, Tai PT, Nguyen TNA, Nghi TN, Nakagawa H, Luong HV, et al. 2,3,7,8-tetrachlorodibenzo-p-dioxin in breast milk increases autistic traits of 3-year-old children in Vietnam. Mol Psychiatry. 2014;19:1220–6.
10. Tai PTNM, Nghi TN, Nakagawa H, Van Luong H, Anh TH, Nishijo H. Effects of perinatal dioxin exposure on development of children during the first 3 years of life. J Pediatr. 2016;175:159–66.
11. Schreck KA, Williams K, Smith AF. A comparison of eating behaviors between children with and without autism. J Autism Dev Disord. 2004;34:433–8.
12. Martins Y, Young RL, Robson DC. Feeding and eating behaviors in children with autism and typically developing children. J Autism Dev Disord. 2008;38(10):1878–87.
13. Tuomisto JT, Pohjanvirta R, Unkila M, Tuomisto J. 2,3,7,8-Tetrachlorodibenzo-p-dioxin-induced anorexia and wasting syndrome in rats: aggravation after ventromedial hypothalamic lesion. Eur J Pharmacol. 1995;293:309–17.

14. Nguyen AT, Nishijo M, Hori E, Nguyen NM, Pham TT, Fukunaga K, et al. Influence of maternal exposure to 2,3,7,8-tetrachlorodibenzo-p-dioxin on socioemotional behaviors in offspring rats. Environ Health Insights. 2013;7:1–14.

15. Nguyen MN, Nishijo M, Nguyen AT, Bor A, Nakamura T, Hori E, et al. Effects of maternal exposure to 2,3,7,8-tetrachlorodibenzo-p-dioxin on parvalbumin- and calbindin-immunoreactive neurons in the limbic system and superior colliculus in rat offspring. Toxicology. 2013;314:125–34.

16. Bor A, Nishijo M, Nishimaru H, Nakamura T, Tran NN, Van Le Q, et al. Effects of high fat diet and perinatal dioxin exposure on development of body size and expression of platelet-derived growth factor receptor β in the rat brain. J Integr Neurosci. 2017;16:453–70.

17. Berridge KC, Ho CY, Richard JM, DiFeliceantonio AG. The tempted brain eats: pleasure and desire circuits in obesity and eating disorders. Brain Res. 2010;1350:43–64.

18. Shott ME, Cornier MA, Mittal VA, Pryor TL, Orr JM, Brown MS, Frank GK. Orbitofrontal cortex volume and brain reward response in obesity. Int J Obes. 2015;39:214–21.

19. Nishijo M, Tran NN, Hideaki N, Etsuro H, Kunio T, Takashi K, et al. Effects of perinatal 2,3,7,8-tetrachlorodibenzo-p-dioxin exposure on development of taste preference in rat offspring. J Addict Res Ther. 22014;5:173. https://doi.org/10.4172/2155-6105.1000173.

20. Hang NM, Saito M, Son LK. Technology selection – principles and progress – for dioxin hotspot remediation in Vietnam. In: The Office of National Steering Committee 33, editor. Proceedings for Vietnamese session in 33rd international symposium on halogenated persistent organic pollutants and POPs –DIOXIN 2013. Hanoi: Office 33; 2013. p.3–6.

21. Wardle J, Guthrie CA, Sanderson S, Rapoport L. Development of the Children's eating behavior questionnaire. J Child Psychol Psychiatry. 2001;42:963–70.

22. Van den Berg M, Birnbaum LS, Denison M, Vito MD, Farland W, Feeley M, et al. The 2005 World Health Organization reevaluation of human and mammalian toxic equivalency factors for dioxins and dioxin-like compounds. Toxicol Sci. 2006;93:223–41.

23. Viana V, Sinde S, Saton JC. Children's eating behavior questionnaire: associations with BMI in Portuguese children. Bri J Nutr. 2008;100:445–50.

24. Sleddens EFC, Kremers SPJ, Thijs C. The Children's eating behaviour questionnaire: factorial validity and association with body mass index in Dutch children aged 6–7. Int J Behav Nutr Phys Act. 2008;5:49.

25. Nadon G, Feldman DE, Dunn W, Gisel E. Association of sensory processing and eating problems in children with autism spectrum disorders. Autism Res Treat. 2011;2011:541926.

26. Miner P, Borkuhova Y, Shimonova L, Khaimov A, Bodnar RJ. GABA-A and GABA-B receptors mediate feeding elicited by the GABA-B agonist baclofen in the ventral tegamental area and nucleus accumbens shell in rats: reciprocal and regional interactions. Brain Res. 2010;1355:86–96.

27. Hays LE, Carpenter CD, Petersen SL. Evidence that GABAergic neurons in the preoptic area of the rat brain are targets of 2,3,7,8-tetrachlorodibenzo-p-dioxin during development. Environ Health Perspect. 2002;110:369–76.

28. Amin S, Moore RW, Peterson RE, Schantz SL. Gestational and lactational exposure to TCDD or coplanar PCBs alters adult expression of saccharin preference behavior in female rats. Neurotoxicol Teratol. 2000;22:675–82.

29. Tsukimori K, Uchin H, Mitoma C, Yasukawa F, Chiba T, et al. Marternal exposure to high levels of dioxins in relation to birth weight in women affected by Yusho disease. Environ Int. 2012;38:79–86.

30. Vreugdenhil HJI, Slijper FME, Mulder PGH, Weisglas-Kuperus N. Effects of perinatal exposure to PCBs and dioxins on play behavior in Dutch children at school age. Environ Health Perspect. 2002;110:A593–8.

31. Remy E, Issanchou S, Chabanet C, Boggio V, Nicklaus S. Impact of adiposity, age, sex and maternal feeding practices on eating in the absence of hunger and caloric compensation in preschool children. Int J Obes. 2015;39:925–30.

32. Kimura S, Endo Y, Minamimae K, Kanzaki S, Hanaki K. Gender differences in childhood food preference: evaluation using a subjective picture choice method. Pediatr Int. 2014;56:389–94.

33. Migraine A, Nicklaus S, Parnet P, Lange C, Monnery-Patris S, Des Robert C, Darmaum D, Flamant C, Amrger V, Roze JC. Effect of preterm birth and birth weight on eating behavior at 2 y of age. Am J Clin Nutr. 2013;97:1270–7.

34. Carper JL, Fisher JO, Birch LL. Young girls' emerging dietary restraint and disinhibition are related to parental control in child feeding. Appetite. 2000;35:121–9.

35. Nordin S, Broman DA, Garvill J, Nyroos M. Gender difference in factors affecting rejection of food in healthy young Swedish adults. Appetite. 2004;43:295–301.

36. Nguyen TNA, Nishijo M, Pham TT, Maruzeni S, Morikawa Y, Tran HA, et al. Maternal risk factors associated with increased dioxin concentrations in breast milk in a hot spot of dioxin contamination in Vietnam. J Expo Sci Environ Epidemiol. 2014;24:489–96.

11

Muscle and tendon morphology alterations in children and adolescents with mild forms of spastic cerebral palsy

Annika Kruse[1], Christian Schranz[2], Markus Tilp[1*] and Martin Svehlik[2]

Abstract

Background: Early detection of changes at the muscular level before a contracture develops is important to gain knowledge about the development of deformities in individuals with spasticity. However, little information is available about muscle morphology in children with spastic diplegic cerebral palsy (CP) without contracture or equinus gait. Therefore, the aim of this study was to compare the gastrocnemius medialis (GM) and Achilles tendon architecture of children and adolescents with spastic CP without contracture or equinus gait to that of typically developing (TD) children.

Methods: Two-dimensional ultrasonography was used to assess the morphological properties of the GM muscle and Achilles tendon in 10 children with spastic diplegic CP (Gross Motor Function Classification System level I–II) and 12 TD children (mean age 12.0 (2.8) and 11.3 (2.5) years, respectively). The children with CP were not restricted in the performance of daily tasks, and therefore had a high functional capacity. Mean muscle and tendon parameters were statistically compared (independent t-tests or Mann-Whitney U-tests).

Results: When normalized to lower leg length, muscle-tendon unit length and GM muscle belly length were found to be significantly shorter ($p < 0.05$, effect size (ES) = 1.00 and 0.98, respectively) in the children with spastic CP. Furthermore, there was a tendency for increased Achilles tendon length when expressed as a percentage of muscle-tendon unit length ($p = 0.08$, ES = − 0.80) in the individuals with CP. This group also showed shorter muscle fascicles (3.4 cm vs. 4.4 cm, $p < 0.01$, ES = 1.12) and increased fascicle pennation angle (21.9° vs. 18.1°, $p < 0.01$, ES = − 1.36, respectively). However, muscle thickness and Achilles tendon cross-sectional area did not differ between groups. Resting ankle joint angle was significantly more plantar flexed (− 26.2° vs. − 20.8°, $p < 0.05$, ES = 1.06) in the children with CP.

Conclusions: Morphological alterations of the plantar flexor muscle-tendon unit are also present in children and adolescents with mild forms of spastic CP. These alterations may contribute to functional deficits such as muscle weakness, and therefore have to be considered in the clinical decision-making process, as well as in the selection of therapeutic interventions.

Keywords: Gastrocnemius medialis, Achilles tendon, Diplegic, Ultrasonography, Muscle fascicle

* Correspondence: markus.tilp@uni-graz.at
[1]Institute of Sports Science, University of Graz, Mozartgasse 14, 8010 Graz, Austria
Full list of author information is available at the end of the article

Background

Cerebral palsy (CP) is a well-recognized, common neuro-developmental disorder in children that describes a "group of permanent disorders of the development of movement and posture, causing activity limitation, that are attributed to non-progressive disturbances that occurred in the developing fetal or infant brain" [1]. CP causes secondary alteration of the musculoskeletal system, e.g., muscle weakness, restricted joint range of motion, and increased joint stiffness [2]; however, the basic mechanisms that lead to these functional deficits are still not clearly understood [3].

Due to their important relation to the functional capacity, recent studies have concentrated on the examination of both the function and the properties of the muscles and tendons in individuals with CP. These studies have reported critical changes within the muscles that cannot be explained by neural changes alone [3]. Consequently, improving the understanding of the alterations in spastic skeletal muscles is of particular importance.

The force-generation capacity of a muscle is, among other things, dependent on its morphological and architectural properties [4], as well as the morphology and the behavior of the corresponding tendon [5, 6]. Since ultrasound (US) imaging is non-invasive, inexpensive, accurately controlled, and accessible in most clinical environments [7], it is often used to examine muscle and tendon properties at a macroscopic level (e.g., fascicle lengths). Recently, US imaging has also been applied to determine the structural alterations of the commonly affected plantar flexors in children with CP [8–15], whereby the gastrocnemius medialis (GM) has often been the muscle of interest due to its functional significance and easy accessibility with US because of both its superficiality and short fascicles [16]. In agreement with studies that have used magnetic resonance imaging [17–19], studies performed with US imaging have reported consistent evidence of reduced muscle size, indicated by, among other things, reduced muscle volume [8, 11, 20, 21], thickness [9, 13], and belly length [8, 11, 15] in children with CP. Some of these alterations, e.g., the reduced muscle volume, have been found in very young children (2 to 5 years of age) [21]. However, studies concerning GM fascicle lengths have delivered inconsistent results, reporting shorter muscle fascicle lengths [9, 14, 22, 23] or no differences [8, 10] in individuals with CP. Investigations of the corresponding fascicle pennation angle have reported no difference between children with CP and typically developing (TD) children [8, 23], as well as between the paretic and non-paretic legs of hemiplegic individuals [9]. The reported inconsistencies might be related to differences in the examination methods of the studies, as well as the high inter-subject variability in children with CP. Furthermore, due to differences in etiology and motor impairment in individuals with CP, the inclusion of individuals with different sub-types (hemiparetic, diparetic) and/or with differences in gross motor function [9, 21, 23, 24] might have hampered the interpretation of the study results.

To date, the Achilles tendon morphological properties have not received much attention, and only a few studies are available that demonstrated increased Achilles tendon length and reduced tendon cross-sectional area in individuals with CP [23, 24]. The functional meaning of these alterations is not clearly understood, but they are considered an adaptation to the altered muscle architecture, to improve function [6]. Nevertheless, these changes may also contribute to muscle weakness [25].

In summary, alterations of the whole GM muscle-tendon unit architecture have been observed in individuals with spastic CP. Most of the previous studies have included severely impaired individuals (Gross Motor Function Classification System level ≥ III) [13], i.e., individuals with plantar flexion contractures [10, 15] and/or equinus gait [14, 24]. However, less information is available about children with spastic CP who do not suffer from contracture or equinus gait. In this context, Barber et al. [21] found reduced muscle volume and physiological cross-sectional area in very young children with CP (aged 2 to 5 years) without contracture, whereby the longer fascicle length and smaller pennation angle differed only at maximum plantar flexion. Furthermore, Wren et al. [24] reported alterations of both the GM muscle and the Achilles tendon (shorter belly length and longer tendon length, respectively) in individuals (~ 8.5 years) without contracture but with dynamic equinus gait. However, it is not well known if and how severely muscle-tendon morphology is altered in children and adolescents with mild forms of spastic CP.

Therefore, the purpose of this study was to examine the GM muscle and Achilles tendon architecture in children with mild spastic CP without muscle contracture or equinus gait, using US imaging, and to compare them to a group of age-matched TD peers. Based on previous results [21, 24], we hypothesized that muscle belly length would be reduced and the Achilles tendon lengthened in this group of children with CP who are not restricted in the performance of daily tasks. Furthermore, we assumed that we would find shorter muscle fascicles [24], as well as reduced muscle thickness [9], in the impaired children, but no differences in the pennation angles between groups.

Methods

Participants

Ten children with spastic diplegic CP (8–16 years; 5 girls and 5 boys) and 12 age-matched TD peers (7 girls and 5 boys) participated in the study. Six of the CP children were graded as GMFCS level I and four as level II. The children had no contracture of the plantar flexors (maximal ankle dorsiflexion ≥5° with knees extended) and did not present with equinus gait nor knee flexion deformities.

The exclusion criteria were other forms of CP than spastic CP, any previous surgery to the plantar flexors, and botulinum toxin application in the last six months. The children included in the present study who had received botulinum toxin A treatment received it nine months or more (range 9 months to 8 years) before the participation. Moreover, five out of the 10 children with spastic CP were botulinum toxin naïve. There were no differences in anthropometric data, e.g., body mass, body height, and lower limb length, between groups (Table 1). All participants were personally informed beforehand about the measurement procedure and parental written consent was obtained. The study was approved by the local ethics committee.

Experimental protocol
All measurements were conducted by an experienced examiner. A standard US imaging system (MyLab60; Esaote S.p.A., Genova, Italy) was used for the image acquisition.

All measurements were made on the leg that demonstrated higher spasticity, as detected by clinical examination (Modified Ashworth scale) in the children with diplegic CP, and on the dominant leg of the TD children.

The lower limb length was first determined by the use of a measuring tape, defined as the distance from the malleolus lateralis to the epicondylus lateralis. For the further GM muscle-tendon unit length and architecture measurements, the children were asked to lie prone on an examination couch, with their feet hanging over the edge and knees fully extended (Fig. 1). US measurements

were repeated three times, and the average values were used for the further analysis.

Resting ankle joint angle determination
The resting ankle angle of each subject was measured by standard goniometry to further determine the Achilles tendon resting length. Therefore, one arm of the goniometer was kept parallel to the sole of the foot, and the other arm was kept in line with the line defined by the participant's malleolus lateralis and epicondylus lateralis. The resting ankle position was defined as the relaxed position of the foot, with no external force applied by the examiner [8].

Length measurements of the muscle-tendon unit
In order to determine the muscle-tendon unit, GM muscle belly, and Achilles tendon length at rest, 3 adhesive tape strips (Fig. 1) were placed on the skin close to predefined landmarks [26]: the most superficial aspect of the medial femoral condyle (Tape 1), the most prominent bulge of the GM (Tape 2), and the muscle-tendon junction of the GM and the Achilles tendon (Tape 3). A measuring tape was used to ascertain the distances between the calcaneus and each tape (distance calcaneus–tape). Subsequently, the US transducer was placed longitudinally over the respective landmarks, and images showing the landmark and the corresponding shadow of the tape in the US image (clearly visible due to its anechoic behavior, Fig. 2) were recorded. To determine the length measurements, a 10 cm linear-array probe (10 MHz; depth 74 mm; LA 923, Esaote, S.p.A) was used, and the focal depth was optimized to allow ease of identification of the structures [27].

Post-processing similar to the approach of Barber et al. [26] was performed by combining both the external

Table 1 Anthropometrics, ankle joint, and muscle-tendon parameters of children with cerebral palsy and typically developing peers

	CP (n = 10)	TD (n = 12)	Effect size
Age (years)	12.0 (2.8)	11.3 (2.5)	
Body mass (kg)	45.2 (19.1)	44.8 (15.5)	
Height (cm)	149.2 (21.2)	152.7 (16.5)	
Lower leg length (cm)	36.2 (6.0)	36.9 (5.3)	
Resting ankle joint angle (°)	−26.2 (5.7)*	−20.8 (4.5)	1.06
MTU length (normalized)[a]	1.06 (0.04)*	1.10 (0.04)	1.00
GM muscle belly length (normalized)[a]	0.53 (0.08)*	0.59 (0.04)	0.98
GM muscle belly length (% of MTU length)	50 (6)	54 (4)	0.80
Achilles tendon length (normalized)[a]	0.53 (0.06)	0.51 (0.05)	−0.37
Achilles tendon length (% of MTU length)	50 (6)	46 (4)	−0.80
Achilles tendon cross-sectional area (mm²)	44.5 (10.6)	52.3 (10.5)	0.74

Values are reported as mean (standard deviation). CP cerebral palsy; TD typically developing; MTU muscle-tendon unit; GM gastrocnemius medialis
[a]normalized to lower leg length
*significantly different from TD, p < .05

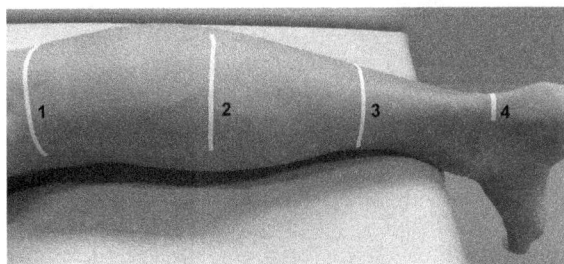

Fig. 1 Measurement setup for the calculation of gastrocnemius medialis muscle and Achilles tendon morphological properties. Numbers 1 and 3 on the lower leg indicate the tape strips used to calculate the muscle belly and tendon length, number 2 shows the tape strip placed as a visual aid to determine 50% of the muscle belly length, and number 4 indicates the tape strip that was utilized as a marker to assess the Achilles tendon cross-sectional area

tape measurements and the length information in the US images, determined by means of Tracker open-source software (version 4.91, http://physlets.org/tracker/). Firstly, the longitudinal distance between the respective landmark and the edge of the shadow of the tape in the US image (Fig. 2, distance) was added to the tape measurement. Secondly, the vertical distance between the upper boundary of the US image and the landmark (Fig. 2, depth) was used to calculate the linear distance from the landmark to the calcaneus with Pythagoras' theorem. With regard to the landmarks (Fig. 2a, b, lateral femoral condyle and muscle-tendon junction), the described procedure allowed us to calculate the muscle-tendon unit length and Achilles tendon length, respectively.

GM muscle belly length was in turn calculated by subtracting the Achilles tendon length from the muscle-

tendon unit length and, therefore, defined as the distance between the medial femoral epicondyle and the GM muscle-tendon junction. Image analysis was conducted for three images, resulting in 3 lengths for each parameter. The mean was defined as the muscle-tendon unit, GM belly, or Achilles tendon length, respectively. All lengths were normalized to lower leg length to account for any differences in body size [24]. Moreover, muscle belly and Achilles tendon length were further expressed as a percentage of muscle-tendon unit length [24].

Measurement of GM muscle architecture and morphology
GM muscle morphological properties were assessed at rest. US images were captured to determine fascicle length, pennation angle, and muscle thickness, whereby the US probe was aligned perpendicular to the deep aponeurosis in order to find the true fascicle plane [28]. Fascicle length (Fig. 3) was defined as the linear distance between the insertion into the deep and superficial aponeurosis [8]. In each of the 3 US images, 3 fascicles that were identifiable throughout their whole length were chosen [14] and manually measured by following their paths in a straight line. As a result, the mean value of 9 fascicles was defined as the subject's GM fascicle length. In contrast to previous studies [10], fascicles were visible over their whole length due to the size of the US probe (10 cm), which allowed direct length measurements without length calculation or use of an extrapolation method. Mean fascicle length was further normalized to the muscle-tendon unit and muscle belly length. The pennation angle (Fig. 3) was defined as the angle between the fascicle selected for length measurement and the deep aponeurosis [29], and was measured for each defined fascicle in each image. GM muscle thickness (Fig. 3) was measured at 50% of the muscle belly as the perpendicular distance between the deep and superficial aponeurosis [9]. In order to find the middle part of the GM muscle belly (50%), tape (Fig. 1) was used as a marker. The mean of 3 thickness values was used in the final analysis. The procedure applied to determine

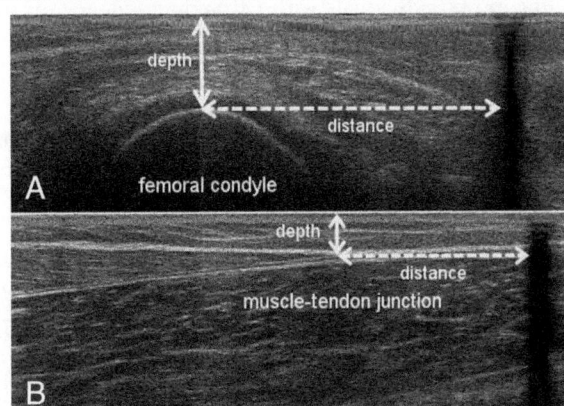

Fig. 2 Ultrasound images used to assess the GM muscle belly and Achilles tendon lengths, based on the US-tape method of Barber et al. 2011. The dashed lines show the distance from the superficial aspect of the condyle (**a**) and the most distal aspect of the muscle-tendon junction (**b**) to the tape (black shadow), whereby the white arrows indicate the US depth

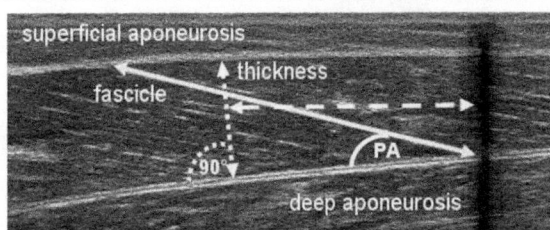

Fig. 3 Ultrasound image of the GM muscle showing determination of muscle thickness (dotted line), fascicle length (solid line), and pennation angle (PA). Muscle thickness was measured at 50% of the muscle belly length (dashed line) determined from the echo of the applied tape (black shadow on the right side)

muscle fascicle length, pennation angle, and muscle thickness has been reported to be highly reliable [9].

Measurement of the Achilles tendon cross-sectional area

To determine the Achilles tendon cross-sectional-area, transverse US images were recorded at the level of the medial malleolus. Therefore, the path from the tip of the malleolus to the tendon action line was quantified and a line was drawn (medio-lateral direction). Owing to the width of the footprint of the transducer (50 mm × 8 mm), a separate line was drawn 4 mm below the first and defined as the measurement position [30]. Similar to the muscle-tendon unit length measurements, an adhesive tape strip was fixed below the second line and used as the lower boundary to locate the selected measurement position (Fig. 1). To enhance the visibility of the tendon boundaries, a stand-off gel pad (SONOKIT soft 200 × 100 × 20 mm; SONOGEL, Bad Camberg, Germany) was placed between the skin surface and the US probe. In contrast to the length measurements, a shorter linear-array transducer (LA 523, Esaote, S.p.A; 10 MHz; 30 mm depth) was used.

The transverse US images of the Achilles tendon cross-sectional area were analyzed using ImageJ software (version 1.48v; National Institutes of Health, USA). The cross-sectional area was manually outlined, excluding the dense connective tissue of the tendon (Fig. 4), and subsequently calculated by the software. Three images were digitized, and the mean value was defined as the cross-sectional area. The mean coefficient of variation for repeated measures was 1.9% [30].

Statistical analysis

All the statistical analyses were performed using SPSS (version 22.0, SPSS Inc., Chicago, III). The level of significance was set to 0.05 for all the tests. Data are presented as means and standard deviations for each group, and independent t-tests were performed to test for differences between groups. Kolmogorov-Smirnov tests were used to test for normal distribution of the data. In the case of the data not being normally distributed, a non-parametric statistical test (Mann-Whitney U-test) was performed. Furthermore, effect sizes (ES, Cohen's d) were calculated, where 0.2 characterizes a small effect, 0.5 a medium effect, and 0.8 a large effect [31].

Results

The resting ankle joint was more plantar flexed (by ~ 5°) in the children with CP compared to the TD children (Table 1). When normalized to lower leg length, muscle-tendon unit length and GM muscle belly length were significantly shorter ($p = 0.02$, respectively) in the children with CP (Table 1). Furthermore, when expressed as a percentage of muscle-tendon unit length, there was a tendency for decreased muscle length and increased tendon length ($p = 0.08$, ES = 0.80 and – 0.80, respectively) in the CP group (Table 1).

GM muscle fascicles at rest were found to be significantly shorter in the children with CP compared to the TD group, in both absolute and normalized terms (ES = 1.12 and 1.42 respectively, Table 2). In addition, the CP group showed a significantly greater GM pennation angle (ES = – 1.36); however, GM muscle thickness did not differ between groups (ES = 0.00). Finally, no significant difference between the children with CP and the TD group could be found in the Achilles tendon cross-sectional area, although we did find a moderate effect (ES = 0.74, Table 1).

Discussion

In this study, we used US imaging to investigate the GM muscle architecture and Achilles tendon properties in 10 children and adolescents with spastic diplegic CP without contracture or equinus gait and 12 TD peers. We found shorter muscle-tendon unit and GM muscle belly lengths in the individuals with CP, and a tendency for increased Achilles tendon length. Furthermore, shorter GM muscle fascicle lengths and increased GM fascicle pennation angle were also present in the CP group.

Muscle architecture crucially determines the amount of force, maximum shortening velocity, excursion of the muscle, and the force that is transmitted to the tendon [32]. Therefore, alterations of these properties may contribute to the reduced force output in individuals with CP. In the present study, we found reduced GM muscle belly lengths in children and adolescents with spastic CP without contracture or equinus gait, which is in good agreement with previous studies in individuals with diplegic and hemiplegic CP [8, 10, 15, 22, 24]. Reduced muscle lengths are commonly thought to be caused by a reduction in muscle fascicle length [33]; however, other explanations, such as a decrease in the mean muscle fiber diameter and, therefore, a shortening of the aponeurosis, have also been put forward [8, 10].

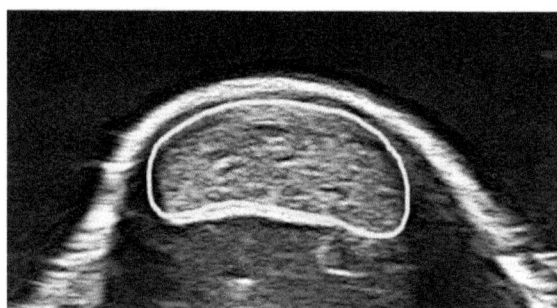

Fig. 4 Transverse US image showing the manually outlined Achilles tendon cross-sectional area (white shape)

Table 2 Muscle morphology of the gastrocnemius medialis in children with cerebral palsy and typically developing children

	CP	TD	Effect size
Fascicle length (cm)	3.4 (1.0)*	4.4 (0.8)	1.12
Fascicle length (normalized to MTU)	0.09 (0.02)**	0.11 (0.02)	1.31
Fascicle length (normalized to muscle belly length)	0.19 (0.04)	0.20 (0.03)	0.29
Pennation angle (°)	21.9 (2.9)**	18.1 (2.7)	−1.36
Muscle thickness (cm)	1.3 (0.4)	1.3 (0.2)	0.00

Values are reported in mean (standard deviation). *CP* cerebral palsy; *TD* typically developing; *MTU* muscle-tendon unit
*significantly different from TD, $p < .05$
**significantly different from TD, $p < .01$

Although fascicle length did not differ between the groups when normalized to muscle belly length, absolute values and lengths normalized to overall MTU were smaller in children with CP therefore confirm previous results [9, 14, 22, 23]. This indicates that reduced GM muscle belly lengths may be a result of reduced fascicle lengths in children with CP. It is widely believed that the reduced fascicle lengths in CP are a result of a loss of serial sarcomeres [19, 34], and studies have consistently shown that sarcomeres in muscles of individuals with CP are longer [35] compared to sarcomeres in normally developed fascicles. In combination with an increased pennation angle, these alterations at the fascicular level will greatly contribute to the decreased force production in children with CP [24, 35].

The determined muscle fascicle pennation angles in the present study were found to be significantly increased in the CP group (TD: 18.1°; CP: 21.9°). This finding is in contrast to other studies [8, 10, 21] that have reported no differences between groups or slightly smaller pennation angles in children with CP. Nevertheless, our finding is in good agreement with the observation of Gao et al. [23], who concluded that, from a geometrical point of view, the pennation angle would increase under similar muscle thickness if a muscle fascicle shortens. Therefore, increases in fascicle pennation angle in children with CP may be an adaptation to a reduction in muscle fascicle length. Our findings support this assumption. Furthermore, recent studies have shown consistent evidence that GM muscle fascicle lengths vary systematically with ankle position [10, 22, 23]. Therefore, we suppose that this increase in fascicle pennation angle may also be related to the more plantar flexed resting ankle joint angle that we found in the CP group. Furthermore, there are several aspects that may explain the different pennation angle values between studies: different measurement locations within the muscle [9], high inter-subject variability for a given age and increases of this angle as a function of age [36], and gender-specific variability of the muscle dimensions [37]. Therefore, a comparison of pennation angle values between studies should be conducted with care.

We further assessed muscle thickness as an approximation of muscle size, due to its high correlation with muscle cross-sectional area [37, 38]. Against our hypothesis, we did not find any difference in muscle thickness between the children with CP and the TD group, which is also in contrast to other studies [9]. However, in contrast to the study of Mohagheghi et al. [9], the analyzed children with CP in the present study were less impaired with regard to motor function, which might have prevented the individuals from showing significant muscle atrophy.

With regard to the Achilles tendon, we found only a tendency for an elongated tendon in children with CP without contracture. Furthermore, we found a smaller (14%) Achilles tendon cross-sectional area in the CP group, but this result was also not statistically significant. Both findings are in line with previous studies that reported significantly longer Achilles tendons [22–24, 39] and significantly smaller tendon cross-sectional areas [23, 39] in more severely impaired children with spastic CP. It has been postulated that a longer and thinner Achilles tendon might be advantageous for energy storage [6] during movement. Therefore, the reported alterations of the tendon may be an adaptation to the altered muscle architecture (e.g. shortening of fascicles) to ensure or keep its function, whereby these structural changes might have a negative influence on joint control and lead to a reduction in muscle force [25]. Nevertheless, the children and adolescents with diplegic CP without contracture or equinus gait showed only a tendency for altered Achilles tendon properties. This finding might be explained by the relatively high activity levels of these individuals, which in turn might have caused a sufficient load to preserve normal tendon structure.

Limitations

This study has several limitations that have to be considered when interpreting the results and/or comparing these results with other studies' outcomes. Firstly, botulinum toxin A treatment within the 6 months before the examination was an exclusion criterion in this study. However, we are aware of some evidence in the literature that botulinum toxin A can introduce structural muscle changes that might last even longer than 6 months [40]. However, research on this topic, especially on humans, is still scarce and the results are inconsistent [40]. Moreover, 5 children out of the 10 did not receive botulinum toxin treatment before the study (Table 3). Therefore, we expect that the observed changes are related to the effects of CP, rather than its treatment with botulinum toxin.

Another aspect that might raise some concerns is the matching of the groups. Despite the fact that we accounted for age, we did not match the groups for sex. Since Kawakami et al. [32] showed that muscle dimensions can vary with sex, we cannot say that this feature did not have an influence on the study outcomes, although the differences between groups were small (50% males vs. 42% females).

Furthermore, we have to note that conventional two-dimensional US imaging has several drawbacks (e.g., operator-dependency [7]), which have to be considered when interpreting the results. The limited dimensions of the transducer do not allow for accessing some important outcome measures such as muscle volume and/or the entire MTU [7]. Due to the fact that two-dimensional US imaging restricts the morphological measurements to one image plane and therefore involve error sources, it is necessary to strictly follow guidelines for the assessments of e.g. fascicle length [28] to increase the repeatability of the measurements. Despite the fact that the described limitations might be overcome by the use of new valid and reliable techniques (e.g. 3-dimensional freehand US imaging [41, 42]), their applicability for the clinical environment still has to be improved [7]. With regard to the procedures used in this study, we can report that all the assessments of muscle and tendon properties between the CP and TD groups were conducted in accordance, so that the possibly occurring errors were similar in both groups, and should therefore not affect the main outcomes of the study.

Additionally, we have to note that we performed the internal reliability analysis only for the assessment of the Achilles tendon cross-sectional area. Therefore, we cannot report on the reliability of the other outcome parameters, such as muscle fascicle length and pennation angle. However, previous studies have shown that the architectural properties of the GM muscle can be reliably assessed with the muscle in a relaxed state, and without formal training of the reviewer [43]. In this study, the measurements were performed by an investigator with two years of experience, and following the guidelines for US assessments [28]. Therefore, we have confidence in our results.

Clinical implications

Muscle architecture is a crucial determinant of muscle force-generating capacity and its excursion [4], whereby muscle fascicle length is the primary determinant of muscle excursion, with shorter muscle fascicles having a reduced range through which they can develop force and power [4]. Furthermore, there is consistent evidence of reduced muscle size, as indicated by reduced muscle volume as well as muscle belly length, in the comparisons between spastic CP and typically developed muscles [e.g. 8, 11, 15, 17, 21]. These architectural features affect the muscle function and contribute to functional deficits such as plantar flexor weakness in individuals with CP. Therefore, to understand the changes in the architecture of spastic muscles is crucial information for planning treatment modalities such as stretching, orthotic management, or even surgery. Our study showed that muscle and tendon morphology is altered even in children with CP without muscle contracture and who are not restricted in their performance of daily tasks. These results may suggest that individuals with mild forms of CP are also at risk of developing contractures. Additionally, such individuals should also be included in interventional studies designed to counteract muscle weakness. Since alterations in GM muscle and Achilles tendon properties could be observed, we further suggest investigating the effects of treatments at both functional and musculo-tendinous levels.

Conclusion

In conclusion, our findings show that architectural and morphological alterations of the GM muscle-tendon unit can also be found in children and adolescents with spastic diplegic CP without contracture or equinus gait. Therefore, we can confirm the previous results in younger individuals and children with CP without contracture but with equinus gait [21, 24]. Beyond the alterations reported for very young children without contracture [21], our findings may implicate deterioration of muscle alteration with growth, even in those children with mild CP.

Table 3 Previous botulinum toxin application (number, past months before study participation) in the medial gastrocnemius in the study participants with mild spastic CP

Subject	Number of injections	Months past from last injection
1	none	–
2	7	9
3	none	–
4	1	9
5	none	–
6	2	96
7	none	–
8	none	–
9	4	72
10	1	84

As morphological properties are the main determinants of function, the observed alterations in muscle and tendon may contribute to functional deficits such as plantar flexor weakness. Reduced GM muscle fascicle lengths and increased fascicle pennation angles in individuals with CP may explain the decreased muscle belly length, as well as elongation of the Achilles tendon. The findings reported in the present study indicate the need to monitor the progression of muscle contracture.

Abbreviations

CP: Cerebral palsy; ES: Effect size; GM: Gastrocnemius medialis; GMFCS: Gross Motor Function Classification System; MTU: Muscle-tendon unit; SPSS: Statistical Package for Social Sciences; TD: Typically developing; US: Ultrasound

Authors' contributions

MS contributed to the design of the study and recruited the study participants. MT contributed to the study design, supervised the data collection, and interpreted the muscle and tendon data, together with MS and AK. AK contributed to the study design, collected the muscle and tendon data, and was responsible for the analysis and interpretation of the outcomes. AK was also a major contributor in the writing of the manuscript. CS contributed to the design of the study, the recruitment of the participants, and the data collection. All authors read and approved the final manuscript.

Competing interests

The authors declare that they have no competing interests.

Author details

[1]Institute of Sports Science, University of Graz, Mozartgasse 14, 8010 Graz, Austria. [2]Department of Paediatric Surgery, Medical University of Graz, Auenbruggerplatz 34, 8036 Graz, Austria.

References

1. Rosenbaum P, Paneth N, Leviton A, Goldstein M, Bax M, Damiano D, et al. A report: the definition and classification of cerebral palsy April 2006. Dev Med Child Neurol. 2007;109:8–14.
2. Barber L, Barrett R, Lichtwark G. Passive muscle mechanical properties of the medial gastrocnemius in young adults with spastic cerebral palsy. J Biomech. 2011;44:2496–500. https://doi.org/10.1016/j.jbiomech.2011.06.008.
3. Lieber RL, Steinman S, Barash IA, Chambers H. Structural and functional changes in spastic skeletal muscle. Muscle Nerve. 2004;29:615–27. https://doi.org/10.1002/mus.20059.
4. Lieber RL, Friden J. Functional and clinical significance of skeletal muscle architecture. Muscle Nerve. 2000;23:1647–66.
5. Lichtwark GA, Wilson AM. Is Achilles tendon compliance optimised for maximum muscle efficiency during locomotion? J Biomech. 2007;40:1768–75. https://doi.org/10.1016/j.jbiomech.2006.07.025.
6. Magnusson SP, Hansen P, Kjaer M. Tendon properties in relation to muscular activity and physical training. Scand J Med Sci Sports. 2003;13:211–23.
7. Cenni F, Schless S-H, Bar-On L, Molenaers G, van Campenhout A, Aertbelien E, et al. Can in vivo medial gastrocnemius muscle-tendon unit lengths be reliably estimated by two ultrasonography methods? A within-session analysis. Ultrasound Med Biol. 2018;44:110–8. https://doi.org/10.1016/j.ultrasmedbio.2017.09.018.
8. Malaiya R, McNee AE, Fry NR, Eve LC, Gough M, Shortland AP. The morphology of the medial gastrocnemius in typically developing children and children with spastic hemiplegic cerebral palsy. J Electromyogr Kinesiol. 2007;17:657–63. https://doi.org/10.1016/j.jelekin.2007.02.009.
9. Mohagheghi AA, Khan T, Meadows TH, Giannikas K, Baltzopoulos V, Maganaris CN. Differences in gastrocnemius muscle architecture between the paretic and non-paretic legs in children with hemiplegic cerebral palsy. Clin Biomech. 2007;22:718–24. https://doi.org/10.1016/j.clinbiomech.2007.03.004.
10. Shortland AP, Harris CA, Gough M, Robinson RO. Architecture of the medial gastrocnemius in children with spastic diplegia. Dev Med Child Neurol. 2002;44:158–63.
11. Fry NR, Gough M, McNee AE, Shortland AP. Changes in the volume and length of the medial gastrocnemius after surgical recession in children with spastic diplegic cerebral palsy. J Pediatr Orthop. 2007;27:769–74. https://doi.org/10.1097/BPO.0b013e3181558943.
12. Shortland AP, Fry NR, Eve LC, Gough M. Changes to medial gastrocnemius architecture after surgical intervention in spastic diplegia. Dev Med Child Neurol. 2004;46:667–73.
13. Ohata K, Tsuboyama T, Haruta T, Ichihashi N, Nakamura T. Longitudinal change in muscle and fat thickness in children and adolescents with cerebral palsy. Dev Med Child Neurol. 2009;51:943–8. https://doi.org/10.1111/j.1469-8749.2009.03342.x.
14. Mohagheghi AA, Khan T, Meadows TH, Giannikas K, Baltzopoulos V, Maganaris CN. In vivo gastrocnemius muscle fascicle length in children with and without diplegic cerebral palsy. Dev Med Child Neurol. 2008;50:44–50. https://doi.org/10.1111/j.1469-8749.2007.02008.x.
15. Fry NR, Gough M, Shortland AP. Three-dimensional realisation of muscle morphology and architecture using ultrasound. Gait Posture. 2004;20:177–82. https://doi.org/10.1016/j.gaitpost.2003.08.010.
16. Barrett RS, Lichtwark GA. Gross muscle morphology and structure in spastic cerebral palsy: a systematic review. Dev Med Child Neurol. 2010;52:794–804. https://doi.org/10.1111/j.1469-8749.2010.03686.x.
17. Noble JJ, Fry NR, Lewis AP, Keevil SF, Gough M, Shortland AP. Lower limb muscle volumes in bilateral spastic cerebral palsy. Brain and Development. 2014;36:294–300. https://doi.org/10.1016/j.braindev.2013.05.008.
18. Elder GCB, Kirk J, Stewart G, Cook K, Weir D, Marshall A, Leahey L. Contributing factors to muscle weakness in children with cerebral palsy. Dev Med Child Neurol. 2003;45:542–50.
19. Oberhofer K, Stott NS, Mithraratne K, Anderson IA. Subject-specific modelling of lower limb muscles in children with cerebral palsy. Clin Biomech. 2010;25:88–94. https://doi.org/10.1016/j.clinbiomech.2009.09.007.
20. Shortland A. Muscle deficits in cerebral palsy and early loss of mobility: can we learn something from our elders? Dev Med Child Neurol. 2009;51(Suppl 4):59–63. https://doi.org/10.1111/j.1469-8749.2009.03434.x.
21. Barber L, Hastings-Ison T, Baker R, Barrett R, Lichtwark G. Medial gastrocnemius muscle volume and fascicle length in children aged 2 to 5 years with cerebral palsy. Dev Med Child Neurol. 2011;53:543–8. https://doi.org/10.1111/j.1469-8749.2011.03913.x.
22. Cheatwood AP, Rethlefsen SA, Kay RM, Wren TA. Changes in medial architecture with spasticity and contracture. Proceedings of the 52nd Annual Meeting of the Orthopaedic Research Society. Chicago; 2006.
23. Gao F, Zhao H, Gaebler-Spira D, Zhang LQ. In vivo evaluations of morphologic changes of gastrocnemius muscle fascicles and Achilles tendon in children with cerebral palsy. Am J Phys Med Rehabil. 2011;90: 364–71. https://doi.org/10.1097/PHM.0b013e318214f699.
24. Wren TA, Cheatwood AP, Rethlefsen SA, Hara R, Perez FJ, Kay RM. Achilles tendon length and medial gastrocnemius architecture in children with cerebral palsy and equinus gait. J Pediatr Orthop. 2010;30:479–84. https://doi.org/10.1097/BPO.0b013e3181e00c80.
25. Maganaris CN, Narici MV, Maffulli N. Biomechanics of the Achilles tendon. Disabil Rehabil. 2008;30:1542–7. https://doi.org/10.1080/09638280701785494.
26. Barber L, Barrett R, Lichtwark G. Validity and reliability of a simple ultrasound approach to measure medial gastrocnemius muscle length. J Anat. 2011; 218:637–42. https://doi.org/10.1111/j.1469-7580.2011.01365.x.
27. Barber L, Barrett R, Lichtwark G. Validation of a freehand 3D ultrasound system for morphological measures of the medial gastrocnemius muscle. J Biomech. 2009;42:1313–9. https://doi.org/10.1016/j.jbiomech.2009.03.005.
28. Benard MR, Becher JG, Harlaar J, Huijing PA, Jaspers RT. Anatomical information is needed in ultrasound imaging of muscle to avoid potentially substantial errors in measurement of muscle geometry. Muscle Nerve. 2009; 39:652–65. https://doi.org/10.1002/mus.21287.
29. Zhao H, Wu YN, Hwang M, Ren Y, Gao F, Gaebler-Spira D, Zhang LQ. Changes of calf muscle-tendon biomechanical properties induced by

passive-stretching and active-movement training in children with cerebral palsy. J Appl Physiol. 2011;111:435–42. https://doi.org/10.1152/japplphysiol. 01361.2010.

30. Kruse A, Stafilidis S, Tilp M. Ultrasound and magnetic resonance imaging are not interchangeable to assess the Achilles tendon cross-sectional-area. Eur J Appl Physiol. 2017;117:73–82. https://doi.org/10.1007/s00421-016-3500-1.

31. Cohen J. Statistical power analysis for the Behavioural sciences. 2nd ed. Hillsdale: Erlbaum Associates; 1988.

32. Moreau NG, Simpson KN, Teefey SA, Damiano DL. Muscle architecture predicts maximum strength and is related to activity levels in cerebral palsy. Phys Ther. 2010;90:1619–30. https://doi.org/10.2522/ptj.20090377.

33. O'Dwyer NJ, Neilson PD, Nash J. Mechanisms of muscle growth related to muscle contracture in cerebral palsy. Dev Med Child Neurol. 1989;31:543–7.

34. Matthiasdottir S, Hahn M, Yaraskavitch M, Herzog W. Muscle and fascicle excursion in children with cerebral palsy. Clin Biomech. 2014;29:458–62. https://doi.org/10.1016/j.clinbiomech.2014.01.002.

35. Mathewson MA, Lieber RL. Pathophysiology of muscle contractures in cerebral palsy. Phys Med Rehabil Clin N Am. 2015;26:57–67. https://doi.org/ 10.1016/j.pmr.2014.09.005.

36. Binzoni T, Bianchi S, Hanquinet S, Kaelin A, Sayegh Y, Dumont M, Jequier S. Human gastrocnemius medialis pennation angle as a function of age: from newborn to the elderly. J Physiol Anthropol Appl Hum Sci. 2001;20:293–8.

37. Kawakami Y, Abe T, Kanehisa H, Fukunaga T. Human skeletal muscle size and architecture: variability and interdependence. Am J Hum Biol. 2006;18: 845–8. https://doi.org/10.1002/ajhb.20561.

38. Bandholm T, Magnusson P, Jensen BR, Sonne-Holm S. Dorsiflexor muscle-group thickness in children with cerebral palsy: relation to cross-sectional area. NeuroRehabilitation. 2009;24:299–306. https://doi.org/10.3233/ NRE-2009-0482.

39. Theis N, Mohagheghi AA, Korff T. Mechanical and material properties of the plantarflexor muscles and Achilles tendon in children with spastic cerebral palsy and typically developing children. J Biomech. 2016;49:3004–8. https:// doi.org/10.1016/j.jbiomech.2016.07.020.

40. Mathevon L, Michel F, Decavel P, Fernandez B, Parratte B, Calmels P. Muscle structure and stiffness assessment after botulinum toxin type a injection. A systematic review. Ann Phys Rehabil Med. 2015;58:343–50. https://doi.org/ 10.1016/j.rehab.2015.06.002.

41. Cenni F, Schless S-H, Bar-On L, Aertbelien E, Bruyninckx H, Hanssen B, Desloovere K. Reliability of a clinical 3D freehand ultrasound technique: analyses on healthy and pathological muscles. Comput Methods Prog Biomed. 2018;156:97–103. https://doi.org/10.1016/j.cmpb.2017.12.023.

42. Barber LA, Read F, Lovatt Stern J, Lichtwark G, Boyd RN. Medial gastrocnemius muscle volume in ambulant children with unilateral and bilateral cerebral palsy aged 2 to 9 years. Dev Med Child Neurol. 2016;58: 1146–52. https://doi.org/10.1111/dmcn.13132.

43. Kwah LK, Pinto RZ, Diong J, Herbert RD. Reliability and validity of ultrasound measurements of muscle fascicle length and pennation in humans: a systematic review. J Appl Physiol. 2013;114:761–9. https://doi.org/10.1152/ japplphysiol.01430.2011.

12

The power of practice: simulation training improving the quality of neonatal resuscitation skills in Bihar, India

Brennan Vail[1]*[iD], Melissa C. Morgan[1,2,3], Hilary Spindler[3], Amelia Christmas[4], Susanna R. Cohen[5] and Dilys M. Walker[3,6,7]

Abstract

Background: Globally, neonatal mortality accounts for nearly half of under-five mortality, and intrapartum related events are a leading cause. Despite the rise in neonatal resuscitation (NR) training programs in low- and middle-income countries, their impact on the quality of NR skills amongst providers with limited formal medical education, particularly those working in rural primary health centers (PHCs), remains incompletely understood.

Methods: This study evaluates the impact of PRONTO International simulation training on the quality of NR skills in simulated resuscitations and live deliveries in rural PHCs throughout Bihar, India. Further, it explores barriers to performance of key NR skills. PRONTO training was conducted within CARE India's AMANAT intervention, a maternal and child health quality improvement project. Performance in simulations was evaluated using video-recorded assessment simulations at weeks 4 and 8 of training. Performance in live deliveries was evaluated in real time using a mobile-phone application. Barriers were explored through semi-structured interviews with simulation facilitators.

Results: In total, 1342 nurses participated in PRONTO training and 226 NR assessment simulations were matched by PHC and evaluated. From week 4 to 8 of training, proper neck extension, positive pressure ventilation (PPV) with chest rise, and assessment of heart rate increased by 14%, 19%, and 12% respectively (all $p \leq 0.01$). No difference was noted in stimulation, suction, proper PPV rate, or time to completion of key steps. In 252 live deliveries, identification of non-vigorous neonates, use of suction, and use of PPV increased by 21%, 25%, and 23% respectively (all $p < 0.01$) between weeks 1–3 and 4–8. Eighteen interviews revealed individual, logistical, and cultural barriers to key NR skills.

Conclusion: PRONTO simulation training had a positive impact on the quality of key skills in simulated and live resuscitations throughout Bihar. Nevertheless, there is need for ongoing improvement that will likely require both further clinical training and addressing barriers that go beyond the scope of such training. In settings where clinical outcome data is unreliable, data triangulation, the process of synthesizing multiple data sources to generate a better-informed evaluation, offers a powerful tool for guiding this process.

Keywords: Neonatal resuscitation, Bihar, India, Simulation Training, Barriers to Care

* Correspondence: brennan.vail@ucsf.edu
[1]Department of Pediatrics, University of California San Francisco, 550 16th Street, 4th Floor, Box 0110, San Francisco, CA 94158, USA
Full list of author information is available at the end of the article

Background

In 2016, 43% of deaths in children under age five globally occurred during the neonatal period [1]. In India, neonatal deaths accounted for 56% under-five deaths [1] and over half of these deaths occurred in only four states: Bihar, Uttar Pradesh, Madhya Pradesh, and Rajasthan [2]. Bihar is a state in eastern India with the highest rural birth rate in the country [3] and the highest multidimensional poverty index in all of South Asia [4]. Nearly one-third of neonatal deaths in Bihar are due to intrapartum related events [5], and yet providers are not adequately trained to perform basic neonatal resuscitation (NR) [6, 7]. Approximately 10% of neonates require tactile stimulation to transition at the time of birth and 3–6% require positive pressure ventilation (PPV) [8]. It is estimated that the effective provision of basic NR could save over 60,000 infants in India alone annually [9].

Although, there are many NR training programs in low- and middle-income countries (LMICs) [10], very few studies have evaluated the impact of such programs on the quality of clinical skills amongst providers with limited formal medical education in rural community settings. One small study evaluating the skills of community health workers in Bangladesh found improvement in initial resuscitation practices (drying, tactile stimulation), neck extension, and mouth-to-mouth ventilation with training, though no statistical analysis was provided [11]. More studies have focused on providers at referral hospitals [12–18]. Results from these studies are variable, with some demonstrating improvements in initial resuscitation [12, 15, 17, 18] and PPV skills [12–17], while others showed no change in initial resuscitation skills [14] or time to initiation of PPV [12, 15]. Several studies assessed skills at one time point and thus could not sufficiently determine the impact of training [19–23]. Others reported only a composite evaluation of skills [24–28], which is less relevant for NR, where outcomes depend on adequate performance of initial steps before proceeding to more complex ones.

This study offers a unique large-scale evaluation of an eight week, in-situ NR training program developed by PRONTO International [29] and implemented in rural primary health centers (PHCs) across Bihar with providers with limited formal medical education. PRONTO training was conducted within a larger maternal and child health quality improvement project called *Apatkaleen Matritva evam Navjat Tatparta* (AMANAT) [30–32]. The specific objectives of this study were 1) to evaluate the impact of PRONTO training on the quality of NR skills in simulated resuscitations; 2) to evaluate the impact of PRONTO training on performance in live deliveries requiring resuscitation of a non-vigorous infant; and 3) to explore obstacles to performance of specific evidence-based practices (EBP) in NR in Bihar.

Methods

Study design and setting

This study employed a mixed methods approach to evaluate the impact of PRONTO training on the quality of NR skills. Quantitative methods were used for the first two objectives and qualitative methods were used for the third objective. The portion of PRONTO simulation training evaluated in this manuscript was conducted at PHCs, where the majority of labor and delivery care in Bihar is provided. Each PHC serves a predominately rural population of ~ 190,000 individuals (number based on monitoring and evaluation data from CARE India [30]). PHCs provide largely preventative health care with limited curative services [33]. The vast majority of obstetric and neonatal care at PHCs is provided by nurses with an Auxiliary Nurse Midwife (ANM) or General Nursing and Midwifery (GNM) qualification, which require 2 and 3.5 years of training after completion of secondary school, respectively [34]. PHCs frequently face staffing shortages, often having only one nurse on duty in the labor room at any given time [33]. PHCs are not staffed with specialists, including pediatricians [33], and, in general, doctors are unavailable to assist in the labor room. Caesarian sections and instrumented deliveries are only performed at higher levels of care and thus require referral out of PHCs [33].

AMANAT and PRONTO interventions

AMANAT is multi-faceted quality improvement project, implemented by CARE India [30] in collaboration with the Government of Bihar, which seeks to improve maternal and child health outcomes in the state using a mentorship model of education [30–32]. AMANAT mentors are nurses with a Bachelor's degree in nursing recruited from across India. Mentees are ANMs and GNMs employed at PHCs.

PRONTO International training consists of in-situ simulations of a variety of neonatal and obstetric emergencies, which are supplemented by teamwork and communication activities, skills stations, and case-based learning [29]. Within AMANAT, PRONTO was responsible for training mentors to teach mentees emergency obstetric and neonatal care. Doctors were not included in the PRONTO training at PHCs as they were not part of the larger AMANAT program at PHCs and were infrequently involved in labor and delivery care in these facilities. Using a train-the-trainer model, PRONTO provided six days of training for mentors on simulation facilitation, team building, communication skills, and debriefing skills before mentoring began, and a four-day refresher training three months into the mentoring period. Over each 8-month phase, mentor pairs rotated between four PHCs, spending one week per month at each PHC conducting simulations. On average, seven NR simulations were conducted at each PHC over the 8 month training cycle.

In the PRONTO curriculum, normal spontaneous vaginal delivery (NSVD) simulations were introduced in week 2 and NR and postpartum hemorrhage (PPH) simulations were introduced in week 3 of training. Notably, bedside mentoring often began earlier, as mentors attended live deliveries during teaching hours with mentees to provide real-time instruction on any complications that arose. Formal assessment simulations were conducted for NSVD, PPH, and NR at weeks 4 and 8 of training. Pre-training assessments were not conducted, providing mentees time to adjust to simulation prior to being evaluated. NR simulations were conducted with the NeoNatalie™ [35] mannequin in situ in the labor rooms where mentees worked. All simulations were video-recorded to enable video-assisted debriefing as well as for programmatic evaluation.

Study population

ANMs/GNMs with labor room duties and interest in the mentoring program were selected for participation as mentees in AMANAT and PRONTO training. This analysis evaluates the clinical NR skills of mentees in both real and simulated deliveries in phases 2 and 3 of AMANAT mentoring conducted between September 2015 and July 2016. During this period, approximately 88% of mentees were ANMs and 12% were GNMs.

Interview participants were mentors who served as simulation facilitators. Twenty mentors, one from each phase 4 mentor pair, were selected for interviews in January 2017 based on the following criteria: 1) mentor was currently employed by AMANAT at the time of interview, and 2) mentor had worked in ≥2 phases of AMANAT (equivalent to 16 months in 8 different PHCs). Two interviewees were unable to participate due to illness and personal travel.

Study procedures
Mentee performance in simulated resuscitations
Evaluation of the quality of mentees' NR skills in simulated resuscitations was based on video-recorded assessment simulations from weeks 4 and 8 of training. At each PHC, mentees were selected by random lottery to participate in the NR assessment simulation for a given week. Assessments were announced but the lottery was conducted immediately prior to simulations. The simulated scenario began with a neonate found apneic while breastfeeding 15 min after birth, progressing to require suctioning, stimulation, and PPV. This simulation was chosen by mentors in place of a simulation beginning with a birth as it involved less set up and was thus easier

to facilitate in high volume PHCs. Additionally, it allowed mentees to focus only on NR during the assessment rather than progressing from NSVD management to NR. Assessment videos were transferred to encrypted USB drives and transported to Patna, the capital of Bihar, where they were uploaded to an encrypted server and transferred to University of California San Francisco (UCSF). Videos were then coded by one of the lead investigators with pediatric clinical experience for pre-defined NR quality indicators selected by a team of clinical and simulation experts at UCSF and the University of Utah. The coder was blinded to time of assessment (week 4 vs. 8 of training). After the completion of coding, indicators least likely to be subject to bias due to simulation artifact were selected for inclusion in the analysis. Variable definitions are provided in Table 1.

Mentee performance in live resuscitations
Mentors attended births occurring in the PHCs during daytime working hours from Monday through Saturday. Mentors were asked to assess mentees' skills immediately after observed live deliveries using a smart phone application based on the OpenDataKit platform [36]. The application asked mentors to subjectively evaluate specific NR skills by indicating if the skill 'went well' or 'needed improvement.' This manuscript only evaluates mentees' performance during live deliveries in which the neonate was non-vigorous.

Table 1 Definition of key variables

Binary variables	
Stimulation	Clinically adequate stimulation performed prior to initiation of PPV
Suction	Suction performed prior to initiation of PPV
Neck extension	Neck extended in the proper sniffing position using towel roll or head tilt
PPV with chest rise	PPV with three consecutive breaths with visible chest rise
PPV rate 40–60 breaths/minute	PPV delivered at a rate of 40–60 breaths per minute
Heart rate assessed	Heart rate assessed at any point during the resuscitation
Time-based variables	
Mentee hands on neonate	Time elapsed between the mother calling for help and the nurse mentee placing hands on the neonate to begin the clinical evaluation
Neonate placed on warmer	Time elapsed between the mother calling for help and the neonate being placed on the warmer to begin the resuscitation
Initiation of PPV	Time elapsed between the mother calling for help and the initiation of PPV
PPV with chest rise	Time elapsed between the mother calling for help and the third consecutive breath of PPV with visible chest rise

PPV positive pressure ventilation

Barriers to evidence-based NR practices

Mentors were interviewed about the barriers to EBP in NR that they had observed mentees facing in PHCs. Study procedures for the qualitative portion of this manuscript have been described in detail in a separate manuscript [37]. In brief, a semi-structured interview guide was developed and piloted with a former AMANAT mentor. A portion of the interview guide asked mentors about each of the following skills before and after training: warming/drying/stimulating, measuring heart and respiratory rates, achieving chest rise during PPV, and performing the resuscitation with adequate urgency. The interview guide allowed the interviewer the flexibility to ask open-ended questions regarding barriers to these skills and to further explore emerging themes. One-on-one interviews were conducted in English by one of the lead investigators in a private room at PHCs. If the interview was conducted outside of business hours or private space was unavailable, the interview was conducted in a private location near the PHC. All interviewees were fluent in English. Interviews were observed by a local Hindi-speaking member of the PRONTO team in case minor phrase translations were required. Interview duration ranged from 45 to 75 min.

After 18 interviews, the interviewer concluded data saturation had been reached as no new barriers to care were being identified. However, this manuscript only presents barriers specifically linked by mentors to one of the skills evaluated in simulated or live resuscitations in an attempt to provide context for quantitative trends. Thus, this manuscript is not an exhaustive exploration of barriers to care, and other barriers that were not explicitly linked to a specific resuscitation skill are explored in a separate manuscript [37].

Analysis

All quantitative analyses were conducted using IBM SPSS Statistics 23 [38].

Mentee performance in simulated resuscitations

Assessment simulations from weeks 4 and 8 of training were paired by PHC. Simulation videos that were corrupt or could not be paired were discarded. Simulations where the mentor stepped in to assist mentees or where the clinical scenario deviated from the assessment scenario were also discarded. The percentage of simulations in which mentees correctly completed key NR tasks, meeting quality indicators, at weeks 4 and 8 of training was compared using McNemar's Test for paired proportions. The median time to mentee completion of key NR tasks at weeks 4 and 8 was compared using the Wilcoxon Signed Rank Test due to violation of the normality assumption of parametric methods.

Mentee performance in live resuscitations

The percentage of live deliveries in which mentors felt mentees adequately performed key NR skills was graphed by week of training. Additionally, the percentage of deliveries in which NR skills 'went well' in weeks 1–3 was compared to weeks 4–8 using the Pearson Chi-Squared Test. Week 3 was chosen as the cut-off because NR simulations were introduced into the PRONTO curriculum at that time. If the expected cell count assumption was violated, a Fisher's Exact Test was substituted.

Barriers to evidence-based NR practices

Audio-recorded interviews were transcribed and analyzed by the interviewer. Qualitative analysis was conducted using the thematic content approach [39, 40], which included 1) data familiarization, 2) identifying codes and then themes, 3) developing a coding scheme and applying it to the data, and 4) refining and organizing codes consistent with the Braun and Clarke approach to thematic analysis [41]. Two interviews (10%) were selected at random for double coding to ensure consistency in identification of key themes.

Results
Mentee performance in simulated resuscitations

A total of 1342 mentees at 160 PHCs participated in phases 2 and 3 of AMANAT/ PRONTO training. A randomly selected subset of these mentees was evaluated in 279 NR assessment simulations, which were video-recorded and coded for quality indicators. This analysis includes 226 (81%) assessment videos, or 113 PHC-matched week 4 and 8 video pairs.

From week 4 to 8 of training, there was a 13.5 percentage-point increase in proper neck extension ($p = 0.01$), a 19.0 percentage-point increase in PPV with visible chest rise ($p < 0.01$), and an 11.6 percentage-point increase in assessment of heart rate during resuscitations ($p < 0.01$). There was no statistically significant change between weeks 4 and 8 in adequate stimulation, suction, or delivery of PPV with the proper rate (Table 2). Additionally, there was no statistically significant change in median time to completion of key NR tasks (Table 3).

Mentee performance in live resuscitations

Mentee performance was evaluated in a total of 3195 live deliveries in phases 2 and 3. Amongst these, 252 (8%) were complicated by birth of a non-vigorous neonate. From early to later weeks of training, the percentage of deliveries in which mentees' identification of non-vigorous neonates, suctioning, and PPV 'went well' increased by 20.7, 25.4, and 22.7 percentage-points respectively (all $p < 0.01$). The percentage of deliveries in which mentors felt mentees performed adequate

Table 2 Percent of simulations in which mentees correctly performed key NR skills at weeks 4 and 8 of training (N = 113 matched pairs)

Key NR skill	N[a]	Week 4	Week 8	Percentage-point change[c]	P-value[d]
		n (%)[b]			
Stimulation	107	38 (35.5)	26 (24.3)	−11.2	0.08
Suction	111	69 (62.2)	78 (70.3)	8.1	0.25
Neck extension	104	78 (75.0)	92 (88.5)	13.5	0.01
PPV with chest rise	100	66 (66.0)	85 (85.0)	19.0	< 0.01
PPV rate 40–60 breaths/min	106	39 (36.8)	52 (49.1)	12.3	0.08
Heart rate assessed	112	97 (86.6)	110 (98.2)	11.6	< 0.01

NR Neonatal resuscitation, PPV Positive pressure ventilation
[a]N = total number of PHC-matched week 4 and 8 simulation pairs in which key NR skill could be evaluated
[b]n = number of week 4 and 8 simulations in which key NR skill was completed % = percent of week 4 and 8 simulations in which key NR skill was completed
[c]Percentage-point difference in completion of key NR skill from week 4 to 8 of training
[d]McNemar's Test of paired proportions

stimulation was high at baseline (94%) and did not change significantly (Table 4). The week-wise trend in these four variables is illustrated in Fig. 1.

Barriers to evidence-based NR practices

High level themes and illustrative quotations of barriers to 1) initial resuscitation, 2) measuring heart and respiratory rates, 3) achieving chest rise during PPV, and 4) performing the resuscitation with adequate urgency are summarized in Table 5.

Initial resuscitation

Prior to training, mentors explained mentees did not understand the clinical significance of the initial steps of resuscitation (warming, drying, stimulating, and suction) and did not know how to properly perform these steps. Rather, they performed traditional practices including holding the neonate upside down, over stimulating, and massaging the chest. Additionally, equipment issues, including the availability of clean, dry cloths precluded effective initial resuscitations.

After training, mentors felt that mentees knew how to perform warm/dry/stim in an evidence-based manner. However, mentors reported that mentees often forgot to perform these initial resuscitation steps in a perceived rush to begin ventilation. On the other hand, mentors felt mentees still did not understand the clinical indications for suctioning and were too quick to jump to this step. Supply issues remained a barrier to initial resuscitation after training. Mentors explained that equipment, including mucus extractors, was often unavailable or disorganized and thus inaccessible when urgently needed.

Measurement of heart and respiratory rates

Mentors explained that prior to training, mentees did not know how to measure vital signs, were inaccurate in their counting, or were unaware of normal parameters and their clinical significance for neonates. This was likely connected to the belief, prior to training, that the management of non-vigorous neonates was the responsibility of doctors. Mentors also explained that mentees' goal in resuscitations was simply to make the baby cry, so vital signs were frequently overlooked.

This goal remained true after training. Mentors reported that mentees frequently forgot to check vital signs because they were too focused on simply making the neonate cry. Nevertheless, mentors felt that mentees understood the significance of vital signs after training. However, they still could not measure them accurately, often because they did not have or could not read a clock.

Table 3 Time to mentee completion of key NR skills in simulation at weeks 4 and 8 of training (N = 113 matched pairs)

Time in seconds to key NR skill	N[a]	Week 4	Week 8	Difference in seconds[c]	P-value[d]
		Median (IQR)[b]			
Mentee hands on neonate	98	9 (6–17)	11 (7–22)	2	0.55
Neonate placed on warmer	105	35 (24–56)	38 (26–62)	3	0.95
Initiation of PPV	106	83 (48–111)	84 (66–114)	1	0.90
PPV with chest rise	58	116 (88–178)	137 (92–195)	21	0.76

NR Neonatal resuscitation, PPV Positive pressure ventilation, IQR Inter-quartile range
[a]N = total number of PHC-matched week 4 and 8 simulation pairs in which key NR skill could be evaluated
[b]Median time in seconds to completion of key NR skill (inter-quartile range)
[c]Difference in median number of seconds to completion of key NR skill from week 4 to 8 of training
[d]Wilcoxon Signed-Rank Test

Table 4 Percent of live deliveries in which mentees successfully completed key NR Skills in the early versus later weeks of training (N = 252)

Key NR skill	Weeks 1–3		Weeks 4–8		Percentage-point change[c]	P-value
	N[a]	n (%)[b]	N[a]	n (%)[b]		
Identification of non-vigorous infant	66	32 (48.5)	156	108 (69.2)	20.7	< 0.01[d]
Warm/dry/stimulate	65	60 (92.3)	144	139 (96.5)	4.2	0.29[e]
Suction	63	27 (42.9)	145	99 (68.3)	25.4	< 0.01[d]
PPV	48	12 (25.0)	109	52 (47.7)	22.7	< 0.01[d]

NR Neonatal resuscitation, *PPV* Positive pressure ventilation
[a]N = number of live deliveries in which performance of NR skill was required and recorded
[b]n = number of live deliveries in which NR skill was successfully completed; % = percent of live deliveries in which NR skill was successfully completed
[c]Difference in percent of live deliveries in which NR skill was completed from early to late weeks of training
[d]Pearson Chi-Squared Test
[e]Fisher's Exact Test

PPV with chest rise

Mentors explained that knowledge of all aspects of PPV, including clinical significance, mask selection, rate of delivery, and assessment of effectiveness was lacking before training. If ventilation was provided, it was often given mouth-to-mouth or by using a self-inflating bag on the mother's abdomen without knowledge of proper technique. Similar to the measurement of vital signs, mentors explained that some mentees believed that doctors were responsible for managing non-vigorous neonates prior to training, which meant they did not initiate ventilation themselves.

After training, mentors felt mentees had accepted the responsibility of providing PPV, but that they continued to have difficulty with mask seal, rhythm, and assessment of PPV effectiveness. Approximately two-thirds of mentors reported observing continued difficulty with neck extension after training, while one-third of mentors felt mentees had mastered this skill. Additionally, mentors reported mentees did not know when to stop PPV for reassessment because mentees did not have or could not read a clock. The availability of ventilation bags and different mask sizes, particularly preterm masks, was identified as a barrier after training-- likely persistent from before training but more frequently identified after PPV became an accepted duty of mentees. Finally, one mentor felt the traditional belief that oxygen was important in addressing respiratory distress was a barrier to performing PPV with self-inflating bags with no oxygen source after training.

Urgency

Mentors explained that mentees did not understand the concept of the golden minute or the significance of achieving effective ventilation within that timeframe prior to training. Additionally, they did not know how to accurately identify non-vigorous neonates requiring resuscitation. Further, mentors explained the traditional practice in Bihar was to patiently wait for neonates to cry, which commonly delayed resuscitations. Other

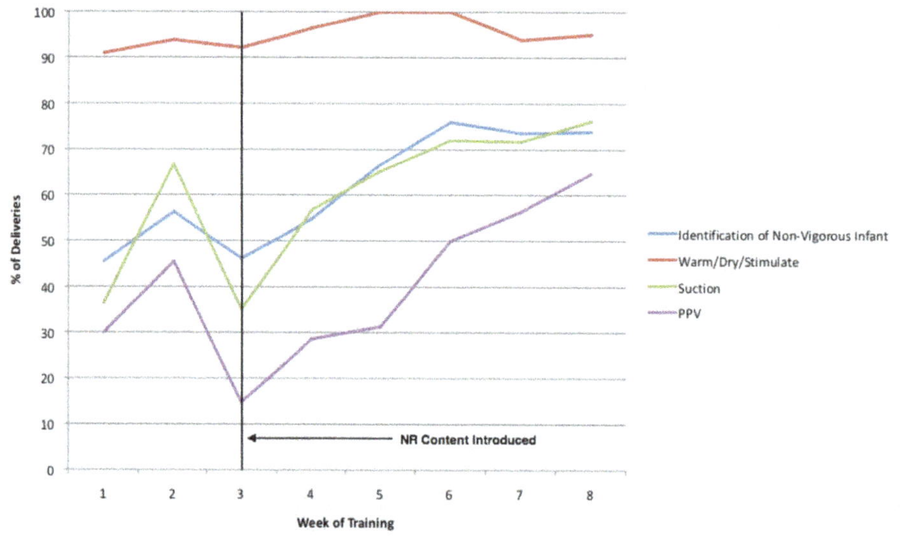

Fig. 1 Trend in the Percent of Live Deliveries in which Mentees Successfully Completed Key NR Skills by Week of Training

Table 5 Barriers to Evidence-Based Practices in Neonatal Resuscitation Before and After Training

Barrier	Before training	After training
Initial resuscitation		
Knowledge	"They were not knowing ok there is a need to stimulate... and they were not knowing ok why they need to dry the baby."	"So much suctioning is there... with the help of drying or stimulating the baby can be saved, but in spite of that they used to go for suctioning... like if baby didn't cry means ok get... sucker, get sucker."
Traditional Practices	"They'll hold the baby upside down, they will shake the baby here and there, they'll beat the baby... but... the proper stimulation they were not aware [that] they should rub the baby back or they should flick [the feet]."	
Equipment	"They used to dry the baby but... not with a clean or dry cloth."	"Baby was [asphyxiated with] thick meconium... suction, all the thing[s] [were] not available and we don't know where they are."
Focus on Later Management		"[Mentees] think that if the baby is not crying, they have to take [the baby] immediately to the warmer, so they forget the stimulation part."
Measurement of heart and respiratory rates		
Knowledge	"Actually before... [mentees] were not knowing ok heart rate and respiration[s] are two different things... then we started teaching them anatomy. Respiration- this is the work of lungs... and heart rate- this is the work of heart."	
Skill		"[Mentees] don't have timers to see or... just for name sake they see... or they don't see it properly... the counting goes here and there. They don't get it accurately."
Equipment		"Some sisters [are] having trouble while checking the heart rate because... watch is not available."
Focus on Later Management	"The goal is the baby should cry. [Mentees] don't see for the respiration rate or for the heart rate, they just see that the baby cries... keep on stimulating so that the baby cries."	"Until [mentees] see the baby [cry], they will give bag and mask, bag and mask. In between... check heart rate, respiratory rate, they were not doing."
Role of MD	"[Mentees] said... 'what's heart rate? How do we check that? That's doctor's thing, they do that with the stethoscope.'"	
PPV with chest rise		
Knowledge	"They were not knowing about the PPV. If any of the [mentees] knew, she was not knowing the correct rhythm... how much time you need to do, how you need to. She only knew ok we need to do."	
Skill	"[Mentees] just pump [the Ambu bag]... according to the baby['s] size they don't use the [correct] mask. Whatever mask they get, they will connect that and they will pump it."	"[Mask] seal is not good for most of the time... and the rhythm also. Some of the mentees, they forget the [ventilation] rhythm also."
Traditional Practices	"Before... in some facilities [mentees] were giving mouth to mouth ventilation... that time they didn't know how to use bag and mask ventilation."	"PPV they are doing but they have more belief in oxygen. If we will put the oxygen... baby will be crying they believe only."
Equipment		"In some PHC we don't have zero [size] mask... we have only one number mask, so it is not as effective, because in preterm baby we can't use the big one."
Role of MD	"Before training [mentees] were not doing [PPV]... they didn't know how to use bag and mask ventilation. They only know... we can't use, doctor has to do."	
Urgency		
Knowledge	"Actually they are not aware what is the effect [of delay]. Until we... know what is the effect, we will not take precaution."	"[Mentees] can't... understand when [the neonates] need resuscitation or not. Sometimes they identify very well but... sometime[s] they waiting for... crying... It's not proper timing."

Table 5 Barriers to Evidence-Based Practices in Neonatal Resuscitation Before and After Training *(Continued)*

Barrier	Before training	After training
Skill	"To cut the cord, to take the baby to the NBCC, and to start [the] resuscitation, it will take more than 5 min they were telling."	"It will take time, especially drying the baby, wiping it, stimulating it, clamping... the cords."
Traditional Practices	"Because their old practice is like... they... will wait, they'll tell, 'Baby will cry now, sister this is normal baby will cry now.'"	"They are thinking it might be crying... they are waiting for some time. But when we are there we are telling them not crying so go fast!"
Equipment		"Golden minute... [mentees] don't have articles for clamping or... they search for suctioning, for mucus extractor... availability is not there in the PHC, so they go outside to get."
Facility Layout		"NBCC is in another room... this is labor room, so next to labor room is NBCC, so that takes [mentees] more than a minute to take the baby from labor room to NBCC."
Maternal Management	"For one to two to three minutes [mentees] will wait... because [until] the placenta is removed, they will concentrate on that. Ok, the placenta is removed, after that they see, ok, baby is not crying. Then they will start with the Ambu."	
Human Resources		"Sometimes only one staff is there for delivery... she will be taking care of the mother and then baby is not crying..."

PPV Positive pressure ventilation, *PHC* Primary health center, *NBCC* Newborn care corner

delays were created by slow cord clamping and performance of the initial NR steps. Finally, mentors described mentees' focus on maternal management as a barrier to timely NR prior to training.

After training, mentors explained mentees were better at identifying non-vigorous neonates and knew about the golden minute; however, some mentors expressed concern some mentees still did not truly understand its clinical significance. Additionally, mentors explained mentees could not read a clock to facilitate timely resuscitations. Regarding skills, mentors explained mentees' inefficiencies in initial resuscitation and cord cutting continued to delay resuscitations after training. One mentor felt that mentees spent too much time trying to seal the mask. Overall, mentors felt more practice performing NR with proper timing was necessary. Other frequently mentioned barriers to urgency that were likely persistent from before training were the traditional practice of patiently waiting for the infant to cry, long distances between labor rooms and the newborn care corners (NBCCs), insufficient staffing, and issues with supply availability, functionality, and organization.

Discussion

PRONTO International's NR simulation training, implemented within the AMANAT quality improvement initiative, had a positive impact on key NR skills amongst ANM/GNM mentees working in rural PHCs across Bihar. Nevertheless, there is room for continued improvement in nearly all NR skills, likely due to the need for additional training as well as significant barriers that

go beyond the scope of clinical skills training. For each of the key skills evaluated in this manuscript-- initial resuscitation, assessment of vital signs, performance of PPV, and urgency in resuscitations-- we present a triangulated discussion of simulation data, live delivery data, and barriers to care identified by mentors in qualitative interviews to facilitate a more nuanced understanding of the positive impacts of PRONTO training and areas for improvement.

Mentees' performance of the initial NR steps, including warming, drying, stimulating, and suctioning, was variable. This is consistent with previously published studies [12, 14]. In interviews, mentors suggested that knowledge of EBPs increased with training. However, there was no significant change in the percentage of simulated NR scenarios in which mentees provided clinically adequate stimulation prior to PPV from week 4 to 8 of training. In observed live deliveries, there was similarly no significant change in stimulation between the early and later weeks of training; although, the rate of stimulation was high at baseline. This knowledge-skill gap may be explained by mentors' observation that mentees frequently forgot initial NR steps in a perceived rush to start PPV. Moreover, the fact that the simulated scenario did not begin with a birth may have also contributed to mentees' relative failure to perform initial steps in simulation compared to live deliveries. Regarding suctioning, there was significant improvement in live deliveries, but not in simulated resuscitations. Despite this improvement in live deliveries, about a quarter of live-born neonates deemed to require suctioning did not receive it during week 8 of training, perhaps due to the supply issues highlighted by mentors.

Assessment of vital signs, including heart rate and respiratory rate, was evaluated only in simulated resuscitations. A significant improvement was observed from week 4 to 8 of training. Mentors explained that vital signs were often not assessed before training due to inadequate knowledge and a prevalent belief that NR was the doctor's responsibility. This suggests the observed change in simulation data, which did not include a true pre-training measurement, may underestimate the impact of training on this skill. Notably, while simulation data captured whether or not mentees checked heart rate, it did not assess the accuracy of heart rate measurements. Mentors explained in interviews that mentees have difficulty reading a clock, suggesting this may be an area for future improvement. This will likely require innovative solutions to help providers identify normal versus abnormal vital signs without the need to count precise rates.

Proper delivery of PPV is the chief focus of many NR trainings. A significant improvement in PPV skills was observed in both simulated and live resuscitations following PRONTO training. Previous studies have similarly reported improvement in PPV skills post-training [12–17]. During week 8, mentees achieved chest rise in 85 and 65% of simulated and live resuscitations, respectively. Other studies report comparable [12, 15] or lower rates of effective PPV [14, 16]. In interviews, mentors explained mentees continued to struggle with mask seal, rhythm, and real time assessment of PPV effectiveness. These observations are supported by the simulation data, which demonstrated no change in the use of the proper rate of PPV following training. Although interviewees disagreed about mentees' ability to perform proper neck extension, a significant improvement in this skill was observed in simulations from week 4 to 8. Mentors felt the persistent PPV knowledge-skill gap was due to insufficient practice as well as lack of availability of functional supplies in PHCs. The need for more practice with longer trainings is not an unfamiliar challenge amongst NR programs in LMICs [42] and the PRONTO training is unique in that it was conducted over 8 months. Nonetheless, given the departure PPV represents from traditional practices in Bihar, interviewees felt even this duration of training was insufficient.

Urgency is another key area for improvement. No significant change was observed in the time to completion of key NR tasks in simulations. In fact, the median time to effective chest rise trended upward non-significantly from week 4 to 8 of training. Other studies have similarly reported both increased and unchanged durations of time to PPV initiation [12, 15]. Nonetheless, mentors described a perceived rush to start ventilation after

training that negatively impacted initial resuscitation measures. The discrepancy between the perceived urgency and true time to completion of key tasks may be related to barriers such as inability to read a clock, distance between labor rooms and NBCCs, and both supply and human resources shortages. Other barriers to urgency identified by interviewees included poor understanding of the true significance of the golden minute and continued performance of traditional clinical practices such as waiting indefinitely for the infant to cry. Timely identification of non-vigorous neonates in live deliveries improved significantly; however, mentees still failed to identify nearly a quarter of live-born neonates deemed non-vigorous by mentors at the end of training.

These results have informed the next iteration of the PRONTO curriculum, which will include greater emphasis on quick identification of non-vigorous neonates, beginning resuscitations with appropriate initial resuscitation measures, recognition of vital sign abnormalities without counting specific rates, and timely initiation of effective PPV. Nevertheless, this study has several limitations. Foremost, due to the unreliable birth registry system in Bihar, there are no reliable clinical outcome data on which to base the impact of this training program. For this reason, we used simulation data as a proxy.

The simulation data lack a true pre-training measurement, which may cause an underestimation of the true impact of training. Nonetheless, this was a conscious choice to allow mentees to adapt to simulation procedures prior to evaluation given their lack of familiarity with this method of learning [42]. The assessment simulation was also not changed between week 4 and 8. However, this is unlikely to have led to an overestimation of the impact of training given the aim of this study was to assess the quality of basic NR skills, which should follow an algorithm that is relatively independent of the clinical scenario in uncomplicated resuscitations. Additionally, simulation data represent the performance of only a subset of mentees who participated in the NR assessment simulations at week 4 and 8 of training. However, as the selection process was random, the impact of selection bias is likely minimal. Finally, this data is based on a single video assessor, which could have introduced interpretation bias. However, the potential for this bias was minimized by blinding the assessor to week of training and by choosing an assessor who was independent from training implementation.

The live birth data represent a convenience sample and could be biased, as data were collected by mentors who were not blind to week of training and who had somewhat limited clinical training themselves, as most were early in their nursing career. Further, live delivery data provide only a binary and subjective assessment of whether key NR steps went well or not. Nevertheless, these data provide the only assessment of performance in live deliveries, as medical record keeping is inconsistent. The investigators felt that a more rigorous assessment of resuscitations in real time would impact clinical care or preclude data collection given the high delivery volume at PHCs.

Qualitative interview data could be influenced by desire of mentors to please the interviewer as well as by any preconceptions mentors may have had about intrapartum or postnatal care in Bihar. We attempted to mitigate these potential biases by clearly stating during the consent process that interviews were not a performance evaluation and by selecting interviewees with at least 16 months of mentoring experience in PHCs. Finally, not all qualitative interview data regarding barriers to care is included in this manuscript. Rather, logistical, cultural, and structural barriers to immediate neonatal care and NR are more fully explored in a separate manuscript [37] and this manuscript only presents barriers explicitly linked by mentors to specific NR skills assessed in simulated and live resuscitations.

Conclusion

PRONTO simulation training conducted within the AMANAT intervention had a positive impact on knowledge and the use of evidence-based NR practices amongst numerous ANMs/GNMs working in rural PHCs throughout Bihar. Nevertheless there is a need for ongoing improvement, which will require addressing many barriers to care that extend beyond the scope of clinical skills training. Data triangulation, incorporating both quantitative and qualitative methodologies, offers a powerful tool for guiding this process in settings such as Bihar where clinical outcome data are unreliable, yet the need for improvement in neonatal care is great.

Abbreviations
ANM: Auxiliary nurse midwife; EBP: Evidence-based practices; GNM: General nursing and midwifery; IQR: Inter-quartile range; LMIC: Low- and middle-income countries; NBCC: Newborn care corner; NR: Neonatal resuscitation; NSVD: Normal spontaneous vaginal delivery; PHC: Primary health center; PPH: Postpartum hemorrhage; PPV: Positive pressure ventilation; UCSF: University of California San Francisco

Acknowledgements
The authors would like to thank the entire CARE India team for their support in facilitating PRONTO International simulation training as part of the AMANAT program throughout Bihar. We would also like to express our sincere appreciation for all phase 2-4 mentors for their commitment to teaching and their willingness to participate in qualitative interviews. Thank you also to the phase 2-4 participates for their commitment to the training and willingness to learn. Special thanks to Rebecka Thanaki, Renu Sharma, and Praicey Thomas for their help in arranging and facilitating qualitative interviews. Lastly, thank you to the entire PRONTO International team for their tireless work throughout implementation and evaluation of the training program.

Funding
This study was funded by the Bill and Melinda Gates Foundation. The funding body had no role in the design of the study; the collection, analysis, and interpretation of data; or in writing the manuscript.

Authors' contributions
BV designed data collection tools, coded all simulation videos, conducted all interviews, performed qualitative and quantitative data analysis, and drafted and revised the manuscript. MM provided clinical expertise and made substantial contributions to the design of data collection tools, data analysis, and manuscript revision. HS was also involved in study design and critical revision of the manuscript. AC was involved in PRONTO curriculum design, supervision of PRONTO training, provided expert local opinion for qualitative analysis, and critically revised the manuscript. SC was involved in PRONTO curriculum design, study design, and made significant contributions during manuscript revision. DW is the principal investigator for the evaluation of PRONTO in Bihar and made significant contributions to all aspects of study design and manuscript preparation. All authors have approved this manuscript for submission.

Competing interests
DW and SC are founding members of PRONTO International and sit on its board of directors. None of the other authors have any conflicts of interest to declare.

Author details
Department of Pediatrics, University of California San Francisco, 550 16th Street, 4th Floor, Box 0110, San Francisco, CA 94158, USA. [2]Maternal, Adolescent, Reproductive, and Child Health Centre, London School of Hygiene and Tropical Medicine, Keppel Street, London WC1E 7HT, UK. [3]Institute for Global Health Sciences, University of California San Francisco, 550 16th Street, San Francisco, CA 94158, USA. [4]PRONTO International, State RMNCH+A Unit, C-16 Krishi Nagar, A.G. Colony, Patna, Bihar 80002, India. [5]College of Nursing, University of Utah, 10 South 2000 East, Salt Lake City, UT 84112, USA. [6]Department of Obstetrics and Gynecology and Reproductive Services, University of California San Francisco, 1001 Potrero Ave, San Francisco, CA 94110, USA. [7]PRONTO International, 1820 E. Thomas Street APT 16, Seattle, WA 98112, USA.

References
1. GBD 2016 Mortality Collaborators. Global, regional, and national under-5 mortality, adult mortality, age-specific mortality, and life expectancy, 1970–2016: a systematic analysis for the Global Burden of Disease Study 2016. Lancet. 2017;390:1084–150.
2. Ministry of Health & Family Welfare Government of India. INAP India Newborn Action Plan. 2014.
3. Registrar General of India. Sample registration system (SRS) statistical report 2013. New Delhi: 2013. Available from: http://www.censusindia.gov.in/vital_statistics/SRS_Reports_2013.html.
4. Oxford Poverty & Human Development Initiative. Multidimensional Poverty Index 2016 Highlights ~ South Asia. University of Oxford. 2016.
5. Dogra V, Khanna R, Jain A, Kumar AM, Shewade HD, Majumdar SS. Neonatal mortality in India's rural poor: findings of a household survey and verbal autopsy study in Rajasthan. Bihar and Odisha J Trop Pediatr. 2015;61(3):210–4.
6. Agrawal N, Kumar S, Balasubramaniam SM, Bhargava S, Sinha P, Bakshi B, et al. Effectiveness of virtual classroom training in improving the knowledge and key maternal neonatal health skills of general nurse midwifery students in Bihar, India: a pre- and post-intervention study. Nurse Educ Today. 2016;36:293–7.
7. Chauhan M, Sharma J, Negandhi P, Reddy S, Sethy G, Neogi SB. Assessment of newborn care corners in selected public health facilities in Bihar. Indian J Public Health. 2016;60(4):341–2.
8. Lee AC, Cousens S, Wall SN, Niermeyer S, Darmstadt GL, Carlo WA, et al. Neonatal resuscitation and immediate newborn assessment and stimulation for the prevention of neonatal deaths: a systematic review, meta-analysis and Delphi estimation of mortality effect. BMC Public Health. 2011;11(Suppl 3):S12.

9. Kamath-Rayne BD, Griffin JB, Moran K, Jones B, Downs A, McClure EM, et al. Resuscitation and obstetrical care to reduce Intrapartum-related neonatal deaths: a MANDATE study. Matern Child Health J. 2015;19(8):1853–63.

10. Reisman J, Arlington L, Jensen L, Louis H, Suarez-Rebling D, Nelson BD. Newborn Resuscitation Training in Resource-Limited Settings: A Systematic Literature Review. Pediatrics. 2016;138(2):e20154490.

11. Dynes M, Rahman A, Beck D, Moran A, Pervin J, Yunus M, et al. Home-based life saving skills in Matlab, Bangladesh: a process evaluation of a community-based maternal child health programme. Midwifery. 2011;27(1):15–22.

12. Ersdal HL, Vossius C, Bayo E, Mduma E, Perlman J, Lippert A, et al. A one-day "helping babies breathe" course improves simulated performance but not clinical management of neonates. Resuscitation. 2013;84(10):1422–7.

13. Couper ID, Thurley JD, Hugo JF. The neonatal resuscitation training project in rural South Africa. Rural Remote Health. 2005;5(4):459.

14. Makene CL, Plotkin M, Currie S, Bishanga D, Ugwi P, Louis H, et al. Improvements in newborn care and newborn resuscitation following a quality improvement program at scale: results from a before and after study in Tanzania. BMC Pregnancy Childbirth. 2014;14:381.

15. Seto TL, Tabangin ME, Josyula S, Taylor KK, Vasquez JC, Kamath-Rayne BD. Educational outcomes of helping babies breathe training at a community hospital in Honduras. Perspect Med Educ. 2015;4(5):225–32.

16. Singhal N, Lockyer J, Fidler H, Keenan W, Little G, Bucher S, et al. Helping babies breathe: global neonatal resuscitation program development and formative educational evaluation. Resuscitation. 2012;83(1):90–6.

17. Carlo WA, Wright LL, Chomba E, McClure EM, Carlo ME, Bann CM, et al. Educational impact of the neonatal resuscitation program in low-risk delivery centers in a developing country. J Pediatr. 2009;154(4):504–8.e5.

18. Kamath-Rayne BD, Josyula S, Rule ARL, Vasquez JC. Improvements in the delivery of resuscitation and newborn care after helping babies breathe training. J Perinatol. 2017;37(10):1153–60.

19. Goudar SS, Somannavar MS, Clark R, Lockyer JM, Revankar AP, Fidler HM, et al. Stillbirth and newborn mortality in India after helping babies breathe training. Pediatrics. 2013;131(2):e344–52.

20. Hoban R, Bucher S, Neuman I, Chen M, Tesfaye N, Spector JM. 'Helping babies breathe' training in sub-Saharan Africa: educational impact and learner impressions. J Trop Pediatr. 2013;59(3):180–6.

21. Jeffery HE, Kocova M, Tozija F, Gjorgiev D, Pop-Lazarova M, Foster K, et al. The impact of evidence-based education on a perinatal capacity-building initiative in Macedonia. Med Educ. 2004;38(4):435–47.

22. Musafili A, EssÉn B, Baribwira C, Rukundo A, Persson L. Evaluating helping babies breathe: training for healthcare workers at hospitals in Rwanda. Acta Paediatr. 2013;102(1):e34–8.

23. Reisman J, Martineau N, Kairuki A, Mponzi V, Meda AR, Isangula KG, et al. Validation of a novel tool for assessing newborn resuscitation skills among birth attendants trained by the helping babies breathe program. Int J Gynaecol Obstet. 2015;131(2):196–200.

24. Bookman L, Engmann C, Srofenyoh E, Enweronu-Laryea C, Owen M, Randolph G, et al. Educational impact of a hospital-based neonatal resuscitation program in Ghana. Resuscitation. 2010;81(9):1180–2.

25. Hosokawa S. Impact of neonatal resuscitation training workshop in Mongolia. Int Med J. 2011;18(2):133–6.

26. McClure EM, Carlo WA, Wright LL, Chomba E, Uxa F, Lincetto O, et al. Evaluation of the educational impact of the WHO essential newborn care course in Zambia. Acta Paediatr. 2007;96(8):1135–8.

27. Opiyo N, Were F, Govedi F, Fegan G, Wasunna A, English M. Effect of newborn resuscitation training on health worker practices in Pumwani hospital Kenya. PLoS One. 2008;3(2):e1599.

28. Woods J, Gagliardi L, Nara S, Phally S, Varang O, Viphou N, et al. An innovative approach to in-service training of maternal health staff in Cambodian hospitals. Int J Gynaecol Obstet. 2015;129(2):178–83.

29. PRONTO International. Available from: http://prontointernational.org [Accessed 20 Feb 2016].

30. CARE India. Available from: https://www.careindia.org [Accessed 20 Feb 2016].

31. Das A, Nawal D, Singh MK, Karthick M, Pahwa P, Shah MB, Mahapatra T. Evaluation of the mobile nurse training (MNT) intervention – a step towards improvement in intrapartum practices in Bihar. India BMC Pregnancy and Childbirth. 2017;17(1):266.

32. Das A, Nawal D, Singh MK, Karthick M, Pahwa P, Shah MB, Mahapatra T, Chaudhuri I. Impact of a nursing skill-improvement intervention on newborn-specific delivery practices: an experience from Bihar. India Birth. 2016;43(4):328–35.

33. Sharma, BP. Rural health statistics. Government of India Ministry of Health and Family Welfare Statistics Division 2015.

34. Indian Nursing Council. Types of Nursing Programs. Available from: http://www.indiannursingcouncil.org/nursing-programs.asp?show=prog-type [Accessed 2 June 2017].

35. Laerdal Medical. NeoNatalie. Available from: https://www.laerdal.com/us/products/simulationtraining/obstetrics-pediatrics/neonatalie/. Accessed 22 Aug 2018.

36. OpenDataKit. Available from: https://opendatakit.org [Accessed 12 May 2017].

37. Vail B, Morgan MC, Dyer J, Chrismas A, Cohen SR, Joshi M, Gore A, Mahapatra T, Walker DM. Logistical, cultural, and structural barriers to immediate neonatal care and neonatal resuscitation in Bihar, India. BMC pregnancy and childbirth. 2017. Under review.

38. IBM Corp. Released 2013. IBM SPSS statistics for Macintosh, version 23.0. Armonk: IBM Corp.

39. Green J, Thorogood N. Qualitative methods for Health Research. 3rd ed. London: SAGE; 2014.

40. Pope C, Mays N. Qualitative research in health care. 2nd ed. London: BMJ Books; 2000.

41. Braun V, Clarke V. Using thematic analysis in psychology. Qual Res Psychol. 2006;3:77–101.

42. Rule ARL, Tabangin M, Cheruiyot D, Mueri P, Kamath-Rayne BD. The call and the challenge of pediatric resuscitation and simulation research in low-resource settings. Simul Healthc. 2017;12(6):402–6.

13

Clinical evaluation of severe neonatal Hyperbilirubinaemia in a resource-limited setting: a 4-year longitudinal study in south-East Nigeria

Chidiebere D. I. Osuorah[1*], Uchenna Ekwochi[2] and Isaac N. Asinobi[2]

Abstract

Background: Neonatal hyperbilirubinaemia is one of the commonest causes of hospital visit in the neonatal period. When severe, it is a leading cause of irreversible neurological and musculoskeletal disability. Prompt recognition and timely interventions are imperative for a drastic reduction in complications associated with severe hyperbilirubinaemia in newborns.

Methods: We report a 4-year descriptive and longitudinal study to determine the causes, clinical presentations and long-term outcomes in newborns admitted for severe neonatal jaundice. Methods: Newborns admitted and managed for severe neonatal jaundice at the Enugu State University Teaching Hospital during a 4-year period were enrolled and followed up for 2 years.

Results: A total of 1920 newborns were admitted during the study period and 48 were managed for severe hyperbilirubinaemia giving an in-hospital incidence rate of 25 (95% CI 18–32) per 1000 admitted newborns. The mean age of onset was 3.4 ± 0.5 days (range 1–8 days) and hospital presentation from time of first notice was 4.3 ± 0.4 days (range 1–9 days). The total and unconjugated admission serum bilirubin ranged from 7.1 to 71.1 (mean 26 ± 2.5 mg/dl) and 4.2 to 46.3 mg/dl (mean 18.3 ± 9.2) respectively. Earliest sign of severe hyperbilirubinaemia in newborns were: refusal to suck (15.2%) and depressed primitive reflexes (24.5%) while the commonest signs included high pitch cry (11.9%), convulsion and stiffness (6.9%) and vomiting (6.3%) in addition to the former signs. The major causes of severe hyperbilirubinaemia were idiopathic (33.3%), sepsis (35.3%), ABO incompatibility (17.6%) and glucose-6-phosphate dehydrogenase (G6PD) deficiency (11.8%). Long-term sequelae on follow-up included delayed developmental milestone attainment, postural deformities, visual and seizure disorders.

Conclusions: There is urgent need for continued education for mothers, families and healthcare workers on the danger newborns with jaundice could face if not brought early to the hospital for timely diagnosis and management.

Keywords: Newborns, Severe hyperbilirubinaemia, Causes, Clinical features, Complications, Enugu

* Correspondence: chidi.osuorah@gmail.com
[1]Child Survival Unit, Medical Research Council UK, The Gambia Unit, Fajara, Banjul, Gambia
Full list of author information is available at the end of the article

Background

Neonatal Jaundice typically results from the deposition of unconjugated bilirubin pigment in the conjunctiva, skin and mucus membranes when there is excessive amount of bilirubin in blood. Hyperbilirubinaemia is defined as a total serum bilirubin level above 5 mg/dL (86 µmol per L) [1]. It is by far the most common reason for hospital presentation in the neonatal follow up clinic [2]. Although majority of newborns that have clinical jaundice in the first week of life recovers without treatment, some cases of hyperbilirubinaemia can however be serious and if not well managed, could results to severe morbidity and mortality [3]. Neonatal hyperbilirubinaemia is considered pathologic if it presents within the first 24 h after birth, the total serum bilirubin level rises by more than 5 mg/dL (85 µmol/L) per day or if the total bilirubin level is higher than 20 mg/dL (340 µmol/L) in term newborns or lower in term newborns with signs and symptoms suggestive of serious illness [1]. Common risk factors for severe hyperbilirubinaemia includes fetal-maternal blood group incompatibility, prematurity, glucose-6-phosphate dehydrogenase deficiency, hepatic diseases and septicaemia [4]. In order to prevent the potential and irreversible complications of severe hyperbilirubinaemia, exchange transfusion which is the most rapid method of lowering serum bilirubin concentrations is used when serum bilirubin reaches critical level and in other cases when serum bilirubin rises despite intensive phototherapy. This descriptive study conducted in the Enugu State University Teaching Hospital (ESUTH) over a 4-year period assessed the incidence, causes and clinical features of severe hyperbilirubinaemia in newborns after birth and followed them up for 2 years for possible complications after discharge from the hospital. It is hoped that findings from this study would aid clinicians in case identification and prompt management of newborns with risk factors for severe hyperbilirubinaemia.

Methods

Study area and site

This was a prospective study carried out in the Neonatal Intensive Care Unit (NICU) of Enugu State University Teaching Hospital (ESUTH). The site is a tertiary health facility that offers specialized medical services and serves as a referral centre to private, general, mission hospitals and other delivery homes within Enugu and the neighbouring states. The NICU offers 24-h services for sick babies born within and outside the hospital within their first 28 days of life. The NICU is manned by consultant neonatologists and resident doctors who are specialists in Paediatrics with further sub-specialist training in neonatology.

Enrolment of newborns into the study

This study was conducted over a period of four years between January 2013 and January 2017. Newborns with severe hyperbilirubinaemia were consecutively enrolled after obtaining an informed consent from their mothers or caregivers. Presence of clinical features that are related to hyperbilirubinaemia and its complications were documented. Results of certain baseline investigations done to ascertain the level and causes of hyperbilirubinaemia were also documented. These include serum bilirubin level, random blood sugar, glucose-6-phosphate dehydrogenase (G6PD) status, blood group, blood culture etc. Other data obtained included age of newborn at onset of jaundice, time of presentation, the number of exchange blood transfusions (EBT) done (i.e. single or double) and the outcome of the index admission (i.e. alive, dead, and left against medical advice). Those that survived were followed up for 2 years in the post-natal clinic. At each visit, they were reviewed to ascertain presence of deficits in milestone development such as motor, postural, visual, hearing and others. Visual and hearing examination was done using clinical assessment methods such as paediatrics visual chart and sound effects. Where abnormalities are noted, further assessment by an audiologist and eye specialist was sought appropriately. Care-givers of newborns that could not present for follow up were contacted on a 3-monthly basis via phones calls. During the call, information on developmental milestones and date attained were explored. They were also asked for presence of postural, visual, hearing and any other concerns they might have regarding their child's growth and development. Where abnormalities were encountered, care-givers were requested to bring the child to the outpatient clinic for further evaluation.

Measures

All aetiologies of jaundice beyond physiologic and breastfeeding or breast milk jaundice are considered pathologic. Features of pathologic jaundice include the appearance of jaundice within 24 h after birth, a total serum bilirubin level higher than 15 mg/dl (256 µmol/L) in preterm newborns and 20 mg/dl (340 µmol/L) in term babies. Others include rise of unconjugated bilirubin by ≥5 mg/dl (85 µmol/L) in 24 h, prolonged jaundice, elevation of the serum conjugated bilirubin level to ≥2 mg/dl (34 µmol/L) and jaundice with evidence of underlying illnesses such as haemolytic conditions, sepsis, liver pathology etc.

Overview of management of severe hyperbilirubinaemia in NICU of ESUTH

Neonatal jaundice occurring after the 2nd day of life in otherwise healthy babies without other symptoms is sent for urgent serum bilirubin estimation to guide further clinical action. As part of the unit protocols, immediate admission is indicated in jaundice occurring in the 1st of life, levels indicative of pathological jaundice (see above), in preterm, in all sick babies and those with identified risk for bilirubin encephalopathy.

After admission, a thorough history is taken documenting the onset and progress of jaundice, duration, gestational age of the baby at delivery and associated symptoms that signifies imminent risk of encephalopathy such as vomiting, refusal to suckle, weakness, abnormal movements, shrill cry, abnormal breathing etc.

A comprehensive physical examination is also done noting the anatomical level of the jaundice, activity of baby, presence of pallor, vital signs and thorough neurological assessment noting the posture, movement, cry, muscle tone and status of the primitive reflexes. Concurrently, basic laboratory investigations to estimate bilirubin level and identify possible causes are done. These tests include; serum bilirubin level (total and direct), haemoglobin level, random blood sugar, maternal and baby's blood group and rhesus status, G6PD status for males, blood film for malaria parasite and size/ shape of the erythrocyte. Further investigations such as blood culture, serum protein coomb's test, serum electrolyte, urine and stool analysis, abdominal ultrasonography and blood gas are also ordered based on the findings in the history, physical examinations and initial laboratory tests.

Generally, three modalities of treatment are available in our centre and these include; i) Pharmacotherapy using phenobarbitone which increases hepatic uptake and metabolism of bilirubin and usually indicated mainly in preterm babies as adjunct therapy in combination with other treatment modalities. ii) Phototherapy for serum bilirubin up to 2/3rd of the critical level for exchange blood transfusion and iii) Exchange blood transfusion (EBT) is the treatment modality of choice for severe hyperbilirubinaemia in cases where serum bilirubin level reaches up to ≥15 mg/dl in preterm babies; ≥ 20 mg/dl in term babies; and a rise of ≥5 mg/dl in 24 h. However, presence of risk factors for bilirubin encephalopathy like acidosis, sepsis, abnormal neurological findings necessitates EBT even at lower serum bilirubin levels. Most times, combination of these treatment modalities is employed except in cases of conjugated hyperbilirubinaemia where phototherapy is avoided because of the risk of the so called 'Bronze Baby Syndrome' See Fig. 1.

Data entry and analysis

The above measures were documented at presentation in the relevant sections of the questionnaire and subsequently transferred into a Microsoft Excel Sheet. Distribution of the measures were categorized into sub-variables and reported in percentages. Enrollees with significant missing information were excluded from the data analysis. Data were analysed using IBM® SPSS version 18.0 (SPSS Inc., Chicago, IL).

Results

Characteristics of newborns with severe hyperbilirubinaemia

Table 1 shows the main characteristics of newborns enrolled for this study. Of the 1920 newborns admitted to the NICU during the study period, 48 were managed for severe hyperbilirubinaemia giving an in-hospital incidence rate of 25 (95% CI 18–32) per 1000 newborns admitted to the unit. Fifteen (31.2%) of these newborns were delivered within ESUTH while the remainder (68.8%) were delivered outside and referred to the hospital. About two-third of the surveyed newborns were male and term deliveries. Twenty (44.4%) were delivered with low birth weight (< 2.5 kg) and double exchange was the modality of EBT used in the management of severe hyperbilirubinaemia in most (73.9%) cases. Table 2 summaries the baseline parameters of newborns admitted for severe hyperbilirubinaemia during the study period.

Causes and clinical features of severe hyperbilirubinaemia in newborns

Table 3 recapitulates possible causes and clinical features of severe hyperbilirubinaemia in newborns surveyed. In over two-third of newborns (33.3%), no aetiology was apparent after both clinical and laboratory evaluation. Sepsis was a co-morbidity in 35.3% of these newborns while G6PD deficiency was the apparent cause in approximately 11.8% of the cases. Of note, 50% (3/6) of the infants with G6PD deficiency used camphor prior to onset of severe hyperbilirubinaeia.

Other probable causes were Rhesus incompatibility (2%) and ABO incompatibility seen between nine mother-infant pairs (17.6%). Blood groups of mothers included [O+] 14 (68.5%), [O-] 1 (4.5%), [A+] 1 (4.5%), [B +] 4 (18.2%) and [AB+] 2 (9.1%) while those of newborns included [O+] 13 (48%), [A+] 6 (24%) and [B+] 6 (24%).

Fever (17%), refusal to suck (15.2%) and depressed primitive reflexes (24.5%) were the commonest clinical manifestations in newborns with severe hyperbilirubinaemia. Of the depressed reflexes seen, suckling was the most common affected 15/39 (38.5%). Other affected reflexes included Moro's reflex 9/39 (23.1), lateral spinal reflex 6/39 and grasp reflex 3/39 (7.7%). There was global areflexia in 10 (20.8%) newborns. Seven of the newborns managed for severe hyperbilirubinaemia died while still on admission giving a case fatality of 14.5% and one was discharged on parent's request against medical advice (Table 1).

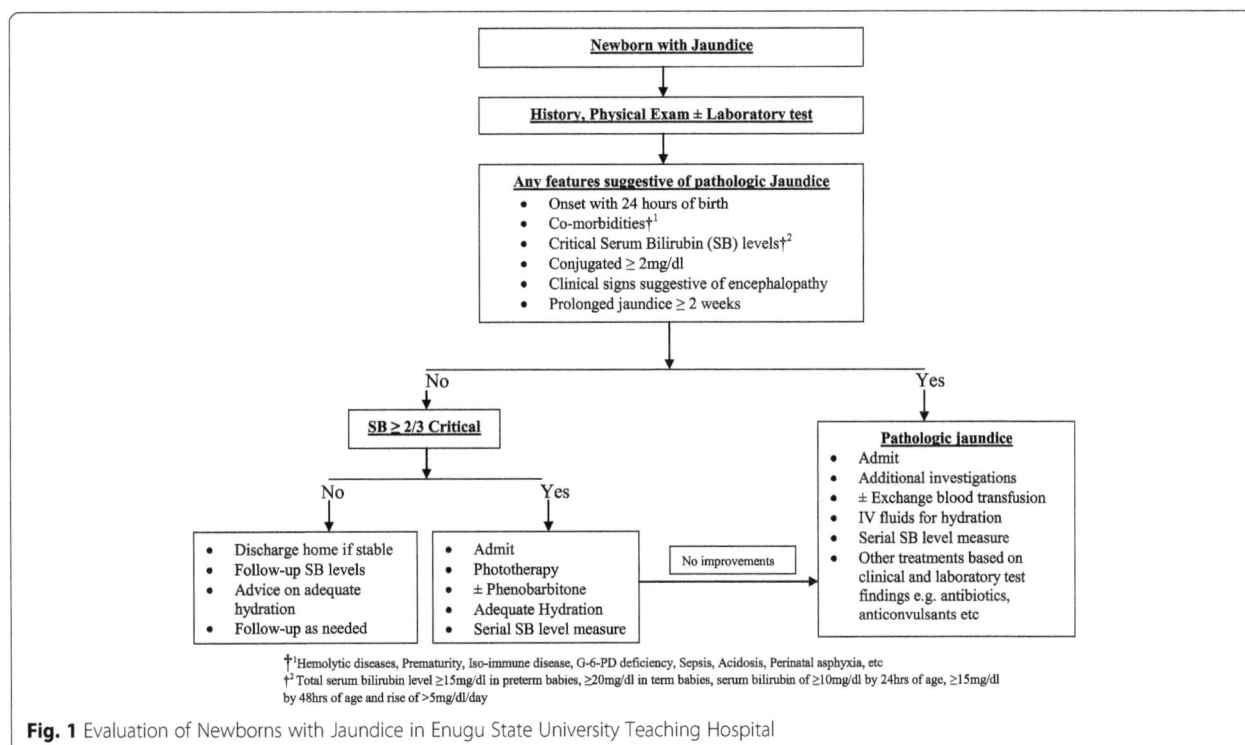

Fig. 1 Evaluation of Newborns with Jaundice in Enugu State University Teaching Hospital

Long-term complications in newborns with severe hyperbilirubinaemia

Newborns managed for severe hyperbilirubinaemia were followed up for approximately 2 years after discharged from the hospital. Over half (25) were lost to follow up due inability to reach parent on phone and/or refusal to attend follow up clinic. Of the 23 remaining newborns successfully followed up, 10 had motor developmental milestone delays which included attainment of neck control between 6 and 12 month, crawling after 1 year, sitting with support at 2 years and walking without support at 2 years. One child had not achieved neck control at the time of follow-up by the age of 2 years. Similarly, six of these children had postural deformity while 4 died before their second birthday (i.e. at 2, 7, 18 and 21 months). Other complications encountered on follow up included visual impairment in one child and seizure disorder in two children. Table 4 shows a cross-tabulation of the complications encountered and some selected demographic characteristics.

Discussion

This study showed a high incidence of severe neonatal hyperbilirubinaemia (25 per 1000 newborns) among neonates in our setting with an incident age range of 1 to 8 days and mean total and unconjugated bilirubin level of 26.0 ± 2.5 and 18.3 ± 9.2 mg/dl. These fit within the parameter for pathological jaundice [1]. The high incidence in our study is comparable to findings from a meta-analysis from 2 different African countries which reported an incidence rate for severe neonatal jaundice of 26.9 and 34.4% in Nigeria and Kenya respectively [5]. These rates are unacceptably high when juxtaposed to the incidence of 1 in 2480 live birth reported in a surveillance study in Canada [6]. The high rate of

Table 1 Demographic characteristics of newborns with severe hyperbilirubinaemia admitted to the Enugu state university teaching hospital

S/N	Characteristic	Variable	Number n	Percentage %
1	Gender (n = 48)	Male	30	62.5
		Female	18	37.5
2	Birth weight (Kg) (n = 45)	< 2.5 kg	20	44.4
		≥ 2.5 kg	25	55.6
3	Gestational Age (Weeks) (n = 45)	Term (≥ 37)	33	68.8
		Pre-term (< 37)	15	31.2
4	Place of birth (n = 48)	Inborn	15	31.2
		Outborn	33	68.8
5	Number of EBT[a1] (n = 46)	Single	12	26.1
		Double	34	73.9
6	Outcome in Hospital (n = 48)	Alive	40	83.3
		Dead	7	14.5
		LAMA[a2]	1	2.2

[a1]EBT exchange blood transfusion
[a2]Left against Medical Advice

Table 2 Baseline parameters of newborns admitted with severe hyperbilirubinaemia in Enugu state university teaching hospital

S/N	Parameters	Mean ± SD	SE	Min value	Max value	Range
1	Birth weight (Kg)	2.7 ± 0.9	0.1	1.2	4.9	3.7
2	Age at onset (days)	3.4 ± 0.5	0.4	1.0	8.0	7.0
3	Time of presentation (days)	4.3 ± 0.4	0.4	1.0	9.0	8.0
4	Total serum bilirubin (g/dl)	26 ± 2.5	2.0	7.1	71.1	64.0
5	Unconjugated serum bilirubin	18.3 ± 9.2	1.7	4.2	46.3	42.1
6	Conjugated serum bilirubin	8.4 ± 8.1	1.5	0.5	25.1	24.6
7	Random blood sugar (mmol/L)	132.7 ± 83.8	16.4	48	450	402

SD for Standard deviation and SE for Standard error

septicaemia in sub-Saharan Africa[7] which was also seen in our study as the commonest comorbidity in newborns with severe hyperbilirubinaemia may account for this wide differences.

The high incidence of clinically significant jaundice seen in our study had no apparent cause in majority of the cases after clinical and laboratory evaluations were done on admission. This complement findings of a similar study in Canada where no cause was identified in 64% of newborns with severe hyperbilirubunaemia [6]. This is approximately twice the proportion of cases with severe hyperbilirubinaemia without an apparent aetiology seen in our study. One plausible explanation might be the lower threshold for diagnosis of sepsis in our setting that accounted for aetiology in more than a third of newborns with severe hyperbilirubinaemia compared to

Table 3 Causes and clinical features of hyperbilirubinaemia in newborns enrolled in Enugu state university teaching hospital

Parameter	Number n[a1]	Percentage %
Causes		
ABO incompatibility	9	17.6
G6PD deficiency[a2]	6	11.8
Sepsis	18	35.3
Rhesus incompatibility	1	2.0
No aetiology seen	17	33.3
Clinical features		
Fever	27	17.0
Convulsion	11	6.9
Refusal to suck	24	15.2
High pitch cry (shrill cry)	19	11.9
Vomiting	10	6.3
Neck retraction	7	4.4
Floppiness (hypotonic)	4	2.5
Stiffness (hypertonic)	11	6.9
Depressed reflexes	39	24.5
Death (while still on admission)	7	4.4

[a1]Multiple causes were noted in some newborns
[a2]G6PD was only tested in male newborns surveyed

0.01% in the referenced study. The other causes of jaundice seen in our study are well known aetiologic factors of severe neonatal jaundice which have been documented in several studies within and outside Nigeria [6–9].

The use of camphor (*Cinnamomum camphora*) also known as naphthalene or moth ball was elicited in the historical assessment of three of the newborns with severe hyperbilirubinaemia in our study. These chemicals are spherical pieces of white solid material containing mostly naphthalene [10]. They are widely used to repel insects especially cockroaches and also as deodorants in some homes in Nigeria. In many instances, mothers place these balls among baby's wears as it is believed to act as a disinfectant as well as an insecticide. Health experts are however of the opinion that like menthol, naphthalene could trigger haemolysis in children that are deficient in G6PD [11]. This was the most likely trigger of haemolysis in 50% of G6PD deficient newborns that presented with severe hyperbilirubinaemia in our study.

The average time of presentation from notice of jaundice by mothers and/or care-giver to admission to the hospital for newborns with severe jaundice recorded in our study was 3.9 to 4.7 days. This delay in presentation to the hospital has previously been reported by the same authors in a study done in the same health facility where it was shown that household (level 1) delays in seeking medical assistance accounted for significant proportion of delays encountered in provision of healthcare to neonates [12]. Additionally, it is possible that the delay in presentation seen in our current study is related to the prevalent belief among most mothers in south-east Nigeria that neonatal jaundice is a trivial disease process which disappears with exposure to sunlight and adequate breast feeding. They therefore only present to hospital when trial of homemade remedies has failed.

Refusal to suck and depressed or absent primitive reflexes were the earliest and commonest clinical presentation see among newborns with severe hyperbilirubinaemia. These may be early signs of bilirubin encephalopathy. Fever was also common in newborns with sepsis. Other common clinical features encountered in these newborns

Table 4 Long-term complication in newborns with severe hyperbilirubinaemia in Enugu state university teaching hospital

S/N	Characteristic	Variable	Motor delays	Postural deformities	Death
			$n = 10$	$n = 6$	$n = 4$
1	Gender	Male	5 (50.0)	4 (66.7)	1 (25.0)
		Female	5 (50.0)	2 (33.3)	3 (75.0)
2	Birth weight (Kg)	< 2.5 kg	4 (40.0)	2 (33.3)	3 (75.0)
		≥ 2.5 kg	6 (60.0)	4 (66.7)	1 (25.0)
3	Gestational Age (Weeks)	Term (≥ 37)	7 (70.0)	5 (83.3)	2 (50.0)
		Pre-term (< 37)	3 (30.0)	1 (16.7)	2 (50.0)
4	Place of birth	Inborn	3 (30.0)	0 (0)	1 (25.0)
		Outborn	7 (70.0)	6 (100)	3 (75.0)

include high pitch cry (shrill cry), convulsion, stiffness and vomiting. These are all well-established signs and symptoms of bilirubin encephalopathy [1]. A case fatality rate of 4.4% was noted among newborns admitted for severe hyperbilirubinaemia in our study which is far higher than the fatality rate of 1.5 recorded in a similar study in Iran [9]. The difference in case fatality between the two studies may be related to the selection of newborns enrolled in both study. While the Iran study recruited and analysed all cases of neonatal jaundice that presented to hospital irrespective of severity, our study focused primarily on newborns with severe hyperbilirubinaemia admitted during the study period. Another study in Iraq which has comparable socio-economic and health indices as our study setting observed a case fatality rate of 21% within 48 h of admission among newborns with severe hyperbilirubinaemia [13]. Unlike our study, this was a retrospective study on newborns with severe hyperbilirubinaemia.

Finally, our study observed neurological sequelae in newborns managed for severe hyperbilirubinaemia after follow-up for 2 years. These included gross motor development abnormalities, postural deformities, seizure disorder and visual impairment. These complications are believed to be caused by damage to the developing brain due to deposition of unconjugated bilirubin. Because of the irreversibility of the damage, every case of jaundice in newborns need aggressive management and close monitoring for signs of worsening severity as documented in this study.

Limitation
The so-called 'Berkson bias' needs to be factored in when interpreting the incidence rate of severe neonatal jaundice seen in this study. Secondly, due to financial and facility constraints we were unable to carry out some more extensive laboratory tests to ascertain other possible causes of severe hyperbilirubinaemia in admitted newborns. Finally, because a significant number of the follow-ups were done over the phone, we cannot with 100% certainty state that the long-term complications encountered in the newborns managed for severe

neonatal jaundice were exclusively due to the disease. Due to recall bias, respondents may have unintentionally omitted important information during follow-up on medical histories of these newborns. Interpretation of the findings of this work should therefore be done in light of these limitations.

Conclusion
The findings of our study show that occurrence of severe hyperbilirubinemia is high and remains a preventable cause of mortality and long-term complications among neonates in south-east Nigeria. Identification of at-risk newborns before discharged together with intensification of efforts among care-givers and healthcare workers in early recognition and timely management could help reduce the burden of this disease on families in particular and the healthcare system in general.

Abbreviations
EBT: Exchange Blood Transfusion; ESUTH: Enugu State University Teaching Hospital; G6PD: Glucose-6-Phosphate Dehydrogenase; NICU: Neonatal Intensive Care Unit

Acknowledgements
The authors wish to thank all the specialist registrars that assisted in data collection during their clinical Neonatal Paediatric posting in the Neonatal Intensive Care Unit. We are also grateful to the highly dedicated staff nurses in the Unit and the Labour ward under the headship of Matron Onovo Priscilla, for their tireless efforts in some study related documentations and heroic efforts in salvaging dying newborns.

Funding
Funding for this study was from equal contributions from all authors. No External funding was received for this study.

Authors' contributions
ODIC and EU conceptualized and designed the study. ODIC drafted the manuscript, analyzed and interpreted the data. EU and ANI supervised the data collection and contributed to the writing of the manuscript. All authors read and approved the final manuscript.

Competing interests
The authors declare that they have no competing interests.

Author details
[1]Child Survival Unit, Medical Research Council UK, The Gambia Unit, Fajara, Banjul, Gambia. [2]Department of Paediatrics, Enugu State University of Science and Technology, Enugu, Enugu State, Nigeria.

References
1. Jaundice and hyperbilirubinemia in the newborn. In: Behrman RE, Kliegman RM, Jenson HB, eds. Nelson Textbook of Pediatrics 16th ed. Philadelphia: Saunders, 2000:511–528.
2. Neonatal Jaundice: Background, pathophysiology and Etiology. Medscape eMedicine 2016. Edited by Thor WR Hansen, Mary L Windle, Brian S Carter and Ted Rosenkrantz.
3. American Academy of Pediatrics. (AAP). Management of hyperbilirubinemia in the newborn infant 35 or more weeks of gestation. Pediatrics. 2004;114(1):297–316.
4. Huang MJ, Kua KE, Teng HC, Tang KS, Weng HW, Huang CS. Risk factors for severe hyperbilirubinemia in neonates. Pediatr Res. 2004;56(5):682–9.
5. Chiara Greco A, Gaston Arnolda J, Nem-Yun Boo C, Iman F, Iskander D, Angela A, Okolo E, Rinawati Rohsiswatmo F, et al. Neonatal jaundice in low- and middle-income countries: lessons and future directions from the 2015 don Ostrow Trieste yellow retreat. Neonatology. 2016;110:172–80.
6. Sgro M, Campbell D, Shah V. Incidence and causes of severe neonatal hyperbilirubinemia in Canada. CMAJ. 2006;175(6):587–90.
7. World Health Organization. Improving the prevention, diagnosis and clinical management of Sepsis Executive Board report EB140/12 140th session 9 January 2017.
8. Olusanya BO, Akande AA, Emokpae A, Olowe SA. Infants with severe neonatal jaundice in Lagos, Nigeria: incidence, correlates and hearing screening outcomes. Trop Med Int Health. 2009;14(3):301–10.
9. Badiee Z. Exchange transfusion in neonatal hyperbilirubinaemia: experience in Isfahan. Iran Singapore Med J. 2007;48(5):421.
10. National Center for Biotechnology Information. PUBCHEM Open Chemistry Database. Available from https://pubchem.ncbi.nlm.nih.gov/compound/camphor.
11. Olowe SA, Ransome-Kuti O. The risk of jaundice in glucose-6-phosphate dehydrogenase deficient babies exposed to menthol. Acta Paediatr Scand. 1980;69(3):341–5.
12. Ekwochi U, Ndu IK, Osuorah CDI, Onah KS, et al. Delays in healthcare delivery to sick neonates in Enugu south-East Nigeria: an analysis of causes and effects. J Public Health. 2015:1–7. https://doi.org/10.1093/pubmed/fdv092.
13. Hameed NN, Na' ma AM, Vilms R, Bhutani VK. Severe neonatal hyperbilirubinemia and adverse short-term consequences in Baghdad, Iraq. Neonatology. 2011;100:57–63.

14

Parental-reported allergic disorders and emergency department presentations for allergy in the first five years of life; a longitudinal birth cohort

Gerben Keijzers[1,2,3*] (iD), Amy Sweeny[1], Julia Crilly[4,5], Norm Good[6], Cate M. Cameron[7,8], Gabor Mihala[9], Rani Scott[8] and Paul A. Scuffham[9]

Abstract

Background: To measure rates of parental-report of allergic disorders and ED presentations for allergic disorders in children, and to describe factors associated with either.

Methods: An existing cohort of 3404 children born between 2006 and 2011 (Environments for Healthy Living) with prospectively collected pre-natal, perinatal and follow-up data were linked to i) nationwide Medicare and pharmaceutical data and ii) Emergency Department (ED) data from four hospitals in Australia. Parental-reported allergy was assessed in those who returned follow-up questionnaires. ED presentation was defined as any presentation for a suite of allergic disorders, excluding asthma. Univariate analysis and multivariate logistic regression were used to descibe risk factors for both parental-reported allergy and ED presentation for an allergic disorder.

Results: The incidence of parental-reported child allergy at 1, 3 and 5 years of age was 7.8, 7.8 and 12.6%, respectively. Independent predictors of parental-report of allergy in multivariate analysis were parental-report of asthma (OR 2.2, 95% CI 1.4–3.4) or eczema (OR 4.3, 95% CI 3.1–6.1) and age > 6 months at introduction of solids (OR 1.3, 95% CI 1.0–1.7). Factors associated with ED presentations for allergy, which occurred in 3.6% of the cohort, were presence of maternal asthma (OR 2.3 95% CI:1.1, 4.9) and child born in spring (OR 1.7, 95% CI 1.1, 2.7).

Conclusions: More than 10% of children up to 5 years have a parental-reported allergic disorder, and 3.6% presented to ED. Parental-report of eczema and/or asthma and late introduction of solids were predictors of parental-report of allergy. Spring birth and maternal asthma were predictors for ED presentation for allergy.

Keywords: Allergy, Anaphylaxis, Birth cohort, Emergency department, Longitudinal study

* Correspondence: Gerben.Keijzers@health.qld.gov.au
[1]Department of Emergency Medicine, Gold Coast University Hospital, 1 Hospital Boulevard, Southport, QLD 4215, Australia
[2]School of Medicine, Bond University, Gold Coast, QLD, Australia
Full list of author information is available at the end of the article

Background

Allergic disorders are common and increasing, especially in children [1]. Allergic disorders consist of a wide spectrum of conditions, including rashes, atopic eczema, and most worryingly anaphylaxis. They represent an immune response to allergens, which are environmental substances that are normally considered harmless [2].

Common known triggers for allergic diseases and/or anaphylaxis include insect stings (especially from the Hymenoptera family of wasps, bees and ants), drugs (especially β-lactam antibiotics), and food (especially nuts, eggs, fish, shellfish and milk) [3]. Allergies seem to be more common in children than in adults, with food allergy prevalence reported between 7 and 10% in children [1].

The cause of the apparent increase in allergic disorders is unclear. Studies on risk factors for the development of allergic disorders have led to a number of meta-analyses of prospective cohort studies [1, 4]. From review articles [5–7] a common emerging theme is that allergic disorders are caused by a complex interrelationship between genetics, environment, and exposures both in-utero and during early infancy [5, 8]. We outline a summary of the literature on risk factors in Additional file 1.

Despite the noted high prevalence of allergic disorders in the community and the mild nature of the majority of allergic disorders, they can occasionally be more severe and anaphylactic reactions can be life-threatening. There are limited data available characterizing patients who present to the Emergency Department (ED) with allergic conditions. One French study [9] reported that allergic disorders represented 1% of all ED presentations, but was conducted nearly 20 years ago and did not report on children less than 10 years of age.

The overall aim of this study was to describe contemporaneous data for allergy presentations to the ED in the first years of life and to provide further understanding of (modifiable) associated risk factors. This study aims to measure the rates of, and describe factors associated with; 1) parental-report of allergy in children, and 2) ED presentations with allergic disorders in children in the first 5 years of life.

Methods

Study design

This study links data on children enrolled in a prospective birth cohort (Environments for Healthy Living [EFHL]: Griffith Birth Cohort study [10], registered *Australian and New Zealand Clinical Trials Registry ACTRN12610000931077*) to data from i) the Emergency Department Information System (EDIS) of four public hospitals, ii) the nationwide Medicare

Benefit Scheme (MBS) and iii) the Pharmaceutical Benefits Scheme (PBS).

Setting

From 2006 to 2011 inclusive, pregnant women from 24 weeks gestation who attended one of the only three public hospitals in the area with a birthing service were enrolled in the EFHL cohort [10]. This area services a population of approximately 800,000 people. A fourth new public hospital ED opened in the area in September 2007. ED data were available for EFHL children for the period from November 2006 to December 2013.

EFHL data

The EFHL dataset included maternal, pregnancy/child, and household data and was collected by self-completed questionnaires by the primary caregiver at enrolment and when their child reached 12 months, 3 and 5 years of age. The baseline survey consisted of 48 self-report items including maternal, household and demographic factors during pregnancy [11]. Parents also provided consent at the time of enrolment to access additional gestational and birth information from hospital perinatal records after the delivery, hospital data and emergency department data.

Study subjects, outcome definition and comparison groups

Study subjects were children born to mothers enrolled in the EFHL study. The primary outcomes of interest included the rate of parental-reported allergic disorders as obtained through questionnaires returned at 1, 3 and 5 years (Table 1), and the rate of ED presentations with an ICD-10 code of allergy or allergic disorder (Fig. 1). Asthma was not included as an allergic disorder. We included 'rash', as an allergic disorder, although other etiologies could be the cause of this diagnosis. As such (sensitivity) analyses were conducted for ED diagnoses of allergy with and without 'rash' included. Mothers or primary caregivers completed the surveys and are hereafter grouped as *parents* for ease of reporting. The one-year questionnaire data was included as source data for potential risk factors (e.g. breast feeding or introduction of solids) for the parental-report of allergy analysis, comparing risk factors amongst children with and without a parental-reported allergy. For the ED presentation analysis, baseline questionnaire data were used to identify risk factors for children with an ED presentation for allergy, compared to children with other ED presentations. For both parental-report and ED presentation analyses, PBS data were utilized. Table 2 summarises the available subjects for both parental-reported allergy analysis and ED presentation analysis.

Table 1 Enrolment into the EFHL cohort study, questionnaire response rates, and consent to Pharmaceutical Benefits Scheme (PBS) linkage

Cohort year	2006	2007	2008	2009	2010	2011	Total
Live births	$n = 631$	$n = 477$	$n = 456$	$n = 628$	$n = 715$	$n = 497$	$n = 3404$
Questionnaire returned at:							
12 months	507 (80.3%)	354 (74.2%)	308 (67.5%)	404 (64.3%)	398 (55.8%)	230 (46.3%)	2201 (64.7%)
3 years	391 (62.0%)	279 (58.5%)	230 (50.4%)	317 (50.5%)	348 (48.8%)		1565 (46.0%)
5 years	271 (42.9%)	196 (41.1%)	181 (39.7%)				648 (19.0%)
Consent given to PBS linkage							
	352 (55.8%)	272 (57.0%)	292 (64.0%)	385 (61.3%)	391 (54.8%)	220 (44.3%)	1912 (56.2%)

EFHL Environments for Healthy Living

Administrative data sources

Table 1 summarizes enrolment and consent timeframes for relevant data sets in this study. The following administrative databases were linked to the EFHL data:

EDIS data

Routinely collected state-wide data from EDIS were extracted from the four public hospitals. This included baseline variables (such as hospital name), ED process variables (i.e. triage category, discharge destination) and clinical variables (i.e. primary presenting complaint and ICD-10 diagnostic codes). The triage scale used in Australia is the Australasian Triage Scale (ATS), a five-tiered scale that categorizes

presentations by urgency, from 1 (immediate review and treatment required) to 5 (treatment/review required within 120 min) [12].

Linkage between EFHL participants and EDIS datasets used a unique identifier and was completed by personnel at the Health Statistics Branch of the Queensland Department of Health, and by the Health Economics and Casemix Unit, Northern NSW Local Health District.

MBS and PBS data

Over half of parents (56%) provided consent to access the Australian government databases of MBS and PBS. Linkage between EFHL and PBS was enabled using participant

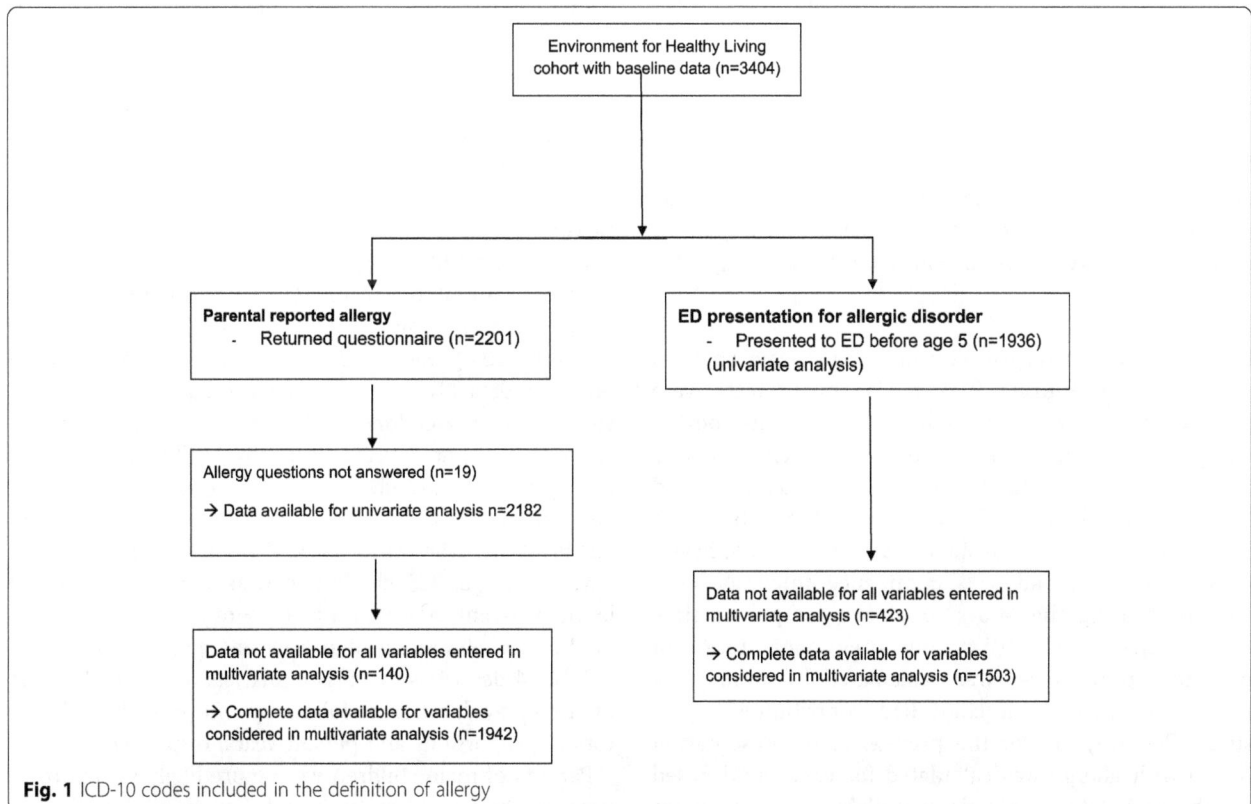

Fig. 1 ICD-10 codes included in the definition of allergy

Table 2 Samples used for analysis of i) self-reported allergy and ii) ED presentation with allergic disorder

ICD-10	Description
J30.1	Hay fever or allergic rhinitis due to pollen
J30.4	Allergic rhinitis, unspecified
J45.0	Allergic rhinitis with asthma or predominantly allergic asthma
J67[a]	Allergic alveolitis and pneumonitis due to inhaled organic dust and particles of fungal, actinomycetic or other origin
K52.2[a]	Allergic gastroenteritis and colitis
L20.0[a]	Atopic dermatitis
L20.8[a]	Atopic dermatitis
L20.9	Atopic dermatitis
L23.0	Allergic contact dermatitis due to metals
L23.9	Allergic contact dermatitis unspecified
L50.0	Allergic urticaria
L50.9	Urticaria, unspecified
R21	Rash and other nonspecific eruptions
T78.0[a]	Anaphylactic shock due to adverse food reaction
T78.2	Anaphylactic shock, unspecified
T78.4	Allergy, NOS
T80.5[a]	Anaphylactic shock due to serum
T88.1	Rash following immunization
T88.6[a]	Anaphylactic shock due to medication properly administered
T88.7	Allergic reaction to medicine properly administered

[a]Although these ICD-10 codes were eligible for inclusion, there were no cases of children in this study with these codes. ICD-10: International Classification of Disease (tenth edition)

Medicare numbers. Linkage to our unique study identifier (ChildID), including manual matching and cleaning of conflicts was completed by Medicare Australia. Only prescriptions supplied prior to presentation date or follow-up time point (1 yr., 3 yr., 5 yr) were counted when comparing medication usage between children with and without allergy.

Statistical analysis

EFHL data was managed with Stata 12.1. Data analyses were undertaken using R [13]. Chi-square tests were used to compare associations between parental-reported allergy and potential risk factors. The presentation rate to ED of children with allergic disorders was calculated based on the whole EFHL cohort ($n = 3404$, Table 1). A p-value of < 0.05 was considered statistically significant. Prevalence rates and 95% confidence intervals were computed using the Mid-p exact test for person-time rates. Person-years (PYs) for prevalence rates of parental-report allergy were calculated by adding the number of years each child had contributed to the study. Person-years for the prevalence of presentation to ED with allergy was calculated for each child based on the last date of ED data available (31 December

2013) minus the child's date of birth, and summed across the cohort. Logistic regression analyses were conducted to identify variables independently associated with parental report of allergy as well as ED diagnosis of allergy (including and excluding 'rash'). For the parental report model, variables significant at a $p < 0.10$ level in the univariate analysis and with complete data on at least 90% of children were considered in a forward stepwise conditional regression model with entry and exit criteria of $p < 0.10$. The same regression technique was used for models determining variables associated with ED presentation for allergy (including and excluding "rash" lead to two separate models). However, because some of the key univariate predictors had > 10% missing data for this model, various models were built on the full sample as well as for subsets with complete data on key variables found to be significant in univariate analysis. Interactions between variables were assessed; significant interactions ($p < .05$) were accounted for in all models. In determining the best model, the number of records, the strength of the associations, the persistence of covariates across models, and the Negelkerke's R square value were considered.

Ethics approval

The Human Research Ethics Committees of both the participating health service districts, and Griffith University approved this study, including linkage of data. For each participant written informed consent was obtained (from the parent or primary caregiver) for completion of a maternal baseline survey, the release of hospital perinatal data related to the birth of their child and linkage of their child's inpatient state hospital records.

Results

Parental-report of allergy in children

Of the 3404 children in EFHL, questionnaire data for at least one time point were available for 2452 unique children (72%), including 2201 children with available one-year data (Table 1). The allergy questions were answered for 2182 children at 1 year, and for 1213 and 627 children at 3 and 5 years, respectively (Table 1). Allergy at any time in the child's life was reported in 7.8% of children at 1 year, in 7.8% of children at 3 years, and in 12.6% of children with 5 years follow-up (Table 3). By 5 years of age, 255 children had an allergy as reported by their parent, representing 10.4% of the starting cohort of children who returned at least one questionnaire.

Table 4 describes univariate analysis of parental report of allergy by duration of follow up and potential risk factors in proportions and person-years, respectively.

Parents of male children were more likely to report allergy in their children at 3 and 5 years (Table 4). The

Table 3 Proportion of children with a parental-report of allergy by age attained, and cumulative prevalence rate of children with parental report of allergy per 1000 person-years

	12 months		3 years		5 years	
	n = 2182		n = 1213		n = 627	
	Person-years =2182		Person-years =4608		Person-years =5862	
	n	(%)	n	%	n	%
Parental reported allergy						
Yes	171	7.8%	93	7.8%	56	12.6%
No	2011	92.2%	1115	92.3%	388	87.4%
Cumulative number of unique children with allergy	171		227		255	
Cumulative prevalence rate per 1000 person-years [95% CI]	78.4 [67.3, 90.8]		49.3 [43.2, 56.0]		43.5 [38.4, 49.1]	

CI confidence interval

cumulative prevalence of allergy for boys over the period was 1.4 times higher than that for girls (Risk Ratio [RR] 1.4 [95% CI 1.2,1.8], Table 4).

Children with three or more other children in the household had a higher risk of allergy compared to children with 0–2 other children in the household (RR = 1.3 [1.0, 1.7], Table 4).

There appeared to be a trend towards lower parental-report of allergy in children who had solids introduced in the first 3 months of life compared to other children, most notable at the 3-year and 5 year time points (Table 4).

At 5 years, parents who were non-smokers during pregnancy reported more allergic disorders in their children than parents who smoked (14.1% vs. 5.6%; $p = 0.03$, Table 4). This finding did not persist when the cumulative rate was considered across all time points (Table 4).

The following (potential risk) factors were not significantly associated with parental-reported allergy in univariate analysis: season of birth, birthweight, maternal education level, household annual income, childcare attendance, breast feeding (ever, and duration), and passive smoking exposure (Table 4).

The logistic regression model considered data on 1942 children; 235 of these had an allergy reported at any time during follow-up. Variables considered in the model were: breast feeding at 12 months, aboriginal or Torres strait island ethnicity (ATSI), birth season, mother's age, mother's education status, other children at home (0,1–2 or 3+), smoking during pregnancy, mother's place of birth, passive smoke exposure, gender, birthweight (< 2500 g and > =2500 g), gestational age (< 37 weeks vs 37+ weeks), age at first food (< 3 months, 3–6 months, 6+ months), child has asthma, child has eczema, and child care (ever) (data not shown). The interaction term of parental-report eczema and parental-report asthma was significant ($p = 0.003$), with a parental-report of asthma or eczema (+/− asthma) significantly associated with parental-report allergy. These variables were thus combined in the model as one variable according to the magnitude of their effect on self-report allergy, with a coding of neither (reference), parental-report of asthma (but

no eczema), and parental-report of eczema (with or without asthma).

The following variables were univariately statistically significantly associated with parental-reported allergy: birthweight (continuous), age at first food, child has asthma, child has eczema, child care (ever). When combined with other potentially predictive variables, Table 5 shows the best model identified included the following significant variables: parental-report of asthma (adjusted Odds Ratio: aOR 2.2, 95% CI 1.4–3.4), parental-report of eczema (aOR 4.3, 95% CI 3.1–6.1) whether the child had attended childcare (aOR 1.4, 95% CI 1.1–1.9), and age of first solid intake > 6 months (aOR 1.3, 95% CI 1.0–1.7).

ED presentations with allergic disorders

There were a total of 5118 ED presentations in this cohort of children aged 0–5 years. Allergic disorders (not including asthma), accounted for 3.6% (182) of these presentations from 160 of the 3404 children in the cohort. The median ED length of stay was 1.9 h. Fifteen children (8.2%) were admitted to hospital; most were assigned an Australian Triage Scale (ATS) category 3 (59%) or 4 (23%), with 14% receiving a more urgent classification (ATS 2; 13% and ATS 1; 1.1%).

Over one-third of presentations (66 of 182) with allergic disorders occurred during the first year of life (Table 6). There were two presentations due to anaphylaxis yielding a prevalence of 0.59 per 1000 PYs for anaphylaxis in the first 5 years of life.

By 12 months of age, 1.8%, of the cohort had presented to ED with an allergic disorder. There was a decreasing cumulative prevalence of allergy presentation to ED, from 19.4 per 1000 person-years to 13.0 per 1000 person years as the children grew older (Table 6). ED presentation with allergy by 1 year of age occurred at a quarter of the rate of parental report of allergy (19.4 per 1000 PY compared to 78.4 per 1000 PY, Tables 3 and 6).

Univariate analysis showed that children who presented to the ED with an allergy during the first 5 years of life were more likely to be born in spring and have a

Table 4 Parental-report of allergy by child's age at follow-up and for all ages combined, and potential risk factors

Characteristic	12 months (n = 2182)			3 years (n = 1213)			5 years (n = 627)			All ages combined		
	Total N	n with allergy	% with allergy	Total N	n with allergy	% with allergy	Total N	n with allergy	% with allergy	Total person-years	Rate ratio	RR [95% CI]
Gender												
Male	1094	93	8.5%	571	56	9.8%*	211	36	17.1%**	2658	69.6	1.4 [1.2,1.8]
Female	1028	74	7.2%	607	37	6.1%	226	19	8.4%	2693	48.3	1.0 (Reference)
Maternal Indigenous status												
Not indigenous	2065	159	7.7%	1177	93	7.9%	433	55	12.7%	5286	58.1	1.0 (Reference)
ATSI	29	4	13.8%	0	0	0.0%	0	0	0.0%	29	138.0	1.8 [0.6, 4.7]
Birthweight												
< 2500 g	59	7	11.8%	33	3	9.1%	0	0	0.0%	125	79.8	1.3 [0.7, 2.5]
≥ 2500 g	1905	160	8.4%	1154	90	7.8%	426	55	12.9%	4212	59.3	1.0 (Reference)
Season of birth												
Summer/Spring	1873	148	7.9%	958	68	7.1%	389	44	11.3%	4568	56.9	1.0 (Reference)
Autumn/Winter	301	22	7.3%	240	25	10.4%	56	12	21.4%	894	66.0	1.2 [0.8, 1.5]
Maternal education												
Did not complete high school	312	29	9.3%	186	21	11.3%	64	7	10.9%	812	70.2	1.2 [0.9, 1.6]
Completed high school	1679	141	8.4%	1000	72	7.2%	380	49	12.9%	4438	59.0	1.0 (Reference)
Household income (annual)												
< $40,000	347	26	7.5%	175	11	6.3%	60	11	18.3%	816	58.8	0.8 [0.7, 1.1]
$40,000 - $70,000	635	47	7.4%	357	25	7.0%	144	15	10.4%	1638	53.1	
≥ $70,000	906	77	8.5%	511	47	9.2%	188	24	12.8%	2303	64.3	1.0 (Reference)
Other children living in household												
0	973	72	7.4%	492	32	6.5%	176	25	14.2%	2310	55.9	1.0 (Reference: 0–2)
1–2	734	47	6.4%	418	33	7.9%	167	18	10.8%	1903	51.5	
3 or more	532	50	9.4%	276	27	9.8%	95	13	13.7%	1273	70.7	1.3 [1.0, 1.7]
Child care attendance (in first year of life)												
Yes	571	52	9.1%	816	62	7.6%	Not applicable			2203	51.7	1.0 (Reference)
No	1575	115	7.3%	380	30	7.9%				2335	62.1	1.2 [0.9, 1.5]
Breast feeding before discharged newborn												
Yes	1072	89	8.3%	524	33	6.3%	204	23	11.3%	2527	57.4	1.2 [0.7, 2.1]

Table 4 Parental-report of allergy by child's age at follow-up and for all ages combined, and potential risk factors (Continued)

Characteristic	12 months (n = 2182)			3 years (n = 1213)			5 years (n = 627)			All ages combined		
	Total N	n with allergy	% with allergy	Total N	n with allergy	% with allergy	Total N	n with allergy	% with allergy	Total person-years	Rate ratio	RR [95% CI]
No	106	5	4.7%	51	5	9.8%	30	3	10.0%	268	48.4	1.0 (Reference)
Not asked	935	72	7.7%	604	55	9.1%	200	29	14.5%	2544	61.3	Not included
Ever breast-fed by 12 months of age												
Yes	2025	160	7.9%	1053	80	7.6%	408	53	13.0%	4946	59.2	1.1 [0.6, 1.9]
No	132	9	6.8%	63	5	7.9%	0	0	0.0%	259	54.1	1.0 (Reference)
Breastfeeding duration												
0–3 months	720	59	8.2%	361	26	7.2%	138	17	12.3%	1718	59.4	1.0 (Reference all < 6 months)
3–6 months	388	31	8.0%	196	9	4.6%	77	9	11.7%	933	52.5	
>6 months	500	36	7.2%	276	27	9.8%	105	19	18.1%	1261	65.0	1.1 [0.9, 1.5]
Age at first consumption of solids												
0–3 months	286	24	8.4%	143	5	3.5%	48	5	10.4%	668	50.9	1.0 (Reference all < 6 months)
3–6 months	1759	139	7.9%	916	76	8.3%	350	42	12.0%	4291	59.9	
>6 months	92	7	7.6%	55	5	9.1%	26	6	23.1%	254	70.9	1.2 [0.8, 1.9]
Smoking during pregnancy												
Yes	423	41	9.7%	247	19	7.7%	89	5	5.6%*	1095	59.4	1.0 [0.8, 1.3]
No	1743	129	7.4%	949	74	7.8%	355	50	14.1%	4350	58.2	1.0 (Reference)
Use of antibiotics (in first year of life)												
None	335	69	20.6%**	232	44	19%***	41	7	17.1%	880	136.4	2.3 [1.6, 3.2][a]
1–4 prescriptions	226	21	9.3%	167	12	7.2%	47	7	14.9%	653	61.2	4.2 [2.3, 8.4][b]
5+ prescriptions	34	4	11.7%	128	5	3.9%	7	1	13.9%	305	32.8	

ATSI Aboriginal or Torres Strait Islander, CI Confidence Interval
[a]Reference group for nil prescriptions vs. 1–4
[b]Reference group for nil prescriptions vs. 5 +
* $p < .05$; **$p < .01$; ***$p < .001$, Reference = reference group

Table 5 Logistic regression results: Variables significantly associated with parental report of allergy by 5 years of age in 1942 children from a birth cohort

Variable	Total children (n)	Self-report allergy (%)	Crude odds ratio (95% CI)	P value	Adjusted odds ratio (95% CI)	P value
Child care status:						
Attended childcare	1283	12.9%	1.4 (1.1, 1.8)	0.017	1.4 (1.1, 1.9)	0.019
Did not attend childcare	994	9.7%	1.0[a]		1.0[a]	
Other self-report conditions:						
Child has neither eczema nor asthma	1742	8.8%	1.0[a]		1.0[a]	<.001
Child has asthma but no eczema	176	16.5%	2.0 (1.3, 3.1)	<.001	2.2 (1.4,3.4)	
Child has eczema (+/− asthma)	248	28.6%	4.1 (3.0, 5.7)	<.000	4.3 (3.1,6.1)	
Age (months) at first food						
< 3 months	68	7.4%	NA	0.07[b]	1.0[ac]	
Between 3 and 6 months	1403	11.3%			1.0[ac]	
6 months and older	635	13.5%			1.3 (1.0, 1.7)[c]	0.05

[a]Reference category
[b]chi-square for linear trend
[c]< 3 and 3–6 months combined as reference group

mother with asthma. (Table 7). These findings persisted in the multivariate analysis as shown in Table 8, with an adjusted odds ratio for ED presentation with allergy (including diagnosis of rash) of 1.7 [95% CI 1.1–2.7] and 2.3 [95% CI 1.1–4.9], respectively. The same variables were found to be independent predictors of similar magnitude if diagnoses of 'rash' were excluded (Table 9).

There were no statistically significant differences in gender, mother's socioeconomic status, the number of children living in the household, breastfeeding duration,

or the age at introduction of solids for children presenting with an allergy compared to other ED presentations (Table 7).

Discussion

This study used prospectively collected antenatal, perinatal and follow-up data from an existing birth cohort to study allergic disorders children under the age of 5 years, including their presentations to ED.

Our study was consistent with the existing literature for several other known risk factors for allergy such as male gender [14], birth in spring [15], co-existent eczema and asthma as well as timing of introduction of solids. Consistent with others we also found no association with breast feeding, parental education or household income [16].

Table 6 Number and cumulative prevalence rate of presentations to ED with an allergic disorder, by age group

Allergic disorder - type	By 12 months, n	by 3 years, n	by 5 years, n
Rash	36	62	70
Allergic reaction, NOS	6	27	40
Urticaria, NOS	8	24	30
Adverse reaction to medication	4	10	11
Allergic contact dermatitis	6	11	16
Allergic rhinitis	1	5	8
Atopic dermatitis	3	3	3
Anaphylaxis	1	1	2
Other	1	2	2
Total presentations, n	66	145	182
Total person-years	3404	9871	14,023
Prevalence per 1000 person-years [95%CI]	19.4 [15.1, 24.5]	14.7 [12.4, 17.2]	13.0 [11.2, 15.0]

ED Emergency Department, CI Confidence Interval, NOS Not otherwise specified

The introduction of solids or potentially allergenic foods has received increased attention recently. While earlier recommendations suggested delayed introduction or avoidance of dairy products, fish and nuts in high-risk infants [17, 18], two recent randomised controlled studies have provided convincing data that early introduction does not cause allergy and may even be protective [19, 20]. Our study was consistent with these latter studies, suggesting an increased risk of allergy with later commencement of solids (Table 5). By virtue of the design of our study, we cannot exclude that this association of delayed solid introduction and allergy could be an example of reverse causation, where families at higher risk introduced solid foods later.

The "Hygiene Hypothesis" [21] proposes that increased incidence in allergies are linked to reduced exposure to microorganisms. Exposure to other children

Table 7 Characteristics of children presenting to ED in the first five years of life: children presenting with allergy compared to all other children presenting

Characteristic	Child with allergy presentation (n = 160)		Child with other ED presentation (n = 1776)	
	n	%	n	%
Gender				
Male	83	52.9%	948	54.2%
Female	74	47.1%	801	45.8%
Maternal Indigenous status				
Not indigenous	151	98.1%	1665	97.8%
ATSI	3	1.9%	37	2.2%
Birthweight				
< 2500 g	3	1.9%	43	2.5%
≥ 2500 g	155	98.1%	1704	97.5%
Season of birth*				
Spring[a]	113	70.6%	1064	59.9%
Summer	13	8.1%	267	15.0%
Autumn	4	2.5%	56	3.2%
Winter	30	18.8%	389	21.9%
Maternal education				
Did not complete high school	41	25.6%	376	21.2%
Completed high school	119	74.4%	1400	78.8%
Household income (annual)				
< $40,000	38	27.9%	335	22.7%
$40,000 - $70,000	40	29.4%	509	34.5%
> $70,000	58	42.6%	632	42.8%
Mother's country of birth				
Australia/ New Zealand	99	61.9%	1069	60.2%
Other	61	38.1%	707	39.8%
Other children living in household				
0	37	35.9%	463	41.4%
1–2	59	57.3%	564	50.4%
3 or more	7	6.8%	91	8.1%
Mother has asthma*				
Yes[b]	9	8.0%	53	3.7%
No	103	92.0%	1365	96.3%
Child care attendance by 1 yr				
Yes	30	27.3%	318	27.0%
No	80	72.7%	861	73.0%
Child care attendance by 3 yrs				
Yes	43	61.4%	590	69.7%
No	27	38.6%	257	30.3%
Breast feeding before discharged newborn				
Yes	87	54.4%	1022	57.5%
No	9	5.6%	117	6.6%
Not asked	64	40.0%	637	35.9%
Breast feeding duration				

Table 7 Characteristics of children presenting to ED in the first five years of life: children presenting with allergy compared to all other children presenting *(Continued)*

Characteristic	Child with allergy presentation (n = 160)		Child with other ED presentation (n = 1776)	
	n	%	n	%
0–3 months	16	25.0%	213	27.8%
3–6 months	16	25.0%	185	24.1%
> 6 months	32	50.0%	369	48.1%
Age at first consumption of solids				
0–3 months	3	2.9%	47	4.1%
3–6 months	70	68.6%	754	65.9%
> 6 months	29	28.4%	344	30.0%
Smoking during pregnancy				
Yes	44	27.8%	460	26.0%
No	114	72.2%	1311	74.0%
Epi-pen prescribed				
none	159	99.4%	1768	99.5%
1+ prescriptions	1	0.6%	8	0.5%
Use of corticosteroids				
none	143	89.4%	1586	89.3%
1+ prescriptions	17	10.6%	190	10.7%
Use of antibiotics				
none	149	92.6%	1613	89.9%
1+ prescriptions	11	7.4%	163	10.1%

ED Emergency Department, *ATSI* Aboriginal or Torres Strait Islander
[a]RR (95% CI) for spring compared to all other seasons = 1.6 (1.1–2.2)
[b]RR (95% CI) for mother with asthma = 2.1 (1.1, 3.9)
*$p < 0.05$

[16, 22] as well as attending day-care [23], have been associated with decrease in allergic disorders. Our study considered these potential exposures, but did not find clear support for this hypothesis in univariate and multivariate modelling.

Parental-report of child allergies occurred at 4 times the level of ED presentation. This is likely explained by the chronic or recurrent nature of certain allergic disorders, such as eczema or atopic dermatitis, which may lead to parents to seek medical attention in the setting of a primary care physician (GP) or outpatient paediatrician, or possibly not seek care at all, rather than attend an ED.

Limitations

Not all parents consented to linkage with the PBS database and loss to follow-up occurred. As a result, the study may have been underpowered to find significant associations for known risk factors, although most point estimates findings were consistent with the existing literature. Also, due to the loss to follow-up, selection bias may have been introduced. Nevertheless, we have no reason to believe children with allergic disorders would have a different rate of loss to follow-up than others. We excluded asthma from our analysis, since our focus was on children between 0 and 5 years where diagnosis of

Table 8 Logistic regression results: Variables significantly associated with ED presentation with allergy (including rash) vs any other condition, by 5 years of age

Variable	Total children (n)	Self-report allergy (%)	Crude odds ratio (95% CI)	P value	Adjusted odds ratio (95% CI)	P value
Season of birth						
Spring	1177	9.6%	1.6 (1.1, 2.3)	0.008	1.7 (1.1, 2.7)	0.011
Other season	759	6.2%	1.0†		1.0[a]	
Mother has asthma						
Yes	62	14.5%	2.3 (1.1,4.7)	0.026	2.3 (1.1,4.9)	0.025
No	1468	7.0%	1.0†		1.0†	

[a]Reference category

Table 9 Logistic regression results. Variables significantly associated with ED presentation with allergy (excluding rash) vs any other condition, by 5 years of age

Variable	Total children (n)	Self-report allergy (%)	Crude odds ratio (95% CI)	P value	Adjusted odds ratio (95% CI)	P value
Season of birth						
Spring	1131	5.9%	1.7 (1.1, 2.7)	0.02	2.2 (1.2, 4.0)	0.011
Other season	738	3.5%	1.0[a]		1.0[a]	
Mother has asthma						
Yes	59	10.2%	2.9 (1.2,6.9)	0.015	3.0 (1.2,7.3)	0.016
No	1419	3.8%	1.0[a]		1.0[a]	

[a]Reference category

asthma is challenging, due to their inability to provide reliable spirometry and the host of competing diagnoses such as bronchiolitis and reactive airway disease [24]. We acknowledge including asthma may have lead to different findings. ED diagnosis of allergy included patients with a diagnosis of 'rash', which accounted for half of the ED presentations in the first year of life for allergy and 40% of all presentations. We did not have approval to access patients' individual medical record and are unable to comment on the exact etiology. A separate audit suggested more than half of these children have an allergic etiology. We conducted a sensitivity analysis by conducting logistic regression with and without patients with 'rash' and found a consistent result. As such we have decided to keep patients with rash in our descriptive analyses. We used ICD-10 coding for ED diagnosis which may have led to misclassification. For example, we noted very few cases of anaphylaxis, although our estimated incidence falls within previously reported ranges [25]. Furthermore, we cannot comment on the accuracy of parental report of allergy. Parental-report is considered a valid measurement for allergy, especially as a follow up measurement for a large cohort where patients are not routinely reviewed by a clinician [26].

Parental-report of allergy was unable to be further subdivided to examine specific drug or food associations. We had access to a detailed baseline database, but not all relevant possible predictors may have been included. Lastly, despite having access to multiple datasets, data entry and linkage may have been incomplete.

Conclusion

In this birth cohort from southeast Queensland, more than 10% of children in the frist 5 years of life had an allergic disorder reported, with 3.6% of the cohort presenting to an ED with an allergic disorder. Parental report of eczema and/or asthma as well as introduction of solids after 6 months of age were significantly associated with parental report of allergy. Spring birth and a mother with asthma were independent predictors for an ED presentation for allergy.

Abbreviations

ATS: Australian Triage Scale; CI: Confidence Interval; ED: Emergency Department; EDIS: Emergency Department Information System; EFHL: Environments for Healthy Living; GP: General Practitioner (Family Doctor); ICD-10: International Classification of Disease – tenth edition; MBS: Medicare Benefit Scheme; NSW: New South Wales; PBS: Pharmaceutical Benefit Scheme; PY: Person year; RR: Relative Risk

Acknowledgements

The research reported in this publication is part of the Griffith Study of Population Health: Environments for Healthy Living (EFHL) (Australian and New Zealand Clinical Trials Registry: ACTRN12610000931077). Core funding to support EFHL is provided by Griffith University. The EFHL project was conceived by Professor Rod McClure, Dr. Cate Cameron, Professor Judy Searle, and Professor Ronan Lyons. We are thankful for the contributions of the Project Manager, and current and past Database Managers. We gratefully acknowledge the administrative staff, research staff, and the hospital antenatal and birth suite midwives of the participating hospitals for their valuable contributions to the study, in addition to the expert advice provided by Research Investigators throughout the project. We also would like to acknowledge Rania Shibl (database manager), Dr. Syed Fasihullah, (Pediatrician, Gold Coast University Hospital), Dr. Stuart Young (Director, Emergency department, Logan Hospital), Dr. Rob Davies (Director, Emergency department, The Tweed Hospital) and Dr. Jae Thone (Gold Coast University Hospital) for the support of this project.

Funding

This research was funded by a Queensland Emergency Medicine Research Foundation grant. This not for profit foundation had no role in methodology, design, data collection and analysis nor in the interpretation of data.Dr. Cameron was supported by a Public Health Fellowship (ID 428254) from the National Health and Medical Research Council.

Authors' contributions

GK: Design, ethics, funding, data interpretation, manuscript preparation, AS: Data analysis and manuscript preparation, JC: Design, ethics, funding, data interpretation, manuscript preparation, NG: Statistical analysis, manuscript review, CC: Design, funding, data interpretation, manuscript review, GM: Cohort data and data linkage manager, manuscript review, RS: Cohort project manager, design, funding, manuscript review, PS: Design, ethics, funding, data interpretation, manuscript preparation. All authors have read and approved the final manuscript.

Competing interests

The authors declare they have no competing interests.

Author details

[1]Department of Emergency Medicine, Gold Coast University Hospital, 1 Hospital Boulevard, Southport, QLD 4215, Australia. [2]School of Medicine, Bond University, Gold Coast, QLD, Australia. [3]School of Medicine, Griffith University, Gold Coast, QLD, Australia. [4]Department of Emergency Medicine, Gold Coast Health, Gold Coast, QLD, Australia. [5]Menzies Health Institute, Gold Coast, QLD, Australia. [6]CSIRO Digitial Productivity/ Australian e-Health

Research Centre, Royal Women's and Children's Hospital, Brisbane, QLD, Australia. [7]Jamieson Trauma Institute, Royal Brisbane & Women's Hospital, Metro North Hospital and Health Service, Herston, QLD, Australia. [8]Menzies Health Institute Queensland, Griffith University, Meadowbrook, QLD, Australia. [9]Menzies Health Institute Queensland, Griffith University, Nathan, QLD, Australia.

References

1. Yang YW, Tsai CL, Lu CY. Exclusive breastfeeding and incident atopic dermatitis in childhood: a systematic review and meta-analysis of prospective cohort studies. Br J Dermatol. 2009;161:373–83.

2. Kay AB. Allergy and allergic diseases. First of two parts. N Engl J Med. 2001;344:30–7.

3. Melville N, Beattie T. Paediatric allergic reactions in the emergency department: a review. Emerg Med J. 2008;25:655–8.

4. Koplin J, Allen K, Gurrin L, Osborne N, Tang ML, Dharmage S. Is caesarean delivery associated with sensitization to food allergens and IgE-mediated food allergy: a systematic review. Pediatr Allergy Immunol. 2008;19:682–7.

5. Sicherer SH, Leung DY. Advances in allergic skin disease, anaphylaxis, and hypersensitivity reactions to foods, drugs, and insects in 2014. J Allergy Clin Immunol. 2015;135:357–67.

6. Kuo CH, Kuo HF, Huang CH, Yang SN, Lee MS, Hung CH. Early life exposure to antibiotics and the risk of childhood allergic diseases: an update from the perspective of the hygiene hypothesis. J Microbiol Immunol Infect. 2013;46:320–9.

7. Lack G. Update on risk factors for food allergy. J Allergy Clin Immunol. 2012; 129:1187–97.

8. Campbell DE, Boyle RJ, Thornton CA, Prescott SL. Mechanisms of allergic disease–environmental and genetic determinants for the development of allergy. Clin Exp Allergy. 2015;45:844–58.

9. Bellou A, Manel J, Samman-Kaakaji H, et al. Spectrum of acute allergic diseases in an emergency department: an evaluation of one years' experience. Emerg Med (Fremantle). 2003;15:341–7.

10. Cameron CM, Scuffham PA, Spinks A, et al. Environments for healthy living (EFHL) Griffith birth cohort study: background and methods. Matern Child Health J. 2012;16:1896–905.

11. Cameron CM, Scuffham PA, Shibl R, et al. Environments for healthy living (EFHL) Griffith birth cohort study: characteristics of sample and profile of antenatal exposures. BMC Public Health. 2012;12:1–11.

12. Australasian College for Emergency Medicine. Policy on the Australasian triage scale. 4th ed; 2013. p. P06. Available from URL: https://acem.org.au/getmedia/484b39f1-7c99-427b-b46e-005b0cd6ac64/P06-Policy-on-the-ATS-Jul-13-v04.aspx. Last Accessed 15 May 2018.

13. R Development Core Team. R: A language and environment for statistical computing. Vienna: R Foundation for Statistical Computing; 2013.

14. Savage J, Johns CB. Food allergy: epidemiology and natural history. Immunol Allergy Clin N Am. 2015;35:45–59.

15. Zeiger R, Heller S, Mellon M, Halsey J, Hamburger R, Sampson H. Genetic and environmental factors affecting the development of atopy through age 4 in children of atopic parents: a prospective randomized study of food allergen avoidance. Pediatr Allergy Immunol. 1992;3:110–27.

16. Schmitz R, Atzpodien K, Schlaud M. Prevalence and risk factors of atopic diseases in German children and adolescents. Pediatr Allergy Immunol. 2012;23:716–23.

17. American College of Allergy A, & Immunology. Food allergy: a practice parameter. Ann Allergy Asthma Immunol. 2006;96:S1–68.

18. Garcia-Ara C, Boyano-Martinez T, Diaz-Pena JM, Martin-Munoz F, Reche-Frutos M, Martin-Esteban M. Specific IgE levels in the diagnosis of immediate hypersensitivity to cows' milk protein in the infant. J Allergy Clin Immunol. 2001;107:185–90.

19. Du Toit G, Roberts G, Sayre PH, et al. Randomized trial of peanut consumption in infants at risk for peanut allergy. N Engl J Med. 2015;372:803–13.

20. Perkin MR, Logan K, Tseng A, et al. Randomized trial of introduction of allergenic foods in breast-fed infants. N Engl J Med. 2016;374:1733–43.

21. Strachan DP. Hay fever, hygiene, and household size. BMJ. 1989;299:1259–60.

22. Koplin JJ, Dharmage SC, Ponsonby AL, et al. Environmental and demographic risk factors for egg allergy in a population-based study of infants. Allergy. 2012;67:1415–22.

23. Boneberger A, Haider D, Baer J, et al. Environmental risk factors in the first year of life and childhood asthma in the central south of Chile. J Asthma. 2011;48:464–9.

24. Khetan R, Hurley M, Neduvamkunnil A, Bhatt JM. Fifteen-minute consultation: AN evidence-based approach to the child with preschool wheeze. Arch Dis Child Educ Pract Ed. 2018;103(1):7–14. https://doi.org/10.1136/archdischild-2016-311254. Epub 2017 Jun 30

25. Piromrat K, Chinratanapisit S, Trathong S. Anaphylaxis in an emergency department: a 2-year study in a tertiary-care hospital. Asian Pac J Allergy Immunol. 2008;26(2–3):121–8.

26. Gunaratne AW, Makrides M, Collins CT. Maternal prenatal and/or postnatal n-3 long chain polyunsaturated fatty acids (LCPUFA) supplementation for preventing allergies in early childhood. Cochrane Database Syst Rev. 2015;7: Cd010085.

15

Feasibility and utility of active case finding of HIV-infected children and adolescents by provider-initiated testing and counselling: evidence from the Laquintinie hospital in Douala, Cameroon

Calixte Ida Penda[1,2*], Carole Else Eboumbou Moukoko[2], Daniele Kedy Koum[1], Joseph Fokam[3,4], Cedric Anatole Zambo Meyong[2], Sandrine Talla[5] and Paul Koki Ndombo[4,6]

Abstract

Background: Universal HIV testing and treatment of infected children remain challenging in resource-limited settings (RLS), leading to undiagnosed children/adolescents and limited access to pediatric antiretroviral therapy (ART). Our objective was to evaluate the feasibility of active cases finding of HIV-infected children/adolescents by provider-initiated testing and counseling in a health facility.

Methods: A cross-sectional prospective study was conducted from January through April 2016 at 6 entry-points (inpatient, outpatient, neonatology, immunization/family planning, tuberculosis, day-care units) at the Laquintinie Hospital of Douala (LHD), Cameroon. At each entry-point, following counseling with consenting parents, children/adolescents (0–19 years old) with unknown HIV status were tested using the Rapid Diagnostic Test (RDT) (Determine®) and confirmed with a second RDT (Oraquick®) according to national guidelines. For children less than 18 months, PCR was performed to confirm every positive RDT. Community health workers linked infected participants by accompanying them from the entry-point to the treatment centre for an immediate ART initiation following the « test and treat » strategy. Statistical analysis was performed, with $p < 0.05$ considered significant.

Results: Out of 3439 children seen at entry-points, 2107 had an unknown HIV status (61.3%) and HIV testing acceptance rate was 99.9% (2104). Their mean age was 2.1 (Sd = 2.96) years, with a sex ratio boy/girl of 6/5. HIV prevalence was 2.1% (44), without a significant difference between boys and girls ($p = 0.081$). High rates of HIV-infection were found among siblings/descendants (22.2%), TB treatment unit attendees (11.4%) and hospitalized children/adolescents (5.6%); $p < 0.001$. Up to 95.4% (42/44) of those infected children/adolescents were initiated on ART. Overall, 487 (23.2%) deaths were registered (122 per month) and among them, 7 (15.9%) were HIV-positive; mainly due to tuberculosis and malnutrition.

Conclusion: The consistent rate of unknown HIV status among children/adolescents attending health facilities, the high acceptability rates of HIV testing and linkage to ART, underscore the feasibility and utility of an active case finding model, using multiple entry-points at the health facility, in achieving the 90–90–90 targets for paediatric HIV/AIDS in RLS.

Keywords: HIV testing, Children, Adolescents, Entry points, MTCT, Cameroon

* Correspondence: idapenda@yahoo.fr
[1]Clinical sciences department, Faculty of Medicine and Pharmaceutical Sciences, University of Douala, PO Box 2071, Douala, Cameroon
[2]HIV Care and Treatment Centre, Laquintinie Hospital of Douala, Douala, Cameroon
Full list of author information is available at the end of the article

Background

Paediatric HIV/AIDS remains a public health priority in children and adolescents worldwide, with 150,000 new infections occurring among children in 2015 [1], with over seventy-nine thousand (79,771) children and adolescents aged 0–19 years were living with HIV and almost half of them were 10 years and older during the same year [1, 2]. Most HIV-infected children are diagnosed late, at an advanced stage of disease progression [2, 3]. This programmatic challenge is of great concern because without antiretroviral therapy (ART), 53% of HIV-positive children die before their second birthday [4]. Thus, challenges in ensuring universal paediatric HIV testing and linkage to care are the driving force in reducing the gap between paediatric coverage and antiretroviral therapy (ART). Out the 1.8 million children living with HIV under the age of 15, only half are on ART worldwide, 20% of them in West and Central Africa in 2015 [5, 6]. Of note, at the time when paediatric ARVs were introduced in Cameroon in 2003, the number of HIV-infected children under 15 years was estimated at 50,334 and 50,284 for those in need of treatment. Though free access to ART (effective since 2007), coupled to progress in the WHO recommendations, has doubled the number of HIV-positive children accessing ART in Cameroon (3114 in 2007 to 6099 [11%] in 2014), the number children in need of ART (51,910 in 2014) remains very high, in the frame of a persistent paediatric HIV incidence nationwide (i.e. 4100 new infections reported in 2015) [7].

Several initiatives to scale up paediatric care have been implemented in recent years: i) the global Elimination Plan of MTCT in 2011 ii) the "Double Dividend" Initiative in 2013 through joint efforts of UNICEF, EGPAF and WHO with the dual goal of ending paediatric HIV epidemic and improving child survival in high HIV prevalence settings; and iii) "Accelerate Children's HIV/AIDS Treatment Initiative" by PEPFAR and UNAIDS [8]. Cameroon has endorsed the UNAIDS strategic 90–90-90 targets: 90% of HIV-infected children and adolescents know their status, 90% of HIV-infected children who know their status are receiving ART and 90% of ART-experienced children have viral suppression [9]. Timely achievement of these targets requires implementing the "Test early, Test closer and Treat earlier" approach for every child and adolescent at all entry points of health facilities [8–10]. Successful implementation of this approach in linking to care warrants an assessment of HIV testing and access to ARVs for children/adolescents living with HIV and to improve quality of supply and demand for services. Our study objective was to ascertain the effectiveness of an active HIV case-finding model in HIV testing and linkages to care of children/adolescents at different entry points of a health facility in a RLS like Cameroon.

Methods

Study design

A cross-sectional and prospective study was conducted at the level of all 6 entry points of children and adolescents' units of the Laquintinie hospital of Douala (LHD) in the Littoral region of Cameroon from January through April 2016. LHD has an Approved Treatment Centre (ATC) for HIV/AIDS day care where in 91% attendees are adults versus 9% children and adolescents. LHD is a centre of excellence for pediatric HIV care, with an active cohort of 452 children and adolescents that represents up to 32% HIV-infected children receiving ART in the Littoral region of Cameroon.

Description of the study site

The HLD has 6 entry points of for pediatric care: (i) Pediatric inpatient unit that includes: Pediatric emergency, general pediatric hospitalizations, nutrition and sickle cell disease unit; (ii) Neonatology unit including premature babies and PMTCT services; (iii) Pediatric outpatient unit; iv) immunization and family planning unit; (v) Tuberculosis Screening and Management Unit (TB unit); and (vi) the day-care hospital/Approved treatment centre (ATC) for people living with HIV (PLWHIV): Adult unit and pediatric unit of care and treatment of PLWHIV. Regarding PMTCT, all of exposed HIV infant in our facility were managed in the PMTCT program. Nevirapine was administered for 6 weeks irrespective of the mode of feeding selected by the mother if she took ART (preferentially TDF + 3TC + EFV) for more than 1 month and for 12 weeks if the mother did not take ART or took them for less than one month.

Sampling method

All children and adolescents aged 0–19 years, of unknown HIV status, or descendants of PLWHIV or siblings of HIV infected children, were consecutively by convenient sampling enrolled during the 4 months study period (January–April 2016). In the absence of real data on the prevalence of paediatric HIV infection for active HIV case finding in Cameroon, a minimum size for the study was calculated using the HIV prevalence of 15.4% based on a systematic review conducted on children and adolescents in sub-Saharan Africa [10], with z at 95% IC (i.e. z = 1.96) and an error rate of 0.05; to determine the minimum sample size using Cochran's formula ($z^2 * p * q / d^2$) [11], given a minimum of 201 children/adolescents for the study.

Model of identification process and the patient flow

We developed a service model to actively look for cases of HIV-infected children and adolescents at all entry points at the LHD (Fig. 1). For every child and adolescent seeking care at any entry point of the LHD, we asked parents or guardians if the child's HIV status was

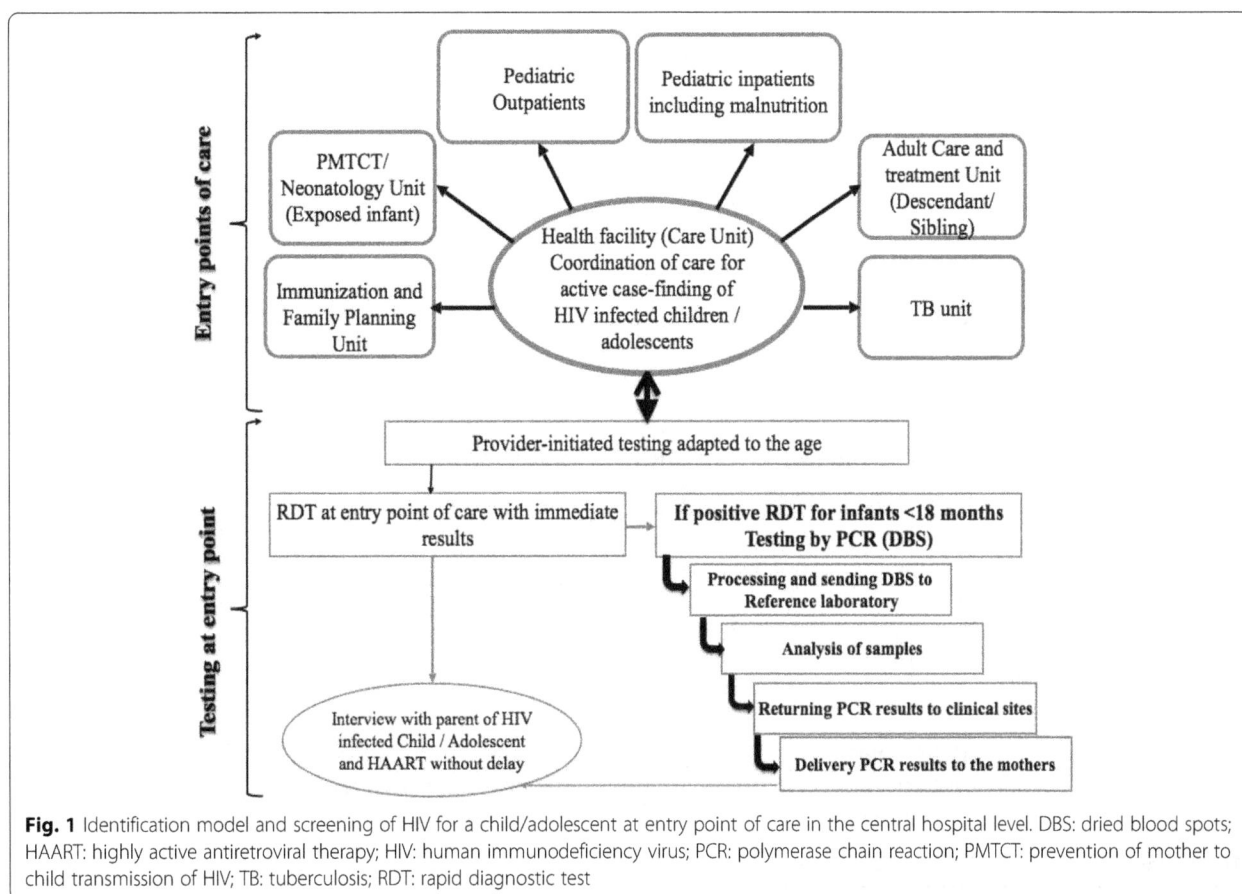

Fig. 1 Identification model and screening of HIV for a child/adolescent at entry point of care in the central hospital level. DBS: dried blood spots; HAART: highly active antiretroviral therapy; HIV: human immunodeficiency virus; PCR: polymerase chain reaction; PMTCT: prevention of mother to child transmission of HIV; TB: tuberculosis; RDT: rapid diagnostic test

known and documented. If the answer was "no", or "I don't know", information on the need for HIV testing was provided to parents by a trained community health worker (CHW) who provided pre-test counselling, written informed consent, onsite HIV testing and result delivery immediately after the post-test counselling. Additionally, all adult PLWHIV attending the ATC of the LHD were asked to take their descendant(s) aged 0–19 years whose HIV status was not known; for HIV-infected children attending the ATC, an active case finding of their siblings was also done. For descendants and siblings, study information was provided to parents during clinic attendance at the level of the waiting room, in order to enhance their motivation in bringing their family members for HIV testing. Then, a family tree of the descendants and siblings was developed from the index patient to determine the number of children and adolescents with unknown HIV status. The parent/guardian then decided on the location for HIV testing of the child or adolescent, who could be either at health facility or home-based. Additionally, HIV status of the mother was sought before carrying out the test of the neonate, infant and child.

The study pre-testing phase consisted of an administration of study tools (closed questions with single or multiple answers) to 20 parents/guardians over a period of one week in order to: (i) assess their understanding and acceptability and (ii) standardize and homogenize the data collection tools at the level of all entry points of the healthcare facility (Fig. 1).

Procedure for HIV screening

Based on a serial algorithm as per the national guidelines for HIV testing (Fig. 2), a rapid diagnostic test (RDT) was offered to consenting parents of participating children, with immediate result delivery, by task shifting from laboratory technicians to trained healthcare providers. Briefly, the first RDT (Determine™ HIV-1/2) was performed using capillary blood from the child/adolescent as per the manufacturer's instructions, with a sensitivity of 100% (98.5–100) and a specificity of 95.8% (93.3–98.4) for HIV-1/2 evaluated locally [12]. After 15 min, the result was provided and post-test counselling done accordingly. In case of a non-reactive HIV result, the child/adolescent has declared HIV-negative (i.e. free of HIV-infection); in case of a reactive HIV result, a second more specific RDT (Oraquick®) was performed as per the manufacturer's instructions, with a sensitivity of 96.7% (94.4–98.9) and a specificity of 100% (98.5–100) to confirm HIV

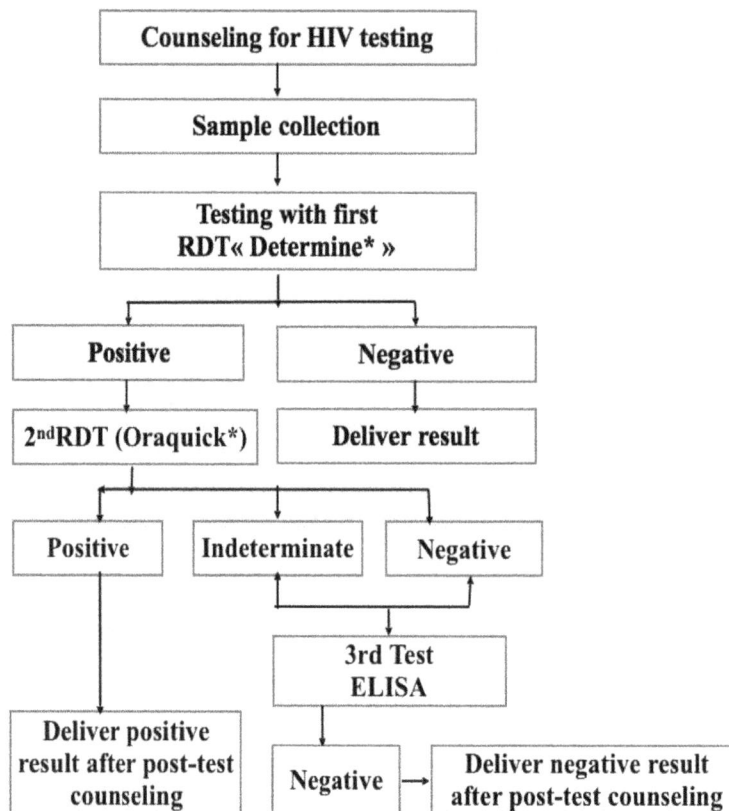

Fig. 2 Screening Algorithm of HIV infection. ELISA: enzyme linked immunosorbent assay; HIV: human immunodeficiency virus; RDT: rapid diagnostic test

infection, as per local assessment [12]. In case of discordant results between the two RDTs, an ELISA test (ELISA" Genscreen™ ULTRA HIV Ag - Ab) was performed as tier breaker following the manufacturer's instructions (i.e to confirm or exclude HIV-infection). Post-test counselling was provided prior to result delivery. In case of a reactive HIV result after RDT in an infant < 18 months, a blood sample was collected from a prick on the heel, toe or finger, directly into a filter paper (Whatman n° 903) for a confirmation of the result by polymerase chain reaction (PCR). Of note, the HIV status of the mothers was sought before carrying out the test of the neonate, infant or child. For HIV-vertically exposed infants of less than 18 months, the serological test reflects the exposure to HIV through their mothers, which requires testing by PCR to either confirm or infirm HIV-infection. For any HIV-positive child/adolescent, CHWs accompanied the concerned from the entry point to the ATC for an immediate initiation on ART according to the strategy of «test and treat». The parents /legal guardians were provided with therapeutic education by a psychosocial agent. Children tested HIV-positive at inpatient services were also initiated on ART and monitored throughout their hospitalization (Fig. 2).

Statistical analyses

Categorical variables were expressed as frequency, while the quantitative variables were presented as means ± Standard deviations (SD) or with 95% interval confidence (IC 95%) if normally distributed. To compare proportions, we used Fisher exact test. Quantitative values were compared using the U-test of Wilcoxon test. Only variables with a p-value ≤ 0.2 in the univariate model were considered for analysis in a multivariate logistic regression model. All statistical analyses were performed using the Stata (version 11SE) and R (version 3.1.1 software). P-value < 0.05 was considered statistically significant.

Results

Basic characteristics and acceptability of HIV testing among study participants

Overall, 3439 interviews were conducted to parents/legal guardians of children/adolescents attending the LHD, and up to 2107 children/adolescents were reported to have an unknown HIV status, indicating a rate of 61.3% unknown HIV infection in this paediatric population (Fig. 3).

Three parental refusals of consent were recorded, among which one each from the in-patient unit, outpatient unit and family tree model, giving 99.9% (2104/2107)

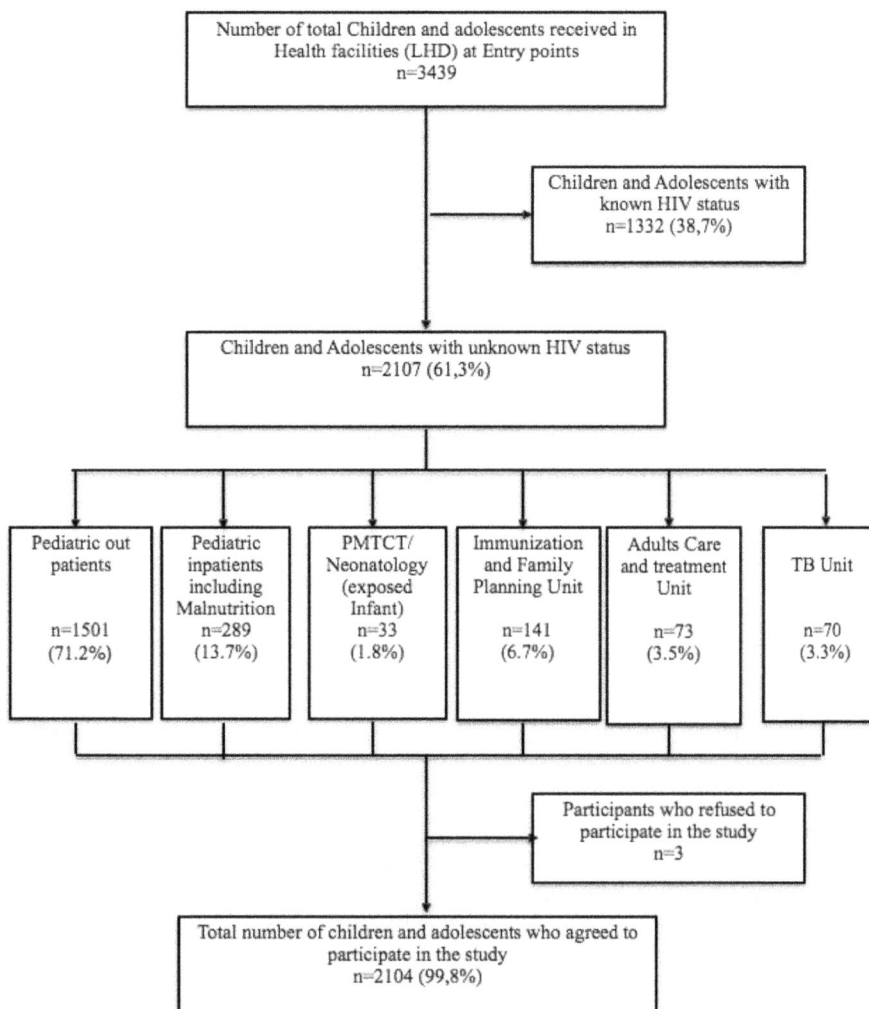

Fig. 3 Flow diagram of child/adolescent enrolled in the Study. HLD: Laquintinie hospital of Douala; HIV: human immunodeficiency virus; PMTCT: prevention of mother to child transmission of HIV; TB: tuberculosis

acceptability rate for enrolment and HIV testing in the entire study population (Fig. 3).

Among 2104 children and adolescents enrolled, the majority came from outpatient unit (71.29%), followed by hospitalized patients (13.69%), as shown in Table 1. Immunization and family planning unit contributed 6.69% of children and adolescents. A comparison of acceptability based on the six entry-points showed no significant difference in performance ($p = 0.090$).

Overall, among 2104 children and adolescents included boys accounted for 54.71% and the boy/girl sex ratio was 6:5 (1151/953) and the mean age of 2.10 (Sd = 2.96) years. The age class 3–6 years of boys was significantly higher compared to that of girls (15.0% vs. 11.2% for girl, $p = 0.015$) (Table 1). No difference was observed between the number of girl and boys patients according to entry point of care. However, the mean age was significantly higher among children enrolled from the family

tree model (5.47 +/-Sd = 4,33) and from the tuberculosis (TB) unit (4.81 + / Sd = 4,50 years), as compared to that of children/adolescents enrolled from in-patient services, ($p = 0.0001$).

HIV prevalence and linkage to ART care according to entry points

Out of 2104 children and adolescents tested for HIV, 44 were diagnosed as HIV-positive, giving an overall prevalence of 2.1% (Table 2). According to entry points, the highest rates of HIV-infection were reported among siblings/descendants, TB unit attendees and hospitalized patients, respectively with 22.2, 11.4 and 5.6%, with statistically significant differences among participants from siblings/descendants, outpatient unit, immunization and family planning ($p \leq 0.001$). Of note, none (0%) of the 141 infants enrolled from the immunization unit was positive,

Table 1 Basic characteristics of the study population by sex and age range

Variables	Girls	Boys	Total	P
Number of participants enrolled: n (%)	953 (45.3)	1.151 (54.7)	2.104 (100.0)	
Entry point of care				
Pediatric Inpatients Unit[*]	116 (12.2)	172 (14.9)	288	1
Pediatric out patient Unit	679 (71.2)	821 (71.3)	1.500	0.121
TB Unit	37 (3.9)	33 (2.8)	70	0.056
Vaccination and Family Planning Unit	71 (7.4)	70 (6.1)	141	0.048
PMTCT/Neonatology Unit	21 (2.2)	12 (1.0)	33	0.010
Adult care and treatment Unit (Descendant/Sibling)	29 (3.0)	43 (3.7)	72	0.898
Mean Age (Sd), years	2.06 (2.95)	2.13 (2.96)	2.10 (2.96)	0.329
[0–3][a]	756 (79.3)	875 (76.0)	1.633 (77.5)	1
[3–6]	95 (10.0)	154 (13.4)	249 (11.8)	0.015
[6–9]	49 (5.1)	67 (5.8)	116 (6.5)	0.391
[9–11]	22 (2.3)	18 (1.6)	40 (1.9)	0.354
[11–15]	25 (2.6)	31 (2.7)	56 (2.7)	0.801
[15–19]	6 (0.6)	6 (0.5)	12 (0.6)	0.801

Data are number and/or proportion (%), unless otherwise indicated; *PMTCT* prevention of mother to child transmission of HIV, *SD* standard deviation, *TB* tuberculosis; [a]: Reference

and only 2 (0.1%) of the 1500 children enrolled from outpatient unit were HIV-positive.

Among the 44 HIV positive children and adolescents, 42 (95.5%) were successfully accompanied by CHWs to the ATC and were all enrolled into care according to the national guidelines for pediatric management of HIV/AIDS. Thus, this gives a very high linkage to care among HIV-positive children/adolescents, with only 4.5% refusal. Prior to ART initiation, two died during hospitalization for malnutrition and TB. Among the 40 HIV-infected children/adolescents who effectively initiated on ART, 5 died subsequently, giving an overall mortality rate of 15.9% (7/44) of HIV positive children/adolescents enrolled in the study (Table 3). In contrast, within the population of HIV-negative children, up to 23.2% (480) mortality rate was reported mainly due to life threatening paediatric emergencies (Table 3). This gives an overall mortality rate of 23.2% (487), resulting to 122 deaths per month.

Discussions

In order to contribute to the global efforts for ending AIDS, we designed and implemented a strategy for universal HIV testing and enrolment to care of all infected children/adolescents in RLS. Our model of multiple entry points to healthcare was highly accepted by parents/legal guardians (> 99%), similar to findings from Uganda (92.8%) and Kenya (82.5%) [11, 13, 14]. These indicate a high success rate of such approach in RLS, which contributes in achieving the 90% HIV diagnosis among children/adolescents with unknown status [9]. In this frame, Provider Initiated Testing and Counselling (PITC) for the children are feasible.

Table 2 Distribution of population according to HIV status at different entry points of care

Entry point of care	HIV status, n (%)			
	HIV Negative 2060 (97.9)	HIV Positive 44 (2.09)	Total 2104	P
Pediatric inpatients Unit[a]	272 (94.4)	16 (5.56)	288	1
Out Pediatric patient Unit	1498 (99.9)	2 (0.1)	1500	< 0.0001
TB Unit	62 (88.6)	8 (11.4)	70	0.078
Immunization and Family Planning Unit	141 (100.0)	0	141	0.004
PMTCT/Neonatology unit	31 (93.9)	2 (6.1)	33	0.905
Adult care and treatment Unit (Descendant/Sibling)	56 (77.6)	16 (22.2)	72	< 0.0001

Data are number and/or proportion (%), unless otherwise indicated; [a]: Reference; *TB* Tuberculosis, *PMTCT* Prevention of mother to child transmission of HIV

Table 3 Mortality in the population of HIV-infected and uninfected children /adolescents

Survival status	Patients						
	HIV Infected		HIV Uninfected		Total		
	n	%	n	%	n	%	P
Died	7	15.9	480	23.2	487	23.2	1
Alive	37	84.1	1580	76.8	1617	76.8	0.85

HIV human immunodeficiency virus, *n* number; %: proportion

Our model of active linkage to care, using CHWs for liaison persons, showed an excellent enrolment into care of HIV-positive children/adolescents (> 95%). Thus, the current model, if well implemented, would contribute in achieving 90% of ART coverage in HIV-infected children/adolescents [9].

Routinely, HIV testing is offered to suspect children or those under the PMTCT program, both accounting for only 10% of children attending consultation and those admitted to the hospital. Of note, the prevalence was low in PMTCT/Neonatology due to maternal exposure to ART, except for children of HIV-infected mother who missed the PMTCT program and were discovered at delivery or postnatal unit (Neonatology). Moreover, task shifting of HIV testing to non-health professionals (CHW), under guardian/parental counselling, significantly reduces waiting time and increases access/acceptability to testing [15].

The mean age of our study population was 2.1 years, higher than those in Bamenda-Cameroon (1.3 year) and in Zambia (1 year) [16, 17]. Nonetheless, these observations altogether indicate late HIV diagnosis in RLS, with high mortality among infected children if untreated [15]. In this model, there is need for ensuring earlier diagnosis and treatment in order to limit HIV-associated mortality [18, 19]. This is crucial for siblings/descendants with unknown HIV status, who often have very late diagnosis (5.47 years in our finding). As previously reported, using family tree as a key to identify unreported children living with HIV and increase paediatric ART would be relevant [10, 15, 20, 21].

HIV prevalence from our study was lower (~ 2%) than those from Malawi and Uganda but higher than that of Kenya [13, 15, 16, 19]; disparities being mainly attributed to varying epidemics in these different geographical settings. HIV prevalence varies by entry point, with a high burden at the TB Unit (11.4%), similar to findings from Ethiopia (14.5%) [22]. TB unit should be considered as a secondary point to catch-up missing cases of paediatric HIV for linkage to care in RLS [22, 23], thus closing the gap in paediatric ART coverage (~ 40 increased fold in Uganda) [24].

The rate of HIV-associated mortality (15.9%) was similar to those in West and Central Africa (16%) in 2014 [25].

However, the high mortality (23.2%) among HIV-negative children was due to late hospital attendance with life threatening emergencies in the frame of malnutrition, TB and encephalopathy. Of note, as a referral centre, the LHD as a referral centre receives cases with clinical complications from primary healthcare facilities and with higher risk of mortality, thereby justifying the surprisingly high mortality rates among HIV-negative children.

A major strength of our findings is the high sensitivity of Determine (100%) used as first RDT and the high specificity of Oraquick (100%) used as second RDT, as reported by Njouom et al. in Cameroon [12], indicating accuracy in identifying the real serological status. However, studies on costing of the current model, that integrates community-based HIV-testing, linkage to care and viral load coverage in pediatric populations, would provide further evidences for policy-making toward ending paediatric AIDS in RLS [1, 9].

Conclusion

A model of HIV testing of children/adolescents at multiple entry points and active linkage to care is feasible and efficient in achieving universal paediatric ART coverage in African RLS. With emphasis on family tree, TB, and/or hospitalised children/adolescents, this model would greatly contribute in achieving the current global targets for paediatric HIV in Cameroon and in other RLS.

Abbreviations
AIDS: Acquired immunodeficiency syndrome; ART: Antiretroviral therapy; ATC: Approved Treatment Centre; CHW: Community health workers; EGPAF: Elizabeth Glaser Pediatric AIDS Foundation; HIV: Human immunodeficiency Virus; LHD: Laquitinie Hospital of Douala; PCR: Polymerase Chain Reaction; PEPFAR: US President Emergency Fund for AIDS Relief; PLWHIV: People Living with HIV; PMTCT: Prevention of Mother-to-Child Transmission; RDT: Rapid Diagnostic Test; RLS: Resource-Limited Settings; TB: Tuberculosis; UNAIDS: Joint United Nations Programme on HIV/AIDS; UNICEF: United Nations Children's Fund; WHO: World health organization

Acknowledgements
We are very grateful to the questionnaire respondents who agreed to participate in this study. We express our gratitude to the LHD wards, EGPAF and Landry Dongmo Tsague Senior HIV/AIDS Specialist/UNICEF Western and Central Africa Regional Office for their support and cooperation during the survey. Statistical analysis and data interpretation were supported by the International Society for Health Research and Training (ISRT-Health), a local Lecturer network.

Funding
The present study was supported by the University of Douala and the Laquintinie Hospital of Douala.

Authors' contributions
CIP, CEEM, DKK, PKN, CAZM and ST designed the study and collected the data. CIP, JF and CEEM analysed and interpreted the data. CIP and JF initiated the manuscript. CEEM, DKK, PKN, CAZM, and ST revised the manuscript. All authors read and approved the final version of the manuscript.

Competing interests
The authors declare that they have no competing interests.

Author details
[1]Clinical sciences department, Faculty of Medicine and Pharmaceutical Sciences, University of Douala, PO Box 2071, Douala, Cameroon. [2]HIV Care and Treatment Centre, Laquintinie Hospital of Douala, Douala, Cameroon. [3]Virology Laboratory, Chantal Biya International Reference Centre for research on HIV/AIDS prevention and management, Yaoundé, Cameroon. [4]Faculty of Medicine and Biomedical Sciences, University of Yaoundé I, Yaoundé, Cameroon. [5]Technical office, Elizabeth Glaser Pediatric AIDS Foundation, LDH, Douala, Cameroon. [6]Mother-Child Centre, Chantal BIYA Foundation, Yaoundé, Cameroon.

References
1. Joint United Nations Programme on HIV/AIDS. UNAIDS. On the Fast-track to an AIDS-Free generation.The incredible journey of the global plan towards the elimination of new HIV infections among children by keeping theirs mothers alive; 2015. https://www.unaids.org/sites/default/files/media_asset/GlobalPlan2016_en.pdf.Geneva. Accessed 18 July 2016.
2. Comité National de lutte contre le SIDA, UNAIDS. Rapport 2015. Estimations et projections sur le VIH et le SIDA au Cameroun. Période: 2010–2020; 2015. http://cnls.cm/sites/default/files/estimation_et_projections_sur_le_vih_et_le_sida_au_cameroun_2010-2020_rapport_2015.pdf. Accessed 18 July 2016.
3. Joint United Nations Programme on HIV/AIDS.UNAIDS. 2015 Progress report on the global plan towards the elimination of new HIV infections among children and keeping their mothers alive; 2015. http://www.unaids.org/sites/default/files/media_asset/JC2774_2015ProgressReport_GlobalPlan_en.pdf.
4. Newell ML, Coovadia H, Cortina-Borja M, Rollins N, Gaillard P, Dabis F. Ghent International AIDS Society (IAS) Working Group on HIV Infection in Women and Children. Mortality of Infected and Uninfected Infants Born to HIV-Infected Mothers in Africa: A pooled analysis. Lancet. 2004;364(9441):1236–43.
5. UNAIDS/UNICEF/WHO Global AIDS Response Progress Reporting and UNAIDS 2016 estimates; 2016. https://www.unicef.org/publications/index_93427.html. Accessed 18 July 2016.
6. United Nations Children's Fund. For every child, end AIDS – seventh stocktaking report. New York: UNICEF; 2016. Accessed 25 July 2017
7. UNAIDS. AIDSinfo. National database. Cameroon. http://www.unaids.org/fr/regionscountries/countries/cameroon. Accessed 25 July 2017.
8. WHO. Global health sector response to HIV, 2000–2015: focus on innovations in Africa: progress report. Geneva; 2016. Accessed 25 July 2017.
9. UNAIDS. Understanding Fast-Track: accelerating action to end the AIDS epidemic by 2030. Geneva; 2015. https://jliflc.com/resources/understanding-fast-track-accelerating-action-to-end-the-aids-epidemic-by-2030/. Accessed 14 Jun 2016.
10. Govindasamy D, Ferrand RA, Wilmore SM, Ford N, Ahmed S, Afnan-Holmes H, Kranzer K. Uptake and yield of HIV testing and counselling among children andadolescents in sub-Saharan Africa: a systematic review. J Int AIDS Soc. 2015;18:20182.
11. Cochran WG. Sampling techniques. 3rd ed. New York (NY): John Wiley and Sons; 1977. Available at https://archive.org/stream/Cochran1977Sampling Techniques_201703/Cochran_1977_Sampling%20Techniques_djvu.txt
12. Njouom R, Ngono L, Mekinda-Gometi DD, Kengne CN, Sadeuh-Mba SA, Marie-Astrid Vernet MA, Tchendjou P, Vernet G. Evaluation of the performances of twelve rapid diagnostic tests for diagnosis of HIV infection in Yaounde, Cameroon. J Virol Meth. 2017;243:158–63.
13. Wanyenze RK, Nawavvu C, Ouma J, Namale A, Colebunders R, Kamya MR. Provider-initiated HIV testing for paediatric inpatients and their caretakers is feasible and acceptable. Tropical Med Int Health. 2010;15(1):113–9. https://doi.org/10.1111/j.1365-3156.2009.02417.x.
14. Muhula S, Memiah P, Mbau L, Oruko H, Baker B, Ikiara G, et al. Uptake and linkage into care over one year of providing HIV testing and counselling through community and health facility testing modalities in urban informal settlement of Kibera, Nairobi Kenya. BMC Public Health. 2016;16(1):373–9.
15. McCollum ED, Preidis GA, Kabue MM, Singogo EBM, Mwansambo C, Kazembe PN, et al. Task shifting routine inpatient pediatric HIV testing improves program outcomes in urban Malawi: a retrospective observational study. PLoS One. 2010;5(3):e9626.
16. Zoufaly A, Hammerl R, Sunjoh F, Jochum J, Nassimi N, Awasom C, et al. High HIV prevalence among children presenting for general consultation in rural Cameroon. Int J STD AIDS. 2014;25(10):742–4.
17. Kankasa C, Carter RJ, Briggs N, Bulterys M, Chama E, Cooper ER, et al. Routine offering of HIV testing to hospitalized pediatric patients at university teaching hospital, Lusaka, Zambia: acceptability and feasibility. JAIDS J Acquir Immune Defic Syndr. 2009;51(2):202–8.
18. Violari A, Cotton MF, Gibb DM, Babiker AG, Steyn J, Madhi SA, Jean-Philippe P, McIntyre JA, CHER study team. Early antiretroviral therapy and mortality among HIV-infected infants. N Engl J Med. 2008;359(21):2233–44.
19. Wachira J, Ndege S, Koech J, Vreeman RC, Ayuo P, Braitstein P. HIV testing uptake and prevalence among adolescents and adults in a large home-based HIV testing program in Western Kenya. J Acquir Immune Defic Syndr. 2014;65(2):e58–66.
20. Lewis Kulzer J, Penner JA, Marima R, Oyaro P, Oyanga AO, Shade SB, et al. Family model of HIV care and treatment: a retrospective study in Kenya. J Int AIDS Soc. 2012;15(1):8–13.
21. Ramirez-Avila L, Noubary F, Pansegrouw D, Sithole S, Giddy J, Losina E, et al. The acceptability and feasibility of routine pediatric HIV testing in an outpatient Clinic in Durban, South Africa. Pediatr Infect Dis J. 2013;32(12):1348–53.
22. Westerlund E, Jerene D, Mulissa Z, Hallström I, Lindtjørn B. Pre-ART retention in care and prevalence of tuberculosis among HIV-infected children at a district hospital in southern Ethiopia. BMC Pediatr. 2014;14:250.
23. UNAIDS. Joint United Nations Programme on HIV/AIDS. Cameroon developing subnational estimates of HIV prevalence and the number of people living with HIV. 2014 Geneva. [http://www.unaids.org/en/resources/documents/2014/2014_subnationalestimatessurvey_cameroon. Accessed 14 June 2016.
24. Luyirika E, Towle MS, Achan J, Muhangi J, Senyimba C, Lule F, et al. Scaling up Paediatric HIV care with an integrated, family-Centred approach: an observational case study from Uganda. PLoS One. 2013;8(8):69548.
25. Dicko F, Desmonde S, Koumakpai S, Dior-Mbodj H, Kouéta F, Baeta N, et al. Reasons for hospitalization in HIV-infected children in West Africa. J Int AIDS Soc. 2014;17:1881.

16

Prevalence and risk factors of testicular microlithiasis in patients with hypospadias: a retrospective study

Michiko Nakamura[1], Kimihiko Moriya[1*] (ID), Yoko Nishimura[1], Mutsumi Nishida[2,3], Yusuke Kudo[2,3], Yukiko Kanno[1], Takeya Kitta[1], Masafumi Kon[1] and Nobuo Shinohara[1]

Abstract

Background: It has been described that the incidence of testicular microlithiasis is high in several congenital disorders which may be associated with testicular impairment and infertility. Several reports have shown that a prepubertal or pubertal hormonal abnormality in the pituitary-gonadal axis was identified in some patients with hypospadias that is one of the most common disorders of sex development. However, exact prevalence or risk factors of testicular microlithiasis in patients with hypospadias have not reported so far. In the present study, to clarify the prevalence and risk factors of testicular microlithiasis in patients with hypospadias, a retrospective chart review was performed.

Methods: Children with hypospadias who underwent testicular ultrasonography between January 2010 and April 2016 were enrolled in the present study. Severity of hypospadias was divided into mild and severe. The prevalence and risk factors of testicular microlithiasis or classic testicular microlithiasis were examined.

Results: Of 121 children, mild and severe hypospadias were identified in 66 and 55, respectively. Sixteen children had undescended testis. Median age at ultrasonography evaluation was 1.7 years old. Testicular microlithiasis and classic testicular microlithiasis were documented in 17 children (14.0%) and 8 (6.6%), respectively. Logistic regression analysis revealed that presence of undescended testis was only a significant factor for testicular microlithiasis and classic testicular microlithiasis. The prevalence of testicular microlithiasis or classic testicular microlithiasis was significantly higher in children with undescended testis compared to those without undescended testis (testicular microlithiasis; 43.8% versus 9.5% ($p = 0.002$), classic testicular microlithiasis; 37.5% versus 1.9% ($p < 0.001$).

Conclusions: The current study demonstrated that the presence of undescended testis was only a significant risk factor for testicular microlithiasis or classic testicular microlithiasis in patients with hypospadias. As co-existing undescended testis has been reported as a risk factor for testicular dysfunction among patients with hypospadias, the current findings suggest that testicular microlithiasis in children with hypospadias may be associated with impaired testicular function. Conversely, patients with isolated HS seem to have lower risks for testicular impairment. Further investigation with longer follow-up will be needed to clarify these findings.

Keywords: Testicular microlithiasis, Hypospadias, Undescended testis, Ultrasonography

* Correspondence: k-moriya@med.hokudai.ac.jp
[1]Department of Renal and Genitourinary Surgery, Hokkaido University
Graduate School of Medicine, North-15, West-7, Kita-Ku, Sapporo 060-8638,
Japan
Full list of author information is available at the end of the article

Background

Hypospadias (HS) is one of the most common disorders of sex development, occurring in 0.52 to 8.2 of every 1000 live male births [1, 2]. Although the exact etiology of HS is unknown in the majority of patients, a multifactorial etiology including genetic, endocrine and environmental factors is considered to be involved in the genesis of this disorder [3]. HS is also considered as one of the symptoms of testicular dysgenesis syndrome (TDS), which was proposed in 2001 [4]. It has been speculated that impaired development of fetal testes could lead to increased risk of undescended testis (UDT), HS, decreased spermatogenesis and testicular cancer [5]. Several reports have shown that a prepubertal or pubertal hormonal abnormality in the pituitary-gonadal axis was identified in some patients with HS from endocrinological point of view [6–10], which is compatible with the concept of TDS.

Testicular microlithiasis (TM) is characterized by multiple, small, uniform-appearing echogenic foci of less than 3 mm without acoustic shadowing in the seminiferous tubules, which may be indicative of degeneration of the testicular parenchyma [11, 12]. Several theories about the origin or causes of TM have been reported, however, the exact etiology of TM still remains unclear [13]. Previous studies have reported an association between TM and testicular germ cell tumors and/or carcinoma in situ [14, 15]. In addition, an association between TM and infertility has been reported [15]. Although real impact of TM in children is still a matter of debate, it has been described in previous reports that the incidence of TM is high in some congenital disorders, such as UDT, Down's syndrome, Klinefelter syndrome, McCune-Albright syndrome and Peuzt-Jeghers syndrome, which may be associated with testicular impairment and infertility [16–20].

Based on these previous reports, TM may be a sign of a future endocrinological abnormality in the pituitary-gonadal axis [6–10] or testicular malignancy among patients with HS as a phenotype of TDS. Therefore, we performed testicular ultrasonography (US) for the screening of testicular abnormalities in patients with HS. Because several reports demonstrated that patients with associated genital anomaly, including UDT, were at higher risk for impaired testicular function [6, 9, 21], we speculated that TM may be identified at a higher rate in such patients. However, the exact prevalence of and TM in patients with HS has not been reported so far.

In the present study, we retrospectively examined the prevalence and the risk factors of TM among children with HS.

Methods

Medical charts of children who visited our hospital for the management or follow-up of HS between January 2010 and April 2016 were retrospectively reviewed. Among them, patients who were born between December 1999 and August 2015, and who underwent on testicular US were included in the present study. Patients with obvious disorders of sex development or with chromosomal abnormalities were excluded. To evaluate and define risk factors of TM in children with HS, the following parameters were assessed with respect to their relation to the prevalence of TM: birth weight, presence of UDT, severity of HS, testosterone administration before HS surgery, and age at US. Severity of HS was divided into mild and severe based on the necessity of transecting urethral plate for correction of chordee deformity according to Koyanagi et al. [22].

TM was defined as 1 or more foci measuring 1 to 3 mm in diameter on testicular US. TM was classified as limited TM (LTM, echogenic foci < 5 /field) or classic TM (CTM, echogenic foci ≥ 5 /field) as reported by Goede et al. [23] (Fig. 1). Among patients with TM, children with CTM in at least one testis were diagnosed with CTM, whereas others were classified as having LTM.

All US evaluation was performed without sedation by sonographers. US evaluations were performed using a PLT-1204BT, a linear probe, 7.2–18 MHz equipped with Aplio™ XG/500 (Toshiba Medical Systems Corp., Tochigi, Japan), a EUP-65, a linear probe 6–14 MHz equipped with HI VISION Avius (Hitachi- Medical, Tokyo, Japan), and a ML6–15, a linear probe 6–15 MHz equipped with Logiq

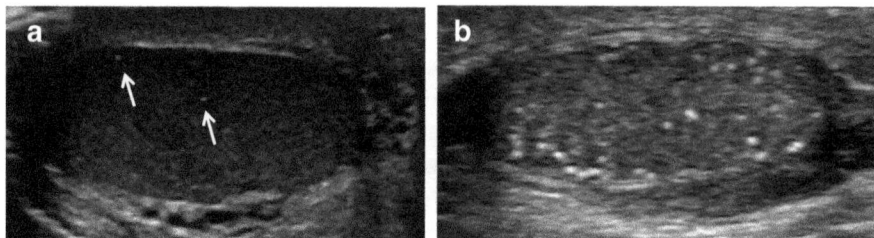

Fig. 1 Representative pictures of LTM and CTM. **a** Limited testicular microlithiasis (arrows) in an 11-year-old boy with hypospadias and undescended testis. Ultrasonography of right testis showed 2 small, uniform-appearing echogenic foci without acoustic shadowing. His left testis also displayed 4 echogenic foci per field. **b** Classic testicular microlithiasis in a 1-year-old boy with hypospadias. Ultrasonography of left testis demonstrated more than 5 echogenic foci per field. Right testis also displayed more than 5 echogenic foci per field

E9 (GE Healthcare, Amersham, UK). If multiple examinations were performed during follow-up, the final assessment findings were evaluated for prevalence and risk factors of TM.

JMP*pro version 12 was used for all statistical analyses. Statistical analyses were performed using logistic regression analysis and Fisher's exact test. $P < 0.05$ was considered significant.

Results

Among 219 children who visited during the study period, 121 children (55.3%) were included in the current study. Patient characteristics are shown in Table 1. Median birth weight was 2456 g, and the number of children with low birth weight (less than 2500 g) was 62. Mild and severe HS were identified in 66 and 55 children, respectively. UDT was observed in 16 patients (bilateral in 11, unilateral in 5). Of those, 4 had mild HS, and 12 had severe HS. Regarding co-existing congenital anomaly, inguinal hernia and heart anomaly were observed in 13 and 8, respectively. Testosterone administration before HS surgery was performed in 94 children. Median age at testicular US was 1.7 years old.

Prevalence of TM and CTM

TM and CTM were documented in 17 children (14.0%) and in 8 children (6.6%), respectively. TM was identified unilaterally in 7, and bilaterally in 10. Among 8 children with CTM, bilateral CTM was identified in 5. In the remaining 3 children, unilateral CTM alone was detected in 1, and CTM on one side and LTM on the other side in 2. No testicular tumors were detected on US in any children.

Risk factors of TM and CTM

Univariate analysis demonstrated that the severe type of HS and presence of UDT were risk factors for TM. On multivariate analyses, presence of UDT was only a risk

factor for TM ($p = 0.006$) (Table 2). Regarding CTM, presence of UDT was only a risk factor on univariate analysis ($p < 0.001$) (Table 3). The incidence of TM or CTM was significantly higher in children with UDT compared with those without UDT (TM; 43.8% versus 9.5% ($p = 0.002$), CTM; 37.5% versus 1.9% ($p < 0.001$)) (Table 4).

Side of TM and UDT (Table 5)

In 11 children with bilateral UDT, unilateral and bilateral TM were observed in 1 and 4, respectively. Among them, CTM in at least one side was identified in 4. Of 5 with unilateral UDT, TM was identified in 2 (both with bilateral CTM). Among 105 children without UDT, unilateral and bilateral TM were observed in 6 and 4, respectively. Of those, CTM in at least one side was observed only in 2.

Discussion

To our knowledge, the current study represented the first report on the prevalence of TM in children with HS. TM and CTM were identified in 14.0 and 6.6%, respectively, of children with HS. Presence of UDT was only a risk factor for TM and CTM.

Previous studies have shown that TM is associated with several conditions, including impaired spermatogenesis, testicular cancer and carcinoma in situ [14, 15]. In asymptomatic adults, the rate of CTM varies from 0.6 to 9% [24, 25]. Recent studies revealed that the prevalence of TM and CTM in asymptomatic boys was 4.2 and 2.4% respectively, and increased with age [23]. The prevalence of TM (14.0%) and CTM (6.6%) in children with HS in the current study seems to be relatively higher compared with that in asymptomatic boys in the previous reports. Although the etiology of HS is considered to be multifactorial, the concept of TDS, which suggests that impaired development of fetal testes could lead to increased risk of HS, has been proposed as one of the causes of HS. Drut et al. proposed that TM may be related with Sertoli cell dysfunction and abnormal embryogenesis during the early stages of testicular development [12]. Wohlfahrt-Veje et al. reported that dysgenetic testes often have an irregular US pattern in which TM may also be visible [5]. The reason for the relatively high prevalence of TM may be due to that children who have such embryological causes of testis anomaly could have been included in the present study.

We demonstrated that the presence of UDT was only a risk factor for TM and CTM. There are several reports of prepubertal or pubertal hormonal abnormalities of the pituitary-gonadal axis in some patients with HS [6–10]. In addition, there are several reports on patients with both HS and UDT, which is a risk factor of TM and CTM as demonstrated in our study, who were at a higher risk for decreased testicular function or impaired spermatogenesis

Table 1 Patient characteristics

	$n = 121$	range
Birth weight (g, median ± SD)	2456 ± 834 (unknown 1)	(472–4048)
Low birth weight (< 2500 g) (pts)	62	
Type of HS (pts)	mild: 66 / severe: 55	
UDT (pts)	16 (unilateral: 5 / bilateral: 11)	
Testosterone administration before surgery (pts)	yes: 94, no: 20 (unknown 7)	
	topical: 67 / systemic: 10 / topical+systemic: 17	
Age at USG (yrs, median ± SD)	1.7 ± 4.0	(0.5–18.2)
TM (pts) (LTM / CTM)	17 (9 / 8)	

Table 2 Risk factors for TM

	Univariate analysis		Multivariate analysis	
	Odds ratio (95% confidence interval)	p value	Odds ratio (95% confidence interval)	p-value
Birth weight (g, median ± SD)	0.44 (0.04–4.09)	n.s.		
Low birth weight (< 2500 g)	0.84 (0.68–4.09)	n.s.		
Severe type of HS	3.40 (1.17–11.35)	0.024*	2.48 (0.79–8.65)	n.s.
UDT	7.39 (2.23–24.55)	0.001*	5.8 (1.68–19.95)	0.006*
Testosterone administration	1.57 (0.39–10.59)	n.s.		
Age at USG	0.28 (0.04–2.52)	n.s.		

*$p < 0.05$

[6, 21]. A number of reports have demonstrated the relationship between TM and impaired spermatogenesis [26–28], although this issue is still controversial [29]. Accordingly, TM in children with HS may be associated with decreased testicular function and/or impaired spermatogenesis. To determine the relationship between TM and testicular function/spermatogenesis in patients with HS, further follow-up with endocrinological evaluations until puberty is necessary.

While the prevalence of TM in patients with HS and without UDT (9.5%) in the current study was slightly higher compared to that in asymptomatic boys (4.2%) reported in the previous literature [23], the prevalence of CTM (1.9%) was almost similar to that in asymptomatic boys (2.4%). Accordingly, patients with isolated HS seem to have lower risks for testicular impairment. On the contrary, although the presence of UDT in patients with HS was demonstrated as a risk factor for TM in the current study or impaired semen quality in the previous report [21], there has been no comparative study focusing on risk of TM or testicular dysfunction between patients with isolated UDT and those with HS and UDT. To clarify the impact of HS in patients with UDT in terms of the risk of TM or testicular dysfunction, additional studies are necessary.

Previous studies reported that the prevalence of primary testicular tumors in patients with TM ranged from 15 to 45% [15, 29]. Thus, there was some concern that TM may lead to testicular cancer at the end of the 1990's. However, two studies revealed that the rate of

Table 3 Risk factors for CTM

	Univariate analysis	
	Odds ratio (95% confidence interval)	p-value
Birth weight (g, median ± SD)	4.26 (0.20–85.70)	n.s.
Low birth weight (< 2500 g)	1.61 (0.38–8.14)	n.s.
Severe type of HS	3.92 (0.86–27.53)	n.s.
UDT	30.90 (6.23–231.37)	< 0.001*
Age at USG	0.19 (0.01–3.62)	n.s.

*$p < 0.05$

TM in the asymptomatic population ranged from 2.4 to 5.6% [24, 25], which is much higher than the prevalence of the lifetime risk of testicular cancer in the general population. Nowadays, it is recognized that TM in adults without known risk factors, such as previous testicular cancer, a history of UDT or testicular atrophy, seems to be a benign condition [19, 24, 25, 30]. Regarding TM detected in childhood, Suominen et al. found 15 patients with neoplasms among 421 pediatric patients (3.6%) by systematic review [31]. They described that TM should be considered a benign condition even in the pediatric age group, but the fact that TM is associated with testicular malignancy (< 5%) cannot be ignored. Although the concept of TDS included symptoms of HS, UDT and testicular cancer [5], as far as we know, there is no report demonstrating that the prevalence of testicular tumors is higher in patients with HS. Although UDT is well-known as a risk factor for testicular malignancy [32], it is obscure whether UDT is also a risk factor for testicular malignancy among patients with HS. Longer follow-up will clarify the exact associations among testicular malignancy, TM and/or UDT in children with HS.

There is some controversy regarding the method and duration of follow-up in patients with TM. In the guidelines produced by the European Society of Urogenital Radiology, the consensus opinion is that the presence of TM alone in the absence of other risk factors is not an indication for regular follow-up in adults [19]. However, this guideline did not mentioned children with HS. At this time, we believe that the follow-up protocol for patients with HS and TM should be determined based on the presence or absence of UDT because the exact risk for testicular malignancy in patients with HS alone remains obscure.

Several limitations of the present study should be addressed. First, this study was conducted in a retrospective

Table 4 Prevalence of TM and CTM

	UDT (+)	UDT (−)	p-value
Prevalence of TM	43.8% (7/16)	9.5% (10/105)	0.002
Prevalence of CTM	37.5% (6/16)	1.9% (2/105)	< 0.001

Table 5 Sides of testicular microlithiasis and undescended testis

	Bilateral UDT $n = 11$	Unilateral UDT $n = 5$	Without UDT $n = 105$
Unilateral TM	1	0	6
CTM	1	0	0
LTM	0	0	6
Bilateral TM	4	2	4
Bilateral CTM:	2	2	1
CTM and LTM	1	0	1
Bilateral LTM	1	0	2

nature and relatively small number of children. Second, there was no control group such as Japanese boys who had no genital disease or isolated UDT. Third, evaluation of chromosomal abnormalities was not performed in all children. Fourth, as children included in the current study were relatively young and because TM sometimes appears later in childhood [23], the true prevalence of TM in patients with HS may be higher than the prevalence in this study. Fifth, as endocrinological examination or semen analysis was not performed in the current study, testicular function could not be compared between patients with and without TM.

Conclusions

TM and CTM were identified in roughly 14.0 and 6.6% of children with HS, respectively. The prevalence of TM and CTM was significantly higher in patients with UDT. As UDT among children with HS has been reported as a risk factor for endocrinological abnormality and/or impaired spermatogenesis, these findings suggest that TM in children with HS may be associated with impaired testicular function. In addition, the prevalence of CTM in patients with isolated HS was almost equal to the previously reported prevalence in asymptomatic boys. Therefore, patients with isolated HS seem to have lower risks for testicular impairment. Further investigation with longer follow-up will be needed to clarify these findings.

Abbreviations
CTM: Classic testicular microlithiasis; HS: Hypospadias; LTM: Limited testicular microlithiasis; TDS: Testicular dysgenesis syndrome; TM: Testicular microlithiasis; UDT: Undescended testis; USG: Ultrasonography

Authors' contributions
MNa collected and analyzed the data and draft the manuscript. KM conceived the study and edit the manuscript. YN collected the data and edit the manuscript. MNi analyzed the data and edit the manuscript. YKu analyzed the data. YKa, TK and MK edit the manuscript. NS supervised this work. All authors have read and approved the final manuscript.

Competing interests
The authors declare that they have no competing interests.

Author details
[1]Department of Renal and Genitourinary Surgery, Hokkaido University Graduate School of Medicine, North-15, West-7, Kita-Ku, Sapporo 060-8638, Japan. [2]Diagnostic Center for Sonography, Hokkaido University Hospital, Sapporo, Japan. [3]Division of Laboratory and Transfusion Medicine, Hokkaido University Hospital, Sapporo, Japan.

References
1. Levitt SB, Reda EF. Hypospadias. Pediatr Ann. 1988;17(1):48–9. 53-44, 57
2. Springer A, van den Heijkant M, Baumann S. Worldwide prevalence of hypospadias. J Pediatr Urol. 2016;12(3):152.e151–7.
3. Marrocco G, Grammatico P, Vallasciani S, Gulia C, Zangari A, Marrocco F, Bateni ZH, Porrello A, Piergentili R. Environmental, parental and gestational factors that influence the occurrence of hypospadias in male patients. J Pediatr Urol. 2015;11(1):12–9.
4. Skakkebaek NE, Rajpert-De Meyts E, Main KM. Testicular dysgenesis syndrome: an increasingly common developmental disorder with environmental aspects. Hum Reprod. 2001;16(5):972–8.
5. Wohlfahrt-Veje C, Main KM, Skakkebaek NE. Testicular dysgenesis syndrome: foetal origin of adult reproductive problems. Clin Endocrinol. 2009;71(4):459–65.
6. Moriya K, Mitsui T, Tanaka H, Nakamura M, Nonomura K. Long-term outcome of pituitary-gonadal axis and gonadal growth in patients with hypospadias at puberty. J Urol. 2010;184(4 Suppl):1610–4.
7. Iwatsuki S, Kojima Y, Mizuno K, Kamisawa H, Umemoto Y, Sasaki S, Kohri K, Hayashi Y. Endocrine assessment of prepubertal boys with a history of cryptorchidism and/or hypospadias: a pilot study. J Urol. 2011;185(6 Suppl):2444–50.
8. Nonomura K, Fujieda K, Sakakibara N, Terasawa K, Matsuno T, Matsuura N, Koyanagi T. Pituitary and gonadal function in prepubertal boys with hypospadias. J Urol. 1984;132(3):595–8.
9. Rey RA, Codner E, Iniguez G, Bedecarras P, Trigo R, Okuma C, Gottlieb S, Bergada I, Campo SM, Cassorla FG. Low risk of impaired testicular Sertoli and Leydig cell functions in boys with isolated hypospadias. J Clin Endocrinol Metab. 2005;90(11):6035–40.
10. Shima H, Ikoma F, Yabumoto H, Mori M, Satoh Y, Terakawa T, Fukuchi M. Gonadotropin and testosterone response in prepubertal boys with hypospadias. J Urol. 1986;135(3):539–42.
11. Backus ML, Mack LA, Middleton WD, King BF, Winter TC, True LD. Testicular microlithiasis: imaging appearances and pathologic correlation. Radiol. 1994; 192(3):781–5.
12. Drut R, Drut RM. Testicular microlithiasis: histologic and immunohistochemical findings in 11 pediatric cases. Pediatr Dev Pathol. 2002;5(6):544–50.
13. Shanmugasundaram R, Singh JC, Kekre NS. Testicular microlithiasis: is there an agreed protocol? Indian J Urol. 2007;23(3):234–9.
14. Meissner A, Mamoulakis C, de la Rosette JJ, Pes MP. Clinical update on testicular microlithiasis. Curr Opin Urol. 2009;19(6):615–8.
15. Sakamoto H, Shichizyou T, Saito K, Okumura T, Ogawa Y, Yoshida H, Kushima M. Testicular microlithiasis identified ultrasonographically in Japanese adult patients: prevalence and associated conditions. Urology. 2006;68(3):636–41.
16. Goede J, Weijerman ME, Broers CJ, de Winter JP, Van der Voort-Doedens LM, Hack WW. Testicular volume and testicular microlithiasis in boys with Down syndrome. J Urol. 2012;187(3):1012–7.
17. Rocher L, Moya L, Correas JM, Mutuon P, Ferlicot S, Young J, Izard V, Benoit G, Brailly-Tabard S, Bellin MF. Testis ultrasound in Klinefelter syndrome infertile men: making the diagnosis and avoiding inappropriate management. Abdom Radiol (NY). 2016;41(8):1596–603.
18. Wasniewska M, Matarazzo P, Weber G, Russo G, Zampolli M, Salzano G, Zirilli G, Bertelloni S. Function ISGfAoGaP: clinical presentation of McCune-Albright syndrome in males. J Pediatr Endocrinol Metab. 2006;19(Suppl 2):619–22.

19. Richenberg J, Belfield J, Ramchandani P, Rocher L, Freeman S, Tsili AC, Cuthbert F, Studniarek M, Bertolotto M, Turgut AT, et al. Testicular microlithiasis imaging and follow-up: guidelines of the ESUR scrotal imaging subcommittee. Eur Radiol. 2015;25(2):323–30.

20. Nishimura Y, Moriya K, Nakamura M, Nishida M, Sato M, Kudo Y, Omotehara S, Iwai T, Wakabayashi Y, Kanno Y, et al. Prevalence and chronological changes of testicular Microlithiasis in isolated congenital undescended testes operated on at less than 3 years of age. Urology. 2017;109:159–64.

21. Asklund C, Jensen TK, Main KM, Sobotka T, Skakkebaek NE, Jorgensen N. Semen quality, reproductive hormones and fertility of men operated for hypospadias. Int J Androl. 2010;33(1):80–7.

22. Koyanagi T, Nonomura K, Yamashita T, Kanagawa K, Kakizaki H. One-stage repair of hypospadias: is there no simple method universally applicable to all types of hypospadias? J Urol. 1994;152(4):1232–7.

23. Goede J, Hack WW, Van der Voort-Doedens LM, Sijstermans K, Pierik FH. Prevalence of testicular microlithiasis in asymptomatic males 0 to 19 years old. J Urol. 2009;182(4):1516–20.

24. Peterson AC, Bauman JM, Light DE, McMann LP, Costabile RA. The prevalence of testicular microlithiasis in an asymptomatic population of men 18 to 35 years old. J Urol. 2001;166(6):2061–4.

25. Serter S, Gümüş B, Unlü M, Tunçyürek O, Tarhan S, Ayyildiz V, Pabuscu Y. Prevalence of testicular microlithiasis in an asymptomatic population. Scand J Urol Nephrol. 2006;40(3):212–4.

26. Aizenstein RI, DiDomenico D, Wilbur AC, O'Neil HK. Testicular microlithiasis: association with male infertility. J Clin Ultrasound. 1998;26(4):195–8.

27. Thomas K, Wood SJ, Thompson AJ, Pilling D, Lewis-Jones DI. The incidence and significance of testicular microlithiasis in a subfertile population. Br J Radiol. 2000;73(869):494–7.

28. Xu C, Liu M, Zhang FF, Liu JL, Jiang XZ, Teng JB, Xuan XJ, Ma JL. The association between testicular microlithiasis and semen parameters in Chinese adult men with fertility intention: experience of 226 cases. Urology. 2014;84(4):815–20.

29. Miller FN, Sidhu PS. Does testicular microlithiasis matter? A review. Clin Radiol. 2002;57(10):883–90.

30. Richenberg J, Brejt N. Testicular microlithiasis: is there a need for surveillance in the absence of other risk factors? Eur Radiol. 2012;22(11):2540–6.

31. Suominen JS, Jawaid WB, Losty PD. Testicular microlithiasis and associated testicular malignancies in childhood: a systematic review. Pediatr Blood Cancer. 2015;62(3):385–8.

32. Møller H, Cortes D, Engholm G, Thorup J. Risk of testicular cancer with cryptorchidism and with testicular biopsy: cohort study. BMJ. 1998; 317(7160):729.

17

Functional profiles of children with cerebral palsy in Jordan based on the association between gross motor function and manual ability

Nihad A. Almasri[1]* ⓘ, Maysoun Saleh[1], Sana Abu-Dahab[2], Somaya H. Malkawi[2] and Eva Nordmark[3]

Abstract

Background: Cerebral palsy (CP) is the most common cause of physical disability in childhood. A major challenge for delivering effective services for children with CP is the heterogeneity of the medical condition. Categorizing children into homogeneous groups based on functional profiles is expected to improve service planning. The aims of this study were to (1) to describe functional profiles of children with CP based on the Gross Motor Function Classification System-Expanded & Revised (GMFCS-E & R) and the Manual Ability Classification System (MACS); and (2) to examine associations and agreements between the GMFCS-E & R and the MACS for all participants then for subgroups based on subtypes of CP and chronological age of children.

Methods: A convenience sample of 124 children with CP (mean age 4.5, SD 2.9 years, 56% male) participated in the study. Children were classified into the GMFCS-E & R and the MACS levels by research assistants based on parents input. Research assistants determined the subtypes of CP.

Results: Thirty six percent of the participants were able to ambulate independently (GMFCS-E & R levels I-II) and 64% were able to handle objects independently (MACS levels I-II). The most common functional profile of children with CP in our study is the *"manual abilities better than gross motor function"*. An overall strong correlation was found between the GMFCS-E & R and the MACS ($r_s = .73$, $p < .001$), the correlations vary significantly based on subtypes of CP and chronological age of children. A very strong correlation was found in children with spastic quadriplegia ($r_s = .81$, $p < .001$), moderate with spastic diplegia ($r_s = .64$, $p < .001$), and weak with spastic hemiplegia ($r_s = .37$, $p < .001$).

Conclusions: The GMFCS- E & R and the MACS provide complementary but distinctive information related to mobility and manual abilities of children with CP. Subtypes of CP and chronological age differentiated functional profiles. Functional abilities of children with CP in Jordan have similar patterns to children with CP in other countries. Functional profiles can inform clinicians, researchers, and policy makers.

Keywords: Gross Motor Function Classification System-Expanded & Revised, Manual ability classification system, Cerebral palsy, Children, Functional profiles, Jordan

* Correspondence: nihadaa@gmail.com
[1]Department of Physiotherapy, School of Rehabilitation Sciences, The University of Jordan, Queen Rania Al Abdallah St, Amman 11942, Jordan
Full list of author information is available at the end of the article

Background

Cerebral palsy (CP) is the most common cause of physical disability in childhood [1]. A major challenge for delivering effective services for children with CP is the heterogeneity of the medical condition. Variety of clinical presentations can be observed in children with CP ranging from children who can ambulate and handle objects independently to children who have severe limitations in mobility and manual abilities further complicated by associated health conditions such as epilepsy and cognitive problems [2]. Therefore, it is useful to categorize children with CP into more homogeneous groups based on their functional profiles. The use of functional profiles in clinical sittings is expected to provide comprehensive description of abilities of children with CP which consequently may improve service planning and research.

Functional profiles of children with CP can be described utilizing functional classifications such as the Gross Motor Function Classification System- Expanded and Revised (GMFCS-E & R) [3, 4] and the Manual Ability Classification System (MACS) [5]. Functional classifications are consistent with the premises of the International Classification of Functioning, Disability, and Health (ICF) [6]. The ICF shifts the health professionals' attention from focusing on primary motor impairments to functional activities and social participation which are considered the optimal outcomes of medical services for children with CP [6]. Functional classifications are useful in setting functional goals and planning services for children with CP in health care systems [3–5].

Associations between the GMFCS-E & R and the MACS allow description of functional profiles of children with CP [7]. The GMFCS-E & R is the first activity-based classification system that was developed to classify children with CP in five levels based on their current performance in gross motor function [3]. Later, the MACS was developed in order to classify manual abilities of children with CP [5]. Both classifications demonstrated acceptable reliability and validity in classifying children with CP and the GMFCS-E & R is reliable to be used in Arabic language [8]. The GMFCS-E & R and the MACS describe different but complementary motor functions and between them, GMFCS-E & R and MACS provide a good description of the functional profiles of children with CP [9]. The associations between the two functional classifications vary based on the subtypes of CP. Previous research found that the strength of associations among the GMFCS-E & R and the MACS based on subtypes of CP were strong to moderate for quadriplegia and hemiplegia and poor to fair for diplegia [10, 7, 11, 12].

Although the GMFCS-E & R and the MACS are available in Arabic language they are not being used in any clinical sittings in Jordan. Health professionals are accustomed to use the traditional impairment-based classification of CP than the functional classifications [13]. Consequently, rehabilitation services for children with CP are focused on treating impairments rather than improving activity and participation of children [13]. For example, physiotherapists who provide services for children with spastic quadriplegia focus on stretching and strengthening more than mobility and activity of daily living training [13]. Utilizing functional profiles might therefore provide a framework to classify children with CP based on their levels of function, and tailor rehabilitation services in Jordan towards outcome that are meaningful to children with CP and their families.

To our knowledge this is the first study in a low-income and middle-income country to describe functional profiles of children with CP based on GMFCS-E & R and MACS. Functional profiles are expected to shift the focus of rehabilitation in Jordan from impairment-based towards function-based services. In addition, functional profiles can be used to guide service planning and to allocate limited resources in areas of major needs of children with CP. We hypothesized that the gross motor function and manual abilities will vary within subtypes of CP and age groups. Variations between the GMFCS-E & R and the MACS by subtypes indicate the need to use functional classifications in addition to motor subtypes to accurately classify children with CP. Variations between the GMFCS-E & R and the MACS based on chronological age of children indicate the presence of a variety of functional abilities supporting the need to use more than one classification system to classify children with CP accurately. The aims of this study; therefore, were to (1) to describe functional profiles of children with CP based on the GMFCS-E & R and the MACS; and (2) to examine associations and agreements between the GMFCS-E & R and the MACS for all participants then for subgroups based on subtypes of CP and chronological age of children.

Methods

Participants

A convenience sample of 124 children 2 to 16 years of age (mean = 4.5, SD = 2.9 years, 56% male) participated in the study. All the participants had a medical diagnosis of CP confirmed by a neuropediatrician. Participant children were recruited from the major public hospital and the major public school in the capital city of Amman where the majority of children with CP receive rehabilitation services. Mothers' of participant children mean age was 35 years (SD = 6.1) and fathers' mean age was 37 years (SD = 7). Forty percent of the mothers and 46% of the fathers reported less than high school educational level. Table 1 presents demographic characteristics of participant children and parents.

This study was approved by the Institutional Review Boards of the University of Jordan Hospital and the Ministry of Health. Participant families were recruited by their

Table 1 Participants' characteristics

Variable (n)	Subcategories	n (%)
Age groups (n = 124)	2–4 years	59(47.6%)
	5–6 years	28(22.6%)
	> 6 years	37(29.8%)
Gender (n = 124)	Male	69 (55.6%)
	Female	55(44.4%)
Comorbidities (n = 123)	Vision impairment	45(36.6%)
	Hearing impairment	4(3.3%)
	Epilepsy/seizures	32(26%)
	Speech impairment	72(58.5%)
	Cognitive impairment	29(23.6%)
Mothers' age (n = 121)		32.5 (SD = 6.1)
Mothers' educational level (n = 123)	Less than high school	49(39.8%)
	Completed high school	38(30.9%)
	College (diploma 2 years)	19(15.4%)
	Graduate degree	15(12.2%)
	Postgraduate degree	2(1.6%)
Fathers' age (n = 122)		37.9 (SD = 7.0)
Fathers' educational level (n = 123)	Less than high school	56(45.5%)
	Completed high school	33(26.8%)
	College (diploma 2 years)	16(13.0%)
	Graduate degree	16(13.0%)
	Postgraduate degree	2(1.6%)

therapists and if they agreed to be contacted, a research assistant called the family and explained the study protocol. Each participating family were required to provide a written consent by one of the parents prior to data collection.

Measures

Gross motor function classification system-expanded and revised (GMFCS-E & R)

The GMFCS [3] was developed to measure functional activities of children with CP. The GMFCS classifies children based on their gross motor function into five levels from Level I (walks without limitation) to Level V (severely limited mobility), as shown in Table 2. The system classifies current performance in daily life with focus on mobility rather than capabilities in standardized environments. The GMFCS was expanded and revised (GMFCS-E & R) [4] to include children with age 0–18 years and to reflect the potential impact of environmental and personal factors on children's mobility. Content validity, inter-rater reliability, and test-retest reliability were established for children with CP [3, 14].

Manual ability classification system (MACS)

The MACS [5] describes children's self-initiated manual ability to handle objects and their need for assistance or

adaptation during daily manual activities. The MACS focuses on performance in home, school, community rather than capability in standardized environment. The MACS classifies children from Level I (handles objects easily and successfully) to Level V (doesn't handle objects and has very limited ability to perform simple actions) as shown in Table 2. Construct validity and inter-rater reliability were established [5].

Procedure

Upon obtaining the written consent, data were collected during the children's visit to receive their physiotherapy treatments in hospital or during physiotherapy sessions in school. The GMFCS-E & R and MACS levels were determined by research assistants who were physiotherapists or occupational therapists with 3 to 5 years of clinical experience with parental input. Research assistants were criterion-tested to classify children reliably prior to data collection. The subtypes of CP were determined by the research assistants according to the topographical distribution and predominant type of motor disorder including: spastic hemiplegia (spasticity in one half of the body), spastic quadriplegia (spasticity in four limbs), spastic diplegia (spasticity in both lower limbs more than both upper limbs), dyskinesia (athetosis, dystonia, chorea), ataxia (hypotonia with dysmetria or poor balance), and unknown type.

Data analysis

Statistical analyses were conducted using the Statistical Package for the Social Sciences (SPSS) for Windows, version 24.0 (SPSS Inc., Chicago, IL, USA). Analyses were performed for the entire sample first followed by subgroups based on the following topographical distribution of motor disorder: spastic diplegia, spastic quadriplegia, spastic hemiplegia, dyskinesia, ataxia, and unknown; and based on the children's chronological age groups: two to less than four years, four to less than six years, and older than six years.

To achieve the first aim of the study descriptive analyses including frequency and cross tabulation of numbers of children in each level of the GMFCS-E & R and the MACS were performed to describe functional profiles.

To achieve the second aim of the study the following statistical tests were performed: (1) associations between GMFCS-E & R and MACS were examined by calculating Spearman's Rho correlation coefficients (r_s) because variables are ordinal. Spearman's Rho coefficient (r_s) was interpreted using the following criteria: $r_s \geq .8$ very strong relationship; $.6 \leq r_s < .8$ strong relationship; $.4 \leq r_s < .6$ moderate relationship; $.2 \leq r_s < .4$ weak relationship; $r_s < .2$ very weak relationship [15]; (2) Levels of agreement between GMFCS-E & R and MACS levels were

Table 2 Summary of GMFCS-E & R and MACS criteria

Level	GMFCS-E & R (Palisano et al., 1997)	MACS (Eliasson et al., 2006)
I	Walks without Limitations	Handles objects easily and successfully
II	Walks with Limitations	Handles most objects but with somewhat reduced quality and/or speed of achievement.
III	Walks Using a Hand-Held Mobility Device	Handles objects with difficulty; needs help to prepare and/or modify activities
VI	Self-Mobility with Limitations; May Use Powered Mobility	Handles a limited selection of easily managed objects in adapted situations
V	Transported in a Manual Wheelchair	Does not handle objects and has severely limited ability to perform even simple actions.

assessed by calculating the non-weighted Kappa statistics. Kappa statistics were interpreted according to Altman criteria where kappa value of <.20 is poor, .21–.40 is fair, .41–.60 is moderate, .61–.80 is good and > .80 is a very good agreement [16]; and (3) Associations were examined based on subtypes of CP and children's chronological age using Wilcoxon signed ranks test and Sign test. A probability level of $p < .01$ was considered statistically significant.

Results

Entire sample

Overall, a strong correlation was found between GMFCS-E & R and MACS levels ($r_s = .73$, $p < .001$) while the agreement between the two classifications was poor (kappa value = .19; SE = .05). Only 9% of the participants were able to ambulate independently and handle objects easily (Level I in both GMFCS-E & R and MACS), whereas 13% have severely limited mobility even with assistive devices and were unable to handle objects (Level V in both GMFCS-E & R and MACS). Of all participants, 36% were able to ambulate independently (GMFCS-E & R Levels I-II) and 64% were able to handle objects independently (MACS Levels I-II). Table 3 shows the distribution of participants across GMFCS-E & R and MACS levels. Fifty seven percent of the participants demonstrated manual abilities better than gross motor function and 34% have been classified into equivalent levels in both classifications (Wilcoxon signed ranks test: $p < .001$, Sign test: $p < .001$).

Groups based on subtypes of CP

Figure 1 shows distribution of children across GMFCS-E & R and MACS levels by CP subtypes. The relationship between GMFCS-E & R and MACS levels is differentiated by subtypes of CP. Specifically, correlations were very strong in children with spastic quadriplegia ($r_s = .81$, $p < .001$), strong in children with ataxia ($r_s = .71$, $p < .001$) and spastic diplegia ($r_s = .64$, $p < .001$), and weak in children with spastic hemiplegia ($r_s = .38$, $p = .12$) and dyskinesia ($r_s = .32$, $p = .54$). None of the participants had a mixed subtype of CP. Overall, poor agreement was found between GMFCS-E & R and MACS levels across different subtypes with kappa values <.2.

Table 4 illustrates concordance between GMFCS-E & R and MACS levels by different CP subtypes and chronological age of children. Only, children with spastic diplegia and spastic quadriplegia demonstrated different profiles of motor function. Seventy percent of children with spastic diplegia and 59% of children with spastic quadriplegia have better manual abilities than gross motor function (Wilcoxon signed ranks test: $p < .001$; Sign test: $p < .001$). However, in children with spastic hemiplegia, dyskinesia, and ataxia the relationships between the GMFCS-E & R and MACS levels were not differentiated significantly based on CP subtypes (Wilcoxon signed ranks test: $p = .24$, .71, .06; Sign test: $p = .58$, .63, .13).

Groups based on chronological age of children

Figure 2 shows distribution of participants across GMFCS-E & R and MACS levels by age groups. The

Table 3 Distribution of the participants across the GMFCS-E & R and the MACS levels

		MACS					Total
		Level I	Level II	Level III	Level IV	Level V	
GMFCS-E & R	Level I	11	5	0	0	0	16 (13.1%)
	Level II	16	9	3	0	0	28 (23.0%)
	Level III	4	10	1	0	0	15 (12.3%)
	Level IV	6	17	10	4	4	41 (33.6%)
	Level V	0	0	3	3	16	22 (18.0%)
Total		37 (30.3%)	41 (33.6%)	17 (13.9%)	7 (5.7%)	20 (16.4%)	122

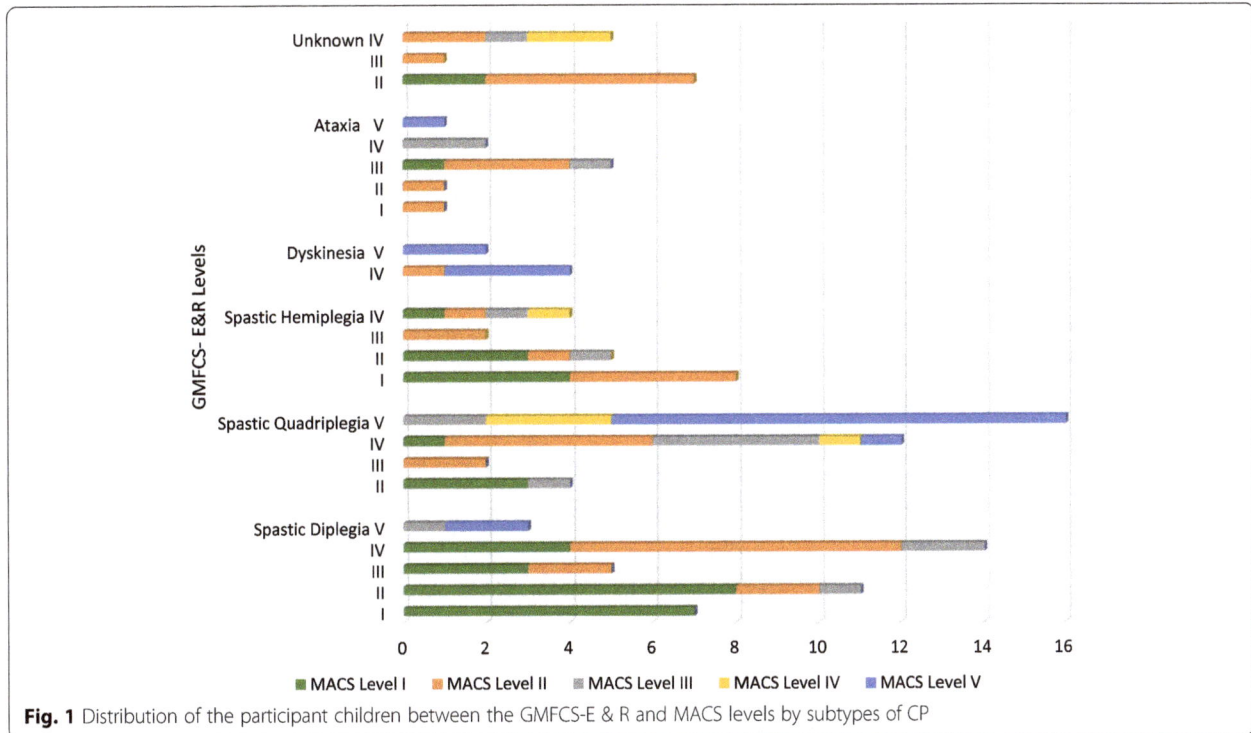

Fig. 1 Distribution of the participant children between the GMFCS-E & R and MACS levels by subtypes of CP

strongest correlation was found between GMFCS-E & R and MACS levels of children at age four to less than six years (r_s = .81, p < .001). The agreement however was poor (kappa value = .21, SE = .10, p < 0.001) with 61% of the children demonstrated manual abilities better than gross motor function (Wilcoxon signed ranks test: p < .001, Sign test: p < .001). Strong correlation was found between GMFCS-E & R and MACS for children older than 6 years (r_s = .78, p < .001), with 83% demonstrating better manual abilities (Wilcoxon signed ranks test: p <

p < .001). A strong correlation was also found (r_s = .73, p < .001) for the youngest age group with fair agreement (kappa value = .31, SE = .08, p < .001). Around 45% of the children were classified into equivalent GMFCS-E & R and MACS levels (Wilcoxon signed ranks test: p = .005, Sign test: p = .052).

Discussion

This is, to our knowledge, the first study that describes functional profiles of children with CP and examines associations between the gross motor functions and the

Table 4 Concordance between the MACS and the GMFCS-E & R levels by subtypes of CP and chronological age groups

	MACS level < GMFCS- E & R level (Manual ability better than gross motor function)	MACS level > GMFCS-E & R level (Gross motor function better than manual ability)	MACS level = GMFCS-E & R level (Manual ability is similar to gross motor function)
Entire sample (n = 122)	69[**] (56.6%)	12[**] (9.8%)	41[**] (33.6%)
Subtype of CP			
Spastic diplegia (n = 40)	28[**] (70.0%)	1[**] (2.5%)	11[**] (27.5%)
Spastic quadriplegia (n = 34)	20[**] (58.8%)	2[**] (5.9%)	12[**] (35.3%)
Spastic hemiplegia (n = 19)	8 (42.1%)	5 (26.3%)	6 (31.6%)
Dyskinesia (n = 6)	1 (16.7%)	3 (50.0%)	2 (33.3%)
Ataxia (n = 10)	6 (60.0%)	1 (10.0%)	3 (30.0%)
Unknown (n = 13)	6 (46.2%)	0 (0.0%)	7 (53.8%)
Chronological age			
2 - > 4 years (n = 58)	22[*](37.9%)	10[*] (17.2%)	26[*] (44.8%)
4 - < 6 years (n = 28)	17[**] (60.7%)	1[**] (3.6%)	10[**] (35.7%)
≥ 6 years (n = 36)	30[**] (83.3%)	1[**] (2.8%)	5[**] (13.9%)

**Wilcoxon signed ranks teat and Sign test significant p < .001
*Wilcoxon signed ranks teat and Sign test significant p < .01

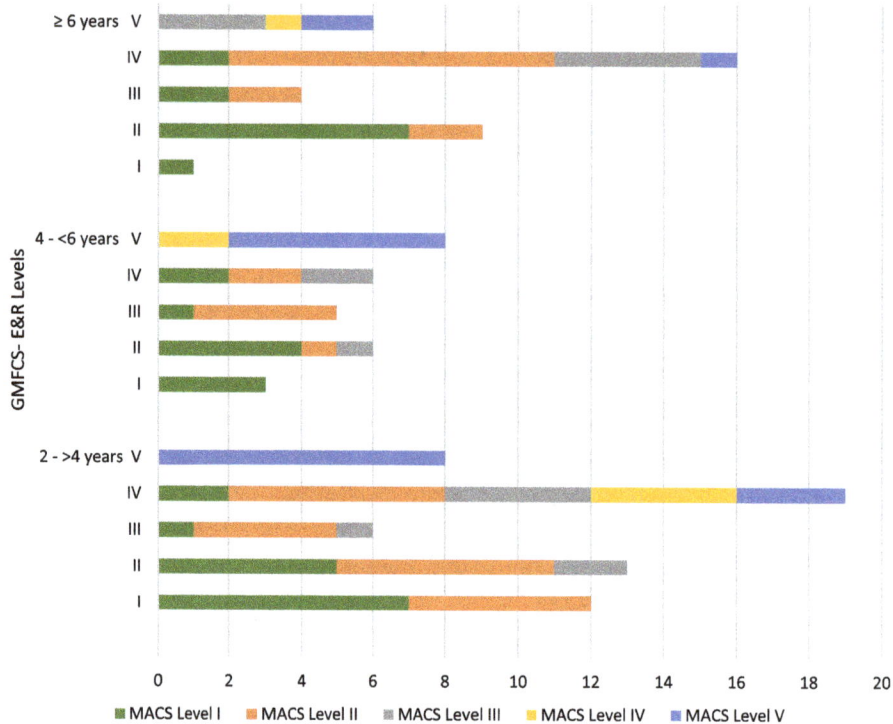

Fig. 2 Distribution of the participant children between the GMFCS-E & R and the MACS levels by chronological age groups

manual abilities in Jordan. The most commonly observed profile was "*manual abilities better than gross motor function*" which was demonstrated by 57% of the participants. Although associations between the GMFCS-E & R and the MACS were very strong in children with spastic quadriplegia and strong in children with spastic diplegia, and very strong in children less than four years and strong in children older than four years; agreements between the two classifications were poor across CP subtypes and chronological age groups indicating related yet diverse functional abilities of children with CP. Different functional profiles were observed and described based on subtypes of CP and chronological age of children.

Examination of functional profiles of children with CP in our study revealed that 53% of the participant children have severe limitation in gross motor functions (I.e., Levels IV and V GMFCS-E & R). This suggested that the majority of children who receive services in the public health care sector in Jordan have severe limitations in the gross motor functions. Describing functional profiles for children with CP in Jordan is expected to inform policy makers about the needs of children and their families. Implications for decision makers are to assure that public health care sector is being equipped to meet the extensive needs of children with severe limitation of function such as: wheelchairs, assistive devices, orthosis, and environmental modifications to enhance their functional activity and participation.

In congruence to research performed in other countries, we found a strong correlation yet poor agreement between the GMFCS-E & R and the MACS [7, 9–12]. This indicates that the two classifications complement each other and describe different types of activities of daily living which are ambulation and manual abilities of children with CP. The utilization of the two classifications by health professionals in Jordan is recommended to provide an accurate description of the functional performance of children with CP. Current rehabilitation practices in Jordan are based on traditional classifications of CP rather than functional classification, with focus on impairment rather than function-based interventions. Using functional classifications in practice is expected to shift the focus of rehabilitation professionals from impairment-based to functional-based practices, consequently, improving outcomes of services.

Functional profiles were differentiated based on subtypes of CP but the observed patterns were not consistent with the subtype's definitions. The most common functional profile of children with diplegia was "*manual abilities better than gross motor function*". This functional profile is consistent with the definition of diplegia, yet 30% of the children demonstrated other functional profiles. Also, the most common functional profile in the group of children with quadriplegia was "*manual abilities better than gross motor function*". Although the term quadriplegia indicates involvement of both upper and lower extremities due to extensive injuries of the sensorimotor areas of the brain [7], 35% of children with spastic quadriplegia had equal fine and gross motor abilities, and 6% had gross motor functions better than manual abilities. These findings suggests that subtypes of CP include children with different functional abilities, highlighting the importance of using more reliable and accurate functional classifications to describe children with CP. A recommendation for health professionals is to combine traditional classifications with more reliable functional classifications when evaluating children with CP to provide comprehensive description of children with CP and guide service planning.

Functional profiles of children were differentiated based on children's chronological age. Forty five percent of children with CP between two and four years of age demonstrated a profile of *"equivalent gross motor and manual abilities"*, whereas 61% of the children between four and six years of age and 83% of children older than six years demonstrated a profile of *"manual abilities better than gross motor function"*. This indicates that children in older age groups demonstrate better manual abilities than gross motor functions. Manual abilities and hand functioning require higher cognitive abilities and motor control than gross motor functions and occur at older ages which might explain increasing percentages of children in advanced manual abilities profiles in older age groups [9]. These findings should be interpreted with caution due to the convenience sampling method used in recruitment; most of the participants were recruited from physiotherapy clinics were children are usually referred due to gross motor function rather than manual abilities limitation. The influence of children's age should be further examined with a population-based sample to confirm our findings.

Applications of functional profiles of children with CP can inform clinicians, researchers, and policy makers in Jordan. Clinicians can use the functional profiles to select appropriate treatment approaches based on child's level of function, and to inform parents and help them to set up goals and plan for their children. For example children with better functional profiles (i.e. better gross motor and fine motor abilities) are more likely to function well in everyday activities in home, school, and community requiring services that are more focused on participation outcomes and integration in the community. Whereas children with limited functional profiles (i.e. profiles of limited gross motor and fine motor abilities) are more likely to demonstrate limitations in activity and require more assistance requiring more intensive treatment plans that focuses on activities of daily living and independency [17, 18]. The use of functional classifications among clinicians can improve communication and coordination of services. Researchers can use

functional profiles in clustering children with CP in homogeneous groups to conduct focused intervention studies. Policy makers can use functional profiles to anticipate needs of children with CP and their families and to insure availability, accessibility, and coordination of services required to fulfill these needs.

This study shows important strengths in that participant children were all classified by criterion tested physio- and occupational therapists with parents' consensus on classifications levels. In addition, participant children had the GMFCS-E & R and the MACS levels determined by the same therapist. The results of the study should be considered in light of some limitations in relation to sample size and selection of participants which might limit generalization of results. This also raises the need for population-based sample to be able to examine the national profiles of children with CP in Jordan and allow for international comparisons.

Conclusions

Health professionals in Jordan are encourage to use both the GMFCS-E & R and MACS in addition to traditional subtypes classification in order to classify children with CP with focus on function rather than impairment. Both the GMFCS-E & R and the MACS provide complementary but distinctive information related to mobility and handling of children with CP, supporting the need to use the two classification to provide comprehensive description of abilities of children with CP. Functional profiles of children with CP provide a practical and easy way for assessment to plan for services, guide provision of interdisciplinary and comprehensive services for children with CP, and enhance communication among professionals who provide services for children with CP and their families in Jordan.

Abbreviations
CP: cerebral Palsy; GMFCS-E & R: Gross Motor Function Classification System Expanded and Revised; ICF: International Classification of Functioning, Disability, and Health; MACS: Manual Abilities Classification System

Acknowledgements
The authors would like to thank the participant families and children for their time and commitment. A special gratitude for the participant sites including Albasheer Hospital, the Cerebral Palsy Foundation, and the University of Jordan Hospital for their support.

Funding
This study is funded by the Scientific Research Support Fund- Ministry of Research and Higher Education- Jordan and by the University Of Jordan Deanship Of Scientific Research.

Authors' contributions
All authors participated in designing the study, NA and MS supervised data collection, NA performed data analysis and prepared the first draft of the manuscript. All authors edited and approved the final manuscript.

Competing interests
The authors declare that they have no competing interests.

Author details
[1]Department of Physiotherapy, School of Rehabilitation Sciences, The University of Jordan, Queen Rania Al Abdallah St, Amman 11942, Jordan. [2]Department of occupational therapy, School of Rehabilitation Sciences, The University of Jordan, Queen Rania Al Abdallah St, Amman 11942, Jordan. [3]Faculty of Medicine, Lund university, P.0. 157, SE-221 00 Lund, Sweden.

References
1. Cans C. Surveillance of cerebral palsy in Europe: a collaboration of cerebral palsy surveys and registers. Dev Med Child Neurol. 2000;42(12):816–24.
2. Rosenbaum P, Paneth N, Leviton A, Goldstein M, Bax M, Damiano D, Dan B. Jacobsson B. A report: the definition and classification of cerebral palsy April 2006. Dev Med Child Neurol Suppl. 2007;109(suppl 109):8–14.
3. Palisano R, Rosenbaum P, Walter S, Russell D, Wood E, Galuppi B. Development and reliability of a system to classify gross motor function in children with cerebral palsy. Dev Med Child Neurol. 1997;39(4):214–23.
4. Palisano RJ, Rosenbaum P, Bartlett D, Livingston MH. Content validity of the expanded and revised gross motor function classification system. Dev Med Child Neurol. 2008 Oct 1;50(10):744–50.
5. Eliasson AC, Krumlinde-Sundholm L, Rösblad B, Beckung E, Arner M, Öhrvall AM, Rosenbaum P. The manual ability classification system (MACS) for children with cerebral palsy: scale development and evidence of validity and reliability. Dev Med Child Neurol. 2006;48(7):549–54.
6. World Health Organization. International classification of functioning, Disability, and Health: ICF. Geneva: World Health Organization; 2001.
7. Hidecker MJ, Ho NT, Dodge N, Hurvitz EA, Slaughter J, Workinger MS, Kent RD, Rosenbaum P, Lenski M, Messaros BM, Vanderbeek SB. Inter-relationships of functional status in cerebral palsy: analyzing gross motor function, manual ability, and communication function classification systems in children. Dev Med Child Neurol. 2012;54(8):737–42.
8. Almasri N, Saleh M. Inter-rater agreement of the Arabic Gross Motor Classification System Expanded & Revised in children with cerebral palsy in Jordan. Disabil Rehabil. 2015;37(20):1895–901.
9. Carnahan KD, Arner M, Hägglund G. Association between gross motor function (GMFCS) and manual ability (MACS) in children with cerebral palsy. A population-based study of 359 children. BMC Musculoskelet Disord. 2007; 8(1):50.
10. Gunel MK, Mutlu A, Tarsuslu T, Livanelioglu A. Relationship among the manual ability classification system (MACS), the gross motor function classification system (GMFCS), and the functional status (WeeFIM) in children with spastic cerebral palsy. Eur J Pediatr. 2009;168(4):477–85.
11. Oskoui M, Majnemer A, Dagenais L, Shevell MI. The relationship between gross motor function and manual ability in cerebral palsy. J Child Neurol. 2013;28(12):1646–52.
12. Majnemer A, Shikako-Thomas K, Shevell M, Poulin C, Lach L, Law M, Schmitz N. Group TQ. The relationship between manual ability and ambulation in adolescents with cerebral palsy. Phys Occup Ther Pediatr. 2013;33(2):243–52.
13. Saleh M, Almasri NA. Cerebral palsy in Jordan: demographics, medical characteristics, and access to services. Child Health Care. 2017;46(1):49–65.
14. Wood E, Rosenbaum P. The gross motor function classification system for cerebral palsy: a study of reliability and stability over time. Dev Med Child Neurol. 2000;42(5):292–6.
15. Campbell, Michael J. Statistics at square two: understanding modern statistical applications in medicine. Hoboken: Blackwell; 2006.
16. Altman DG. Practical statistics for medical research. Boca Raton: CRC press; 1990.
17. Mutlu A, Akmese PP, Gunel MK, Karahan S, Livanelioglu A. The importance of motor functional levels from the activity limitation perspective of ICF in children with cerebral palsy. Int J Rehabil Res. 2010;33(4):319–24.
18. Rosenbaum P, Stewart D. The World Health Organization International Classification of Functioning, Disability, and Health: a model to guide clinical thinking, practice and research in the field of cerebral palsy. In Seminars in Pediatr Neurol. 2004;11(1):5–10. WB Saunders

18

Cultural adaptation and harmonization of four Nordic translations of the revised Premature Infant Pain Profile (PIPP-R)

Emma Olsson[1,2]* , Agneta Anderzén-Carlsson[3], Sigríður María Atladóttir[4,5], Anna Axelin[6], Marsha Campbell-Yeo[7,8], Mats Eriksson[9], Guðrún Kristjánsdóttir[4,5], Emilia Peltonen[6], Bonnie Stevens[10,11], Bente Vederhus[12] and Randi Dovland Andersen[13,14]

Abstract

Background: Preterm infants are especially vulnerable to pain. The intensive treatment often necessary for their survival unfortunately includes many painful interventions and procedures. Untreated pain can lead to both short- and long-term negative effects. The challenge of accurately detecting pain has been cited as a major reason for lack of pain management in these non-verbal patients. The Premature Infant Pain Profile (PIPP) is one of the most extensively validated measures for assessing procedural pain in premature infants. A revised version, PIPP-R, was recently published and is reported to be more user-friendly and precise than the original version. The aims of the study were to develop translated versions of the PIPP-R in Finnish, Icelandic, Norwegian, and Swedish languages, and to establish their content validity through a cultural adaptation process using cognitive interviews.

Methods: PIPP-R was translated using the recommendations from the International Society for Pharmacoeconomics and Outcomes Research and enhanced with cognitive interviews. The respondent nurse was given a copy of the translated, national version of the measure and used this together with a text describing the infant in the film to assess the pain of an infant in a short film. During the assessment the nurse was asked to verbalize her thought process (thinking aloud) and upon completion the interviewer administered probing questions (verbal probing) from a structured interview guide. The interviews were recorded, transcribed, and analyzed using a structured matrix approach.

Results: The systematic approach resulted in translated and culturally adapted versions of PIPP-R in the Finnish, Icelandic, Norwegian and Swedish languages. During the cultural adaptation process several problems were discovered regarding how the respondent understood and utilized the measure. The problems were either measure problems or other problems. Measure problems were solved by a change in the translated versions of the measure, while for other problems different solutions such as education or training were suggested.

Conclusions: This study have resulted in translations of the PIPP-R that have content validity, high degree of clinical utility and displayed beginning equivalence with each other and the original version of the measure.

Keywords: Neonatal, Pain, Pain assessment

* Correspondence: miniemma@hotmail.com
[1]Department of Pediatrics, Faculty of Medicine and Health, Örebro University Hospital, S-701 85 Örebro, Sweden
[2]Faculty of Medicine and Health, School of Medical Sciences, Örebro University, Örebro, Sweden
Full list of author information is available at the end of the article

Background

Preterm infants, delivered weeks and often months early, are especially vulnerable to pain. All their bodily systems, including the nervous system, are immature. While their pain-signaling pathways are present and fully functional, their pain inhibitory systems are still underdeveloped, causing their pain to be prolonged and increased [1]. The intensive treatment often necessary for their survival includes many painful interventions and procedures. A recent Dutch study reported that infants in the neonatal intensive care unit (NICU) underwent a mean of 11.4 (SD 5.7) painful procedures per day [2], findings consistent with a recent systematic review of epidemiological studies [3]. Sadly, pain-relieving interventions were associated with fewer than half of these procedures [3].

The challenges of accurately detecting pain in these non-verbal patients has been cited as a major reason for lack of pain management in this population [4]. While over 40 infant pain measures have been published, their validity varies widely, adding to the difficulties of accurate pain assessment, especially in preterm infants [5]. Clinical use of insufficiently validated measures poses a risk to patient safety as they may result in both under- and over-assessment of pain. Under-assessment may cause unnecessary pain and suffering, as untreated pain in an infant can lead to both short- and long-term negative consequences including physiologic instability and altered development of the neurological, somatosensory and stress response systems [6] and poorer brain development [7]. Repeated exposure to pain may also lower the infants' pain thresholds and increase sensitivity to subsequent pain [1] an effect that can persist after the neonatal period [8–10].

Over-assessment of pain, i.e. assuming that the patient is in pain while he/she is not, may lead to unnecessary use of pain-relieving medication with their potentially negative side effects [11]. Pharmacological treatments should be used selectively during the neonatal period because of the infants' immature drug metabolism and elimination. The use of opioids increases the risk of respiratory depression and may also affect neurodevelopment [12, 13]. These vulnerabilities emphasize the importance of valid and effective assessment of pain in this patient group in order to both minimize pain and the risks associated with pharmacological treatment of pain [14, 15].

The Premature Infant Pain Profile (PIPP) is one of the most extensively validated measures for assessing procedural pain in premature infants [15, 16]. PIPP is currently being used in clinical practice in several Nordic NICUs. A revised version, PIPP-R, was recently published and is reported to be more user-friendly and precise than the original version [17, 18].

In accordance with the COSMIN taxonomy [19] face and content validity are two aspects of content validity. Both face and content validity are judgment-based, qualitative evaluations. While face validity concerns whether the PIPP/PIPP-R looks like a good reflection of the construct pain, construct validity is an evaluation of whether the PIPP/PIPP-R is an adequate representation of the construct pain concerning relevance and comprehensiveness. Content validity of the PIPP/PIPP-R was established during the construction of the PIPP measure [16]. In addition, content validity also needs to be addressed for all translated versions of the measure, as their validity is dependent upon how the translation and cultural adaptation were carried out [20]. Content validity should be assessed by those who are going to use the scale [21], for example through cognitive interviews where future users of the scale explain their understanding and use of the measure [20]. When establishing content validity of a translated measure, the translation needs to maintain fidelity towards the original version [22]. A systematic cultural adaptation ensures that the original meaning and content is retained in the translated versions of the measure [23]. Measure equivalence is a prerequisite for valid comparisons between data collected with different language versions of a measure [24]. Performing a parallel and collaborative translation and cultural adaptation of several language version of the measure simultaneously helps ensure beginning equivalence across the translated versions and between the translated versions and the original version. In that regard, this collaborative process will support future collaborative research involving the PIPP-R.

Translation and cultural adaptation is a necessary first step towards clinical implementation of the revised version of the PIPP in the Nordic countries. As such, the aims of this study were to develop translated versions of the PIPP-R in Finnish, Icelandic, Norwegian, and Swedish languages, and to establish their content validity and beginning equivalence through a cultural adaptation process using cognitive interviews.

Methods

Study design

The study followed the methodology recommended by the International Society For Pharmacoeconomics and Outcomes Research (ISPOR) Task Force for Translation and Cultural Adaptation [20]. An existing study protocol developed based on ISPOR methodology and enhanced with cognitive interviews [25] was modified for this study. For an overview of the translation and cultural adaptation process, see Fig 1.

The authors of the original PIPP-R granted permission to translate PIPP-R and the work was done in collaboration with them.

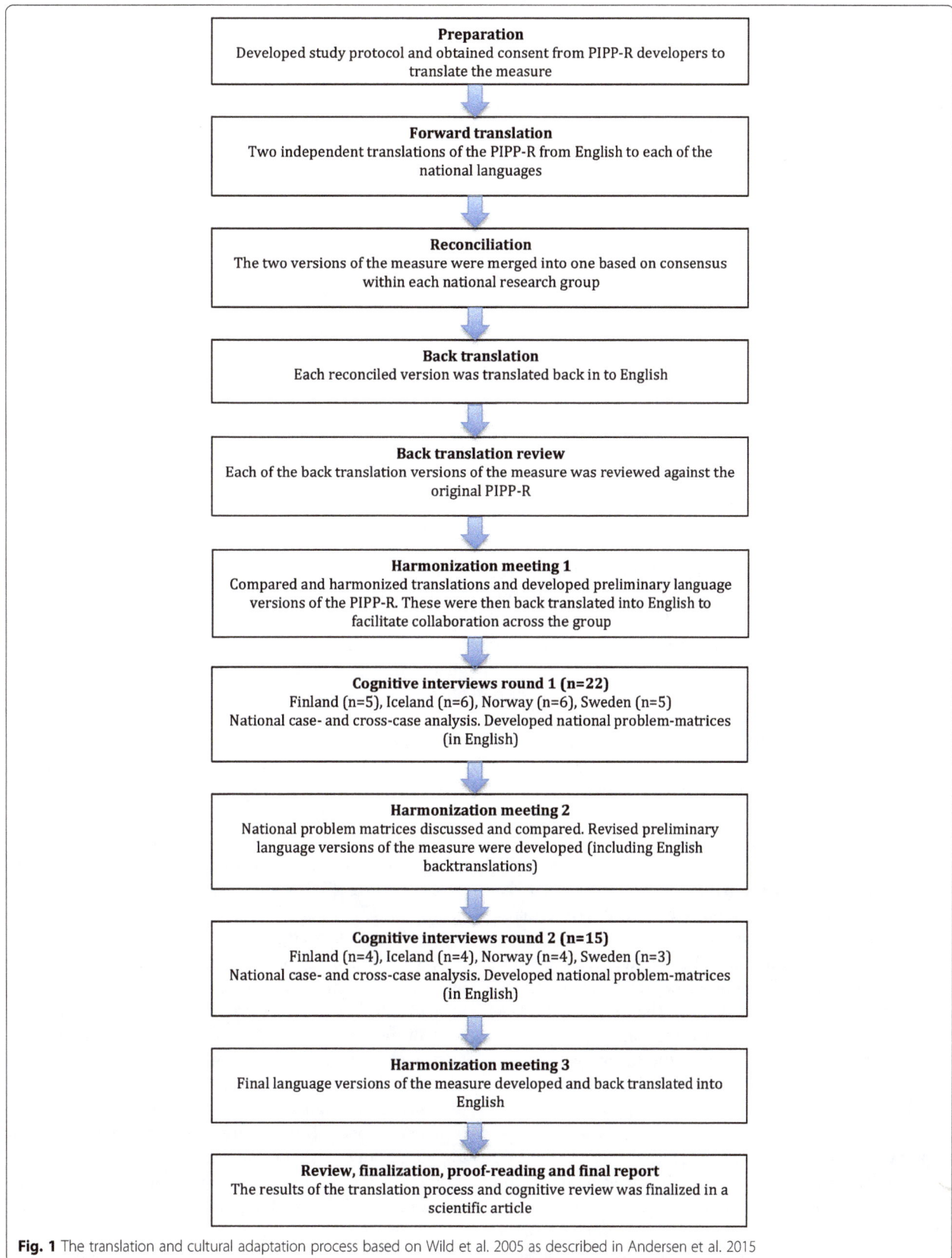

Fig. 1 The translation and cultural adaptation process based on Wild et al. 2005 as described in Andersen et al. 2015

PIPP-R

PIPP-R is a multidimensional pain assessment measure. It consists of three behavioral indicators (brow bulge, eye squeeze, and naso-labial furrow), two physiological indicators (heart rate and oxygen saturation), and two contextual indicators (corrected gestational age and behavioral state) that modify the score. The assessment starts with a 15 s baseline measurement of the heart rate and oxygen saturation and the infants' corrected gestational age and behavioral state are noted. Changes in physiological and behavioral indicators are then assessed during the first 30 s of the painful procedure. If there is a response in the physiologic and behavioral variables during the procedure, scores for corrected gestational age and behavioral state are added. These contextual variables weight greater points for the more immature infants and the infants in quiet sleep state since it is well known that these infants react with less vigorous pain cues [18]. Each indicator is scored from zero to three points and summed into a total pain intensity score ranging from zero to 21 points.

Translation procedure

The process, which was performed during 2015, started with a forward translation in which two independent translations of the PIPP-R were performed in each country, one by the national investigator with extensive knowledge of neonatal pain assessment and one by a certified translator. The two versions of the measure were then merged into one, through consensus within each national group. The respective reconciled versions were then back-translated by a native English-speaking health care professional or a certified translator blinded to the original scale. All translators were bilingual and translated into their native language. Each back-translated version of the measure was reviewed against the original PIPP-R, any discrepancies examined against the reconciled version, and appropriate revisions were made on national level. During a meeting with all members of the group (harmonization meeting 1), the four preliminary versions of the PIPP-R were compared and harmonized with each other and with the original PIPP-R measure. Back-translated English versions of the preliminary measures were used during the meetings to make comprehension and comparison possible within the research group.

Cognitive interviews

The cultural adaptation of the national versions of the PIPP-R was carried out using cognitive interviews as described by Andersen et al. [25]. Originally, cognitive interviewing aims to understand how respondents understand, process and answer questions and also to identify potential problems with survey questions. The

process often starts with the respondents "thinking aloud," recounting everything they think about while completing a task. The investigator can also use verbal probing, asking the respondents to paraphrase questions, define meanings of different items, or explain their answers [26]. Andersen and colleagues (2014) modified this approach for use with observational pain scales.

A structured interview guide was developed for the cognitive interviews by two of the national researchers (EO and RDA). It included training of the participant in the think-aloud method and an introduction to the PIPP-R, followed by a section where the respondent used the think-aloud method to describe their understanding of the PIPP-R measure and a set of structured questions about how the respondent understood each item of the PIPP-R. Finally, the respondent was given the opportunity to add anything that had not been brought up earlier. The same national researchers (EO and RDA) each carried out one pilot interview to test the interview guide and small adjustments were made. The interview guide was then translated into the different languages by the national investigators in each country.

Sample and setting

A total of 37 nurses with a minimum of one year of NICU experience and fluent in the target national language were recruited and agreed to be interviewed. A purposeful sampling procedure was used to include a diverse group of nurses in regard to age, education, clinical experience, and experience with structured pain assessment measures. The participating nurses had between 1 and 33 years of NICU experience, and 15 of them had a specialist education. While all had access to pain assessment measures at their unit, just over half reported using them (see Table 1). None of them had previous experience using PIPP-R.

Data collection procedure

Following informed consent, the respondent participated in a cognitive interview that was recorded and transcribed verbatim. The respondent nurse was given a copy of the translated PIPP-R and was instructed to read it through and familiarize herself with the measure. Subsequently, the respondent was asked to use the PIPP-R to assess pain from a short film showing an infant exposed to a painful procedure (the same film was used for all respondents) and an accompanying written text describing the infant in the film. The respondent was asked to verbalize her thought process while completing the assessment (thinking aloud), and upon completion of the assessment the interviewer used probing questions from the structured interview guide (verbal probing). The aim of the interviews was to identify any

Table 1 Demographic information about the included nurses

Participants in each country (round 1+ round 2)	Finland $n = 9$ (5 + 4)	Iceland $n = 10$ (6 + 4)	Norway (n = 10) (6 + 4)	Sweden ($n = 8$) (5 + 3)
Level of education	RN – 7 Specialist nurse – 2	RN – 6 Specialist nurse – 4	RN – 6 Specialist nurse – 3	RN – 2 Specialist nurse - 6
Clinical NICU experience (years)	1.5–13.5 (median 3.5)	1.5–24 (median 8.5)	1–33 (median 16.3)	2–22 (median 11.5)
Experience with pain assessment	9	9	10	8
Access to pain assessment instrument at unit	9	9	10	8
Received training in how to use instrument at unit	7	4	9	6
Use pain assessment instrument in daily work	4	0	10	8

problems in the understanding and application of the measure. One researcher performed the interviews in Finland, Iceland, and Sweden respectively, while two researchers performed the interviews in Norway.

Data were collected and analyzed in two rounds during 2016. The first round comprised 22 interviews (five in Finland, six in Iceland, six in Norway, and five in Sweden) and the second round 15 interviews (four in Finland, four in Iceland, four in Norway, and three in Sweden). The interviews lasted from 38 min to 66 min.

Data analysis
The interview data were analyzed using Miles and Huberman's [27] approach to data analysis using matrices and case- and cross-case analyses. A predefined problem matrix was developed with a set of organizational categories including the items on the PIPP-R (change in heart rate, decrease in oxygen saturation, brow bulge, eye squeeze, naso-labial furrow, corrected gestational age and behavioral state), the title of the measure, the scoring instructions, use of film and the overall use of the measure. Problems perceived by either the respondents or the interviewers during the interviews were entered in the matrix together with suggested strategies from the researchers for solving the problems.

After each round of interviews, the national data was independently analyzed in the national language by the national researcher. Each participant was considered a case and a single-case analysis was conducted after each interview. Data from national single-case problem matrices were compiled into one cross-case matrix, condensed and refined. The cross-case matrices were translated into English and the translated versions discussed in two harmonization meetings (one after each interview round) with all researchers present. After the first round of interviews, the researchers identified problems that required adjustment in the preliminary translated versions of the PIPP-R. These were discussed during the second harmonization meeting, and the developers of the measure were consulted about the

proposed changes described below. Revisions were made and the revised versions of the respective measure where then used in the second round of interviews. A final cross-country, cross-case matrix was developed and provided an overview of all problems identified in the study.

Results
This systematic approach resulted in translated and culturally adapted versions of the PIPP-R pain assessment measure in the Finnish, Icelandic, Norwegian, and Swedish languages. During the cultural adaptation process several problems were discovered regarding how the respondents understood and utilized the measure. The problems can be divided into two categories: measure problems and other problems. Measure problems were solved by a change in the translated versions of the measure, while for the other problems different solutions such as education or training were suggested. Measure problems were further divided into the two sub-categories: problems related to the original version of the measure and problems related to the translated versions of the measure. The respective problems will be described below and are visualized in Table 2.

Problems related to the original version of the measure
Before the first interview round a few inaccuracies were discovered in the published original version of the PIPP-R [18] and these were adjusted for in all the translated versions. In the categorization of gestational age, the symbol > had been used instead of ≥, and as a result neonates born at 36 weeks' gestation did not fit into any of the categories. In step 2 of the scoring instructions the phrase "maximal heart rate" was used, although the indicator says "change in heart rate" to allow scoring of both an increase and a decrease in heart rate. Finally, "gestational age" was missing from the equation in step 4 and was therefore added.

In the indicator "oxygen saturation," respondents found the use of the word oxygen to describe both oxygen saturation and oxygen supply confusing. To clarify this, the abbreviation "SaO2" (oxygen saturation) was

Table 2 Problems and solutions found during the cultural adaptation process

Problems found	Solution	Finland	Iceland	Norway	Sweden
Problems related to the original version of the scale					
The application of the scale were not understood	Title clarification	X	X	X	
The word oxygen used to describe both oxygen supply and oxygen saturation	Wording changes to distinguish between SaO2 and FiO2	X	X	X	X
Scale uses both "corrected gestational age" and "gestational age" which respondents found confusing.	Changed to "corrected gestational age" throughout the scale	X	X	X	X
Unclear in step 2 which time frame that should be used for assessment	Clarification which 30 s that are to be used	X	X	X	X
The term "vital sign" is not explained in the scale	Changed to "physiological indicators"	X		X	X
In step 3 unclear when to include score for corrected GA and behavioral state	Clarifications on when these factors should be included	X	X	X	X
Unclear time frame for when to give points for additional oxygen	Clarification that it is the first 30 s that are to be assessed		X	X	X
Problems related to the translated versions of the scale					
Baseline not a familiar term	Change of wording			X	X
Not understanding the facial indicator "Brow Bulge"	Change of wording				X
Not understanding the facial indicator "Naso-labial furrow"	Change of wording	X	X	X	X
Explanatory word for the different categories (eg minimal, maximal) not making sense	Change of wording	X	X		
Problems that can be solved with education and training					
Unclear if you should assess baseline behavioral state once or several times	Education and training	X			
Unclear if it is duration or intensity of pain that is to be assessed	Education and training	X	X	X	X
Difficult to assess several parameters at the same time	Education and training	X	X	X	X
Would like a guiding instruction for the acquired pain score/a pain algorithm	Education and training	X	X	X	X
Uses mean heart rate/oxygen saturation instead of highest/lowest	Education and training		X		
The "+" sign before each scoring category is confusing	Education and training		X		
Difficulties distinguishing between the different behavioral states categories	Education and training		X	X	X
Unsure about how to assess a decrease in heart rate	Education and training			X	X
Difficult to understand how to score if fiO2 is increased	Education and training			X	
Scores for the time when the reaction occurs and not the duration of the reaction	Education and training			X	
Difficult to separate "Brow bulge" from "Eye squeeze" since they are highly correlated	Education and training			X	

The described problems were found in the language versions marked with "X"

added to the indicator, and in the + 3 score box the abbreviation FiO2 (fraction of inspired oxygen) was used to indicate any additional, delivered oxygen. The original measure used both the terms "gestational age" and "corrected gestational age" to describe the infant's age at the time of the assessment; several respondents were confused about whether this meant that the infant's age at birth (gestational age) was to be reported or the infant's age at the time for the procedure (corrected gestational age). ".. *I thought that gestational age meant the gestational age the baby was when it was born and not the*

gestational age the baby is now" (I3). All translated versions were revised to use "corrected gestational age" consistently.

In step 2 of the scoring instructions respondents expressed uncertainty about the time frame for the assessment. "*It says here 'after the procedure'. To my way of thinking it would be natural to score the child also during the procedure*" (N4). The phrase "observe infants for 30 seconds after the procedure" was changed into "observe infants during the first 30 seconds of the procedure".

The term "vital signs" in the original PIPP-R was used to describe heart rate and oxygen saturation, but because behavioral state was mentioned in the same sentence, some of the respondents thought this was also included in the vital signs. "*So I guess I would count those three (heart frequency, oxygen saturation and baseline behavioral state) as vital signs*" (S3). The term "physiological indicators" was thus chosen instead of "vital signs" in all versions except the Icelandic to make it clearer that oxygen saturation and heart rate were intended. In Icelandic the term "vital signs" is used in health care and well understood and was therefor kept in it's original form. In step 3 of the scoring instructions "score for corrected gestational age and behavioral state if the sub-total score >0," respondents did not understand when to give points for corrected gestational age and baseline behavioral state and when not to. All versions were clarified with the instruction "calculate *only* if the sub-total score is >0."

Problems related to the translated versions of the measure

This sub-category comprised misunderstandings of the translation of certain words or phrases. A direct translation of the word "baseline" was not a well-known expression in Norway and Sweden so it was replaced with various, more idiomatic versions of "before the procedure." "*I'm thinking it is often a bit difficult to know what the baseline is in comparison to when you observe and how you are supposed to – it has to be an average over some time*" (N6). The translation of the different facial indicators also proved difficult to understand in several of the countries. "*Naso-labial furrow.. What is that? Is it here?*" [Points to midline of upper lip] (I2). "Naso-labial furrow" was thus changed in all languages to a more descriptive phrase such as "furrow from nostril to corner of mouth" (Icelandic version) to enhance understanding, and "brow bulge" was changed to "frowning eye brows" in the Swedish version.

The explanatory words for assigning an indicator score for the different facial indicators were questioned in Iceland and Finland during the first round of interviews and a different set of descriptive scoring words were used in the second round. "*The option of 'much' seems to be missing from the indicator score. There is 'moderate' and then comes 'maximal'*" (F5). Abbreviations used in the original version of the measure, (e.g. BS for behavioral state) did not have equivalents in the target languages and were written out instead "*My first question would be what are the GA and BS indicator scores?*" (F1).

In the second round of interviews there were notably fewer measure problems and the only issue that led to a change was one nurse's belief that she should give points for any additional oxygen given at any time before or during a procedure even if the procedure lasted longer than the 30-s assessment period. The scoring instructions for step 2 "if an infant requires an increase in oxygen at any time before or during the procedure" did not specify the time frame and was clarified to read "before or during *the first 30 seconds* of the procedure".

Problems that can be solved with education and training

All other issues identified did not require a change in the measure and will most likely be solved with appropriate education, training and access to a scoring manual. Some of these problems differed between countries, while some were apparent in all versions. For example, many of the respondents were conflicted about whether it was the duration or the intensity of pain that should be assessed and reported. PIPP-R uses both a descriptive word for pain in each scoring category for the facial indicators (none, minimal, moderate, or maximal) but also a time reference (< 3, 3–10, 6–8, or > 8), which was confusing for most of the respondents. "*I am having a bit of trouble with the seconds. How long it [the reaction] is actually present. But maybe rather how strong the reaction is*" (S6). Respondents from all countries acknowledged having difficulty with assessing multiple indicators at the same time, something that will probably become easier with education and training. Nurses also wanted to know what to do with the score and asked for a pain management algorithm (i.e. what score represents pain and when should pain-relieving treatments be used).

Discussion

We translated and culturally adapted the PIPP-R pain assessment measure to Finnish, Icelandic, Norwegian, and Swedish through an international collaboration. During the translation we discovered that the respondents had a range of different problems understanding the measure as intended. Some problems were related to the original version of the measure and most were solved by clarifying the different aspects of the measure that were not understood correctly. The problems related to the translations of the measure mainly were unfamiliar words or phrases not commonly used in the various national settings. The use of different words and phrases elucidated these issues. This highlights the importance of not only translating a measure but also using a thorough translation and cultural adaptation process to preserve the meaning of the items in the measure [23, 28]. A simple direct translation procedure would not have sufficiently addressed the linguistic and cultural differences that were discovered during the work in this study.

This project was done in collaboration with the developers of the original measure [18]. This made it possible to go back to them for information about the intended use of the PIPP-R when questions arose. The PIPP-R, as well as any pain assessment measure, should be accompanied by adequate education and training before it is incorporated into clinical practice; research has shown that education can improve the use of pain assessment measures [29]. Many of the issues identified in this study will be eliminated through training and consistent education before the translated versions of the measure are used in clinical settings. A great deal of discussion was generated by the information in the scoring boxes for the facial indicators. The seemingly conflicting instructions of both intensity and duration of pain lead to discussions in the group about possibly removing the describing word from the measure. In consultation with the intention of the original measure, to be used both in clinical and research settings, this was considered as too much of a change to the published PIPP-R. A systematic on-line learning program has been developed for the PIPP-R that will probably solve this and many other issues.

A strength of this study was the simultaneous translation and harmonization process where the four translations of the PIPP-R were harmonized with both the original version of the measure [18] and with each other. Some of the problems we found were apparent in several of the translated versions, making it more likely that those problems were related to the original version of the measure and not a result of the translation. Through systematic comparisons across the different translated versions and between the translated versions and the original version we have laid the groundwork for further equivalence testing between scores obtained with the different language versions of the PIPP-R, an important requirement when these measures are used in research across countries [24].

The collaborative process resulted in beneficial discussions and diverse views of the different problems. The results of collaborative research may be more robust because of the different strengths and specialties in the group [30]. Having a team working together in different countries and with different native languages could be demanding but potential problems were reduced having English as a common language and by frequent meetings online and in person throughout the process. The results of this study are based on a rigorous translation and cultural adaptation process, which included cognitive nterviews with a total of 37 neonatal nurses with a wide variety of experience. All of them had access to pain assessment measures, but none had previous experience with the PIPP-R. This made it possible for them to have an unbiased opinion about the measure and few preconceived assumptions. Although all the nurses had access to a pain assessment measure, just over half of them reported using it in their daily practice. This is worrying because the use of pain assessment measures in this sensitive and non-verbal population is highly recommended [6]. This reported percentage might also be an over-estimation because of potential response bias [31]; nurses might have

wished to create a positive impression by stating that they used pain assessment measures more frequently than they actually did. The PIPP-R was designed to enhance feasibility and feasible measures are more likely to be used [18]. We believe this study have resulted in translations of the PIPP-R with good content validity, good feasibility and beginning equivalence to the original version of the measure, all of which support the clinical utility of the measure. Assumptions regarding equivalence and clinical utility of the measure need to be tested in further studies.

While considerable time has been spent on the development of pain assessment measures to assess infant pain, less emphasis has been placed on the clinical utility of these tools. This oversight may have contributed to the lack of consistent pain assessment and management and the wide variation in practice uptake across neonatal units worldwide. Future work in this area should ensure that emphasis is placed not only on ensuring the validity and reliability of pain assessment tools but also their clinical utility. Ensuring measures are systematically translated; including appropriate evaluation is an important component that should not be overlooked. Efforts should be made to translate and culturally adapt the learning program for PIPP-R so that health care professionals will be able to use the translated versions of the measure with appropriate comprehension and knowledge of how to use the measure. Future studies should also conduct psychometric testing and cross-cultural equivalence testing of the translated versions of the measure.

Why nurses choose not to use available pain assessment measures in their daily practice is another important area that requires deeper understanding.

Conclusions

This study have resulted in translations of the PIPP-R that have content validity, high degree of clinical utility and displayed beginning equivalence with each other and to the original version of the measure.

Abbreviations
FiO2: Fraction of Inspired Oxygen; ISPOR: International Society for Pharmacoeconomics and Outcomes research; NICU: Neonatal Intensive Care Unit; PIPP: Premature Infant Pain Profile; PIPP-R: Premature Infant Pain profile - revised; SaO2 : Oxygen saturation

Authors' contributions
All authors made substantial contributions to conception and design, analysis and interpretation of data. Translation and back-translation as well as the cognitive interviews and the preliminary analyses of them were done

respectively in Finland (AA, EP), Iceland (SMA, GK), Norway (RDA, BV) and Sweden (EO, AAC, ME). BS and MCY provided calibration with the original and updated English version of the instrument. Final analysis of the interviews and compilation of the language instruments were done together by all authors who also revised the manuscript and approved its final version.

Competing interests

The authors declare that they have no competing interests.

Author details

[1]Department of Pediatrics, Faculty of Medicine and Health, Örebro University Hospital, S-701 85 Örebro, Sweden. [2]Faculty of Medicine and Health, School of Medical Sciences, Örebro University, Örebro, Sweden. [3]University Health Care Research Center, Faculty of Medicine and Health, Örebro University, Örebro, Sweden. [4]Faculty of Nursing, University of Iceland, Reykjavik, Iceland. [5]Neonatal Intensive Care Unit, Lanspitali University Children's Hospital, Reykjavik, Iceland. [6]Department of Nursing Science, University of Turku, Turku, Finland. [7]School of Nursing, Faculty of Health Professions and Departments of Pediatrics, Psychology & Neuroscience, Dalhousie University, Halifax, Canada. [8]Centre for Pediatric Pain Research, IWK Health Centre, Halifax, Canada. [9]Faculty of Medicine and Health, School of Health Sciences, Örebro University, Örebro, Sweden. [10]Lawrence S Bloomberg, Faculty of Nursing, University of Toronto, Toronto, Canada. [11]Department of Nursing, The Hospital for Sick Children, Toronto, Canada. [12]Department of Pediatrics, Haukeland University Hospital, Bergen, Norway. [13]Department of Child and Adolescent Health Services, Telemark Hospital, Skien, Norway. [14]Department of Neurobiology, Care Sciences and Society, Karolinska Institutet, Stockholm, Sweden.

References

1. Fitzgerald M. The development of nociceptive circuits. Nat Rev Neurosci. 2005;6(7):507–20.
2. Roofthooft DW, Simons SH, Anand KJ, Tibboel D, van Dijk M. Eight years later, are we still hurting newborn infants? Neonatology. 2014;105(3):218–26.
3. Cruz MD, Fernandes AM, Oliveira CR. Epidemiology of painful procedures performed in neonates: a systematic review of observational studies. Eur J Pain. 2016;20(4):489–98.
4. Allegaert K, Tibboel D, Naulaers G, Tison D, De Jonge A, Van Dijk M, et al. Systematic evaluation of pain in neonates: effect on the number of intravenous analgesics prescribed. Eur J Clin Pharmacol. 2003;59(2):87–90.
5. Hatfield LA, Ely EA. Measurement of acute pain in infants: a review of behavioral and physiological variables. Biol Res Nurs. 2015;17(1):100–11.
6. Committee On F, Newborn SOA, Pain M. Prevention and Management of Procedural Pain in the Neonate: An Update. Pediatrics. 2016;137(2): e20154271.
7. Brummelte S, Grunau RE, Chau V, Poskitt KJ, Brant R, Vinall J, et al. Procedural pain and brain development in premature newborns. Ann Neurol. 2012;71(3):385–96.
8. Buskila D, Neumann L, Zmora E, Feldman M, Bolotin A, Press J. Pain sensitivity in prematurely born adolescents. Arch Pediatr Adolesc Med. 2003; 157(11):1079–82.
9. Grunau RV, Whitfield MF, Petrie JH. Pain sensitivity and temperament in extremely low-birth-weight premature toddlers and preterm and full-term controls. Pain. 1994;58(3):341–6.
10. Vederhus BJ, Ge E, Natvig GK, Markestad T, Graue M, Halvorsen T. Pain tolerance and pain perception in adolescents born extremely preterm; 2012. p. 1528–8447.
11. McGrath PJ, Stevens BJ, Walker S, Zempsky WT. Oxford textbook of paediatric pain. Oxford: Oxford University Press; 2014.
12. Davidson A, Flick RP. Neurodevelopmental implications of the use of sedation and analgesia in neonates. Clin Perinatol. 2013;40(3):559–73.
13. Dong C, Anand KJ. Developmental neurotoxicity of ketamine in pediatric clinical use. Toxicol Lett. 2013;220(1):53–60.
14. Walter-Nicolet E, Annequin D, Biran V, Mitanchez D, Tourniaire B. Pain management in newborns: from prevention to treatment. Paediatr Drugs. 2010;12(6):353–65.
15. Stevens B, Johnston C, Taddio A, Gibbins S, Yamada J. The premature infant pain profile: evaluation 13 years after development. Clin J Pain. 2010;26(9): 813–30.
16. Stevens B, Johnston C, Petryshen P, Taddio A. Premature infant pain profile: development and initial validation. Clin J Pain. 1996;12(1):13–22.
17. Gibbins S, Stevens BJ, Yamada J, Dionne K, Campbell-Yeo M, Lee G, et al. Validation of the premature infant pain profile-revised (PIPP-R). Early Hum Dev. 2014;90(4):189–93.
18. Stevens BJ, Gibbins S, Yamada J, Dionne K, Lee G, Johnston C, et al. The premature infant pain profile-revised (PIPP-R): initial validation and feasibility. Clin J Pain. 2014;30(3):238–43.
19. Mokkink LB, Terwee CB, Patrick DL, Alonso J, Stratford PW, Knol DL, et al. The COSMIN study reached international consensus on taxonomy, terminology, and definitions of measurement properties for health-related patient-reported outcomes. J Clin Epidemiol. 2010;63(7):737–45.
20. Wild D, Grove A, Martin M, Eremenco S, McElroy S, Verjee-Lorenz A, et al. Principles of good practice for the translation and cultural adaptation process for patient-reported outcomes (PRO) measures: report of the ISPOR task force for translation and cultural adaptation. Value Health. 2005;8(2):94–104.
21. de Vet HCW, Terwee CB, Mokkink LB, Knol DL. Measurement in medicine. A practical guide. Cambridge: Cambridge University Press; 2011.
22. Sperber AD. Translation and validation of study instruments for cross-cultural research. Gastroenterology. 2004;126(1Suppl1):S124–S8.
23. Sousa VD, Rojjanasrirat W. Translation, adaptation and validation of instruments or scales for use in cross-cultural health care research: a clear and user-friendly guideline. J Eval Clin Pract. 2011;17(2):268–74.
24. Eremenco SL, Fau CD, Arnold BJ, Arnold BJ. A comprehensive method for the translation and cross-cultural validation of health status questionnaires. Eval Health Prof. 2005;28:0163–2787.
25. Andersen RD, Jylli L, Ambuel B. Cultural adaptation of patient and observational outcome measures: a methodological example using the COMFORT behavioral rating scale. Int J Nurs Stud. 2014;51(6):934–42.
26. Drennan J. Cognitive interviewing: verbal data in the design and pretesting of questionnaires. J Adv Nurs. 2003;42(1):57–63.
27. Miles MB, Huberman AM. Qualitative data analysis : an expanded sourcebook. Thousand Oaks, CA: Sage; 1994.
28. Hilton A, Skrutkowski M. Translating instruments into other languages: development and testing processes. Cancer Nurs. 2002;25(1):1–7.
29. Drake G, Williams AC. Nursing education interventions for managing acute pain in hospital settings: a systematic review of clinical outcomes and teaching methods. LID - S1524-9042(16)30215-6 [pii] LID - https://doi.org/10.1016/j.pmn.2016.11.001. Pain Manag Nurs. 2016:1532–8635.
30. O'Keefe LC, Frith KH, Barnby E. Nurse faculty as international research collaborators. Nurs Health Sci. 2016;19(1):119–25.
31. Kemmelmeier M. Cultural differences in survey responding: issues and insights in the study of response biases. Int J Psychol. 2016;51(6):439–44.

19

Nutritional status, dental caries and tooth eruption in children: a longitudinal study in Cambodia, Indonesia and Lao PDR

Jed Dimaisip-Nabuab[1,11], Denise Duijster[2,3]*, Habib Benzian[4], Roswitha Heinrich-Weltzien[5], Amphayvan Homsavath[6], Bella Monse[1], Hak Sithan[7], Nicole Stauf[8], Sri Susilawati[9] and Katrin Kromeyer-Hauschild[10]

Abstract

Background: Untreated dental caries is reported to affect children's nutritional status and growth, yet evidence on this relationship is conflicting. The aim of this study was to assess the association between dental caries in both the primary and permanent dentition and nutritional status (including underweight, normal weight, overweight and stunting) in children from Cambodia, Indonesia and Lao PDR over a period of 2 years. A second objective was to assess whether nutritional status affects the eruption of permanent teeth.

Methods: Data were used from the Fit for School - Health Outcome Study: a cohort study with a follow-up period of 2 years, consisting of children from 82 elementary schools in Cambodia, Indonesia and Lao PDR. From each school, a random sample of six to seven-year-old children was selected. Dental caries and odontogenic infections were assessed using the World Health Organization (WHO) criteria and the pufa-index. Weight and height measurements were converted to BMI-for-age and height-for-age z-scores and categorized into weight status and stunting following WHO standardised procedures. Cross-sectional and longitudinal associations were analysed using the Kruskal Wallis test, Mann Whitney U-test and multivariate logistic and linear regression.

Results: Data of 1499 children (mean age at baseline = 6.7 years) were analyzed. Levels of dental caries and odontogenic infections in the primary dentition were significantly highest in underweight children, as well as in stunted children, and lowest in overweight children. Dental caries in six to seven-year old children was also significantly associated with increased odds of being underweight and stunted 2 years later. These associations were not consistently found for dental caries and odontogenic infections in the permanent dentition. Underweight and stunting was significantly associated with a lower number of erupted permanent teeth in children at the age of six to seven-years-old and 2 years later.

Conclusions: Underweight and stunted growth are associated with untreated dental caries and a delayed eruption of permanent teeth in children from Cambodia, Indonesia and Lao PDR. Findings suggest that oral health may play an important role in children's growth and general development.

Keywords: Dental caries, Tooth eruption, Underweight, Overweight, Growth, Children

* Correspondence: D.Duijster@acta.nl
[2]Department of Social Dentistry, Academic Centre for Dentistry Amsterdam, Gustav Mahlerlaan 3004, 1081LA Amsterdam, The Netherlands
[3]Department of Epidemiology and Public Health, University College London, Torrington Place 1-19, London WC1E 6BT, UK
Full list of author information is available at the end of the article

Background

The relationship between children's oral health and general health has become a research subject of growing interest. Dental caries, the most prevalent childhood disease worldwide, commonly remains untreated [1]. Accumulating evidence indicates that dental caries negatively affects children's nutritional status and growth [2]. Yet, the nature of this relationship remains controversial, both in terms of the direction and its underlying mechanisms. According to recent systematic reviews, some studies reported an association between dental caries and underweight (low Body Mass Index (BMI)-for-age), stunting (low height-for-age) and failure to thrive, whereas other studies found that dental caries was associated with overweight; or they suggested that there is no relationship [3–5].

Evidence supporting a relationship between dental caries and underweight primarily comes from studies conducted in low- and middle-income countries (LMICs), where severity of dental caries is high [6–9]. Children with high caries levels both in the primary and permanent dentition had significantly lower BMI-for-age, and treatment of severely decayed teeth has been associated with an increased rate of weight gain [2]. Several mechanisms have been postulated to explain this relationship, including the direct effect of dental caries on children's eating ability and nutritional intake [10], as well as indirect effects of chronic dental inflammation on children's growth via metabolic and immunological pathways [11]. An opposite theory is that undernutrition (underweight and stunting) could predispose a person to dental caries. Chronic undernutrition has been associated with disturbed dental development, including enamel defects (hypoplasia) and delayed eruption of the primary teeth [12, 13]. However, evidence of the effect of undernutrition on the formation and eruption of permanent teeth is less substantial.

A relationship between dental caries and overweight was more apparent in studies conducted in Europe and the United States [3, 4, 14–16]. Notably, these studies often included samples in which underweight children were underrepresented [3]. In all probability, the mechanisms underlying this relationship follow a different pathway; dental caries and overweight are most likely associated because they have dietary risk factors in common that are both cariogenic and obesogenic, such as a sugar-rich diet [4, 17].

Based on the conflicting findings in the literature, Hooley et al. [3] and Li et al. [5] suggested that dental caries and BMI might be related in a non-linear U-shaped pattern, with caries levels being higher in both children with low and high BMI. There is a lack of studies that have tested this hypothesis, since there are few analyses that covered the full range of anthropometric measurements including underweight, normal weight and overweight (weight status), as well as stunting. In Southeast Asia, dental caries levels are among the highest worldwide, with a prevalence ranging between 79 to 98% in six-year-old children [18, 19]. Undernutrition remains a major public health concern in most countries of the region, yet obesity is also on the rise due to socioeconomic development, globalization and related shifts in dietary intake and physical activity patterns through the nutrition transition [20]. This coexistence of both childhood underweight and overweight, also termed as the 'double burden of malnutrition', allows analysis of possible non-linear associations between oral health and nutritional status. Hence, the aim of this study was to assess the relationship between dental caries in both the primary and permanent dentition and nutritional status (as indicated by weight status and stunting) in children from Cambodia, Indonesia and Lao People's Democratic Republic (Lao PDR), over a period of 2 years. A second objective was to assess whether nutritional status affects the eruption of permanent teeth.

Methods

Fit for school – Health outcome study

This study used data from the Fit for School - Health Outcome Study (FIT-HOS), conducted from 2012 to 2014 [21]. The study was originally designed to evaluate the effect of the Fit for School (FIT) programme, which is an integrated Water, Sanitation and Hygiene (WASH) and school health programme to improve child health. It implements evidence-based interventions in public primary schools, including daily group handwashing with soap and toothbrushing with fluoride toothpaste, biannual deworming, and the construction of group washing facilities [22, 23].

The FIT-HOS was a longitudinal cohort study with a follow-up period of 2 years. The cohort consisted of children recruited from 82 public elementary schools - 20 schools in Cambodia, 18 schools in Indonesia, and 44 schools in Lao PDR. Half of the schools in each country ($n = 41$) implemented the FIT programme and the other 41 schools implemented the regular government health education curriculum and biannual deworming as part of the respective national deworming programmes. Per school, a random selection of six to seven-year-old children (6.00 to 7.99 years of age) was drawn from the list of enrolled grade-one students. Baseline data of the children were collected in 2012, and the same children were re-examined 24 months later in 2014. Full details of the study procedures, the selection of schools and the power calculation are described in a previous publication [21]. For the purposes of this study, children were evaluated as one cohort, disregarding the type of school they attended (FIT programme or regular programme).

Data collection

In each country, a team of local researchers performed data collection on the school ground. For calibration and standardisation purposes, the research teams underwent 3 days of training prior to data collection.

Clinical dental examination

Clinical dental examinations were performed by four calibrated dentists in the schoolyard or inside a classroom. Dental caries status was scored following the World Health Organization (WHO) Basic Methods for Oral Health Surveys 4th edition [24], using mouth mirrors with illumination (Mirrorlite) and a CPI-ball-end probe. The dt/DT-index was used to score untreated dental caries, by calculating the sum of decayed (d/D) teeth (t/T). The pufa/PUFA-index was used to measure odontogenic infections as a result of untreated dental caries, which scores the presence of teeth with open pulp (p/P), ulceration (u/U), fistula (f/F) and abscesses (a/A) [25]. For both indexes, lowercase letters refer to primary teeth, and uppercase letters refer to permanent teeth. The number of erupted permanent teeth was scored by counting all permanent teeth that had erupted, which was defined as 'any permanent tooth surface that had pierced the alveolar mucosa'. Kappa-scores for inter-examiner reliability of the dentists ranged from 0.73 to 0.97 (mean $k = 0.87$) for dt/DT and from 0.58 to 1.00 (mean $k = 0.78$) for pufa/PUFA.

Anthropometric measurement

Two trained nurses obtained children's weight and height measurements, using standards described by Cogill [26]. Weight was measured to the nearest 0.1 kg using a SECA digital weighing scale. Standing height was measured to the nearest 0.1 cm using a microtoise. The equipment was calibrated at the start of each day and after every 10th child. Children wore light clothes and no shoes during measurement. Measurements were obtained in duplicate, and the average of two measurements was reported. BMI was calculated as weight/height^2 (kg/m^2). Weight and height data were subsequently converted to BMI-for-age z-scores and height-for-age z-scores with the WHO AnthroPlus software, which uses the WHO Growth reference 2007 [27]. Z-scores allow comparison of an individual's weight, height or BMI, adjusted for age and sex relative to a reference population, expressed in standard deviations (SDS) from the reference mean. Cut-offs for BMI-for-age z-scores were used to categorize children's weight status into underweight (< – 2 (SDS), normal weight (≥ -2SDS & ≤ 2SDS) and overweight (> 2SDS). Stunting was defined as a height-for-age z-score < -2SDS; scores ≥-2SDs were classified as 'not stunted' [28].

Sociodemographic interview

Sociodemographic information was collected from the children through an interview-administered questionnaire in the respective native language. Demographic information included sex and date of birth, which were cross-checked with the school records. Data on television (TV) ownership, car/motorcycle ownership and number of siblings were collected as proxy indicators of socioeconomic status (SES).

These variables have been described as useful proxy measures of SES in LMICs by Howe et al. [29]. Children were asked whether they have a TV at home, and whether they have a car or motorcycle at home, with response options 'yes' and 'no'. The number of siblings was assessed by combining two questions: 'How many brothers do you have?' and 'How many sisters do you have?'

Data analysis

Data were analyzed using STATA 14 (Stata Corp, College Station, Texas, USA). A P-value of ≤0.05 was regarded as significant. Complete case analysis was used to handle missing data. Data were analyzed for each country separately.

The association between dental caries status and odontogenic infections (in further reference: dental caries) and nutritional status was assessed cross-sectionally and longitudinally. First, cross-sectional associations were tested between [i.] dt and pufa and nutritional status at baseline at age 6 to 7 years (age 6–7), and [ii.] DT and PUFA and nutritional status at follow-up at age 8 to 9 years (age 8–9), using the Kruskall Wallis test for weight status and the Mann Whitney U-test for stunting. Permanent teeth generally start to erupt at the age of 6 years, which means that children's dentition at baseline mainly consisted of primary teeth, while children's dentition at follow-up also included permanent teeth. Second, multivariate logistic regression with stepwise backward selection was performed to assess the longitudinal association between dental caries at baseline (dt, DT, pufa and PUFA at age 6–7) and [i.] underweight at follow-up (age 8–9) (reference category = no underweight), and [ii.] stunting at follow-up (age 8–9) (reference category = not stunted). The regression models were adjusted for sociodemographic factors, number of primary and permanent teeth at baseline and type of school (FIT programme or regular programme).

The association between nutritional status and the number of permanent teeth was assessed cross-sectionally at baseline (age 6–7) and at follow-up (8–9), using the Kruskal Wallis test for weight status and Mann Whitney U-test for stunting. Multivariate linear regression with stepwise backward selection was performed to test the longitudinal association between nutritional status at baseline (age 6–7) and the number of permanent teeth at follow-up (age 8–9). The regression model was adjusted for sociodemographic factors and type of school.

Results

Description of the study sample

A total of 1847 children participated in the baseline study – 624 children in Cambodia, 570 in Indonesia and 653 children in Lao PDR. Of those, 76.6% ($n = 478$), 85.3% ($n = 486$) and 81.0% ($n = 535$) were followed-up after 2 years, respectively. Dropout children did not significantly differ from those who were followed-up in terms of their dental caries status and nutritional status at baseline. The mean time interval between baseline and follow-up was 23.88 ± 0.27 months.

The mean age of all children at baseline was 6.7 ± 0.5 years (range 6.0–8.0 years) and 50.2% were boys. The prevalence of underweight and overweight was 7.6% and 7.4% in children at baseline, and 10.2% and 12.3% in children at follow-up, respectively. More than a quarter of children were stunted (30.2% at baseline and 26.2% at follow-up). On average, the number of erupted permanent teeth per child was 5.8 ± 2.8 at baseline and 12.4 ± 3.4 at follow-up. At baseline, the prevalence of dental caries and odontogenic infections in the primary dentition was 94.4% and 69.2%, respectively. Children had a mean dt of 8.4 ± 4.7 and a mean pufa-score of 2.5 ± 2.7. At follow-up, the prevalence of dental caries in the permanent teeth was 41.2% with a mean DT of 0.7 ± 1.2, and the prevalence of odontogenic infections was 7.2% with a mean PUFA of 0.1 ± 0.4. The characteristics of the study samples in the respective countries are described in Table 1.

The association between dental caries and nutritional status

Table 2 shows the cross-sectional associations between dental caries and nutritional status. In Cambodia and Indonesia, dt and pufa were significantly associated with weight status at age 6–7: the mean dt and pufa scores where highest in underweight children and lowest in overweight children. These associations were not observed in Lao PDR. No associations were found between DT or PUFA and weight status at age 8–9, except in Cambodia where the mean DT was again significantly highest in underweight children and lowest in overweight children.

In all three countries, a higher mean dt was significantly associated with stunting at age 6–7. In Indonesia, stunted children also had significantly higher levels of pufa at age 6–7, but not in Cambodia and Lao PDR. No significant associations between DT and PUFA and stunting at age 8–9 were found.

Table 3 shows the association between dental caries at age 6–7 and underweight at age 8–9. In Cambodia, higher dt and DT at age 6–7 were significantly associated with increased odds of being underweight at age 8–9, after adjustment for age, sex, the number of permanent teeth and stunting. In Lao PDR the same direction of association was found, but only for dt, while Indonesia showed no association between dt or DT and underweight.

The association between dental caries at age 6–7 years and stunting at age 8–9 years is presented in Table 4. In Indonesia and Lao PDR, a higher dt at age 6–7 was significantly associated with higher odds of being stunted at age 8–9, after adjustment for age, number of

permanent teeth, weight status, car/motorcycle ownership and geographical location. The same association was found in Cambodia for DT instead of dt.

The association between nutritional status and the number of erupted permanent teeth

The cross-sectional association between nutritional status and the number of erupted permanent teeth is shown in Table 5. In Indonesia and Lao PDR, weight status at age 6–7 and at age 8–9 were significantly associated with the number of erupted permanent teeth: the mean number of erupted permanent teeth was lowest in underweight children and highest in overweight children. In all countries, stunted children had significantly fewer erupted permanent teeth than children with normal height-for-age, both at age 6–7 and age 8–9 (except in Indonesia at age 8–9).

Table 6 shows the longitudinal association between nutritional status and the number of erupted permanent teeth. In all three countries, underweight at age 6–7 (except in Cambodia) and stunting at age 6–7 were significantly associated with a lower number of erupted permanent teeth at age 8–9, after adjustment for age, sex, and geographical location.

Discussion

This study investigated the relationship between nutritional status and untreated dental caries, as well as status of eruption of permanent teeth in a community-based sample of children from Cambodia, Indonesia and Lao PRD over a period of 2 years. Findings showed that untreated dental caries in children was significantly associated with underweight and stunted growth. Generally, levels of untreated dental caries in the primary dentition were highest in underweight children, as well as in stunted children, and lowest in overweight children. Untreated dental caries in six to seven-year old children was also significantly associated with increased odds of being underweight and stunted 2 years later. Yet, no consistent associations between dental caries in the permanent dentition and weight status or stunting were found. Hence, the findings of this study did not support the hypothesis of Hooley et al. [3] and Li et al. [5] which suggested that dental caries is associated with both low and high BMI in a U-shaped pattern.

Discussion of findings related to dental caries and nutritional status

Findings of the current study affirm the results of a number of previous studies, which demonstrated an inverse relationship between dental caries and nutritional status in children [7, 9, 30–33]. These studies have in common that their study population consisted of children with a high caries experience and high caries risk. Most of the studies were conducted in LMICs where

Table 1 Characteristics of the study sample in Cambodia, Indonesia, Lao PDR

	Cambodia		Indonesia		Lao PDR	
	Baseline (n = 624)	Follow-up (n = 478)	Baseline (n = 570)	Follow-up (n = 486)	Baseline (n = 653)	Follow-up (n = 535)
	n (%)	n (%)	n (%)	n (%)	n (%)	n (%)
Gender						
Boys	308 (49.4)	245 (51.3)	295 (51.8)	249 (51.2)	325 (49.8)	272 (50.8)
Girls	316 (50.6)	233 (48.7)	275 (48.3)	237 (48.8)	328 (50.2)	263 (49.2)
Age (years)						
Baseline | Follow-up						
6 to < 7 | 8 to < 9	516 (82.7)	393 (82.2)	388 (68.1)	337 (69.3)	426 (65.2)	358 (66.9)
7 to < 8 | 9 to < 10	108 (17.3)	85 (17.8)	182 (31.9)	149 (30.7)	227 (34.8)	177 (33.1)
Geographical location						
Rural	378 (60.6)	309 (64.6)	–	–	214 (32.8)	187 (35.0)
Urban	246 (39.4)	169 (35.4)	570 (100.0)	486 (100.0)	439 (67.2)	348 (65.1)
Number of siblings[a]						
1 or no siblings	–	144 (30.1)	–	253 (52.3)	–	199 (37.2)
2 siblings	–	137 (28.7)	–	143 (29.6)	–	187 (35.0)
3 or more siblings	–	197 (41.2)	–	88 (18.2)	–	149 (27.9)
TV ownership[a]						
No	–	58 (12.2)	–	3 (0.6)	–	23 (4.3)
Yes	–	418 (87.8)	–	481 (99.4)	–	508 (95.7)
Car / motorcycle[a] ownership						
No	–	72 (15.1)	–	330 (68.2)	–	41 (7.7)
Yes	–	406 (84.9)	–	154 (31.8)	–	492 (92.3)
Weight status						
Underweight	53 (8.7)	67 (14.3)	45 (7.9)	37 (7.6)	41 (6.4)	46 (8.8)
Normal weight	539 (87.9)	375 (80.1)	443 (78.1)	337 (69.6)	566 (88.2)	434 (82.5)
Overweight	21 (3.4)	26 (5.6)	79 (13.9)	110 (22.7)	35 (5.5)	46 (8.8)
Stunting						
No	410 (66.9)	318 (68.2)	480 (84.8)	401 (83.5)	381 (59.4)	365 (69.5)
Yes	203 (33.1)	148 (31.8)	86 (15.2)	79 (16.5)	261 (40.7)	160 (30.5)
	mean ± sd	mean ± sd	mean ± sd	mean ± sd	mean ± sd	mean ± sd
Number of permanent teeth	5.4 ± 2.7	12.1 ± 3.4	6.0 ± 2.6	12.6 ± 3.0	6.0 ± 3.0	12.6 ± 3.8
dt	9.8 ± 4.5	6.7 ± 3.6	8.2 ± 4.5	5.0 ± 3.4	7.3 ± 4.8	4.4 ± 3.5
DT	0.2 ± 0.6	1.1 ± 1.4	0.1 ± 0.5	0.5 ± 0.9	0.3 ± 0.8	0.6 ± 1.1
pufa	2.6 ± 2.4	2.8 ± 2.1	3.2 ± 3.1	2.7 ± 2.3	1.9 ± 2.4	1.9 ± 1.9
PUFA	0.0 ± 0.1	0.1 ± 0.4	0.0 ± 0.0	0.1 ± 0.4	0.0 ± 0.1	0.1 ± 0.4

[a]Measured at follow-up
Number of missing values at baseline: anthropometric data, n = 25; dental data, n = 8
Number of missing values at follow-up: anthropometric data, n = 21; dental data, n = 16

dental caries is highly prevalent and commonly untreated, or they included children requiring dental rehabilitation under general anesthesia. This may suggest that the severity of dental caries (the number of caries lesions and caries activity) plays a role in the direction and nature of its relationship with nutritional status. For example, Benzian et al. [8] found that odontogenic infections as a result of untreated decay (pufa/PUFA > 0) was a stronger determinant of low weight in children than dental caries experience (number of decayed, missing and filled teeth (dmft/DMFT > 0)). In the current study, only 1.7% and 6.3% of caries lesions in the primary teeth and permanent teeth respectively were filled or extracted, and most caries lesions concerned decay

Table 2 Dental caries and odontogenic infections according to weight status and stunting in children from Cambodia, Indonesia and Lao PDR at age 6–7 years and at age 8–9 years

	Dental caries (mean ± sd)				Odontogenic infections (mean ± sd)			
	Underweight	Normal weight	Overweight	P^a	Underweight	Normal weight	Overweight	P^a
	dt at baseline (age 6–7)				pufa at baseline (age 6–7)			
Cambodia (n = 53 | 538 | 21)	11.7 ± 4.7	9.6 ± 4.4	8.6 ± 4.2	0.004	3.1 ± 2.4	2.5 ± 2.4	1.7 ± 2.2	0.033
Indonesia (n = 45 | 441 | 79)	9.3 ± 5.0	8.3 ± 4.4	6.3 ± 4.5	< 0.001	3.6 ± 2.9	3.3 ± 3.1	2.5 ± 3.1	0.007
Lao PDR (n = 41 | 562 | 35)	8.8 ± 5.2	7.2 ± 4.8	6.5 ± 4.4	0.094	1.8 ± 2.1	1.8 ± 2.3	2.1 ± 3.2	0.997
	DT at follow-up (age 8–9)				PUFA at follow-up (age 8–9)			
Cambodia (n = 67 | 372 | 26)	1.4 ± 1.4	1.1 ± 1.3	0.7 ± 1.2	0.030	0.1 ± 0.5	0.1 ± 0.4	0.1 ± 0.3	0.985
Indonesia (n = 37 | 335 | 109)	0.9 ± 1.3	0.6 ± 0.9	0.4 ± 0.8	0.176	0.2 ± 0.6	0.1 ± 0.4	0.1 ± 0.3	0.751
Lao PDR (n = 45 | 427 | 46)	0.8 ± 1.1	0.6 ± 1.1	0.5 ± 1.0	0.537	0.1 ± 0.3	0.1 ± 0.4	0.1 ± 0.3	0.987
	Not stunted	Stunted		P^b	Not stunted	Stunted		P^b
	dt at baseline (age 6–7)				pufa at baseline (age 6–7)			
Cambodia (n = 409 | 203)	9.6 ± 4.3	10.2 ± 4.8		0.058	2.5 ± 2.3	2.6 ± 2.5		0.992
Indonesia (n = 478 | 86)	7.9 ± 4.4	9.6 ± 4.6		0.002	3.0 ± 3.0	4.1 ± 3.6		0.010
Lao PDR (n = 377 | 261)	6.9 ± 4.8	7.8 ± 4.9		0.018	1.8 ± 2.2	1.9 ± 2.5		0.666
	DT at follow-up (age 8–9)				PUFA at follow-up (age 8–9)			
Cambodia (n = 316 | 147)	1.1 ± 1.4	1.0 ± 1.3		0.496	0.1 ± 0.4	0.1 ± 0.2		0.316
Indonesia (n = 399 | 79)	0.5 ± 0.9	0.7 ± 1.1		0.485	0.1 ± 0.4	0.1 ± 0.5		0.867
Lao PDR (n = 357 | 160)	0.7 ± 1.2	0.5 ± 0.9		0.294	0.1 ± 0.5	0.1 ± 0.3		0.820

[a]Kruskall Wallis Test, [b] Mann Whitney U-Test

Table 3 The association between dental caries and odontogenic infections at age 6–7 years and underweight at age 8–9 years of children in Cambodia, Indonesia and Lao PDR

	Cambodia (n = 467[a])		Indonesia (n = 478[a])		Lao PDR (n = 522[a])	
	OR (95% CI)	P	OR (95% CI)	P	OR (95% CI)	P
Weight status at follow-up (age 8–9): no underweight (reference), underweight						
dt (baseline)	1.09 (1.02; 1.16)	0.010			1.09 (1.02; 1.16)	0.011
DT (baseline)	1.75 (1.15; 2.66)	0.009				
Number of permanent teeth (baseline)	0.84 (0.74; 0.95)	0.007	0.82 (0.70; 0.96)	0.015	0.85 (0.75; 0.96)	0.011
Sex						
Boys	1				1	
Girls	0.27 (0.15; 0.50)	< 0.001			0.08 (0.03; 0.22)	< 0.001
Age (baseline)						
6 < 7 years	1		1			
7 < 8 years	2.29 (1.08; 4.83)	0.030	3.97 (1.84; 8.59)	< 0.001		
Stunting (follow-up)						
No			1			
Yes			2.79 (1.32; 5.89)	0.007		

Logistic regression
Variables in the model: dt at baseline, DT at baseline, pufa at baseline, PUFA at baseline, number of primary teeth at baseline, number of permanent teeth at baseline, sex (boys, girls), age group at baseline (6 to < 7 years, 7 to < 8 years), geographical location (urban, rural), number of siblings (1 or no siblings, 2 siblings, 3 or more siblings), TV ownership (no, yes), car/motorcycle ownership (no, yes), stunting at follow-up (no, yes), FIT programme (no, yes)
'1' refers to the reference category: no underweight (BMI: SDS ≥ −2)
[a]Number of children with missing values of variables in the model: Cambodia, n = 11, Indonesia, n = 8, Lao PDR, n = 13

Table 4 The association between dental caries and odontogenic infections at age 6–7 years and stunting at age 8–9 years of children in Cambodia, Indonesia and Lao PDR

	Cambodia ($n = 467^{a}$)		Indonesia ($n = 478^{a}$)		Lao PDR ($n = 521^{a}$)	
	OR (95% CI)	P	OR (95% CI)	P	OR (95% CI)	P
Stunting at follow-up (age 8–9): not stunted (reference), stunted						
dt (baseline)			1.07 (1.01; 1.13)	0.003	1.05 (1.01; 1.09)	0.025
DT (baseline)	1.67 (1.14; 2.43)	0.008				
Number of permanent teeth (baseline)	0.74 (0.67; 0.82)	< 0.001	0.89 (0.79; 1.00)	0.044	0.82 (0.76; 0.89)	< 0.001
Age (baseline)						
6 < 7 years	1		1		1	
7 < 8 years	3.62 (2.02; 6.51)	< 0.001	3.01 (1.69; 5.37)	< 0.001	2.27 (1.44; 3.57)	< 0.001
Weight status (follow-up)						
Underweight	1		1		1	
Normal weight	0.60 (0.34; 1.06)	0.079	0.44 (0.21; 0.94)	0.034	0.77 (0.40; 1.48)	0.431
Overweight	0.13 (0.03; 0.62)	0.011	0.10 (0.03; 0.33)	< 0.001	0.16 (0.04; 0.59)	0.006
Geographical location						
Rural					1	
Urban					0.56 (0.37; 0.85)	0.006
Car/motorcycle ownership						
No	1					
Yes	0.48 (0.27; 0.87)	0.015				

Logistic regression

Variables in the model: dt at baseline, DT at baseline, pufa at baseline, PUFA at baseline, number of primary teeth at baseline, number of permanent teeth at baseline, sex (boys, girls), age group at baseline (6 to < 7 years, 7 to < 8 years), geographical location (urban, rural), number of siblings (1 or no siblings, 2 siblings, 3 or more siblings), TV ownership (no, yes), car/motorcycle ownership (no, yes), weight status at follow-up (underweight, normal, overweight), FIT programme (no, yes)

'1' refers to the reference category: not stunted (Height: SDS ≥ − 2)

[a]Number of children with missing values of variables in the model: Cambodia, $n = 13$, Indonesia, $n = 8$, Lao PDR, $n = 14$

with advanced progression into the dentine. Therefore, only active caries (dt/DT) was considered in the analysis (rather than dmft/DMFT), which may explain why this study found a stronger association between dt/DT and underweight or stunting in multivariate regression analyses.

There are several explanations of how severe untreated dental caries may be associated with underweight and poor growth in children. Untreated caries can cause pain and discomfort, which negatively affects children's ability to eat and sleep [9, 17, 34]. Limited ability to eat could lead to poor appetite and reduced nutritional intake, while disturbance of sleep could impair the secretion of growth hormones [35]. Indirectly, chronic inflammation as a result of severe caries with pulpitis could affect growth via immune and metabolic responses. Inflammatory cytokines, for example interleukin-1, can inhibit erythropoiesis, leading to chronic anaemia as a result of suppressed erythrocyte production and haemoglobin levels [36–38]. Inflammation may also contribute to undernutrition through increased metabolic demands and impaired nutrient absorption [11]. Evidence for the mechanisms being causal comes from Acs et al. [39] and the Weight Gain Study [40], which showed a significant increase in weight gain ("catch-up growth") after extraction

of severely decayed teeth in underweight children. However, two randomized-controlled trial in Saudi-Arabia could not confirm these findings [41].

In affluent populations, the relationship between dental caries and nutritional status is likely of a different nature. Studies in industrialized countries have demonstrated positive associations between BMI and dental caries, particularly in the permanent dentition [4, 14–16]. Both diseases have dietary and sociodemographic risk factors in common, which likely underlie the association. As Hooley et al. [3] pointed out, the development of dental caries in affluent populations might be progressing more slowly because of better oral hygiene, higher fluoride exposure and access to oral healthcare. Hence, measurement of dental caries in studies from industrialized countries often included initial enamel lesions or dentine lesions without pulpitis, as well as filled and extracted teeth (rather than untreated caries only), making comparison of results between low, middle and high income countries challenging.

Surprisingly, no significant associations with regards to dental caries in the permanent dentition were found in this study, except in Cambodia. The probable reason for this is that the permanent teeth had just erupted in children at baseline at the age of 6 to 7 years, which means

Table 5 Number of permanent teeth according to weight status and stunting in children from Cambodia, Indonesia and Lao PDR at age 6–7 years and at age 8–9 years

Country (n in weight categories)	Number of permanent teeth (mean ± sd)			
	Underweight	Normal weight	Overweight	p^a
	Baseline (age 6–7)			
Cambodia (n = 53 | 538 | 21)	5.08 ± 2.59	5.38 ± 2.75	5.71 ± 2.81	0.599
Indonesia (n = 45 | 441 | 79)	5.53 ± 2.47	5.78 ± 2.48	7.32 ± 2.76	< 0.001
Lao PDR (n = 41 | 562 | 35)	5.44 ± 2.67	5.96 ± 2.96	7.49 ± 3.02	0.008
	Follow-up (age 8–9)			
Cambodia (n = 67 | 372 | 26)	11.99 ± 3.23	12.09 ± 3.45	12.69 ± 3.96	0.604
Indonesia (n = 37 | 335 | 109)	11.97 ± 2.76	12.28 ± 2.87	13.69 ± 3.32	< 0.001
Lao PDR (n = 45 | 427 | 46)	11.20 ± 3.70	12.53 ± 3.62	14.67 ± 4.18	< 0.001
	Not stunted	Stunted		p^b
	Baseline (age 6–7)			
Cambodia (n = 409 | 203)	5.84 ± 2.76	4.43 ± 2.44		< 0.001
Indonesia (n = 478 | 86)	6.11 ± 2.59	5.20 ± 2.28		0.003
Lao PDR (n = 377 | 261)	6.69 ± 2.96	5.03 ± 2.70		< 0.001
	Follow-up (age 8–9)			
Cambodia (n = 316 | 147)	12.62 ± 3.38	10.99 ± 3.36		< 0.001
Indonesia (n = 399 | 79)	12.68 ± 3.01	12.14 ± 3.09		0.206
Lao PDR (n = 357 | 160)	13.14 ± 3.75	11.36 ± 3.42		< 0.001

[a]Kruskall Wallis Test, [b] Mann Whitney U-Test

that there was little time in the study for caries to develop in the permanent dentition. The low levels of DT and PUFA at follow-up at the age of 8 to 9 years may have resulted in too little variance to establish significant associations. Previous studies that did find an association between underweight and dental decay in the permanent dentition included children who were at least 3 years older [7, 8, 33]. A probable reason why significant associations could be demonstrated in Cambodia is that the prevalence of dental caries was substantially higher in Cambodia than in Indonesia and Lao PDR. This could potentially be explained by worse general conditions of living and hygiene, which could have affected children's oral health. Another potential explanation is that the implementation quality of the Fit for School programme (including the toothbrushing activity and exposure to fluoride toothpaste) was poorer in Cambodia as compared to the other two countries.

Discussion of findings related to nutritional status and the eruption of permanent teeth

The current study also presented evidence for a relationship between nutritional status and the number of erupted permanent teeth. Underweight and stunted children had a delayed eruption of permanent teeth compared to children of normal weight and height, while overweight children showed an accelerated eruption. These findings confirm those of others [13, 42, 43]. Impaired dental

development and underweight or stunting likely have common risk factors. For example, nutritional deficiency, including protein-energy malnutrition, may impair dental development via similar mechanisms of influencing skeletal and physical development. Hence, delayed permanent tooth eruption may be one of the manifestations of chronic nutritional deficiencies, making it a valuable indicator of poor overall development in children. The development of permanent teeth follows a sequence over a long period of time, which already starts before or soon after birth. There is evidence that undernutrition during the susceptible stages of tooth development, particularly during a child's early years, can lead to enamel hypoplasia, making teeth more susceptible to demineralization and dental caries [12, 44]. This suggests that bidirectional effects may exist between undernutrition and dental caries, whereby undernutrition increases the risk of dental caries and vice versa.

Strengths and limitations

The findings of this study should be interpreted in view of their strengths and limitations. Strengths of the current study were the large community-based sample of children from Cambodia, Indonesia and Lao PDR, the inclusion of both dental caries and odontogenic infections, as well as the full spectrum of anthropometric measurements, and the use of standardized methods to assess oral health and nutritional status by calibrated

Table 6 The association between weight status and stunting at age 6–7 years and the number of permanent teeth at age 8–9 years of children in Cambodia, Indonesia and Lao PDR

	Cambodia (n = 464[a])		Indonesia (n = 480[a])		Lao PDR (n = 516[a])	
	(95% CI)	P	(95% CI)	P	(95% CI)	P
Number of permanent teeth						
Weight status (baseline)						
Underweight			Reference		Reference	
Normal weight			0.55 (−0.38; 1.48)	0.247	0.52 (−0.68; 1.73)	0.393
Overweight			1.94 (0.81; 3.07)	0.001	2.98 (1.25; 4.72)	0.001
Stunting (baseline)						
No	Reference		Reference		Reference	
Yes	−1.67 (−2.30; −1.04)	< 0.001	−0.87 (−1.60; −0.14)	0.019	−2.22 (−2.83; −1.62)	< 0.001
Sex						
Boys	Reference		Reference		Reference	
Girls	−1.35 (−1.96; −0.74)	< 0.001	1.07 (0.57; 1.57)	< 0.001	−0.75 (−1.35; −0.14)	0.015
Age (baseline)						
6 < 7 years	Reference		Reference		Reference	
7 < 8 years	1.96 (1.13; 2.73)	< 0.001	2.00 (1.45; 2.56)	< 0.001	2.59 (1.97; 3.21)	< 0.001
Geographical location						
Rural	Reference					
Urban	0.77 (0.13; 1.40)	0.018				

Linear regression

Variables in the model: weight status at baseline (underweight, normal weight, overweight), stunting at baseline (no, yes), sex (boys, girls), age group at baseline (6 to < 7 years, 7 to < 8 years), geographical location (urban, rural), number of siblings (1 or no siblings, 2 siblings, 3 or more siblings), TV ownership (no, yes), car/motorcycle ownership (no, yes), FIT programme (no, yes)

[a]Number of children with missing values of variables in the model: Cambodia, n = 14, Indonesia, n = 6, Lao PDR, n = 19

examiners. Yet, comparison of our results with previous research should be made with caution, since non-uniform parameters have been used in the literature to assess nutritional status, including continuous BMI or BMI z-scores or classifications according to WHO references, the 2000 Center for Disease Control and prevention (CDC) growth charts [45] or national references. An important limitation of the study is that no causal inferences are allowed, since the study had only a short follow-up period of 2 years. Furthermore, the study findings are limited to children who attend primary schools. According to data of the World Bank, school enrollment rates of primary school-aged children varied from 92.9 to 97.4% in Cambodia, Indonesia and Lao PDR in 2012 [46]. Hence, a small percentage of children who do not go to school at all could not be represented in the current study sample, yet these children may differ in terms of health and socioeconomic characteristics from those who do attend school.

Data on socioeconomic factors were collected through measurement of TV ownership, car/motorcycle ownership and number of siblings as proxy indicators for SES. Although asset-based measures and family size can be useful proxy indicators for SES in LMICs, they were collected from young children via self-reporting. Possible limitations with regard to the reliability and validity of

their response and the socioeconomic data in this study should be kept in mind. Furthermore, this study did not account for a number of other potentially relevant confounders, such as dietary factors, poverty and living conditions. Cambodia, Indonesia and Lao PDR have been experiencing a nutrition transition as a result of economic development and globalization over the last decades [47]. This transition describes a rapid shift in dietary patterns and energy expenditure, which is partially associated with an increased accessibility to nutrient-poor foods that are high in saturated fats and sugars [20]. Particularly the increasing availability and affordability of sugary foods and drinks, also for families from lower SES, pose children at higher risk of developing both dental caries and poor nutritional status. School feeding programmes that provide sugar-rich foods to undernourished children may also contribute to the development of dental caries. To the authors' knowledge, none of the schools that participated in the study implemented a feeding programme dyring the course of the study, but in nearly all schools children can buy fast food and unhealthy snacks on the school ground. Future studies should include the aforementioned factors, using additional methods of data collection, to explore the potential mechanisms underlying the relationship between oral and nutritional health.

Conclusions

This study found that untreated dental caries in the primary dentition was associated with underweight and stunted growth in children from Cambodia, Indonesia and Lao PDR. These associations were not found for dental caries in the permanent dentition. The study also provided evidence that underweight and stunting was associated with a delayed eruption of permanent teeth. These findings suggest that oral health may play an important role in children's growth and general development. Both dental caries and delayed tooth eruption are likely related to chronic rather than acute episodic undernutrition, given the associations found with low BMI-for-age and height-for-age over a period of 2 years.

Findings of this study have important public health implications. In the context of achieving the Sustainable Development Goals [48], in particular goal 2 'zero hunger' to end all forms of malnutrition and goal 3 'good health and well-being', it is of high importance that the underlying determinants of undernutrition and poor development are addressed. Severe dental caries is one of those determinants, which can be effectively tackled through simple, evidence-based and cost-effective measures. These include oral urgent care (often involving tooth extractions) to treat dental infections and address pain and suffering, and promoting the availability and use of fluoride toothpaste to prevent further caries progression and onset of new caries lesions. This should be combined with strategies to reduce the exposure and intake of sugars for effective caries prevention. The Philippines and other contries of the region have already introduced a taxation on sugar-sweetened beverages and regulations on food available in schools [49], which are first steps in the comprehensive prevention and control of non-communicable diseases through upstream policy changes. Promoting good oral health and addressing untreated tooth decay should be among the priority choices in health promotion planning to improve the development and well-being of millions of children that are underweight worldwide.

Abbreviations
BMI: Body mass index; CDC: Center for disease control and prevention; dmft/DMFT: Number of decayed, missing and filled primary/permanent teeth; dt/DT: Number of decayed primary/permanent teeth; FIT: Fit for School; FIT-HOS: Fit for School – Health Outcome Study; Lao PDR: Lao People's Democratic Republic; pufa/PUFA: Number of primary/permanent teeth with pulp involvement, ulcerations, fistula and abscesses; SDS: Standard deviations; WASH: Water, Sanitation and Hygiene; WHO: World Health Organization

Acknowledgements
The authors would like to thank the Cambodian Ministry of Education, Youth and Sports, the Cambodian Ministry of Health, the Provincial Education Office of West Java, the Indonesian Ministry of Health, the West Java School Health Team, the Bandung Health Office, the Lao PDR Ministry of Education and Sports, the Lao PDR Ministry of Health for their support and cooperation. The authors thank Ayphalla Te, Rigil Munajat and Bouachanh Chansom for the logistical support. The authors aregrateful to all examiners and field staff who supported the data collection and study logistics, as well as the principals, teachers, parents and children in participating schools for their time.

Funding
This study was financially supported by funds from the Deutsche Gesellschaft für Internationale Zusammenarbeit (GIZ) GmbH, GIZ Office, Manila, PDCP Bank Centre, V.A. Rufino cor. L.P. Leviste Str, Makati, Metro Manila, Philippines. No funding was received for writing the scientific paper.

Authors' contributions
Leading investigators of the study: HB, AH, BM, HS, SS, KKH. Conception, design and study protocol: HB, AH, BM, HS, NS, SS. Study implementation and data collection: JDN, DD, BM. Statistical analysis: JDN, DD, RHW, KKH. Interpretation of study findings: JDN, DD, HB, RHW, BM, KKH. Drafting of the initial manuscript: JDN, DD. Read and approved the final version of the manuscript: JDN, DD, HB, RHW, AH, BM, HS, NS, SS, KKH.

Competing interests
The authors declare that they have no competing interests.

Author details
[1]Deutsche Gesellschaft für Internationale Zusammenarbeit (GIZ), L.P. Leviste corner Rufino Street, Makati City, Metro Manila, Philippines. [2]Department of Social Dentistry, Academic Centre for Dentistry Amsterdam, Gustav Mahlerlaan 3004, 1081LA Amsterdam, The Netherlands. [3]Department of Epidemiology and Public Health, University College London, Torrington Place 1-19, London WC1E 6BT, UK. [4]Department of Epidemiology and Health Promotion, WHO Collaborating Center for Quality Improvement and Evidence-based Dentistry, College of Dentistry, New York University, 433 First Avenue, New York, NY 10010, USA. [5]Department of Preventive Dentistry and Pediatric Dentistry, University Hospital Jena, Friedrich Schiller University Jena, Bachstraße 18, 07743 Jena, Germany. [6]Faculty of Dentistry, University of Health Sciences Ministry of Health, 7444 Mahosot Rd, Vientiane, Lao People's Democratic Republic. [7]Department of Preventive Medicine, Ministry of Health, 151-153 Kampuchea Krom Avenue, Phnom Penh, Cambodia. [8]The Health Bureau Ltd., Whiteleaf Business Center, 11 Little Balmer, Buckingham MK18 1TF, UK. [9]Department of Dental Public Health, Faculty of Dentistry, Padjadjaran University, Sekelda Selatan I, Bandung, Indonesia. [10]Institute of Human Genetics, University Hospital Jena, Friedrich Schiller University Jena, Am Klinikum 1, 07740 Jena, Germany. [11]Department of Epidemiology and Biostatistics, College of Public Health, University of the Philippines, 625 Pedro Gil St, Ermita, Manila, Philippines.

References
1. Kassebaum NJ, Smith AGC, Bernabé E, Fleming TD, Reynolds AE, Vos T, Murray CJL, Marcenes W. Global, regional, and national prevalence, incidence, and disability-adjusted life years for oral conditions for 195 countries, 1990–2015: a systematic analysis for the global burden of diseases, injuries, and risk factors. J Dent Res. 2017;96:380–7.
2. Sheiham A. Dental caries affects body weight, growth and quality of life in pre-school children. Br Dent J. 2006;201:625–6.
3. Hooley M, Skouteris H, Boganin C, Satur J, Kilpatrick N. Body mass index and dental caries in children and adolescents: a systematic review of literature published 2004 to 2011. Syst Rev. 2012;1:57.
4. Hayden C, Bowler JO, Chambers S, Freeman R, Humphris G, Richards D, et al. Obesity and dental caries in children: a systematic review and meta-analysis. Community Dent Oral Epidemiol. 2013;41:289–308.
5. Li LW, Wong HM, Peng SM, McGrath CP. Anthropometric measurements and dental caries in children: a systematic review of longitudinal studies. Adv Nutr. 2015;6:52–63.
6. Alvarez JO. Nutrition, tooth development, and dental caries. Am J Clin Nutr. 1995;61(Suppl 1):410–6.
7. Narksawat K, Tonmukayakul U, Boonthum A. Association between nutritional status and dental caries in permanent dentition among primary schoolchildren aged 12–14 years, Thailand. Southeast Asian J Trop Med Public Health. 2009;40:338–44.
8. Benzian H, Monse B, Heinrich-Weltzien R, Hobdell M, Mulder J, van Palenstein Helderman W. Untreated severe dental decay: a neglected determinant of low body mass index in 12-year-old Filipino children. BMC Public Health. 2011;11:558.

9. Alkarimi H, Watt RG, Pikhart H, Sheiham S, Tsakos G. Dental caries and growth in school-age children. Pediatrics. 2014;133:616–23.

10. Anderson HK, Drummond BK, Thomson WM. Changes in aspects of children's oral-health-related quality of life following dental treatment under general anesthesia. Int J Paediatr Dent. 2004;14:317–25.

11. Stephensen CB. Burden of infection on growth failure. J Nutr. 1999; 129(Suppl 2):534–8.

12. Psoter WJ, Reid BC, Katz RV. Malnutrition and dental caries: a review of the literature. Caries Res. 2005;39:441–7.

13. Psoter W, Gebrian B, Prophete S, Reid B, Katz R. Effect of early childhood malnutrition on tooth eruption in Haitian adolescents. Community Dent Oral Epidemiol. 2008;36:179–83.

14. Hong L, Ahmed A, McCunniff M, Overman P, Mathew M. Obesity and dental caries in children aged 2–6 years in the United States: National health and nutrition examination survey 1999–2002. J Public Health Dent. 2008;68:227–33.

15. Ismail AI, Sohn W, Lim S, Willem JM. Predictors of dental caries progression in primary teeth. J Dent Res. 2009;88:270–5.

16. Gerdin EW, Angbratt M, Aronsson K, Eriksson E, Johansson I. Dental caries and body mass index by socio-economic status in Swedish children. Community Dent Oral Epidemiol. 2008;36:459–65.

17. Sheiham A, Watt RG. The common risk factor approach: a rational basis for promoting oral health. Community Dent Oral Epidemiol. 2000;28:399–406.

18. Monse B, Benzian H, Araojo J, Holmgren C, van Palenstein Helderman W, Naliponguit EC, Heinrich-Weltzien R. A silent public health crisis: untreated caries and dental infections among 6- and 12-year-old children in the Philippine National Oral Health Survey 2006. Asia Pac J Public Health. 2015;27:2316–25.

19. Duangthip D, Gao SS, Lo EC, Chu CH. Early childhood caries among 5- to 6-year-old children in Southeast Asia. Int Dent J. 2016; https://doi.org/10.1111/idj.12261.

20. World Health Organization. The double burden of malnutrition. Policy brief. Geneva: World Health Organization; 2017.

21. Duijster D, Monse B, Dimaisip-Nabuab JM, Djuharnoko P, Heinrich-Weltzien R, Hobdell MH, Kromeyer-Hauschild K, Kunthearith Y, Mijares-Majini MCC, Siegmund N, Soukhanouvong P, Benzian H. 'Fit for school' – a school-based water, sanitation and hygiene programme to improve child health: results from a longitudinal study in Cambodia, Indonesia and Lao PDR. BMC Public Health. 2017;17:302.

22. Monse B, Naliponguit E, Belizario V, Benzian H, van Palenstein Helderman W. Essential health care package for children – the 'fit for school' program in the Philippines. Int Dent J. 2011;60:85–93.

23. Monse B, Benzian H, Naliponguit E, Belizario V, Schratz A, van Palenstein Helderman W. The fit for school health outcome study: a longitudinal survey to assess health impacts of an integrated school health programme in the Philippines. BMC Public Health. 2013;13(256)

24. World Health Organization. Oral health surveys basic methods. 4th ed. Geneva: WHO; 1997.

25. Monse B, Heinrich-Weltzien R, Benzian H, Holmgren C, van Palenstein Helderman W. PUFA – an index of clinical consequences of untreated dental caries. Community Dent Oral Epidemiol. 2010;38:77–82.

26. Cogill B. 2003 revised edition anthropometric indicators measurement guide. Washington DC: Academy for Educational Development; 2003.

27. de Onis M, Onyango AW, Borghi E, Siyam A, Nishida C, Siekmann J. Development of a growth reference for school-aged children and adolescents. Bull World Health Organ. 2007;85:660–7.

28. World Health Organization [http://www.who.int/growthref/who2007_bmi_for_age/en/.] Accessed 4 July 2016.

29. Howe LD, Galobardes B, Matijasevich A, Gordon D, Johnston D, Onwujekwe O, et al. Measuring socio-economic position for epidemiological studies in low- and middle-income countries: a methods of measurement in epidemiology paper. Int J Epidemiol. 2012;41:871–86.

30. Acs G, Lodolini G, Kaminsky S, Cisneros GJ. Effect of nursing caries on body weight in a pediatric population. Pediatr Dent. 1992;14:302–25.

31. Cameron FL, Weaver LT, Wright CM, Welbury RR. Dietary and social characteristics of children with severe tooth decay. Scott Med J. 2006;51:26–9.

32. Sheller B, Churchill SS, Williams BJ, Davidson B. Body mass index of children with severe early childhood caries. Pediatr Dent. 2009;31:216–22.

33. Delgado-Angulo EK, Hobdell MH, Bernabe E. Childhood stunting and caries increment in permanent teeth: a three and a half year longitudinal study in Peru. Int J Paediatr Dent. 2013;23:101–9.

34. Duijster D, Sheiham A, Hobdell MH, Itchon G, Monse B. Associations between oral health-related impacts and rate of weight gain after extraction of pulpally involved teeth in underweight Filipino children. BMC Public Health. 2013;13:533.

35. van Cauter E, Plat L. Physiology of growth hormone secretion during sleep. J Pediatr. 1996;128:32–7.

36. Means RT Jr. Recent developments in the anemia of chronic disease. Curr Hematol Rep. 2003;2:116–21.

37. Schroth RJ, Levi J, Kliewer E, Sellers EA, Friel J, Kliewer E, Moffatt ME. Vitamin D status of children with severe early childhood caries: a case-control study. BMC Pediatr. 2013;13:174.

38. Bansal K, Goyal M, Dhingra R. Association of severe early childhood caries with iron deficiency anemia. J Indian Soc Pedod Prev Dent. 2016;34:36–42.

39. Acs G, Shulman R, Ng MW, Chussid S. The effect of dental rehabilitation on the body weight of children with early childhood caries. Pediatr Dent. 1999;21:109–13.

40. Monse B, Duijster D, Sheiham A, Grijalva-Eternod CS, van Palenstein Helderman W, Hobdell MH. The effects of extraction of pulpally involved primary teeth on weight, height and BMI in underweight Filipino children. A cluster randomized clinical trial. BMC Public Health. 2012;12:725.

41. Alkarimi HA, Watt RG, Pikhart H, Jawadi AH, Sheiham A, Tsakos G. Impact of treating dental caries on schoolchildren's anthropometric, dental, satisfaction and appetite outcomes: a randomized controlled trial. BMC Public Health. 2012;12:706.

42. Heinrich-Weltzien R, Zorn C, Monse B, Kromeyer-Hauschild K. Relationship between malnutrition and the number of permanent teeth in Filipino 10- to 13-year olds. Biomed Res Int. 2013;2013:205950.

43. Must A, Phillips SM, Tybor DJ, Lividini K, Hayes C. The association between childhood obesity and tooth eruption. Obesity Silver Spring. 2012;20:2070–4.

44. Alvarez JO, Navia JM. Nutritional status, tooth eruption and dental caries: a review. Am J Clin Nutr. 1989;49:417–26.

45. Centers for Disease Control and Prevention. Use of World Health Organization and CDC Growth Charts for Children Aged 0–59 Months in the United States. MMWR. 2010;59:1–15.

46. World Bank. [https://data.worldbank.org/indicator/SE.PRM.NENR.] Accessed 22 June 2018.

47. Lipoeto NI, Geok Lin K, Angeles-Agdeppa I. Food consumption patterns and nutrition transition in South-East Asia. Public Health Nutr. 2013;16:1637–43.

48. UNDP. Support to the implementation of the sustainable development goals. United Nations Development Programme, 2016.

49. Reeve E, Thow AM, Bell C, Engelhardt K, Gamolo-Naliponguit EC, Go JJ, Sacks G. Implementation lessons for school food policies and marketing restrictions in the Philippines: a qualitative policy analysis. Glob Health. 2018;14:8.

20

Multi-professional meetings on health checks and communication in providing nutritional guidance for infants and toddlers in Japan: a cross-sectional, national survey-based study

Midori Ishikawa[1*] (iD), Kumi Eto[2], Mayu Haraikawa[3], Kemal Sasaki[5], Zentaro Yamagata[6], Tetsuji Yokoyama[1], Noriko Kato[1,7], Yumiko Morinaga[8] and Yoshihisa Yamazaki[4]

Abstract

Background: Health personnel must provide continuous support in response to problematic results from health checks of infants and toddlers (hereinafter "infant[s]"). Among this support, it is important for health personnel to provide nutritional guidance to families as a collaborative effort between the staff from multiple disciplines and community organizations. This study aimed to clarify the factors affecting collaboration with community organizations in providing nutritional guidance to families following health checks for infants in Japan.

Methods: The design of this study consisted of a cross-sectional, multilevel survey. A self-administered questionnaire was mailed to all municipalities (1741 towns and cities) in Japan to be completed by the person responsible for nutrition advice. The research was performed in August 2015. We obtained 988 valid responses (response rate of 56.7%).

To identify the factors that affect the collaboration with community organizations in providing nutritional guidance, we determined how municipalities responded to infants needing support (five items), how municipalities evaluated health guidance (five items), the number of distributed maternal and child health handbooks, and the number of infants who received follow-up evaluations.

Results: The results of multivariate analyses showed that the factors related to successful community collaboration in providing nutritional guidance included holding a multi-professional staff meeting after health checks (post-conference; odds ratio [OR], 2.34; $P = 0.001$); following up children suspected of having developmental and mental disabilities or delays before entering elementary school (OR, 1.77; $P = 0.0004$); and considering dental caries data from dental checkups in providing health guidance (OR, 1.56; $P = 0.003$).

Conclusions: Holding a multi-professional meeting after infant health checks (post-conference) was strongly associated with community collaboration in providing nutritional guidance for infants.

Keywords: Infant health checks, Nutritional guidance, Community collaboration, Multi-professional meeting, Japan

* Correspondence: ishikawa.m.aa@niph.go.jp
[1]Department of Health Promotion, National Institute of Public Health, 2-3-6 Minami, Wako, Saitama 351-0197, Japan
Full list of author information is available at the end of the article

Background

In Japan's maternal and child health (MCH) policy, *Healthy Parents and Children 21 (Second Phase)*, the collaboration between the municipality and stakeholders in the community (e.g., kindergartens, preschools, child welfare facilities) is required to provide ongoing support for children and parents in need of health and nutritional care guidance [1]. By using a multi-professional approach—in which experts collaborate to meet the needs of the infant and parent—the appropriate quality of healthcare support can be provided [2, 3]. For example, there are cases of parents being unwilling to acknowledge concerns about the delayed development of their child based on the results of health checks. Parents may refuse to accept the guidance provided by public health nurses about their child's development. Other issues involve children having an unbalanced diet. In such cases, dietitians are expected to provide nutritional guidance while considering the needs of the children and parents [2, 4]. Community collaboration may be required to properly respond to infants and parents needing support, health evaluation, and nutritional guidance. It is therefore important to provide nutritional guidance based on the results of infant health checks and as a collaborative effort between multi-professional staff and community organizations.

One study evaluating infant health status in the United States showed that positive weight change is related to an effective network of community collaborations [5]. Access to quality childcare services using community resources on the results of infant health status assessments is also important in improving parental behavior and reducing the need for emergency medical care for infants [6, 7]. However, no studies in Japan have investigated this topic.

In Japan, infant health checks are required by the Maternal and Child Health Law [8]. The main purpose of infant health checks and health guidance is to clarify explicit and potential health concerns and to support parents and children in dealing with these concerns [8, 9]. In 2015, the participation rate for health checks was 95.6% for infants aged 3–4 months, 95.7% for those aged 1.6 years, and 94.3% for those aged 3 years [10].

Before or after health checks in Japan, a multi-professional meeting is convened by health staff to identify health concerns (a "pre-/post-conference"). Although this form of conference is not a mandate of the designated country, this form has been adopted for information sharing among staff to connect health checks and health guidance for children in municipalities. At the pre-conference, the staff discuss pre-established concerns about each child. At the post-conference, the children who require follow-up evaluations are confirmed. In some cases, continuous support (follow-up) [11, 12], as well as

the provision of nutritional guidance in conjunction with community collaborations, may be required. In such cases, it is important to share information about infant health checks with community organizations. This sharing allows deciding the best approaches to support children and parents, evaluate responses to their needs, and assess the outcomes of those activities [5]. However, few studies have investigated factors that affect the ability of health personnel and community organizations to collaborate on providing nutritional guidance to families [13]; moreover, no studies have addressed this topic in Japan.

This survey aimed to clarify the proportion of municipalities in Japan cooperating with communities in providing nutritional guidance to families whose infants received health checks, and to identify the factors related to collaboration with community organizations in providing nutritional guidance.

Methods

Study municipalities and procedure

This study was a cross-sectional survey of all 1741 municipalities in Japan. We used a self-administered questionnaire to determine whether infant health checks were being carried out and whether health and nutritional guidance was being provided. A copy of the questionnaire was mailed to each municipality. The department responsible for nutritional guidance following infant health checks was asked to complete the questionnaire. The director of the department then returned the questionnaire by mail or fax.

This research was performed in August 2015. In total, 1172 municipalities completed the questionnaire (response rate of 67.3%). Only questionnaires with complete responses to the items included in our analysis were considered valid, providing 988 valid questionnaires for analysis (response rate of 56.7%).

Measurement

The questionnaire items included indicators of existing policy measures and guidelines [1, 2, 14, 15] of the Ministry of Health, Labour and Welfare; these guidelines were used in a national nutrition survey of preschool children [16]. The reliability of the items was previously confirmed [17–19].

The dependent variable was whether community collaboration is involved in providing guidance on infant nutrition. The survey respondents were asked: "Does your municipality provide nutritional guidance or education targeting infants and parents in collaboration with any organizations or groups, such as nursery schools, kindergartens, welfare facilities, or related agencies in the community, and do you evaluate those activities?" [18]. Health personnel were asked to choose an answer from the following categories: 1) We collaborate with community organizations and evaluate the activities; 2) We collaborate with community organizations but do not evaluate the activities; and 3) We do not collaborate with any organization. We designated municipalities that answered either 1 or 2 as the collaborating group and those that answered three as the non-collaborating group.

We expected certain factors to be associated with such collaboration, including methods for carrying out infant health checks, methods for determining how to respond to infants and parents needing support (five items), and methods for evaluating health guidance (five items). We also asked about potential confounding factors related to infant health checks. They included the annual number of distributed Mother and Child Health (MCH) handbooks, the annual number of infants who received a follow-up and municipality category by number of children eligible for health checks at 3 years old.

These items were chosen because they are important indicators of the health and nutrition of infants in Japan, and there are clear differences between municipalities. A copy of the MCH Handbook is provided for all pregnant women and provides a consistent health and information-provision record during pregnancy, delivery, and early years of child rearing. At every infant health check, information related to health and nutritional status are entered in the handbook, to determine suitable follow-up.

A previous study using the same data reported the validity of the municipality categories for the geographical area, the population size, and the number of children eligible for health checks at 3 years old [19]. However, the report did not show the relationship between the municipality category and community collaboration on nutritional guidance for infants. We therefore included whether category was related to the collaboration items, as a possible confounding factor.

The Appendix shows the five items addressing "how staff responded to infants and parents needing support" and "the evaluation of health guidance." The possible answers were yes or no.

Statistical analysis

To determine the response to infants and parents needing support (five items) and methods used to evaluate health guidance (five items), we performed an analysis comparing the answers of the collaborating and non-collaborating municipalities to the survey items about the methods used. We analyzed the results using the Cochran–Mantel–Haenszel test. Using

correspondence analysis, we analyzed the relationships between the 11 items (one item on collaborating with community organizations; five items on determining responses to infants and parents; and five items on evaluating health guidance).

We performed univariate analysis for each factor using a logistic regression model based on the results of the correspondence analysis. The analyzed factors were those that were expected to be associated with collaboration in nutritional guidance: implementing a pre-conference; sharing medical records; sharing verbal information with responsible staff; implementing a post-conference; providing feedback to public health nurses and related organizations; evaluating health guidance for parents; using dental caries data in health guidance; evaluating health guidance and follow-up; and providing follow-up evaluations for infants before or after beginning elementary school.

To identify factors important for community collaboration, we performed stepwise logistic regression using the following variables: holding pre-conferences; sharing medical records; sharing verbal information with staff; holding post-conferences; providing feedback to public health nurses and related organizations; evaluating health guidance for parents; using dental caries information in health guidance; evaluating health guidance and follow-up; and providing follow-up evaluations for children who have entered or not entered elementary school. These data were adjusted for the annual number of distributed MCH handbooks, the annual number of infants who received follow-up evaluations, and the annual number of 3-year-olds who underwent health checks (model 1).

Statistical analysis was conducted using SAS software, version 9.2 (SAS Institute, Inc., Cary, NC, USA). A P value of < 0.05 was considered statistically significant.

Results

Table 1 shows the comparison between community collaboration to provide nutritional guidance with distribution of MCH Handbook, number of infants who received follow-up, and municipality category by number of children eligible for health checks at 3 years old. The proportion of municipalities that collaborated with community organizations in providing nutritional guidance based on infant health checks (collaborating group) was 69.5%. The proportion that did not collaborate with any community organizations (non-collaborating group) was 30.5%. There were no significant differences between the two groups for the annual number of MCH handbooks distributed, the annual number of infants who received follow-up and

Table 1 Comparison between community collaboration in providing nutritional guidance with distribution of MCH Handbook, number of infants who received follow-up, and municipality category by number of children eligible for health checks at 3 years old

		Collaborating group		Non-collaborating group		
		no	%	no	%	
		687	69.5	301	30.5	p
		mean	SD	mean	SD	
Number of distributions of MCH Handbook/year		693.7	1703.9	698.4	1197.5	0.240
Number of infants who received follow-up/year		58.3	140.7	70.0	164.5	0.899
Municipality category by scale of number of subjects to health checks for 3-year-old children		no	%	no	%	
I < 8	I	11	1.6	10	3.3	0.239
8 ≤ II < 54	II	119	17.3	43	14.3	
54 ≤ III < 391	III	301	43.8	123	40.9	
39 ≤ IV < 2916	IV	218	31.7	106	35.2	
2916 ≤ V	V	38	5.5	19	6.3	

n = 988

p for homogeneity between 2 groups by Cochran-Mantel-Haenszel

the municipality category by number of children eligible for health checks at 3 years old.

Table 2 shows the relationship between community collaboration to provide nutritional guidance for infants and parents, decisions on how staff responded to infants and parents needing support (five items), and methods used to evaluate health guidance (five items).

Collaborating municipalities were more likely to implement a pre-conference ($P = 0.014$) and a post-conference ($P < 0.001$) and to provide feedback to public health nurses ($P = 0.023$). The collaborating group also consisted of more municipalities that evaluated health guidance for parents ($P = 0.002$), used dental caries information in health guidance ($P = 0.001$), followed up children prior to elementary school ($P = 0.001$), and evaluated the relevance of health guidance and follow-ups ($P = 0.005$).

Figure 1 maps the results of the correspondence analysis for the relationships between community collaboration in providing nutritional guidance, decisions on the response to infants and parents needing support, and evaluation of health guidance. Items on the evaluation of health guidance were closer to community collaboration in provision of nutritional guidance than items on determining the response to infants and parents. A post-conference was closely associated with community collaboration in providing nutritional guidance in items addressing decisions on the response to infants and parents needing support. The positions of the pre-conference and post-conference were far apart, which indicates that these conferences might have different roles.

Using logistic analysis

Table 3 shows the factors in the health check activities that were related to successful community collaboration in nutritional guidance. Following normalization (Model 1), these factors included the following: having a pre-conference (odds ratio [OR] = 1.45; 95% confidence interval [CI]: 1.08–1.94; $P = 0.014$), having a post-conference (OR = 2.82; 95% CI: 1.72–4.61; $P < 0.001$), providing feedback to public health nurses and related stakeholders (OR = 1.54; 95% CI: 1.11–2.15; $P = 0.010$), evaluating health guidance for parents needing support (OR = 1.70; 95% CI: 1.22–2.37; $P = 0.002$), using data about dental caries in health guidance (OR = 1.82; 95% CI: 1.37–2.42; $P < 0.001$), following up children before they began elementary school (OR = 2.01; 95% CI: 1.48–2.73; $P < 0.001$), and evaluating the relevance of health guidance (OR = 1.58; 95% CI: 1.14–2.18; $P = 0.005$).

In the multivariate analysis, the factors related to successful community collaboration in nutritional guidance included the following: having post-conferences (OR = 2.34; 95% CI: 1.39–3.94; $P = 0.001$), following up children before they entered elementary school (OR = 1.77; 95% CI: 1.29–2.43; $P = 0.0004$), and using data on dental caries in health guidance (OR = 1.56; 95% CI: 1.16–2.10; $P = 0.003$).

Discussion

Factors related to community collaboration in nutritional guidance

In this study, community collaboration in providing nutritional guidance was strongly related to the implementation of a multi-professional meetings after health checks (post-conferences). This finding is consistent with previous

Table 2 Relationship between community collaboration in nutritional guidance for infants and parents, decisions on how staff responded to infants and parents needing support, and methods used to evaluate health guidance

		Collaborating group		Non-collaborating group		$n = 988$
		no	%	no	%	
		687	69.5	301	30.5	p
How staff responded to infants and parents needing support (5 items)						
Implement a pre-conference	Yes	510	74.2	200	66.5	0.014
	No	177	25.8	101	33.6	
Share medical records	Yes	458	66.7	203	67.4	0.812
	No	229	33.3	98	32.6	
Share verbal information with responsible staff	Yes	426	62.0	181	60.1	0.577
	No	261	38.0	120	39.9	
Implement a post-conference	Yes	654	95.2	264	87.7	<.0001
	No	33	4.8	37	12.3	
Provide feedback to public health nurses and related organizations	Yes	547	79.6	220	73.1	0.023
	No	140	20.4	81	26.9	
Methods used to evaluate health guidance (5 items)						
Evaluate health guidance for parents	Yes	195	28.4	57	18.9	0.002
	No	492	71.6	244	81.1	
Use dental caries data in health guidance	Yes	316	46.0	97	32.2	<.0001
	No	371	54.0	204	67.8	
Provide follow-up evaluations for infants before beginning elementary school	Yes	272	69.6	74	24.6	<.0001
	No	415	60.4	227	75.4	
Provide follow-up evaluations for infants after beginning elementary school	Yes	11	1.6	4	1.3	0.747
	No	676	98.4	297	98.7	
Evaluate health guidance and follow-up	Yes	206	30.0	64	21.3	0.005
	No	481	70.0	237	78.7	

p for homogeneity between 2 groups by Cochran-Mantel-Haenszel

reports in which sharing information among staff enabled professionals to both create a shared vision, strong leadership, and broad collective goals and to clarify strengths and priorities for developing and launching projects [20]. The importance of selecting the most appropriate approach to create a collaboration has been reinforced by health data and reliable information showing the results of environmental and behavioral change [21]. If staff are unable to share child health information, then it will be unclear whether a particular response or approach is appropriate [22]. It is necessary to confirm why some municipalities do not conduct post-conferences. Post-conferences may help to establish a better system for health checks and nutritional improvement for infants.

Multidisciplinary collaboration for nutritional support in the community

In Japan, health checks are used to make an accurate assessment of the needs of infants and their parents.

Parents may continue to experience difficulties and require support throughout their child's early years [2, 16]. It is therefore important to establish a system that enables continuous support of infants and parents in the community [2, 21, 23].

According to Japan's national infant nutritional survey, an unbalanced diet (including snacks and soft drinks) leads to dietary issues in children. The proportion of children with such diets is significantly higher in low-income households [16]. Other studies have reported a relationship between the consumption of sugary drinks and poor eating behavior among infants and children [24–26].

One of the main objectives of community collaboration is to monitor the progress of infants and parents who require particular support in certain areas, including nutrition [21]. A multi-sectorial approach is required to address various dimensions of maternal and child healthcare, including environmental health [27].

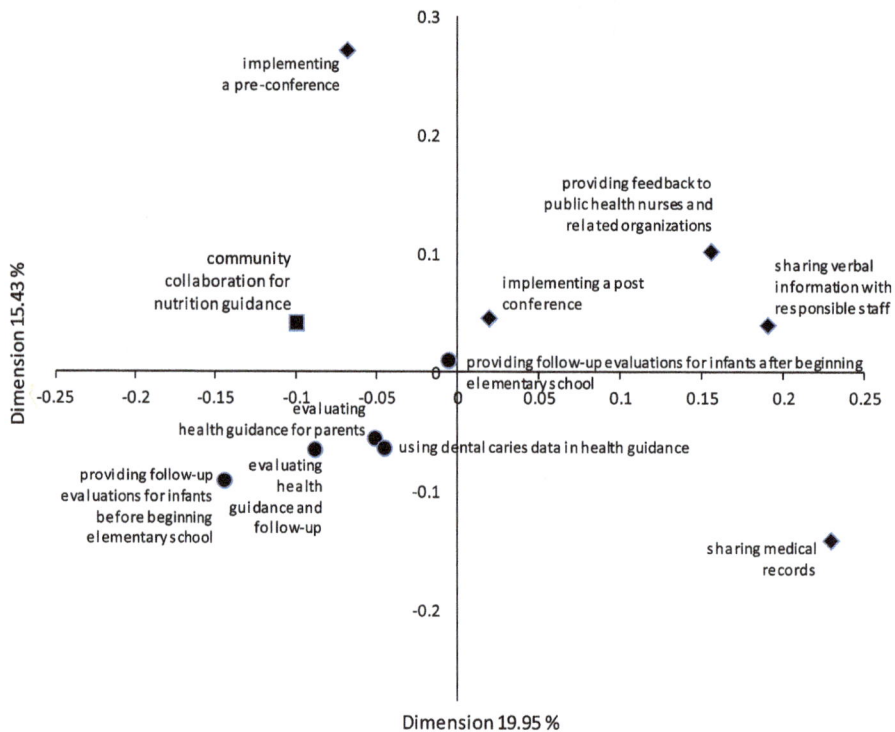

Fig. 1 Relationships between "community collaboration for nutritional guidance", and items on "how staff responded to infants and parents needing support" and "methods used to evaluate health guidance", from the correspondence analysis. Key: ♦: How staff responded to infants and parents needing support (5 items); ●: Methods used to evaluate health guidance (5 items)

Health professionals such as dietitians can then be involved in deciding whether further assistance is necessary or whether the issues have been resolved with the support provided [2, 5]. It is important that staff from multiple health disciplines and community groups are involved in discussions about infants and parents at post-conferences, as this involvement enables a consensus on the need for monitoring, continued support, or follow-up evaluations with home visits [6, 23].

This study found that the factors strongly related to community collaboration in providing nutritional guidance included sharing information about infant dental checkups and the results of follow-up activities before children entered elementary school. Sharing this information will lead to ongoing support throughout the child's education [10]. The life course perspective is a critical addition to this work: it highlights the importance of ensuring that infants and children live in supportive community environments that will foster optimal health, development, and well-being throughout their lives [3, 7].

It is important to develop long-term support systems for infants and parents by sharing information, especially about food and nutrition, between community organizations such

as nursery schools, pediatric clinics, kindergartens, child welfare facilities, associations for the promotion of better dietary habits, community cafeterias for children, and other governmental and non-governmental organizations [10].

This study had some limitations. First, its cross-sectional design suggests that no causal relationships can be inferred, such that reverse causation or simple correlation could account for the observations. Second, the final response rate of 56.7% was relatively low. The questionnaire was not administered to individuals, and it covered a broad range of disciplines; moreover, staff operating in different fields may have responded differently to certain items. Local government staff may also have the lacked time to complete the questionnaire during working hours and, in particular, to obtain a consensus from other staff members. Characteristics of municipalities that did not respond (around one third in total) were almost the same as those that did, including population size (small, medium and large population). One of the reasons why some municipalities did not respond may have been because that they have no full-time staff in charge of nutrition. During the study period, several municipalities responded to explain that they only

Table 3 Factors in health check activities that are related to successful community collaboration in nutritional guidance, assessed by logistic analysis

item		Model 1[a]				Stepwise			$n = 988$
		OR	95% CI		p	OR	95% CI		p
How staff responded to infants and parents needing support (5 items)									
Implement a pre-conference	Yes	1.45	1.08	1.94	0.014	1.22	0.89	1.66	0.212
	No	1.00				1.00			
Share medical records	Yes	1.01	0.74	1.38	0.949				
	No	1.00							
Share verbal information with responsible staff	Yes	1.13	0.85	1.52	0.405				
	No	1.00							
Implement a post-conference	Yes	2.82	1.72	4.61	<.0001	2.34	1.39	3.94	0.001
	No	1.00				1.00			
Provide feedback to public health nurses and related organizations	Yes	1.54	1.11	2.15	0.010				
	No	1.00							
Methods used to evaluate health guidance (5 items)									
Evaluate health guidance for parents	Yes	1.70	1.22	2.37	0.002				
	No	1.00							
Use dental caries data in health guidance	Yes	1.82	1.37	2.42	<.0001	1.56	1.16	2.10	0.003
	No	1.00				1.00			
Provide follow-up evaluations for infants before beginning elementary school	Yes	2.01	1.48	2.73	<.0001	1.77	1.29	2.43	0.000
	No	1.00				1.00			
Provide follow-up evaluations for infants after beginning elementary school	Yes	1.19	0.37	3.76	0.772				
	No	1.00							
Evaluate health guidance and follow-up	Yes	1.58	1.14	2.18	0.005				
	No	1.00							

[a]Model 1: Adjusted for category of subject in 3-year-old infant health examinations, number of Mother Child Handbooks distributed per year, and number of infants followed up per year

OR Odds ratio, CI Confidence interval

had part-time staff responsible for nutritional guidance, so could not cooperate. In future surveys, it will be necessary to consider the investigation method to ensure that municipalities are not excluded because of the employment situation of staff in charge of providing nutritional guidance. Responses to the survey may also have been limited to municipalities that actively conduct health checks. A follow-up study using face-to-face interviews with health workers should be considered. Fourth, our analysis was restricted to items that could apply to all municipalities. Future investigations should examine whether the response options are unique to Japan. Municipal income was not included as a confounding factor in this survey, but should be included in a future study.

Despite these limitations, this study found relationships between community collaboration in providing nutritional guidance and the implementation of post-conferences, the follow-up evaluation of children suspected of having developmental and mental difficulties before they enter elementary school, and the use of dental checkup results in health guidance for parents and their children. The results of this study are significant because very few studies to date have examined the links between nutritional guidance and infant health checks.

Conclusions

This study found that sharing information in a multi-professional meeting following infant health checks (a post-conference) was strongly associated with successful community collaboration in providing nutritional guidance. It highlights the importance of ensuring that infants and children live in supportive community environments that will foster optimal health, development, and well-being throughout their lives.

Appendix

Table 4 Items of questionaiire on factors to be associated with community collaboration in nutritional guidance for infants and parents

How staff responded to infants and parents needing support (5 items)

Do you share information with staff from different disciplines at meetings before health checks (pre-conference)?

Do you share medical record information?

Do you verbally share information with responsible public health staff?

Do you share information with staff from different disciplines at meetings after health checks (post-conference)?

Do you provide feedback on infant health information to the public health nurse responsible for the area of residence and related stakeholders?

Methods used to evaluate health guidance (5 items)

Do you evaluate the relevance of health guidance for parents who are having difficulties raising their child?

Do you use data about dental caries from dental health checks in health guidance?

Do you follow up children who are suspected of having developmental or mental disabilities or delays before entering elementary school?

Do you follow up children suspected of having developmental or mental disabilities or delays after entering elementary school?

Do you evaluate the relevance of health guidance and follow-ups, including for children who are not unhealthy but where there is some cause for concern?

Abbreviations
CI: Confidence interval; MCH: maternal and child health; MHLW: Ministry of Health, Labour and Welfare; OR: Odds ratio; SD: Standard deviation

Acknowledgements
This study was supported by the Japan Agency for Medical Research and Development Grants and Health and Labour Sciences Research Grants, Japan. We also thank the municipalities who participated in this study.

Funding
This study was supported by the Japan Agency for Medical Research and Development Grants (H27–28 16gk0110010j1002) and Health and Labour Sciences Research Grants (H29Sukoyaka-Ippan 003). This research did not receive any specific grant from funding agencies in the commercial, or not-for-profit sectors.

Authors' contributions
MI designed the study, collected and analyzed the data and drafted the manuscript; KE, MH, KS, ZY, KN, YM and YY conceived and designed the study, collected the data and helped draft the manuscript; and TY helped analyze the data and draft the manuscript. All authors have read and approved the final version of the manuscript and agree with the order of presentation of the authors.

Competing interests
The authors declare that they have no competing interests.

Author details
[1]Department of Health Promotion, National Institute of Public Health, 2-3-6 Minami, Wako, Saitama 351-0197, Japan. [2]Faculty of Nutrition, Kagawa Nutrition University, 3-9-21 Chiyoda, Sakado, Saitama 350-0288, Japan. [3]Department of Child Studies, Faculty of Child Studies, Seitoku University, 550 Iwase, Matsudo, Chiba 271-8555, Japan. [4]Child Health Center, Aichi Children's Health and Medical Center, 426-7, Morioka, Obu, Aichi 474-8710, Japan. [5]Department of Food and Health Sciences, Jissen Women's University, 4-1-1 Osakaue, Hino, Tokyo 191-8510, Japan. [6]Faculty of Medicine, University of Yamanashi, 1110 Shimokato, Chuo, Yamanashi 409-3898, Japan. [7]Present Address: Department of Early Childhood Care and Education, Jumonji University, 2-1-28 Sugasawa, Niizashi, Saitama 352-8510, Japan. [8]Faculty of Medicine, School of Nursing Public Health Nursing, Kagawa University, 1750-1, Ikenobe, Miki, Kita, Kagawa 761-0793, Japan.

References
1. Ministry of Health, Labour and Welfare (MHLW): Healthy Parents and. Children 21(second), 2015(in Japanese) http://www.mhlw.go.jp/file/06-Seisakujouhou-11900000-Koyoukintoujidoukateikyoku/0000067539.pdf#search=%27%E5%81%A5%E3%82%84%E3%81%8B%E8%A6%AA%E5%AD%9021%E7%AC%AC%E4%BA%8C%E6%AC%A1%27. Accessed 5 Sep 2017.
2. Study group on health checkup and health guidance for maternal and child health through multi-occupational cooperation (SGHC): Standard health checkup and health guidance in infant and early childhood. 2015 (in Japanese) http://www.mhlw.go.jp/file/06-Seisakujouhou-11900000-Koyoukintoujidoukateikyoku/tebiki.pdf. Accessed 5 Sep 2017.
3. Shrimali P, Luginbuhl J, Malin C, Flournoy R, Siegel A. The building blocks collaborative: advancing a life course approach to health equity through multi-sector collaboration. Maternal Child Health J. 2014;18:373–9.
4. Mustila T, Keskinen P, Luoto R. Behavioral counseling prevent childhood obesity-study protocol of a pragmatic trial in maternity and child health care. BMC Pediatr. 2012;12(93) https://doi.org/10.1186/1471-2431-12-93.
5. Darnell AJ, Barile JP, Weaver SR, Harper CR, Kupermine GP, Emshoff JG. Testing effects of community collaboration on rates of low infant birthweight at county level. Am J Community Psychol. 2013;51:398–406. https://doi.org/10.1007/s10464-012-9559-x.
6. Dodge KA, Goodman WB, Murphy RA, O'Donnell K, Sato J, Guptill S. Implementation and randomized controlled trial evaluation of universal postnatal nurse home visiting. Am J Public Health. 2014;104:S143 https://doi.org/10.2105/AJPH.2013.301361.
7. Komro KA, Tobler AL, Delisile AL, O'Mara RJ, Wagenaar AC. Beyond the clinic; improving cild health through evidemce^based community development. BMC Pediatr. 2013;13(72) https://doi.org/10.1186/1471-2431-13-172.
8. Ministry of Health, Labour and Welfare (MHLW). Maternal and Child Health Act (in Japanese) http://law.e-gov.go.jp/htmldata/S40/S40HO141.html Accessed 5 Aug 2017.
9. Kuo DZ, Houtrow AJ, Arango P, Kuhthau KA, Simmons JM, Neff JM. Family-centered care: current applications and future directions in pediatric health care. Matern Child Health J. 2014(12):297–305 https://doi.org/10.1007/s10995-011-0751-7.
10. Ministry of Health, Labour and Welfare (MHLW). Report on Regional Public Health Services and Health Promotion Services 2015 (in Japanese) http://www.mhlw.go.jp/toukei/saikin/hw/c-hoken/15/dl/kekka1.pdf. Accessed 5 Sep 2017.
11. Nakamura Y. Maternal and child health handbook in Japan. Int Med Comm. 2010;53:259–65.
12. Takeuchi J, Sakagami Y, Perez R. The mother and child health handbook in Japan as a health promotion tool. Global Pediatric Health. 2016; https://doi.org/10.1177/2333794X16649884.
13. Martin KS, Wolff M, Lonczak M, Chambers M, Cooke C, Whitney G. Formative research to examine collaboration between special supplemental nutrition program for women, infants, and children and head start programs. Matern Child Health J. 2014;18:326–32.
14. Ministry of Health, Labour and Welfare (MHLW). Report on the Study Group on the ideal way to foster children's health through food and nutrition 2004; 13 (in Japanese) http://www.mhlw.go.jp/stf/seisakunitsuite/bunya/0000134208.html Accessed 5 Sep 2017.
15. Ministry of Health, Labour and Welfare (MHLW). Maternal and Child Health Handbook, Japan (in Japanese) http://www.mhlw.go.jp/stf/seisakunitsuite/bunya/kodomo/kodomo_kosodate/boshi-hoken/kenkou-04.html Accessed 5 Sep 2017.
16. Ministry of Health, Labour and Welfare (MHLW). Report on National nutrition survey on preschool children.2016 (in Japanese) http://www.mhlw.go.jp/stf/seisakunitsuite/bunya/0000134208.html. Accessed 5 Sep 2017.
17. Takahashi N, Haraikawa M, Niimi S, Eto K, Ishikawa M, Kato N, et al. Characteristics of concerns about maternal and childhood nutrition which

was described by nutrition educating staff in municipal maternal and child health activities-an analysis of open-ended question on pregnant women, infants, and children. Japanese J Public Health. 2016;63:569–77.

18. Eto K, Ishikawa M, Takahashi N, Haraikawa M, Niimi S, Sasaki K, et al. Implementation status and contents of nutritional guidance for infants and young children in municipalities in Japan. J Health Welf Stat. 2017;64:27–34 (in Japanese).

19. Sasaki K, Niimi S, Yamagata Z, Sato T, Akiyama C, Ogura K, et al. A nationwide survey on the subject age of 3-year old child health checkup. J Health Welf Stat. 2016;63:8–13 (in Japanese).

20. Aquino R, Oliveira NF, Barreto ML. Impact of the family health program on infant mortality in Brazilian municipalities. Am J Public Health. 2009;99:87–93 https://doi.org/10.2105/AJPH.2007.127480.

21. Bosch SO, Duch H. The role of cognitive stimulation at home in low-income preschoolers' nutrition. Physical activity and body mass index. BMC Pediatr. 2017;17(178) https://doi.org/10.1186/s12887-017-0918-5.

22. Olson BH, Horodynski M, Herb HB, Iwanski KC. Health professionals' perspectives on the infant feeding practices of low income mothers. Maternal Child Health Journal. 2010;14:75–85.

23. Martin MA, Rothschild SK, Lynch E, Christoffel K, Pagan MM, Rodriguez JL, et al. Addressing asthma and obesity in children with community health workers: proof-of-concept intervention development. BMC Pediatr. 2016;16(198) https://doi.org/10.1186/s12887-016-0745-0.

24. Sogabe R, Maruyama R, Nakamura F, Tsuchiya R, Inoue M, Goseki M: Development of oral function and eating habits of infants living in a city area of Japan; In relation to results of dental health examinations of infants aged 14 months at public health centers. *Japanese Journal of Public Health.* 2010, 57: 641–648. doi: https://doi.org/10.11236/jph.57.8_641

25. Okubo H, Miyake Y, Sasaki S, Tanaka K, Hirota Y. Early sugar-sweetened beverage consumption frequency is associated with poor quality of later food and nutrient intake patterns among Japanese young children: the Osaka Maternal and Child Health Study. Nutr Res. 2016;36:594–602 https://doi.org/10.1016/j.nutres.2016.01.008.

26. Ueno Y. Saeki K, Yoshimura S: the relationship between tooth eruption and ingestion of 15 food items among children aged 18-20 months. Japanese J Public Health. 2017;64:143–9 https://doi.org/10.11236/jph.64.3_143.

27. Horii N, Habi O, Dangana A, Maina A, Aizouma S, Charbit Y. Community-based behavior change promoting child health care: a response to socio-economic disparity. J Health, Promot Nutri. 2016;35:12 https://doi.org/10.1186/s41043-016-0048-y.

21

Effectiveness of weekly cell phone counselling calls and daily text messages to improve breastfeeding indicators

Archana Patel[1,2], Priyanka Kuhite[2], Amrita Puranik[2]* (iD), Samreen Sadaf Khan[2], Jitesh Borkar[2] and Leena Dhande[1]

Abstract

Background: Every year, nearly one million deaths occur due to suboptimal breastfeeding. If universally practiced, exclusive breastfeeding alone prevents 11.6% of all under 5 deaths. Among strategies to improve exclusive breastfeeding rates, counselling by peers or health workers, has proven to be highly successful. With growing availability of cell phones in India, they are fast becoming a medium to spread information for promoting healthcare among pregnant women and their families. This study was conducted to assess effectiveness of cell phones for personalized lactation consultation to improve breastfeeding practices.

Methods: This was a two arm, pilot study in four urban maternity hospitals, retrained in Baby Friendly Hospital Initiative. The enrolled mother-infant pairs resided in slums and received healthcare services at the study sites. The control received routine healthcare services, whereas, the intervention received weekly cell phone counselling and daily text messages, in addition to counselling the routine healthcare services.

Results: 1036 pregnant women were enrolled (518 - intervention and 518 - control). Rates of timely initiation of breastfeeding were significantly higher in intervention as compared to control (37% v/s 24%, $p < 0.001$). Pre-lacteal feeding rates were similar and low in both groups (intervention: 19%, control: 18%, $p = 0.68$). Rate of exclusive breastfeeding was similar between groups at 24 h after delivery, but significantly higher in the intervention at all subsequent visits (control vs. intervention: 24 h: 74% vs 74%, $p = 1.0$; 6 wk.: 81% vs 97%, 10 wk.: 78% vs 98%, 14 wk.: 71% vs 96%, 6 mo: 49% vs 97%, $p < 0.001$ for the last 4 visits). Adjusting for covariates, women in intervention were more likely to exclusively breastfeed than those in the control (AOR [95% CI]: 6.3 [4.9–8.0]).

Conclusion: Using cell phones to provide pre and postnatal breastfeeding counselling to women can substantially augment optimal practices. High rates of exclusive breastfeeding at 6 months were achieved by sustained contact and support using cell phones. This intervention shows immense potential for scale up by incorporation in both, public and private health systems.

Keywords: Breastfeeding counselling, Cell phone counselling, Exclusive breastfeeding, Infant nutrition, Lactation, Infant and young child feeding, Post-natal counselling, Maternal health

* Correspondence: puranikamrita@yahoo.co.in
[2]Lata Medical Research Foundation, Nagpur, Maharashtra 440022, India
Full list of author information is available at the end of the article

Background

Every year, suboptimal breastfeeding is responsible for around 800,000 under 5 child deaths globally [1]. It has been found to be the second largest risk factor for children under 5 years with 47.5 million disability-adjusted life years lost in the year 2010 [2]. Universal practice of exclusive breastfeeding has the potential to avert 11.6% of under -5 deaths [1]. All-cause neonatal mortality could be reduced by 22.3%, just by timely initiation of breastfeeding (defined by the World Health Organization as putting the newborn to the breast within 1 h of birth). Timely initiation of breastfeeding has the potential to save 250,000 newborns in India alone [3]. Infants who have delayed initiation of breastfeeding (initiation of breastfeeding > 1 h after birth) have 33% greater risk of neonatal mortality when compared to those with timely initiation of breastfeeding [4]. Exclusive breastfeeding protects against ear infections, allergies, anaemia in infants and has large 'programming' effects on risks for hypertension, hypercholesterolemia, obesity, cancer, autoimmune disease, and cognitive function later in life [5, 6].

Suboptimal feeding causes malnutrition which accounts for 10% of the global disability adjusted life years for under five children and 50% of the mortality [7]. Thus, in 2001, World Health Organization, after reviewing available evidence, made a global recommendation that all infants should be breastfed exclusively for 6 months and continue until 24 months. Breastfeeding should be supplemented with semi-solid or complementary foods after 6 months of age, as growth faltering may start with lack of timely initiation of complementary feeding [8–10]. Despite the known advantages of breastfeeding and timely initiation of complementary feeding, the Indian National Family Health Survey 2005–06 reported timely initiation of breastfeeding rates of 24.5%, exclusive breastfeeding rates at 6 months of 46.4%, and only 56.7% of 6–9 month old being fed complementary foods [11].

In India, there is an increase in the number of women delivering in hospitals due to a government monetary incentive scheme but the health staff has limited counselling skills for infant and young child feeding. Studies have shown that all infant and young child feeding indicators are better in women who adhere to their scheduled antenatal visits where they may have received breastfeeding related counselling during these visits [12]. A meta-analysis of individual peer counselling for the promotion of exclusive breastfeeding showed that the odds of exclusive breastfeeding in mothers receiving lactation counselling were substantially higher in the neonatal period (15 studies; odds ratio [OR] 3.45, 95% CI (2.20–5.42), $p < 0.0001$; random effects) and at 6 months of age (9 studies; 1.93, 95% CI (1.18–3.15), $p < 0.0001$) [13]. However, individualized counselling at health centres or by home visits, is expensive and not feasible in a populous, low income country, like India. Cultural barriers restrict women from leaving their households for at least 6 weeks after delivery and when required they need to be escorted by a care-giver to the facility.

In India, nearly all households including those below the poverty line have at least one cell phone. Given the extensive usage of cell phones, it is now possible to use it for health promotion and bringing about behavioural changes among the pregnant women and their families [14, 15]. Health workers can not only use cell phones to counsel pregnant women but also use the short text message system to send reminders and health promotional messages. Breastfeeding practices can also be enhanced through cell phone counselling. It can provide opportunity for early detection of breastfeeding problems, preventing of erroneous guidance by family members, friends, or health professionals, and, reduce the need to visit a hospital. We conducted a study to assess the effectiveness of using cell phones for personalized lactation counselling to improve exclusive breastfeeding rates. The aim of this study was to evaluate the effectiveness of text messages and counselling using cell phones as they are ubiquitous, even in the lower socio-economic strata of the urban population. Other forms of communications such as landlines, smart phones, internet, laptops etc. are not available in these poor households. The secondary objectives were to assess rates of timely initiation of breastfeeding, timely initiation of complementary feeding, pre-lacteal feeding, bottle feeding, infant hospitalization, satisfaction with the lactation counselling received and infant weight. We also evaluated the cost-effectiveness of cell phones to increase exclusive breastfeeding rates at 6 months of infant's age.

Methods

Trial design, settings and location

This was a two arm, hospital-based pilot study conducted in four urban, public, maternity hospitals in Nagpur, India from August 2010 – to June 2012. This pilot study was conducted to understand the effectiveness of weekly cell phone counselling and daily text messages meant for pregnant and lactating women attending antenatal care and infant immunization clinics at these hospitals. This pilot will be essential to design a larger cluster randomized control trial to be implemented in rural India.

Eligibility criteria

The participating hospitals (two in intervention and two in control) had to have annual deliveries of above 5000 and catered to women belonging to poor socio-economic background. Women in their third trimester (32–36 weeks), registered for antenatal clinics, planning to deliver at the same hospital and willing to give follow up till 6 months of infant age were considered eligible. An informed consent was obtained from all eligible women. Women with presence of complications in pregnancy that could affect exclusive breastfeeding such as severe anemia (Hb < 6 g/dL), at the risk of eclampsia or pre-eclampsia, consuming drugs contraindicated in pregnancy or HIV positivity were excluded. A record of all women screened, consented and attrition was maintained, including those ineligible and the reasons for not participating in the study.

Randomization

Standardized Baby Friendly Hospital Initiative re-training was imparted by certified instructors to healthcare providers at all the four hospitals using the 'Breastfeeding Promotion Network of India' curriculum. The hospitals were then randomized to intervention (cell phone counselling + Baby Friendly Hospital Initiative re-training) and control (Baby Friendly Hospital Initiative re-training only) by the toss of a fair coin.

Description of the intervention

Cell phone counselling was provided by certified lactation counsellors once a week, starting in the third trimester of pregnancy until a week after the infant was 6 months old. These counsellors were auxiliary nurse midwives with additional training for counselling over the phone. They provided advice on importance of antenatal care, iron-folic acid supplementation, maternal nutrition, appropriate infant and young child feeding practices, avoiding of pre-lacteal feeds (additional liquid supplements prior to initiation of breastfeeding), how to deal with problems regarding breastfeeding and infant immunizations. The counsellors also facilitated seeking of care at the hospitals if the mother or infant reported ill. Additionally, women received a text message daily, in the regional language to augment appropriate feeding practices. These women were also provided cell phones, seven free recharge vouchers and subsidized prepaid calling cards. Also, they could call the counsellors as and when needed, using a speed dial facility. During the study, if a mother lost her study cell phone, she was asked to use her personal or family cell phone.

The counsellors were trained to manage their counselling logs for scheduling their weekly calls and sending daily health promotional bulk text messages.

Implementation and data collection

Prior to randomization, the baseline exclusive breastfeeding rates at the participating hospitals were assessed at delivery; 6, 10, 14 weeks postpartum. The rates of exclusive breastfeeding 24 h post delivery were 71.8% in the intervention and 72.3% in the control; similarly, at 6 weeks the rates were 52.8% versus 64.3%, at 10 weeks 52% versus 65% and at 14 weeks they were

40.3% versus 57.6% respectively. Data were collected by independent, trained data collectors from the enrolled women at the study hospitals. These data collection visits coincided with the woman's antenatal care and child immunization visits. Data were collected at the following time points – registration (visit 1), a week after registration (visit 2), within 24 h of delivery (visit 3) and at 6 weeks (visit 4), 10 weeks (visit 5), 14 weeks (visit 6) post delivery of a live birth. The last two visits were at 6 months (visit 7) and a week after 6 months (visit 8). At registration information on socio-demographic details and preliminary health status were collected. At visit 2, information was collected on maternal illness, whether routine breastfeeding advice has been received and if breast examination has been done. In visit 3, data regarding mode of delivery, birth outcome, place of delivery, infant anthropometry, breastfeeding initiation, pre-lacteal feeds given along with their reasons, maternal or infant illnesses that prolonged hospitalization were obtained. In post-natal visits (4, 5, 6, 7 and 8) data were collected on breastfeeding practices, infant immunization and initiation of complementary feeding. Maternal satisfaction was noted, in both arms, by using a pictorial Likert scale. Random unannounced home visits in 5% of the intervention sample were conducted by data collectors to assess exclusive breastfeeding and inquire from family members about presence of infant formula or bottle in the household.

Cost data collection

The health care costs incurred by the healthcare provider and patients were collected using micro–costing techniques. These costs were measured at enrollment, at delivery and on any subsequent hospitalization (maternal or infant). The costs of cell phones, caller plan subscription, text messages, dialed calls and recharge were recorded. The time and salaries of lactation counsellors, costs of health facility visits and hospitalizations were noted. The variable costs, i.e., direct medical (defined as cost of service, investigations and medication), direct non-medical (defined as cost of travel, food, living outstation etc.) and indirect costs (defined as wages lost during hospital visits) of the two study arms, were measured. The protocol driven costs were excluded from cost calculations. The mean differences in costs and the predictors of total cost were analyzed. The incremental cost-effectiveness of the two study arms was assessed as the incremental total cost of intervention per percentage increase in exclusive breastfeeding.

Outcomes

The primary outcome was exclusive breastfeeding rates at delivery, and postnatal 6, 8, 10, 14 weeks, 6 months and a week after 6 months. It was assessed using the standard World Health Organization's 24-h recall questionnaire.

An infant receiving only breastmilk and no supplemental liquids or solid foods other than vitamins, minerals supplements, medicines or *Janamghuti* (herbal supplement) in last 24 h was considered to be exclusively breastfed. Other outcomes assessed were timely initiation of breastfeeding (breastfeeding the infant within an hour of birth), pre-lacteal feeds (additional liquid supplements prior to initiation of breastfeeding), neonatal outcomes, bottle feeding rates (use of bottle with nipple / teat), timely initiation of complementary foods (initiation of semi-solid foods after completion of 6 months of infant's age), infant hospitalizations (any hospitalization more than 24 h related to an illness), infant weight (unclothed weight to the nearest 10 g), maternal satisfaction and incremental cost-effectiveness.

Sample size

We anticipated a total of 1036 mothers-infant dyads (518 per group i.e. 259 per cluster) would participate in the trial, based on the cluster sample size calculation and analysis plan (PASS 2007 software) to achieve 80% power and 5% two-sided alpha to detect an absolute difference between the group proportions of 0.15 (46% exclusive breastfeeding in control group under null hypothesis and 61% under the alternative hypothesis). The test statistic used was the two-sided Z test (unpooled) and the intra cluster correlation coefficient was 0.008.

Data analysis

All the analyses were performed in STATA version 11.2, STATACorp, 4905, Lakeway drive, College Stations, Texas, United States of America. These analyses were conducted at the mother-infant dyad level, for both intervention and control arms (unclustered analyses). The primary analyses compared the prevalence of exclusive breastfeeding in children at 6 months using Pearson's chi-square tests and 95% confidence intervals for the group differences. We used generalized linear mixed models for non-continuous outcomes (logistic mixed models for binary outcomes - percentage of exclusive breastfeeding). Modelling analyses examined the primary outcome variable taking into account the repeated measurements within children (time) as random effect and all co factors as fixed effects. Variables that may have had impact on the outcome based on a review of the literature were selected as covariates and adjusted for in the models.

Cost analysis was done by calculating the mean costs of cell phone use, counselling, the facility visits and inpatient stay if any. A robust boot-strap method was used to obtain the incremental cost effectiveness ratio. A re-sampling to 100,000 observations was done. Group differences in mean cost of the study arms were assessed using Student's t-test after normalizing the data. For the incremental cost-effectiveness, the numerator was the difference in the predicted

total costs and the denominator was the difference in effects such as the number of not exclusively breastfeeding avoided i.e. number of inappropriate practices that were avoided by an incremental cost of using cell phones.

Results

We screened 2938 pregnant women from the four hospitals and a total of 1037 were enrolled, of which 518 were assigned to the control group and 519 to the intervention group (Fig. 1).

After randomization of the study sites, baseline characteristics of women enrolled in the study were compared. Rates of low BMI (mother's), Other Backward Classes (castes), age of mother (21–30 years), primigravida, decision making ability, advice received on breastfeeding at least once during antenatal period (by doctor or nurse), iron–folic acid supplementation, breast examination done by a doctor and advice from relatives were higher in control group as compared to the intervention. On the other hand, Muslim population, maternal education less than 10th grade, age of mother (< 21 years), infrequent exposure to mass media, ability to visit health facility alone, mean level of hemoglobin, mean number of antenatal visits and ownership of personal cell phones were higher in the intervention group (Table 1).

Exclusive breastfeeding

Comparable proportion of women in control and intervention were exclusively breastfeeding their infants within 24 h of delivery, with significant increase at subsequent visits in intervention. The rates of exclusive breastfeeding were sustained above 95% at all visits in the cell phone group but dropped from 81% at 6 weeks to 48.5% at 6 months in the control group. The distribution of women exclusively breastfeeding at each visit is shown in Fig. 2.

On multivariable analyses, significantly higher adjusted odds ratio was observed for exclusive breastfeeding was 6.30 (95% CI: 4.93, 8.03) in the cell phone intervention group when adjusted for the following covariates: mother's age, BMI, religion, caste, education, age at marriage, household wealth index, exposure to mass media, household decision making power, parity, obstetric complications, possessing a personal cell phone, number of antenatal clinic visits, mode of delivery, place of delivery, sex of baby and low birth weight. Thus, each woman who received the intervention was six times more likely to exclusively breastfeed her infant for six months in comparison to those women who received standard healthcare services.

Overall, there were 506 out of 1031 women (49%) (control: 350/513; 68.2% and intervention: 156/518; 30.1%) that reported some reason for not exclusively breastfeeding at any given time point, starting from 24 h after delivery till 6 months of infant age. The intervention group had the highest rates of not

Visits	4 clusters randomly assigned	

At screening → 1211 women approached in 2 Control clusters | 1727 women approached in 2 Intervention clusters

693 excluded
- 31 - not between 32 to 36 gestational period
- 501 - not willing to deliver & follow up at study site
- 28 - presence of severe anemia or lab evidence of sickle cell anemia
- 110 - presence of eclampsia/pre-eclampsia
- 18 - receiving contraindicated medicine during BF
- 5 - HIV +ve

1208 excluded
- 330 - not between 32 to 36 gestational period
- 734 - not willing to deliver & follow up at study site
- 15 - presence of severe anemia / lab evidence of sickle cell anemia
- 91 - presence of eclampsia / pre-eclampsia
- 16 - receiving contraindicated medicine during BF
- 7 - HIV +ve
- 15 - declined to participate

At third trimester (Visit 1) → 518 pregnant women enrolled | 519 pregnant women enrolled

5 Excluded
- 4 - Lost to follow up
- 1 - Child death

2 Excluded
- 1 - HIV +ve
- 1 - Lost to follow up

At third trimester (Visit 2) → 513 women were expected / 309 Interviewed / 56 delivered / 148 missed visit | 517 women were expected / 397 Interviewed / 47 delivered / 73 missed visit

1 Excluded
- 1 - Lost to follow up

Within 24 hrs. after delivery (Visit 3) → 513 mother-infant dyads interviewed / 1 - Twin delivery | 518 mother-infant dyads interviewed / 1 - Twin delivery

21 excluded
- 6 - Moved out of study area
- 10 - Lost to follow up
- 5 - Child death

15 excluded
- 2 - Moved out of study area
- 3 - Lost to follow up
- 10 - Child death

At 6th week after delivery (Visit 4) → 492 mother-infant dyads interviewed | 503 mother-infant dyads interviewed

4 excluded
- 4 - Lost to follow up

4 excluded
- 2 - Moved out of study area
- 2 - Lost to follow up

At 10th week after delivery (Visit 5) → 488 mother-infant dyads interviewed | 499 mother-infant dyads interviewed

3 excluded
- 2 - Lost to follow up
- 1 - Child death

4 excluded
- 1 - Withdrawal of consent
- 3 - Lost to follow up

At 14th week after delivery (Visit 6) → 485 mother-infant dyads interviewed | 495 mother-infant dyads interviewed

9 excluded
- 4 - Moved out of study area
- 4 - Lost to follow up
- 1 - Child death

13 excluded
- 2 - Withdrawal of consent
- 3 - Moved out of study area
- 6 - Lost to follow up
- 2 - Child death

At 6th month after delivery (Visit 7) → 476 mother-infant dyads interviewed | 482 mother-infant dyads interviewed

7 excluded
- 1 - Moved out of study area
- 6 - Lost to follow up

At one week and 6th month after delivery (Visit 8) → 476 mother-infant dyads interviewed | 475 mother-infant dyads interviewed

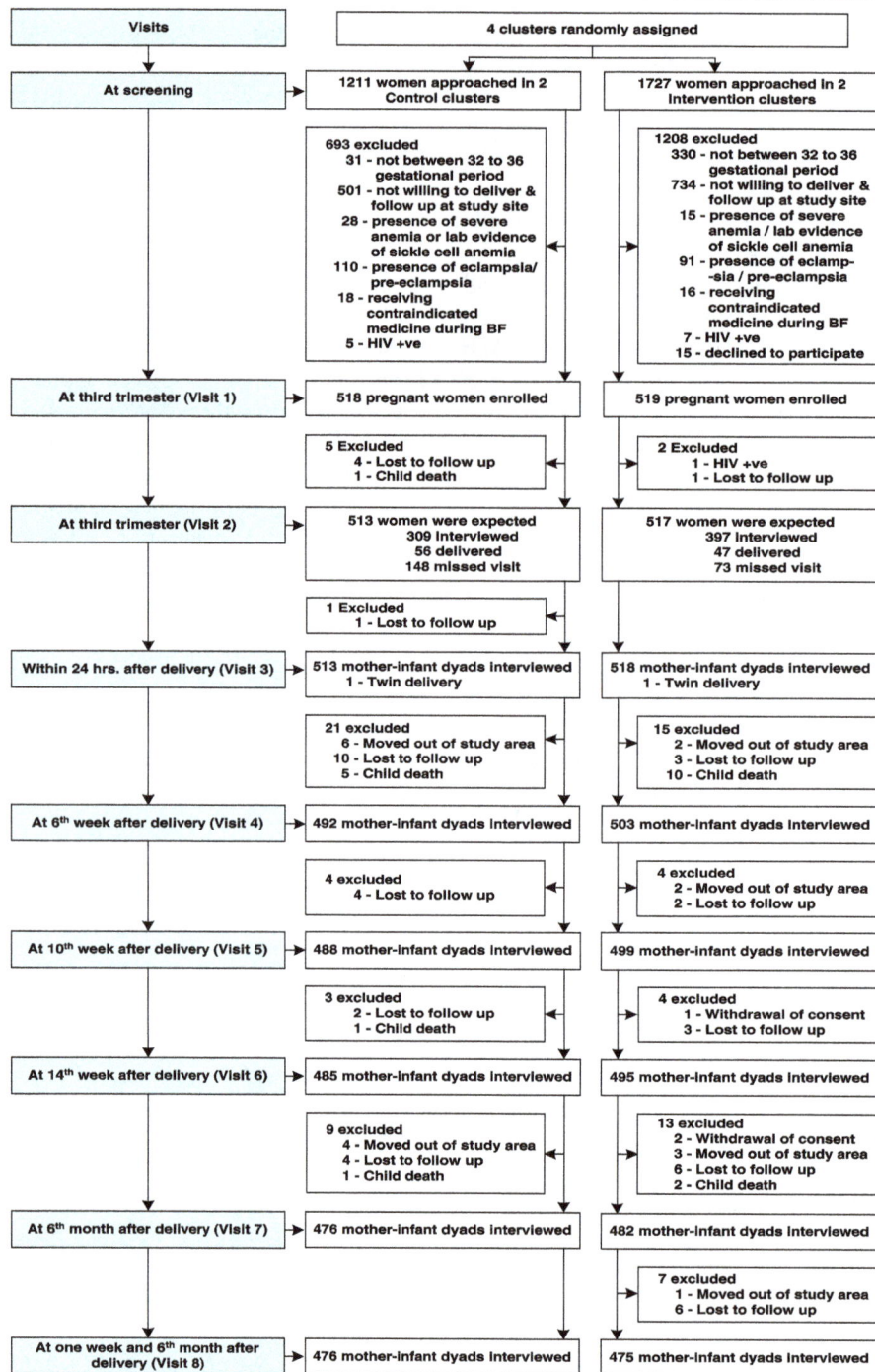

Fig. 1 Flow chart of study recruitment and attrition

exclusive breastfeeding on the first visit after delivery. The reasons were: woman's choice to substitute breastmilk in 205/1031; 19.9% (control: 194/513; 37.8% vs. intervention: 11/518; 2.1%, $p < 0.001$), perceived insufficient breastmilk secretions in 129/1031; 12.5% (control: 88/513; 17.2% vs. intervention: 41/518; 7.9%, $p < 0.001$) and prescription of infant formula by physicians in 131/1031; 12.7% (control: 85/513; 16.6% vs. intervention: 46/518; 8.9%, $p < 0.001$). Infant illness was reported in 77/1031; 7.5% (control: 45/513; 8.8% vs. intervention: 32/518; 6.2%) of cases of mothers not exclusively breastfeeding, whereas, maternal illness was reported in only 8/1031; 0.8% (control: 5/513; 1.0% vs. intervention: 3/518; 0.6%) of cases.

Table 1 Baseline characteristics of intervention and control arms post randomization

Maternal characteristics	Control (N = 518)		Intervention (N = 519)	
	N	%	n	%
Mothers age (y)	518		518	
<=24	285	55.1	264	50.9
25–30	201	38.7	213	41.0
>=31	32	6.2	41	7.9
Mother's BMI (kg/m^2)	518		518	
≤ 18.5	48	9.3	26	5.0
> 18.5	470	90.8	492	95.0
Religion	518		519	
Hindu	367	70.9	331	63.8
Muslim	68	13.1	156	30.1
Christian	4	0.8	1	0.2
Sikh	1	0.2	0	0.0
Buddhist	77	14.8	31	6.0
Others	1	0.2	0	0
Caste	518		519	
Other backward classes(OBC)	199	38.3	206	39.7
Scheduled castes(SC)	106	20.4	67	12.9
Scheduled tribes(ST)	100	19.3	52	10.0
Others	114	22	194	37.4
Mother can read	518		519	
Yes	514	99.0	493	95.0
Mother can write	518		519	
Yes	513	98.8	499	96.2
Maternal education (y)	518		519	
< 10	86	16.6	127	24.5
10–12	277	53.4	239	46.1
> 12	156	30.1	153	29.5
Age at marriage (y)	518		517	
< 21	210	40.5	235	45.5
21–30	305	59.0	280	54.2
> 30	3	0.6	2	0.4
Working hours per day (Mean ± SD)	10	6.6 ± 3.5	22	4.4 ± 2.1
Household Wealth index	517		518	
Poorest	95	18.4	112	21.6
Poorer	116	22.4	94	18.2
Middle	136	26.3	127	24.5
Richer	85	16.4	75	14.5
Richest	85	16.4	110	21.2
Exposure to mass media	518		519	
Not at all/At least once a week	47	9.1	84	16.2
Almost everyday	471	90.9	435	83.8

Table 1 Baseline characteristics of intervention and control arms post randomization (Continued)

Maternal characteristics	Control (N = 518)		Intervention (N = 519)	
	N	%	n	%
Number of decisions participant make	518		519	
0	107	20.6	156	30.1
1–2	170	32.8	153	29.5
3–4	57	11.0	35	6.7
5–7	184	35.7	175	33.7
Allowed to visit market places	513		518	
Alone	12	2.3	35	6.8
With someone else/Not at all	501	97.7	483	93.2
Allowed to visit health facility	513		518	
Alone	10	2.0	36	7.0
With someone else/Not at all	503	98.1	482	93.1
Allowed to go outside the village / community	513		518	
Alone	6	1.2	16	3.1
With someone else/Not at all	507	98.9	502	96.9
Is she a primi gravida?	513		517	
Yes	287	56.0	256	49.5
Period of gestation (weeks) according to LMP (Mean ± SD)	510	33.8 ± 1.4	495	33.9 ± 1.3
Number of ANC visits attended (Mean ± SD)	516	6.1 ± 2.3	519	7.9 ± 3.6
She takes iron and folic acid supplementation	513		518	
Yes	461	89.9	432	83.4
She takes calcium supplementation	513		518	
Yes	428	83.4	431	83.2
Number of the tetanus immunization doses received (Mean ± SD)	514	2 ± 0.1	515	2 ± 0.2
Received advice on breastfeeding at least once during antenatal period	518		517	
Yes	125	24.1	51	9.9
Received the advice on breastfeeding from Doctor	518		517	
Yes	76	14.6	17	3.3
Received the advice on breastfeeding from Nurse	518		517	
Yes	36	6.9	4	0.8
Received the advice on breastfeeding from Social worker	518		517	
Yes	7	1.4	6	1.2
Received the advice on breastfeeding from Relative	518		517	
Yes	42	8.1	22	4.3
Breast examination done by Doctor /Nurse	518		517	
Yes	24	4.6	9	1.7

Table 1 Baseline characteristics of intervention and control arms post randomization (Continued)

Maternal characteristics	Control (N = 518)		Intervention (N = 519)	
	N	%	n	%
Breast problem on examination	518		516	
a) Flat nipple	1	0.2	1	0.2
b) Inverted Nipple	1	0.2	0	0.0
She breastfed her previous children	220		266	
Yes	180	81.8	218	82.0
Any obstetrics complication	518		515	
Yes	5	1.0	10	1.9
Any infections during pregnancy	518		515	
Yes	5	1.0	5	1.0
Any systemic illness[a]	517		515	
Yes	0	0.0	3	0.6
Hemoglobin level (g/dL)	518	9.9 ± 0.6	517	10.6 ± 0.9
Cell Phone Information				
Family have a phone	518		517	
Yes	503	96.9	505	97.7
Family have a Landline phone	513		515	
Yes	28	5.5	29	5.6
She is having cell phone for personal use	518		517	
Yes	215	41.4	243	47.0

[a]Any systemic illness was defined as any health related status or condition that was previously diagnosed by the physician and documented evidence for the same was present with the participant such as heart condition (congenital heart disease, rheumatic heart disease, Ischemic heart disease etc.), blood pressure, diabetes mellitus, UTI etc.)

Timely initiation of breastfeeding, pre-lacteal feeds and neonatal outcomes

Rates of initiation of breastfeeding within an hour of birth were significantly higher in the intervention compared to the control (36.9% v/s 23.6% $p < 0.001$). Reasons reported by the women for delayed initiation of breastfeeding were: caesarean section (419/1031; 40.6%); delayed mother-baby contact due to late shifting of the baby with the mother (294/1031; 28.5%); infant illness (86/1031; 8.3%); infant had poor suck (30/1031; 2.9%); perceived insufficient breastmilk secretions (26/1031; 2.5%); breast related problems (6/1031; 0.6%); choice of the woman to substitute breastmilk (5/1031; 0.5%) and maternal illness (1/1031; 0.1%). The rates of pre-lacteal feeds were similar in both groups (intervention: 19%, control: 18%). A comparison of mother and newborn characteristics at birth between control and intervention is explained in Table 2.

Bottle feeding

The bottle feeding rates were negligible in the intervention group in the first 6 months whereas a steady increase, from 5.7% at 6 weeks to 18.3% at 6 months, was observed in the control cluster (Fig. 3).

Timely introduction of complementary foods

Inappropriate introduction of complementary foods was observed in 26.9% in the control and only 0.4% in the intervention. In the intervention, nearly all the infants were introduced complementary foods appropriately (after completing 6 months) (99.6%).

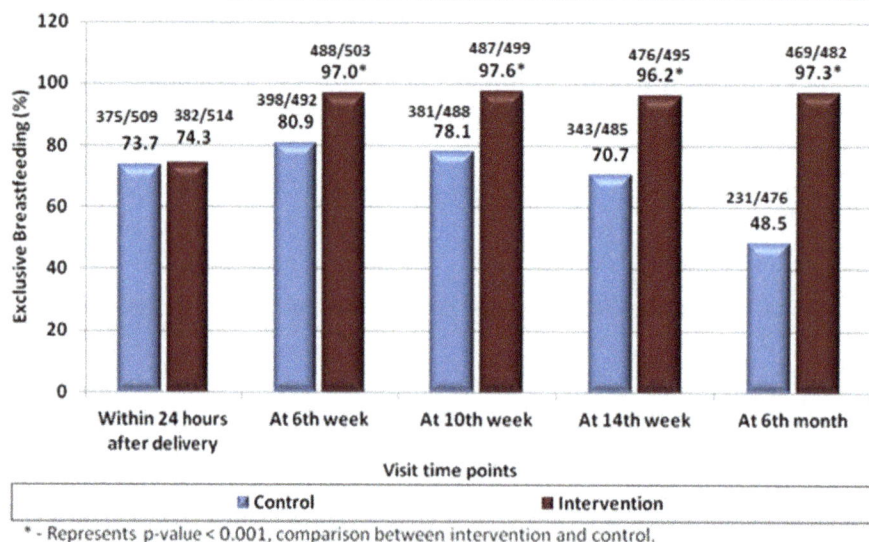

Fig. 2 Rates of exclusive breastfeeding intervention v/s control

Table 2 Comparison of maternal and newborn characteristics within 24 h of delivery

Child characteristics	Control (N = 513)		Intervention (N = 518)	
	N	%	N	%
Mode of Delivery	513		518	
Normal	280	54.6	311	60.0
Lower Segment Caesarean Section	230	44.8	202	39.0
Forceps/Assisted delivery	3	0.6	5	1.0
Place of Delivery	513		517	
Hospital	506	98.6	512	98.8
Home	5	1.0	5	1.0
Other	2	0.4	0	0.0
Status of Mother within 24 h	500		515	
Alive and well	499	99.8	514	99.8
Alive and sick	1	0.2	1	0.2
Maternal death	0	0.0	0	0.0
Present pregnancy outcome	513		518	
Single	511	99.6	516	99.6
Twin	2	0.4	2	0.4
Triplets or more	0	0.0	0	0.0
Birth Outcome	512		518	
Live birth	510	99.4	514	99.2
Fresh Still birth	1	0.2	2	0.4
Macerated SB	1	0.2	2	0.4
Sex of the baby	511		517	
Male	256	49.9	268	51.7
Status of baby within 24 h	511		516	
Alive and well	454	89.2	496	96.1
Alive and sick	53	10.4	16	3.1
Neonatal death	2	0.4	3	0.6
Low birth weight	503		517	
Yes	106	21.1	102	19.7
Gestational age	504	39.3 ± 1.3	493	39.4 ± 1.8
Baby cried immediately after birth	511		515	
Yes	476	93.1	503	97.7
Was resuscitation of new born required	505		513	
Not required	469	92.9	503	98.1
With bag & mask	25	5.0	3	0.6
Intubation required	2	0.4	2	0.4
Not Known	9	1.8	5	1.0

Infant hospitalization

The rates of infant hospitalization (neonatal intensive care unit admissions) were significantly lower in the intervention at visit 3 (12.5% v/s 6.8% $p < 0.01$). These rates were similar between both groups from visit 4 (6 weeks postnatal) till the last visit, with an exception of visit 7 where rates of hospitalization were greater in the intervention. (visit 4: 4.27% vs 5.77%, $p = 0.28$; visit 5: 1.02% vs 0.8%, $p = 0.72$; visit 6: 1.03% vs 1.62%, $p = 0.42$; visit 7: 1.26% vs 3.11%, $p = 0.05$; visit 8: 0.21% vs 0.84%, $p = 0.18$ in control vs intervention, respectively).

Infant weight

The mean weight of babies at delivery was similar in both groups, but infants in the intervention group weighed significantly more than those in the control group at each subsequent visit (control vs intervention: visit 3, at birth: 2726 g vs 2730 g, $p = 0.87$; visit 4, at 6 weeks: 4085 g vs 4296 g, $p < 0.001$; visit 5, at 10 weeks: 4941 g vs 5204 g, $p < 0.001$; visit 6, at 14 weeks: 5710 g vs 5893 g, $p < 0.001$; visit 7, 6 months: 7183 g vs 7396 g, $p = 0.026$; visit 8, 6mo + 1 week: 7183 g vs 7396 g, $p = 0.02$).

Maternal satisfaction with breastfeeding counselling

In the intervention, 92.3% of the women were completely satisfied with breastfeeding counselling provided by the lactation counsellors over cell phones. It was reported by 93% women from the intervention that the information received by them was helpful. In the control, only 36% of women were completely satisfied with the breastfeeding counselling provided by the health care provider and 31% felt that all the information they received regarding breast-feeding was helpful.

Costs effectiveness

The average total cost incurred by all the subjects in the study from third trimester to 1 week and 6 months after delivery was Rs.4687.

The point estimate of incremental cost-effectiveness ratio showed that it was costlier [5603; 95%CI (5587, 5619)] to receive cell phone counselling (Table 3). The bootstrap estimate of the total mean cost of intervention group i.e. of cell phone counselling group [Rs. 6077; 95% CI (6074, 6080) versus Rs.3282; 95%CI (3279, 3284)] was more and the effect size i.e. proportion of exclusive breastfeeding at 6th month after delivery was significantly larger [0.95; 95%CI (0.95, 0.95) versus 0.42; 95%CI (0.42, 0.42)].

Discussion

This is the first trial using cell phones for breastfeeding counselling in India. We found that our cell phone intervention resulted in substantially higher rates of exclusive breastfeeding from the infant's birth till 6 months of age. There were significant improvements in rates of initiation of breastfeeding as well as complementary feeding. Significant reductions in bottle feeding rates, from birth till a week after 6 months of age were also observed. Rates of pre-lacteal feeding were similar amongst both

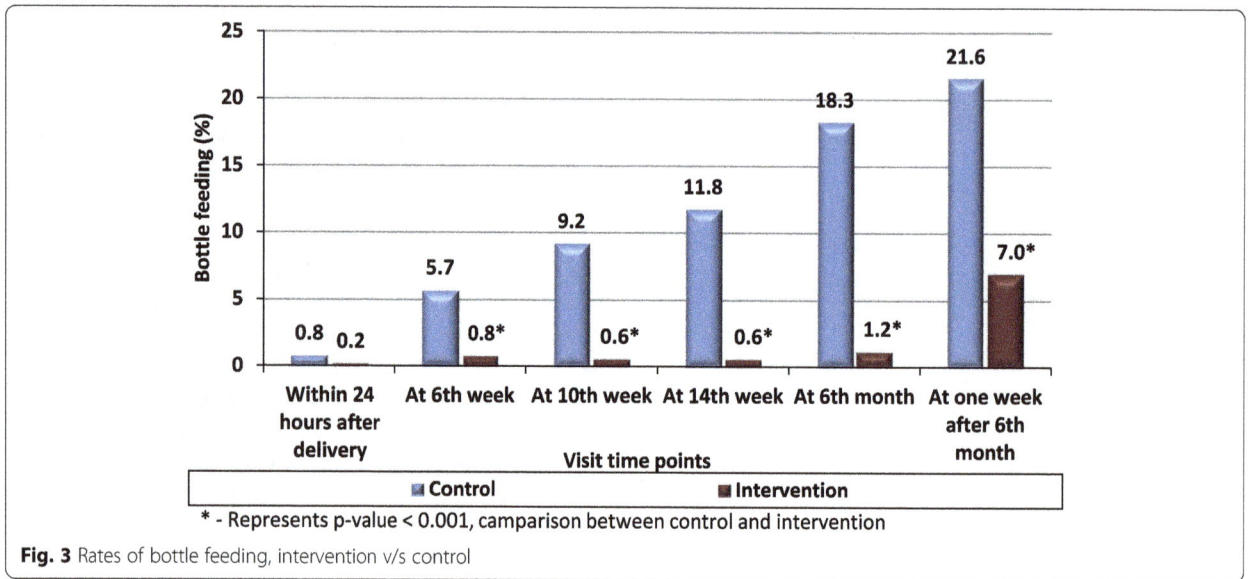

Fig. 3 Rates of bottle feeding, intervention v/s control

the groups. The intervention was also associated with lower rates of infant hospitalization within 24 h of delivery, increased maternal satisfaction and resulted in significantly better infant weight at all visits after birth.

The National Family Health Survey III (2005–2006) reported that 23.4% newborns had timely initiated breastfeeding (soon after birth) and only 50% of the infants (between 0 to 5 months) were exclusively breastfed [15]. Our study showed higher rates of exclusive breastfeeding at all the post-natal visits until 6 months in intervention and control arms. Exclusive breastfeeding rates in the intervention were remarkably high, over 95% in all the visits, as compared to the control in which only 48.5% of infants were exclusively breastfed. A recent systematic review concluded that, any pre and postnatal breastfeeding promotion strategy, increased exclusive breastfeeding rates by nearly 6 folds as compared to no intervention being provided [16]. Our intervention had a retention rate higher than that reported by a Cochrane review, where 50.9% of those receiving the intervention had stopped any breastfeeding by 6 months as opposed to 55.5% in the control (unweighted percentage) [17].

The remarkable improvement in exclusive breastfeeding rates observed during this study can be attributed to the frequency of support provided to the lactating mothers by daily text messages and weekly counselling calls made by the counsellors. The intervention may have also affected exclusive breastfeeding rates through other causal pathways. Prompt support received from the lactation counsellors, prevents the women from accepting incorrect advice given by their family members or friends. Also, during any illnesses, timely advice provided by the counsellors could limit further deterioration of their health which may otherwise impede breastfeeding. The frequent reinforcement of standard feeding recommendations by the lactation counsellors sustains, enables, and improves exclusive breastfeeding.

The control group too showed rates of exclusive breastfeeding higher than the national estimates. This increase can be attributed to the baby friendly hospital initiative retraining conducted for health providers at both control and intervention hospitals. Reasons observed for not adhering to exclusive breastfeeding (in both arms) were woman's choice to supplement breast milk with other feeds; perceived insufficiency of breastmilk secretions and lastly prescription of infant formula by doctors. These reasons are amenable to frequent counselling and could be adequately addressed by the lactation counsellors resulting in excellent rates of exclusive breastfeeding in the intervention. Despite presence of the Infant Milk Substitute Act,

Table 3 Summary results of 100,000 bootstrap re-sampled observations of cost and effects

Variable	Mean	Std. Err.	[95% Conf. Interval]
Cost in Control group	3281.69	1.15	(3279.43, 3283.94)
Cost in Intervention group	6077.17	1.60	(6074.03, 6080.29)
Proportion of exclusive breastfeeding in Control	0.42	0.00	(0.42, 0.42)
Proportion of exclusive breastfeeding in Intervention	0.95	0.00	(0.95, 0.95)
ICER	5603.36	8.20	(5587.29, 5619.43)

rates of prescribing infant formula by a health practitioner continued to be higher in the control as compared to the intervention. This change may be attributed to the increased awareness of the women towards harmful effects of these supplements, as a result of frequent counselling.

High rates of exclusive breastfeeding noted in our study could also be a result of the Hawthorne effect. An attempt was made to mitigate this by conducting unannounced home visits in a sub-sample of mothers of the intervention arm. However, none of the home visits revealed that women practiced a behavior contrary to what they reported. The Hawthorne effect cannot be completely eliminated as these home visits were conducted in a sub sample.

The rates of timely initiation of breastfeeding were significantly higher in the intervention at 37% as compared to 24% in the control. Despite pre-natal counselling, the rates were much below the desired target of Millennium Development Goal of 50% [18]. These rates are dependent on behavior of hospital staff and less reliant on what the mother may desire as a result of her counselling. Therefore, prenatal cell phone counselling failed to have a desired impact. A major reason for the low rates of initiation was delayed shifting of the baby to the mother (28.5%) causing lower rates of skin to skin contact and noncompliance of essential newborn care recommendations [19]. This delayed shifting predominantly occurred in women who were delivered by caesarean section (40.6%), a known deterrent to timely initiation of breastfeeding [10, 20].

Cell phone counselling did not have an impact on reducing pre-lacteal feeds as changing family traditional practices over a short period of counselling, mostly directed at the mother, may not be sufficient [21].

The bottle-feeding rates were higher in the control with women starting to bottle feed their babies as soon as 6 weeks after birth. This occurrence was consistent with reports from other studies that have shown women with inadequate postnatal breastfeeding support, have a decline in exclusive breastfeeding rates and are at an increased risk of bottle feeding at about 6 weeks [22]. Face to face or cell phone counselling has shown to reduce bottle feeding rates and effectively increase duration of breastfeeding [16]. This study also showed that mothers appropriately started semi-solid foods after 6 months as a result of weekly cell phone counselling and daily text messages. Mothers from the control arm had inappropriately initiated complementary foods i.e. before 6 months further lowering exclusive breastfeeding rates to 46%. Similar studies have reported that sustained encouragement, confidence building and reassurance of mothers regarding the adequacy of their milk, both in terms of nutrition and quantity, has restricted the use of any other form of feeding beside breastfeeding till 6 months of infant age [23]. A women's confidence in the adequacy of their feeds tends to erode in absence

of sustained counselling and support, resulting in additional feeding earlier than 6 months due to family and peer pressure [24].

Over 93% of the women were satisfied with the weekly cell phone counselling they received, translating into high adherence to exclusive breastfeeding. Nutritional sufficiency of exclusive breastfeeding along with appropriate initiation of complementary feeding were also evident as weight gain of infants in the intervention was significantly better as compared to control. Similar results were reported by Thakur in Bangladesh in low birth weight babies [25, 26].

Lower rates of hospitalization into the neonatal intensive care unit (NICU) within the first 24 h of delivery in the intervention group may have resulted due to timely telephonic consultations received just around delivery. Women perhaps reported promptly to the hospitals, which may have resulted in better intra-partum care and fewer rates of neonatal resuscitation. This shows that cell phone counselling had a favorable impact on the health care seeking behavior at the time of delivery. Subsequently, the rates of infant hospitalization were similar in both groups.

The cost effectiveness analysis showed that, for a cost of Rs.5603 (approximately, 127 dollars) a 50% improvement in exclusive breastfeeding (at 6 months) can be achieved. The cost in terms of 'years of life saved', as a result of improvement of exclusive breastfeeding, estimated using the Markov model, was not within the scope of this study. This intervention, though being marginally costlier, has twice the potential to improve exclusive breastfeeding as compared to the existing healthcare services. It was found cost effective when compared with the World Health Organization's CHOICE (CHOosing interventions that are Cost Effective) thresholds for low income countries [27]. For India the cost effectiveness threshold is equivalent to 1345 dollars that is the gross domestic product, per capita in year 2010 [28]. In comparison to this, our intervention costs below 130 dollars per mother–infant dyad.

This is one of the first trials where cell phones were used for lactation counselling to improve optimal feeding practices soon after birth. The impact of intervention on exclusive breastfeeding was adjusted for the differences in baseline characteristics. Therefore, the large and significantly beneficial impact of cell phone counselling, on breastfeeding indicators was not likely by chance. This was a pragmatic effectiveness trial that leveraged on the services of existing hospital staff therefore has potential to scale up in low resource setting. The cost-effectiveness assessment helped to inform investments needed for promotion of infant and young child feeding at these health facilities.

The limitation of the study was that it was an unblinded pilot study of only four clusters. This can potentially bias the results due to imbalances in baseline characteristics that may impact exclusive breastfeeding. However, the intervention arm had lower baseline rates of exclusive breastfeeding and other characteristics that may positively influence rates of exclusive breastfeeding. We adjusted for these imbalances by using generalized linear mixed model. We acknowledge that there were other unobserved differences between the hospitals and so residual confounding may remain.

Another limiting factor was that the intervention was not designed to assess the effectiveness of different frequencies of contact with the women, on exclusive breastfeeding. Ascertaining optimal frequency of contact needed to observe a similar improvement in exclusive breastfeeding rates was beyond the scope of this study. However, it has been noted that, if a woman is not provided prompt assistance, within few days, she is likely to adopt alternative inappropriate feeding practices. Other implementation challenges such as switched off phones, discharged phones, rejected calls or unanswered calls, calls received by someone other than the enrolled women and loss of cell phones were also encountered during the study.

Conclusions

In conclusion, we found lactation counselling using cell phones proved to be a very useful tool for frequent and sustained support to pregnant and lactating mothers. It alleviates the need for hospital visits and face to face counselling. This intervention can be successfully implemented in low resource settings by training nurse midwives who can potentially communicate with large number of beneficiaries. This health care delivery system is now particularly relevant as the use of cell phones in Indian households is nearly universal. It needs further evaluation prior to scale up and incorporation into the public as well as private health systems.

Abbreviations
ANC: Antenatal Care; BMI: Body Mass Index; DALYs: Disability Adjusted Life Years; Hb: Hemoglobin; HIV: Human Immunodeficiency Virus; ICER: Incremental cost effectiveness ratio

Acknowledgements
This study (Trial registration number: CTRI/2011/06/001822, available on: http://www.ctri.nic.in/Clinicaltrials/pmaindet2.php?trialid=3060) was funded by the World Bank- SARDM (South Asia Region Development Marketplace) and the Alive and Thrive initiative by The Bill and Melinda Gates Foundation. We would like to acknowledge the timely support provided by the funding organizations during the implementation and dissemination of the study results. The authors would like to acknowledge the efforts of Dr. Yamini Pusdekar in providing constructive inputs for editing this manuscript and Mr. Amber Abhijeet Prakash for conducting additional end-line analyses. We would also like to appreciate the hard work by Ms. Smita Puppalwar for management and co-ordination of the research activity. We would like to thank the participating hospitals for extending timely cooperation: Indira Gandhi Government Medical College, Nagpur; Matru Sewa Sangh Hospital – Buldi and Mahal; Daga Memorial Hospital, Nagpur. We are also thankful to all mother – infant dyads and their families that were a part of this study.

Funding
This trial was initially funded by World Bank- SARDM (South Asia Region Development Marketplace Grant ID - 806410) and subsequently by Alive and Thrive initiative, *The Bill and Melinda Gates Foundation* (Grant ID – 09-000076-AT10-4LMR).

Authors' contributions
AP designed and conceptualized the intervention. AP, LD, PK and SK designed the study tools and training material. AP, PK, SK, AP were involved in data collection, analysis and drafted the manuscript. JB was responsible for formal data analysis. All authors critically reviewed the manuscript before submission and approved the final manuscript. All authors accept the final responsibility for the paper.

Competing interests
The authors declare that they have no competing interests.

Author details
[1]Department of Pediatrics, Indira Gandhi Government Medical College, Nagpur, Maharashtra 440018, India. [2]Lata Medical Research Foundation, Nagpur, Maharashtra 440022, India.

References
1. Black RE, et al. Maternal and child undernutrition and overweight in low-income and middle-income countries. Lancet. 2013;382:427–51.
2. Lim SS, Vos T, Flaxman AD, et al. A comparative risk assessment of burden of disease and injury attributable to 67 risk factors and risk factor clusters in 21 regions, 1990–2010: a systematic analysis for the global burden of disease study 2010. Lancet. 2012;380(9859):2224–60. https://doi.org/10.1016/S0140-6736(12)61766-8.
3. Edmond KM, Zandoh C, Quigley MA, et al. Delayed breastfeeding initiation increases risk of neonatal mortality. Pediatrics. 2006;17:e380–e38. https://doi.org/10.1542/peds.2005-1496.
4. Smith ER, Hurt L, Chowdhary R, et al. Delayed breastfeeding initiation and infant survival: a systematic review and meta-analysis. Plos. 2016. https://doi.org/10.1371/journal.pone.0180722.
5. Horta BL, Bahl R, Martines JC, Victora CG, editors. Evidence on the long-term effects of breastfeeding: systematic reviews and meta-analysis. Geneva: World Health Organization; 2007.
6. Caulfield LE, de Onis M, Blossner M, Black RE. Undernutrition as an underlying cause of child deaths associated with diarrhea, pneumonia, malaria, and measles. Am J Clin Nutr. 2004;80:193–8.
7. WHO. The optimal duration of exclusive breastfeeding: a systematic review. WHO/FCH/01.23. Geneva: WHO; 2002. Ref Type: Report
8. Bhutta ZA, Ahmed T, Black RE, Cousens S, Dewey K, et al. What works? Interventions for maternal and child undernutrition and survival. Lancet. 2008;371:417–40.
9. Dewey KG, Brown KH. Update on technical issues concerning complementary feeding of young children in developing countries and implications for intervention programs. [erratum appears in Food Nutr Bull. 2003 Jun;24(2):239]. Food & Nutrition Bulletin. 2003;24:5–28.
10. Patel A, Badhoniya N, Khadse S, Senarath U, Agho KE, Dibley MJ. Infant and young child feeding indicators and determinants of poor feeding practices in India: secondary data analysis of National Family Health Survey 2005–06. Food Nutr Bull. 2010;31(2):314–33.
11. International Institute for Population Sciences (IIPS) and Macro International. 2007. National Family Health Survey (NFHS-3), 2005–06: India: Volume I, Mumbai: IIPS.
12. Sudfeld CR, Fawzi WW, Lahariya C. Peer support and exclusive breastfeeding duration in low and middle income countries – a systematic review and Meta – analysis. PLoS One. 2012. https://doi.org/10.1371/journal.pone.0045143.
13. Joo N-S, Kim B-T. Mobile phone short message service messaging for behavior modification in a community based weight control programme in Korea. J Telemed Telecare. 2007;13(8):416–20.
14. Wei J, Hollin I, Kachnowski S. A review of the use of mobile phone text messaging in clinical and healthy behavior interventions. J Telemed Telecare. 2011;17(1):41 8.

15. Arnold F, Parasuraman S, Arokiasamy P, Kothari M. Nutrition in India. National Family Health Survey (NFHS-3), India, 2005 - 06. Mumbai; Calverton: International Institute for Population Sciences; ICF Macro; 2009.

16. Imdad A, Yakoob MY, Bhutta ZA. Effect of breastfeeding promotion interventions on breastfeeding rates, with special focus on developing countries. BMC Public Health. 2011. https://doi.org/10.1186/1471-2458-11-S3-S24.

17. Renfrew MJ, Mc Cormick FM, Wade A, Quinn B, Dowswell T. Support for healthy breastfeeding mothers with healthy term babies. Cochrane Database Syst Rev. 2012. https://doi.org/10.1002/14651858.CD001141.pub4.

18. World Health Organization, UNICEF.Global Nutrition Targets 2025: Breastfeeding policy brief. 2014, WHO/NMH/NHD/147.

19. Global strategy for infant and young child feeding. Geneva: World Health Organization. 2003; http://apps.who.int/iris/bitstream/10665/42590/1/9241562218.pdf. Accessed 27 Jan 2018.

20. Patel A, Bucher S, Pusdekar Y, et al. Rates and determinants of early initiation of breastfeeding and exclusive breast feeding at 42 days postnatal in six low and middle-income countries: a prospective cohort study. Reprod Health. 2015. https://doi.org/10.1186/1742-4755-12-S2-S10.

21. McKenna KM, Shankar RT. The practice of Prelacteal feeding to newborns among Hindu and Muslim families. J Midwifery Womens Health. 2009. https://doi.org/10.1016/j.jmwh.2008.07.012.

22. Gangal P. Breast crawl, initiation of breastfeeding by breast crawl, UNICEF Maharashtra, Mother Support and Training Coordinator, BPNI. 2007; Published by: unicef.org/india, http://www.breastcrawl.org/pdf/breastcrawl.pdf. Assessed 27 Jan 2018.

23. Kushwaha KP, Sankar J, Sankar MJ, et al. Effect of peer counselling by mother support groups on infant and young child feeding practices: the Lalitpur experience. PLoS One. 2014. https://doi.org/10.1371/journal.pone.0109181.

24. Haider R, Saha KK. Breastfeeding and infant growth outcomes in the context of intensive peer counselling support in two communities in Bangladesh. Int Breastfeed J. 2016. https://doi.org/10.1186/s13006-016-0077-6.

25. Thakur SK, Roy SK, Paul K, and Ferdous S. Effect of counselling on appropriate exclusive breastfeeding on weight gain of low-birth weight babies. Poster presentation. 12th ASCON 2009. Published by ICDDRB.

26. Piwoz EG, Huffman SL, Quinn VJ. Promotion and advocacy for improved complementary feeding: can we apply the lessons learned from breastfeeding? Food Nutr Bull. 2003. https://doi.org/10.1177/156482650302400103.

27. Woods B, Revill P, Sculpher M, Claxton K. Country-Level Cost-Effectiveness Threshholds: Initial Estimates and the Need for Further Research. Value in Health. 2016. https://doi.org/10.1016/j.jval.2016.02.017

28. World Integrated Trade Solution (WITS), World Bank Group India GDP per capita constant. 2010 US$, 2005–2010. Available at: https://wits.worldbank.org/CountryProfile/en/Country/IND/StartYear/2005/EndYear/2010/I ndicator/NY-GDP-PCAP-KD. Accessed 18 May 2018.

22

Predictors of breastfeeding duration in a predominantly Māori population in New Zealand

Kathy M. Manhire[1,2*], Sheila M. Williams[3], David Tipene-Leach[1,2], Sally A. Baddock[4], Sally Abel[5], Angeline Tangiora[1], Raymond Jones[1] and Barry J. Taylor[1]

Abstract

Background: Although breastfeeding duration in New Zealand's indigenous Māori is shorter than in non-Māori, we know little about barriers or motivators of breastfeeding in this community. The aim of this analysis was to identify predictors for extended duration of breastfeeding amongst participants drawn from predominantly Māori communities in regional Hawke's Bay.

Methods: Mother/baby dyads were recruited from two midwifery practices serving predominantly Māori women in mostly deprived areas, for a randomised controlled trial comparing the risks and benefits of an indigenous sleeping device (*wahakura*) and a bassinet. Questionnaires were administered at baseline (pregnancy) and at one, three and six months postnatal. Several questions relating to breastfeeding and factors associated with breastfeeding were included. The data from both groups were pooled to examine predictors of breastfeeding duration.

Results: Māori comprised 70.5% of the 197 participants recruited. The median time infants were fully breastfed was eight weeks and Māori women were more likely to breastfeed for a shorter duration than New Zealand European women with an odds-ratio (OR) of 0.45 (95% CI 0.24, 0.85). The key predictors for extended duration of breastfeeding were the strong support of the mother's partner (OR = 3.64, 95% CI 1.76, 7.55) or her mother for breastfeeding (OR = 2.47, 95% CI 1.27, 4.82), longer intended duration of maternal breastfeeding (OR = 1.02, 95% CI 1.00, 1.03) and being an older mother (OR = 1.07, 95% CI 1.02, 1.12). The key predictors for shorter duration of breastfeeding were pacifier use (OR = 0.28, 95% CI 0.17, 0.46), daily cigarette smoking (OR = 0.51, 95% CI 0.37, 0.69), alcohol use (OR = 0.54, 95% CI 0.31, 0.93) and living in a more deprived area (OR 0.40, 95% CI 0.22, 0.72).

Conclusions: Breastfeeding duration in this group of mainly Māori women was shorter than the national average. Increasing the duration of breastfeeding by these mothers could be further facilitated by ante and postnatal education involving their own mothers and their partners in the support of breastfeeding and by addressing pacifier use, smoking and alcohol use.

Keywords: Infant nutrition, Lactation, Maternal knowledge, Pacifier

* Correspondence: kmanhire@eit.ac.nz
[1]Department of Women's and Children's Health, Dunedin School of Medicine, University of Otago, Dunedin, New Zealand
[2]Faculty of Education, Humanities and Health Sciences, Eastern Institute of Technology, Hawke's Bay, New Zealand
Full list of author information is available at the end of the article

Background

Breastfeeding, including the consumption of expressed breast milk, is the normative standard for infant feeding and nutrition [1] and is significant in the prevention of disease in later life [2, 3] particularly where breastfeeding is exclusive and lasts for at least six months [4]. In New Zealand, Māori women generally live in more deprived and low income circumstances and have a shorter duration of breastfeeding than non-Māori and reducing this disparity among the indigenous population is a major focus for the New Zealand Ministry of Health [5]. Therefore, understanding the barriers and motivators to extended breastfeeding among Māori is important.

A range of demographic factors are known to affect breastfeeding duration. These include maternal age [6], socioeconomic status [7], ethnicity [8] and cultural group or indigeneity [9]. Factors known to extend breastfeeding include maternal breastfeeding knowledge and beliefs [10, 11], maternal intention to breastfeed [12] and family support for breastfeeding behaviour [7]. On the other hand, those associated with a shorter duration of breastfeeding include factors, such as maternal smoking [13, 14], maternal alcohol use [15] and maternal depression [16, 17], and the use of a pacifier [18, 19]. The effect of the early introduction of baby to solids is unclear, needing both a definition of 'early' and being clearly differentiated from introduction of formula [20, 21].

A number of qualitative studies in New Zealand have examined motivators for and barriers to extended breastfeeding duration among Māori women. One study found factors that extended breastfeeding among young Māori mothers included maternal perception of breastfeeding as natural and easy, early stage breastfeeding support, being determined to breastfeed despite adversity and informed decision-making around the use of infant formula [22]. Negative influences on breastfeeding from two larger qualitative studies with Māori mothers and whānau (extended family) included: difficulty establishing early breastfeeding, insufficient professional support, the perception of inadequate milk supply and the need to return to work [23]; the lack of culturally pertinent breastfeeding information, confusion about the impacts on the baby when smoking during breastfeeding, uncertainty about the safety of bedsharing and a perceived lack of acceptability of breastfeeding in public [24]. Some commentators have argued that the breakdown in whānau breastfeeding norms and low Māori breastfeeding rates are attributable to the impacts of colonization, including the influence of mid twentieth century infant welfare programmes encouraging the use of infant formula [25].

This paper adds to these qualitative findings by reporting on results from a recent quantitative study which enables us to identify and quantify predictors for extended breastfeeding in a sample of predominantly Māori women from more deprived communities in New Zealand.

Methods

Healthy mother/baby dyads from singleton pregnancies were recruited between June 2011 and April 2013 from two midwifery practices supporting predominantly Māori families in areas of Hawke's Bay, most of which had a high New Zealand deprivation index score [26]. At the prenatal visit they were entered into a two arm, randomised controlled trial comparing the risks and benefits of an indigenous infant sleep device, the *wahakura* (a 36 × 72 cm flax bassinet), and a stand-alone bassinet. A baseline survey was completed in pregnancy with further surveys at one, three and six months postnatally. The complete methodology, including recruitment strategy and sample size for breastfeeding, has been published previously [27].

Data were collected by a local Māori researcher using machine readable questionnaires (HP TeleForm ©2014 Hewlett-Packard Development Company, L.P.). The one and three month questionnaires were completed as face-to-face interviews with the babies' mothers and the six-month questionnaire was administered by telephone. Participants were given a NZ $25 voucher on completion of each of the three and six month interviews.

Self-identified ethnicity and a range of other demographic data were collected at baseline as were questions about the mother's intention to breastfeed ('do you plan to breastfeed' and 'to what age do you plan to exclusively breastfeed') and her knowledge of breastfeeding ('recommended age for exclusive breastfeeding' and 'recommended age for introduction of solids'). The survey also included a question about whether the mother herself was breastfed as a baby.

In the three postnatal surveys, questions relating to breastfeeding behaviour, including the use of expressed breast milk, were asked; ('currently breastfeeding your baby for any time' and 'currently fully breastfeeding your baby'). Supplementary questions enquired about the age at which babies 'stopped breastfeeding,' 'stopped fully breastfeeding,' 'had any milk or food that was not breast milk' and when they 'began solids'. This information allowed the breastfeeding practice to later be reclassified as: exclusive (breastmilk and prescribed medicines from birth); full (breastmilk and minimal water/water-based drinks or prescribed medicines in the last 48 h); partial (breastmilk and solid or semi-solid food which may include infant formula or non- human milk); and no breastmilk at all [28]. There were open questions about the type of food and solids given to babies. Questions relating to sleep location (shared parents' bedroom and shared mother's bed), maternal sleep quality and quantity (on a 4 point scale) [29] and a question about pacifier (dummy) use, ('Did baby use dummy in the past week?') were also asked at these times.

At both the baseline and one month surveys, participants were asked about how supportive ('strongly supportive, supportive, neutral, not supportive, not at all supportive') their partner, and also their mother would be or was of them breastfeeding their baby. At one month questions were also asked about tobacco use (tobacco smoking status and daily use) and alcohol consumption ('on the days when you drink alcohol, how many drinks do you usually have?') As we have no information about the frequency of alcohol consumption we limited the analysis to alcohol use at one month. Maternal depression (Edinburgh Postnatal Depression Scale score > 10) was asked about using the Edinburgh Postnatal Depression Scale (EPDS) [30] at baseline, and then at three and six months.

Statistical analyses

The proportional-odds cumulative logit model was used to analyze most of the data [31]. This provides an odds-ratio or, in this case, a proportional-odds (OR) which compares, in a cumulative way, people who are in groups greater than k versus those who are in groups less than or equal to k, where k is the level of the response variable. This can be interpreted as for a one unit change in the predictor variable, the odds for cases in a group that is greater than k versus less than or equal to k are the proportional-odds times larger. The data was analyzed using a Stata (Stata Statistical Software: Release 13) procedure, which provides a check of the underlying assumptions for proportional-odds models. As some variables, for instance the use of a pacifier, were collected in the same way at all three postnatal interviews, we used a logistic model which accounted for the time varying covariates [31].

Ethics approval to conduct this study was granted by the New Zealand Central Region Ethics Committee (CEN/10.12.054). All participants were provided with a written Participant Information sheet and a Consent Form to be signed.

Results

One hundred and ninety-seven mother/baby dyads were recruited out of 600 eligible mothers giving a recruitment rate of 33%. Seventy percent self-identified as Māori and two-thirds were from quintile five areas, those with highest deprivation index score [27]. The retention rate at six months was 88%.

The frequency of full, partial and no breastfeeding and the age of the infant at the time of the one, three and six month surveys, alongside information about the frequency of feeding 'foods not breast milk' and the 'introduction of solids' can be seen in Table 1. Notably, by one month over half (53.3%) were having 'food not breast milk' and some (4.9%) were having 'solids introduced'. The open questions revealed that 'food other than breast milk' was mainly some form of infant formula and the 'solids introduced' included Weetbix, Farex, baby rice or yoghurt. By three months, those foods included canned baby food, mashed vegetables, pureed fruit and custard and, in the case of one baby, strawberries dipped in chocolate. Although foods such as avocado, biscuits, and chewed sausage were given to one or two babies before six months, the majority of babies were given baby cereal, canned food or mashed fruit or vegetables.

Because the mothers were asked about the timing of stopping fully or partially breastfeeding their infants as well as the timing of the introduction of foods other than breast milk, we were able to estimate that the median time the infants were breast fed was eight weeks (IQR 3–20). As the age at assessment did not match the nominated times of one, three and six months we estimated the frequency of exclusive, fully and partial breastfeeding at four, 13 and 26 weeks. Table 1 shows that three-quarters of the sample were having some breastmilk at both the one month assessment (75.8%)

Table 1 Mean assessment age, frequency of breastfeeding/other foods and estimated breastfeeding prevalence at 4, 13 and 26 weeks

Assessment	1 month N = 182	3 month N = 183	6 month n = 173
Age at assessment (days) Mean (sd)	51 (25)	108 (29)	203 (33)
Breastfeeding	n (%)	n (%)	n (%)
Full	92 (50.5)	66 (36.0)	28 (16.2)
Partial	46 (25.3)	49 (26.8)	52 (30.1)
None	44 (24.2)	72 (39.3)	93 (53.7)
Food not breast milk introduced	97 (53.3)	114 (62.3)	154 (89.3)
Solids introduced	9 (4.9)	42 (22.9)	166 (93.4)
Reclassification of breastfeeding [a]	4 weeks	13 weeks	26 weeks
Exclusive	75 (40.1)	35 (18.7)	0
Full	31 (16.6)	28 (15.0)	29 (15.5)
Partial	33 (17.7)	44 (23.5)	53 (28.3)
None	48 (25.7)	80 (42.8)	105 (56.1)

[a]Based on information gained at the 1, 3 and 6 month interviews

and at the reclassified four weeks (74.6%). Of these, 40.1% were exclusively breastfeeding and this fell to 20% by 13 weeks and to zero by 26 weeks. Full breastfeeding fell from 56.6 to 15.5% over that time period.

For further analysis the sample was divided into four groups related to the length of time they were fully breastfed: babies who were breastfed for less than four weeks (n = 95), babies breastfed for four weeks or more but less than 13 weeks (n = 31), babies breastfed for 13 weeks or more but less than 26 weeks (n = 33) and babies still fully breastfeeding at the age of 26 weeks (n = 28). We used the proportional-odds ratio (OR) to estimate the association between these four breastfeeding groups and a number of important demographic and social characteristics of the mothers and babies. These are shown in Table 2. The proportional-odds for maternal age indicates that older mothers were more likely to breastfeed their babies for longer (OR = 1.07; 95% CI 1.02, 1.12); that mothers living in a more deprived neighbourhood were likely to breast-feed their baby for a shorter period than those living in a more advantaged neighbourhood (OR = 0.40; 95% CI 0.22, 0.72) and that non-Māori women breastfed their babies for longer than Māori (OR = 2.22; 95% CI 1.17, 4.21). Babies heavier at birth were also more likely to be breastfed for longer the odds-ratio for a 100 g difference in birthweight was OR = 1.07 (95% CI 1.01,1.13). Mothers level of education, having a partner, number of children, gender of child, mode of birth, knowledge of *iwi* (tribal) origin, and being randomized to receive a wahakura were not related to breastfeeding duration.

Table 3 shows frequencies, or in some cases the means (sd), of baseline variables for the four 'fully breastfeeding' time periods. The majority (92%) indicated they planned to 'exclusively breastfeed' and gave a planned duration of breastfeeding. Half planned to breastfeed for 24 weeks (IQR, 24–48) and the length of time they planned to breastfeed was positively associated with the duration breastfeeding (OR = 1.02, 95% CI 1.00, 1.03). The median for both questions asking about 'the recommended time for exclusive breastfeeding' of 48 weeks (IQR, 24–52) and the 'introduction of solids' of 24 weeks (IQR, 20–24), indicated that although breastfeeding knowledge was reasonable it was not predictive of breastfeeding duration.

Before the birth of the child, 92% of mothers planned to breastfeed and the odds ratio for the duration of breastfeeding was strong (OR = 15; 95% CI 2, 118) but imprecise. Having a strongly supportive partner at the baseline interview (OR = 2.42; 95% CI 1.15, 5.11) was predictive of extended duration of breastfeeding. While there was trend for a similar support of breastfeeding by the mother of the participants to be predictive, this was not statistically significant. 'Being breastfed as a baby' was not associated with breastfeeding patterns.

At one month, having a 'strongly supportive partner' (OR = 3.64; 95% CI 1.76, 7.55) and a 'strongly supportive mother' (OR = 2.37; 95% CI 1.27, 4.82) was associated with extended breastfeeding. 'Fatigue' and 'having others care for the baby' was not. Both maternal smoking and the use of alcohol were associated with shorter duration of breastfeeding and the proportional-odds for the trend across the smoking categories was significant (OR = 0.51; 95% CI 0.37, 0.69; $p < 0.001$) (Table 4).

Data collected at all three postnatal surveys divided into the four breastfeeding groups mentioned above is shown in Table 5. To demonstrate the frequency for sleep place, bed sharing, pacifier use and sleep quantity and quality we employed a statistical model which allowed for time dependent covariates. The fourth group (mothers fully breastfeeding at 26 weeks) was censored, that is, not included in the analysis. Analysis showed that use of a pacifier was strongly associated with shortened periods of breastfeeding (OR = 0.28 95% CI 0.17, 0.46). Sleep place, bedsharing, maternal sleep and 'possible depression' were not associated with breastfeeding duration.

Discussion

In this study we showed that in a predominantly Māori population drawn largely from deprived communities, the key predictors for extended duration of breastfeeding were the strong support for breastfeeding of the woman's partner and her mother at one month postnatal, an intended duration of breastfeeding and being an older mother. Interestingly, whilst antenatal breastfeeding support by the participant's mother was not predictive, support by the partner was, and although antenatal planning to breastfeed was a strong predictor, it was almost universal and therefore too imprecise to be useful. The key predictors for shorter duration of breastfeeding were pacifier use, daily cigarette smoking and increasing number of cigarettes per day, alcohol use and living in a more deprived area. Māori women were more likely to breastfeed for a shorter duration than non-Māori women.

We found the breastfeeding was extended by the strong support (for breastfeeding) of the woman's partner and her mother, a higher intended duration of breastfeeding and being an older mother. Other studies have also identified the importance of partner and mother support for the duration of breastfeeding [12, 32] and family, peer and partner support for a pregnant woman's intention to breastfeed [7]. New Zealand qualitative studies of infant feeding decisions by young Māori women indicate that, while mothers perceived breastfeeding as natural, easy, normal and healthy, it was "early stage breastfeeding support" in particular that was crucial to the development and maintenance of breastfeeding [22, 24]. We also found that breastfeeding duration increased with maternal age; in this case, year by year from 25 years to 29 years,

Table 2 Means and frequency for demographic and birth variables for four 'fully breastfeeding' groups

	Full breastfeeding stopped before 4 weeks N = 95	Full breastfeeding stopped at/after 4 weeks but before 13 weeks N = 31	Full breastfeeding stopped at/after 13 weeks but before 26 weeks N = 33	Full breastfeeding stopped at/after 26 weeks N = 28	OR (95% CI)	p
Mothers mean age (sd)	25.1 (6.05)	26.1 (6.09)	27.8 (6.43)	28.8 (6.55)	1.07 (1.02, 1.12)	0.002
Mothers education	n (%)	n (%)	n (%)	n (%)		
Completed year 11	48 (56)	16 (19)	13 (15)	9 (10)		
Completed year 13	20 (51)	5 (13)	8 (21)	6 (15)		
Some tertiary qual	27 (44)	10 (16)	12 (19)	13 (21)	1.34 (0.99, 1.82)[b]	0.060
Has partner						
No	9(9)	2 (6)	2(6)	2 (7)		
Yes	86 (91)	29 (94)	31 (94)	26 (93)	1.43 (0.50, 4.04)	0.758
Number of children						
0	23 (24)	12 (39)	9 (27)	3 (11)		
1	25 (26)	7 (23)	15 (45)	11 (39)		
2	22 (23)	5 (16)	7 (21)	8 (29)		
3 or 4	25 (26)	7 (23)	2 (6)	6 (21)	0.91 (0.74,1.14)[b]	0.415
NZDEP						
1–8	19(22)	5(16)	14(62)	14(50)		
9,10	74 (78)	26 (84)	19 (58)	14 (50)	0.40 (0.22, 0.72)	0.003
Maternal ethnicity						
Maori	73 (77)	23 (74)	18 (55)	17 (61)	1.00	
European/other	15 (16)	7 (23)	11 (33)	9 (32)	2.22 (1.17, 4.21)	0.014
Pacific Island	7 (7)	1 (3)	4 (12)	2 (7)	1.43 (0.51, 4.04)	0.501
Knows iwi (tribe)						
No	67(91)	20(92)	17 (11)	14 (18)		
Yes	7 (9)	24 (8)	2 (89)	3/ (82)	0.68 (0.24, 1.97)	0.484
Sex of infant						
Boy	46(48)	28(58)	16(48)	14(50)		
Girl	49 (52)	13 (42)	17 (52)	14 (50)	0.93 (0.54, 1.60)	0.799
Babies birth wgt (g) (mean)(sd)	3405 (445)	3843 (442)	3599 (499)	3600 (666)	1.07 (1.01, 1.13)	0.016[a]
Mode of delivery						
Normal	67 (71)	22 (71)	26 (79)	22 (79)		
Assisted	4 (4)	2 (6)	1 (3)	2 (7)	1.17 (0.34, 4.06)	0.810
Caesarean Section	24 (25)	7 (23)	6 (18)	4 (14)	0.65 (0.33, 1.27)	0.203
Randomised to wahakura						
No	48(51)	15(48)	18(55)	9(32)		
Yes	47(49)	16 (52)	15 (45)	19 (68)	1.33 (0.78, 2.28)	0.298

Proportional odds models were used to analyse the data
[a]The odds ratio is based on a difference in birthweight of 100 g
[b]The proportional odds model fitted as a trend across categories for the number of children

contrary to results of a study from the United States with deprived inner city teen mothers [33].

We note that our study participants reported a median duration of full breastfeeding of only eight weeks, with only 18.7% exclusively breastfeeding at 13 weeks. These figures are lower than those reported nationally in New Zealand and far lower than the recommended "exclusive breastfeeding until six months of age" [28]. We propose

Table 3 Means or frequency for breastfeeding planning, antenatal breastfeeding support, sleep quantity/quality for four 'fully breastfeeding' groups

	Full breastfeeding stopped before 4 weeks N = 95	Full breastfeeding stopped at/after 4 weeks but before 13 weeks N = 31	Full breastfeeding stopped at/after 13 weeks but before 26 weeks N = 33	Full breastfeeding stopped at/after 26 weeks N = 28	OR (95% CI)	p
Days before birth of child Mean (sd))	47 (25)	47 (24)	50 (23)	55 (25)		0.391
Plan to feed baby	n (%)	n (%)	n (%)	n (%)		
No	14 (18)	0 (0)	1 (4)	0 (0)		
Yes	81 (82)	31 (100)	32 (96)	28 (100)	15 (2, 118)	0.009
Plan to breastfeed (weeks) Mean (sd)[a]	29 (22)	34 (20)	40 (27)	41 (24)	1.02 (1.00,1.03)	0.012
Breast fed as baby						
Yes	68 (72)	20 (65)	24 (73)	22 (79)		
No	17 (18)	6 (19)	4 (12)	3 (11)	1.41 (0.66, 3.00)	0.368
Unsure	10 (11)	5 (16)	5 (15)	3 (11)	1.13 (0.51, 2.51)	0.758
Partner support (antenatal)						
Neutral/no support	23 (27)	6 (21)	4 (13)	2 (8)		
Strongly supportive	63 (73)	23 (79)	27 (87)	24 (92)	2.42 (1.15, 5.11)	0.02
Mother support (antenatal)						
Neutral/no support	25 (26)	7 (22)	7 (21)	2 (7)		
Strongly supportive	70 (74)	24 (77)	26 (79)	26 (93)	1.87 (0.96, 3.66)	0.067
Sleep Quantity Mean (sd)	2.6 (0.78)	2.8 (0.73)	2.4 (0.87)	2.6 (0.80)	1.01 (0.72. 1.42)	0.939
Sleep Quality Mean (sd)	2.8 (0.66)	2.9 (0.72)	2.9 (0.61)	2.9 (0.68)	1.22 (0.81, 1.83)	0.349

Proportional odds models were used to analyse the data
[a]Based on 66 participants in first group, 29 in the second, 24 in the third and 23 in the fourth

that the very early introduction of solids that we have described played a role in this poor outcome. Our finding that 5% of mothers had introduced solids by one month is also of concern given the growing body of evidence relating early introduction of solids to a range of later life health issues, notably obesity [34, 35].

We found Māori ethnicity to be a negative predictor of breastfeeding duration, but we think that this is unlikely to be a factor per se; rather, it is a part of the complex web linking ethnicity, deprivation and cigarette smoking, the latter being of high prevalence in the Māori community. This is one of New Zealand's 'hard-to-change' public health issues particularly amongst pregnant Māori women [36]. Tobacco use is known to be more prevalent in more deprived communities [37] and deprivation is a known predictor of early

discontinuation of breastfeeding, interacting strongly with other socio-demographic factors, including age, education and ethnicity [7]. Maternal smoking and socio-economic status were both negative predictors for breastfeeding duration in our study. We also confirmed the dose relationship shown by others [38], that heavier smokers breastfeed for shorter periods. Whilst there may be physiological explanations for the relationship between smoking and breastfeeding, there are also complex psycho-social reasons [13], not least of which is mothers' perceived risk of harm to their baby through tobacco's toxic and addictive substances in their breast milk [14]. In response, some women stop breastfeeding if smoking cessation is too difficult. This same behaviour has also been found amongst Māori women [24].

Table 4 Means or frequency for breastfeeding support and smoking at 1 month for four 'fully breastfeeding' groups

	Full breastfeeding stopped before 4 weeks $N = 95$	Full breastfeeding stopped at or after 4 weeks but before 13 weeks $N = 31$	Full breastfeeding stopped at or after 13 weeks but before 26 weeks $N = 33$	Full breastfeeding stopped at or after 26 weeks $N = 28$	OR (95% CI)	p
Age (days) at 1 m interview (Mean) (sd)	54 (29)	52 (28)	48 (17)	46 (15)		0.101
Breastfeeding support	n (%)	n (%)	n (%)	n (%)		
Strong partner support						
Neutral/no support	31/89 (45)	6/31 (19)	4/33 (12)	2/27 (7)		
Strongly supportive	58/89 (65)	25/31 (81)	29/33 (88)	25/27 (93)	3.64 (1.76, 7.55)	0.001
Strong mother support						
Neutral/no support	30/90 (33)	6(31 (19)	9/33 (28)	1/27 (4)		
Strongly supportive	60/90 (67)	25/31 (81)	24/33 (72)	26/27 (96)	2.47 (1.27, 4.82)	0.008
Others helped mother care for baby last night						
No	80/91 (88)	25/31 (19)	27/33 (22)	22/27 (81)		
Yes	11/91 (12)	6/31 (19)	6/33 (18)	5/27 (19)	1.50 (0.73, 3.11)	0.272
Fatigue (mean)(sd)	7.2 (4.59)	6.1 (2.67)	7.2 (5.56)	6.1 (4.79)[a]	0.97 (0.91, 1.03)	0.324
Maternal smoking						
None	37 (41)	21 (68)	25 (76)	21 (78)		
Occasional	9 (10)	0 (0)	2 (6)	1 (4)		
Daily	45 (49)	10 (32)	6 (18)	5 (19)	0.51 (0.37, 0.69)[b]	< 0.001
Alcohol use						
No	31/90 (48)	18 (58)	20/33 (61)	14/27 (56)		
Yes	59/90 (62)	13/31 (42)	13/33 (39)	13/27 (44)	0.54 (0.31, 0.93)	0.026

Proportional odds models were used to analyse the data

[a]Based on 91 participants in first group, 31 in the second, 33 in the third and 27 in the fourth

[b]Fitted as a trend across the categories

Our study suggests that alcohol use may reduce breastfeeding duration. Infants are known to have decreased milk intake after their mothers have consumed alcohol [39]. Additionally, it is suggested that women might believe it better to stop breastfeeding if they drink alcohol in order not to harm baby [13] in the fashion suggested above for smoking. We also found pacifier use to be a very strong negative predictor of breastfeeding duration. While a meta-analysis investigating the protective effect of pacifiers for sudden infant death syndrome, found that the later use of a pacifier (after 4 weeks of age) did not impact on long term breastfeeding rates [40], other studies have noted that early and frequent, but not occasional, pacifier use shortens breastfeeding duration [18, 19, 41]. Our findings therefore support New Zealand's stance to not promote pacifier use for the prevention of sudden infant death [42] as breastfeeding is protective of sudden unexpected death of an infant [43].

Breastfeeding education [44], in particular breastfeeding education for fathers [45], has been shown to enhance breastfeeding duration. However, despite evidence of reasonable breastfeeding knowledge amongst our participants, we did not demonstrate an association between knowledge of breastfeeding and duration of breastfeeding. Similarly, while being breastfed as a baby has been found to extend breastfeeding [46], we found no such association in our study. Others have found bedsharing to be a predictor of increased duration of breastfeeding [47] but we did not, and nor did a study in an inner city low income community in the United States of America [48]. In our study however, there were only small numbers bedsharing, given that participants were provided a wahakura or bassinet and asked to use it, but it could also be that bedsharing in this more deprived demographic is motivated by other factors rather than facilitation of breastfeeding. In a similar fashion, we did not find in this analysis that being assigned a wahakura extended breastfeeding duration as we did in our previous

Table 5 Frequency for sleep place, bed-sharing, dummy use, sleep quantity and quality and depression against duration of 'full breastfeeding'

	Breast feeding from birth N = 182	Still Breast feeding from 4 weeks or more N = 90	Still Breast feeding 13 weeks or more N = 61	Still Breast feeding 26 weeks or more N = 28	OR (95% CI)	p
	n (%)	n (%)	n (%)	n (%)		
Shared parent bedroom[a]	161 (82)	70 (78)	44 (72)	21 (75)	0.75 (0.42, 1.33)	0.324
Shared mother's bed[a]	16 (9)	13 (14)	8 (13)	3 (11)	0.64 (0.33, 1.23)	0.179
Used dummy[a]	68 (37)	19 (21)	7 (11)	1 (4)	0.28 (0.17, 0.46)	< 0.001
Sleep quantity and	2.5 (0.65)	2.7(0.61)	2.7 (0.65)	2.5 (0.69)	0.91 (0.64, 1.29)	0.609
sleep quality (4 pt. scale)[a]	3.2 (0.54)	3.2 (0.51)	3.2 (0.60)	3.3 (0.70)	1.14 (0.74, 1.75)	0.549
'Possible depression' [b] (10+ on the EPDS)	65 (33)	10 (11)	4 (15)	2 (7)	0.92 (0.54, 1.57)	0.758

Cumulative odds models were used to analyse the data
[a]using data collected at all three postnatal assessments
[b]using data collected at baseline and 3 and 6 months

study [49]. This may be due to the more complex breastfeeding history collected and analyzed for this paper. Lastly, we found no association of depression in pregnancy with duration of breastfeeding although a systematic review of the literature [50] noted the association of depression during pregnancy and in the postpartum period with a shorter duration of breastfeeding.

The main strength of this study despite the low response rate was that it succeeded in recruiting a large sample of predominantly Māori women from deprived communities who we know are often reluctant to participate in research [51] particularly given the invasive nature of the full study, with cameras in the bedroom. Secondly, retention in the study was high, with 88% of those recruited still participating at the six-month interview. Thirdly, the breastfeeding history collected at each assessment was quite detailed and thus meant that the extent and length of breastfeeding could be robustly investigated. The reliability of data collected by phone at six months remains high as the research nurse had a well-established relationship with the participant.

Its main weakness, the possibility of recall bias around the breastfeeding duration, is offset somewhat by this study having used more than one question to identify behaviors, such as the use of 'food not breast milk' and 'the introduction of solids', rather than a simple 24 h food recall. Although our sample was not entirely Māori and Māori breastfeeding duration was shown to be shorter than non-Māori, we are assuming the predictors of breastfeeding duration described here are still relevant for a Māori population. Lastly, although the data is now five years old, the findings are relevant as the duration of breastfeeding in New Zealand has remained static since that time [52].

Conclusion

This study of mainly Māori women from a relatively deprived community in New Zealand identified a shorter breastfeeding duration than other New Zealand women and confirmed the known negative predictors of breastfeeding duration, maternal smoking, alcohol consumption, pacifier use, and the early consumption of solids. Strong maternal and partner support of the mother was the strongest positive predictor of extended breastfeeding duration. Antenatal and postnatal education that includes the mothers and the partners of pregnant women and focuses on the identified predictors could be an effective strategy to increase breastfeeding in this population.

Abbreviations
CI: Confidence intervals; IQR: Interquartile range; OR: Proportional odds ratio

Funding
Funding was obtained from the Health Research Council of New Zealand (Ref 10/477) and a University of Otago Research Grant. The funders had no role in study design, or in the collection, analysis, and interpretation of data, or in the writing of the report or the decision to submit the article for publication.

Authors contributions
BT and DTL were responsible for the initial concept of the project and, with SB, SW, SA, KM, AT and RJ, participated in the design of the study. AT collected the data and RJ coordinated the study along with DTL, SB and BT. SW designed and completed the analysis. BT, SB, DTL, SA and KM contributed to interpretation of the data. SW and KM drafted the manuscript with reviewing and editing assistance from SB, SA, BT and DTL. All authors read and approved the final manuscript.

Competing interests

The authors declare that they have no competing interests.

Author details

[1]Department of Women's and Children's Health, Dunedin School of Medicine, University of Otago, Dunedin, New Zealand. [2]Faculty of Education, Humanities and Health Sciences, Eastern Institute of Technology, Hawke's Bay, New Zealand. [3]Department of Preventive & Social Medicine, Dunedin School of Medicine, University of Otago, Dunedin, New Zealand. [4]School of Midwifery, Otago Polytechnic, Dunedin, New Zealand. [5]Kaupapa Consulting Ltd, Napier, Napier, New Zealand.

References

1.   Eidelman AI, Schanler RJ, Johnston M, et al. Breastfeeding and the use of human milk. Pediatrics. 2012;129:e827–41.

2.   Smith JP, Harvey PJ. Chronic disease and infant nutrition: is it significant to public health? Public Health Nutr. 2010;14:279–89.

3.   Fewtrell M. Long-term benefits of breastfeeding. Curr Paediatr. 2004;14(4): 559–66.

4.   Horta B, Victora C. Long-term effects of breastfeeding-a systematic review. Geneva, Switzerland: World Health Organisation; 2013.

5.   Ministry of Health. National Strategic Plan of Action for Breastfeeding, 2008–2012. National Breastfeeding Advisory Committee of New Zealand's advice to the director-general of health. Wellington: Ministry of Health; 2009.

6.   Whipps MD. Education attainment and parity explain the relationship between maternal age and breastfeeding duration in US mothers. J Hum Lact. 2017;33:220–4.

7.   Persad MD, Mensinger JL. Maternal breastfeeding attitudes: association with breastfeeding intent and socio-demographics among urban Primiparas. J Community Health. 2008;33:53–60.

8.   Thulier D, Mercer J. Variables associated with breastfeeding duration. J Obstet Gynecol Neonatal Nurs. 2009;38:259–68.

9.   Dodgson JE, Duckett L, Garwick A, Graham BL. An ecological perspective of breastfeeding in an indigenous community. J Nurs Scholarsh. 2002;34:235–41.

10.   Cernadas JMC, Noceda G, Barrera L, Martinez AM, Garsd A. Maternal and perinatal factors influencing the duration of exclusive breastfeeding during the first 6 months of life. J Hum Lact. 2003;19:136–44.

11.   Manhire KM, Hagan AE, Floyd SA. A descriptive account of New Zealand mothers' responses to open-ended questions on their breastfeeding experiences. Midwifery. 2007;23:372–81.

12.   Meedya S, Fahy K, Kable A. Factors that positively influence breastfeeding duration to 6 months: a literature review. Women and Birth. 2010;23:135–45.

13.   Amir LH, Donath SM. Does maternal smoking have a negative physiological effect on breastfeeding? The epidemiological evidence. Birth. 2002;29:112–23.

14.   Goldade K, Nichter M, Nichter M, Adrian S, Tesler L, Muramoto M. Breastfeeding and smoking among low-income women: results of a longitudinal qualitative study. Birth. 2008;35:230–40.

15.   Giglia RC. Alcohol and lactation: an updated systematic review. Nutrition & Dietetics. 2010;67:237–43.

16.   Dunn S, Davies B, McCleary L, Edwards N, Gaboury I. The relationship between vulnerability factors and breastfeeding outcome. J Obstet Gynecol Neonatal Nurs. 2006;35:87–97.

17.   Dennis C-L, McQueen K. Does maternal postpartum depressive symptomatology influence infant feeding outcomes? Acta Paediatr. 2007;96:590–4.

18.   Howard CR, Howard FM, Lanphear B, deBlieck EA, Eberly S, Lawrence RA. The effects of early pacifier use on breastfeeding duration. Pediatrics. 1999; 103:e33.

19.   Kramer MS, Barr RG, Dagenais S, et al. Pacifier use, early weaning, and cry/fuss behavior: a randomized controlled trial. JAMA. 2001;286:322–6.

20.   Hornell A, Hofvander Y, Kylberg E. Solids and formula: association with pattern and duration of breastfeeding. Pediatrics. 2001;107

21.   Haiek L, Gauthier D, Brosseau D, Rocheleau L. Understanding breastfeeding behavior: rates and shifts in patterns in Québec. J Hum Lact. 2007;23:24–31.

22.   Gosman H. What influences infant feeding Deecisions for Maori mothers aged 15–24 years? Master of nursing thesis. New Zealand: Eastern Institute of Technology, Hawke's Bay; 2015.

23.   Manaena-Biddle H, Waldon J, Glover M. Influences that affect Maori women breastfeeding. Breastfeeding Review. 2007;15:5–14.

24.   Glover M, Waldon J, Manaena-Biddle H, Holdaway M, Cunningham C. Barriers to best outcomes in breastfeeding for Māori: Mothers' perceptions, Whānau perceptions, and services. J Hum Lact. 2009;25:307–16.

25.   Glover M, Cunningham C. Hoki ki te ukaipo: reinstating Māori infant care practices to increase breastfeeding rates. In: Infant feeding practices: a Cross-Cultural. Perspective. School of Public Health, La Trobe University, Australia. Pub:Springer, New York, 2011

26.   Atkinson J, Salmond C, Crampton P. NZDep2013 index of deprivation. Ministry of Health: New Zealand; 2014.

27.   Tipene-Leach D, Baddock S, Williams S, et al. Methodology and recruitment for a randomised controlled trial to evaluate the safety of wahakurafor infant bedsharing. BMC Pediatr. 2014;14:240.

28.   Ministry of Health. Food and Nutrition Guidelines for Healthy Pregnant and Breastfeeding Women. A background paper. Ministry of Health. In: Wellington; 2006.

29.   Taylor B, Heath A-L, Galland B, et al. Prevention of overweight in infancy (POI.Nz) study: a randomised controlled trial of sleep, food and activity interventions for preventing overweight from birth. BMC Public Health. 2011;11

30.   Cox JL, Holden JM, Sagovsky R. Detection of postnatal depression. Development of the 10-item Edinburgh postnatal depression scale. Br J Psychiatry. 1987;150:782–6.

31.   Jenkins SP. East estimation methods for discrete-time duration models. Oxf Bull Econ Stat. 1995;57:129–36.

32.   Rempel L, Rempel J. Partner influence on health behavior decision-making: increasing breastfeeding duration. J Soc Pers Relat. 2004;21:92–111.

33.   Alexander A, O'Riordan MA, Furman L. Do breastfeeding intentions of pregnant inner-city teens and adult women differ? Breastfeed Med. 2010;5: 289–96.

34.   Papoutsou S, Savva S, Hunsberger M, et al. Timing of solid food introduction and association with later childhood overweight and obesity: the IDEFICS study. Maternal & Child Nutrition. 2017:e12471.

35.   Huh SY, Rifas-Shiman SL, Taveras EM, Oken E, Gillman MW. Timing of solid food introduction and risk of obesity in preschool-aged children. Pediatrics. 2011;127:e544.

36.   Glover M, Kira A. Pregnant Māori smokers' perception of cessation support and how it can be more helpful. J Smok Cessat. 2012;7

37.   Kleinschmidt I, Hills M, Elliott P. Smoking behaviour can be predicted by neighbourhood deprivation measures. J Epidemiol Community Health. 1995;49:S72.

38.   SM D, LH A. The relationship between maternal smoking and breastfeeding duration after adjustment for maternal infant feeding intention. Acta Paediatr. 2004;93:1514–8.

39.   Mennella JA, Pepino MY, Teff KL. Acute alcohol consumption disrupts the hormonal milieu of lactating women. The Journal of Clinical Endocrinology & Metabolism. 2005;90:1979–85.

40.   Hauck F, Omojokun O, Siadaty M. Do pacifiers reduce the risk of sudden infant death syndrome? A meta-analysis. Pediatrics. 2005;116:e716.

41.   Scott JA, Binns CW, Oddy WH, Graham KI. Predictors of breastfeeding duration: evidence from a cohort study. Pediatrics. 2006;117:e646.

42.   Ministry of Health and Child and Youth Mortality Review Committee. Preventing sudden unexpected death in infancy: Information for the health practitioner. 2007.

43.   Hauck F, Thompson J, Tanabe K, Moon R, Vennemann M. Breastfeeding and reduced risk of sudden infant death syndrome: a meta-analysis. Pediatrics. 2011;128:103–10.

44.   Stuebe AM, Bonuck K. What predicts intent to breastfeed exclusively? Breastfeeding knowledge, attitudes, and beliefs in a diverse urban population. Breastfeed Med. 2011;6:413–20.

45.   Susin LRO, Giugliani ERJ, Kummer SC, Maciel M, Simon C, Da Silveira LC. Does parental breastfeeding knowledge increase breastfeeding rates? Birth. 1999;26:149–56.

46.   Di Manno L, Macdonald JA, Knight T. The intergenerational continuity of breastfeeding intention, initiation, and duration: a systematic review. Birth. 2015;42:5–15.

47. Blair PS, Heron J, Fleming PJ. Relationship between bed sharing and breastfeeding: longitudinal, population-based analysis. Pediatrics. 2010;126:e1119.

48. Brenner RA, Simons-Morton BG, Bhaskar B, Revenis M, Das A, Clemens JD. Infant-parent bed sharing in an inner-city population. Arch Pediatr Adolesc Med. 2003;157:33–9.

49. Baddock SA, Tipene-Leach DC, Williams SM, et al. Wahakura versus bassinet for safe infant sleep: a randomized trial. Pediatrics. 2017; Jan:e20160162. https://doi.org/10.1542/peds2016-0162.

50. Dias CC, Figueiredo B. Breastfeeding and depression: a systematic review of the literature. J Affect Disord. 2015;171:142–54.

51. Parry O, Bancroft A, Gnich W, Amos A. Nobody home? Issues of respondent recruitment in areas of deprivation. Crit Public Health. 2001;11:305–17.

52. Royal New Zealand Plunket Society Breastfeeding Data: Analysis of 2010–2015 data 2017;11–14. Retrieved from: https://www.plunket.org.nz/news-and-research/research-from-plunket/plunket-breastfeeding-data-analysis/.

23

High rate of antibiotic resistance among pneumococci carried by healthy children in the eastern part of the Democratic Republic of the Congo

Archippe M. Birindwa[1,2,3,5*] (iD), Matilda Emgård[1], Rickard Nordén[1], Ebba Samuelsson[1], Shadi Geravandi[1], Lucia Gonzales-Siles[1], Balthazar Muhigirwa[2], Théophile Kashosi[3], Eric Munguakonkwa[2], Jeanière T. Manegabe[2], Didace Cibicabene[2], Lambert Morisho[2], Benjamin Mwambanyi[2], Jacques Mirindi[2], Nadine Kabeza[2], Magnus Lindh[1], Rune Andersson[1,4] and Susann Skovbjerg[1]

Abstract

Background: Pneumococcal conjugate vaccines have been introduced in the infant immunisation programmes in many countries to reduce the rate of fatal pneumococcal infections. In the Democratic Republic of the Congo (DR Congo) a 13-valent vaccine (PCV13) was introduced in 2013. Data on the burden of circulating pneumococci among children after this introduction are lacking. In this study, we aimed to determine the risk factors related to pneumococcal carriage in healthy Congolese children after the vaccine introduction and to assess the antibiotic resistance rates and serotype distribution among the isolated pneumococci.

Methods: In 2014 and 2015, 794 healthy children aged one to 60 months attending health centres in the eastern part of DR Congo for immunisation or growth monitoring were included in the study. Data on socio-demographic and medical factors were collected by interviews with the children's caregivers. Nasopharyngeal swabs were obtained from all the children for bacterial culture, and isolated pneumococci were further tested for antimicrobial resistance using disc diffusion tests and, when indicated, minimal inhibitory concentration (MIC) determination, and for serotype/serogroup by molecular testing.

Results: The pneumococcal detection rate was 21%, being higher among children who had not received PCV13 vaccination, lived in rural areas, had an enclosed kitchen, were malnourished or presented with fever (*p* value < 0.05). The predominant serotypes were 19F, 11, 6A/B/C/D and 10A. More than 50% of the pneumococcal isolates belonged to a serotype/serogroup not included in PCV13.

Eighty per cent of the isolates were not susceptible to benzylpenicillin and non-susceptibility to ampicillin and ceftriaxone was also high (42 and 37% respectively). Almost all the isolates (94%) were resistant to trimethoprim-sulphamethoxazole, while 43% of the strains were resistant to ≥3 antibiotics.

(Continued on next page)

* Correspondence: birindwaarchippe@gmail.com;
archippe.muhandule.birindwa@gu.se
[1]Department of Infectious Diseases, Institute of Biomedicine, University of Gothenburg, Gothenburg, Sweden
[2]Panzi Hospital, Bukavu, Democratic Republic of the Congo
Full list of author information is available at the end of the article

(Continued from previous page)

Conclusions: Our study shows alarmingly high levels of reduced susceptibility to commonly used antibiotics in pneumococci carried by healthy Congolese children. This highlights the importance of local antibiotic resistance surveillance and indicates the needs for the more appropriate use of antibiotics in the area. The results further indicate that improved living conditions are needed to reduce the pneumococcal burden, in addition to PCV13 vaccination.

Keywords: *Streptococcus pneumoniae*, Antibiotic resistance, DR Congo, Nasopharyngeal carriage, Children, PCV13

Background

Streptococcus pneumoniae, or the pneumococcus, is a leading bacterial cause of death in young children worldwide, mainly due to pneumonia [1, 2]. The bacterium is also an important pathogen in other community-acquired respiratory infections, including acute *otitis media*, and in invasive infections, such as meningitis and sepsis.

Pneumococcal infections are estimated to cause 11% of all deaths in children less than 5 years of age worldwide, with a disproportionate number of these deaths in low- and middle income countries [3]. In sub-Saharan Africa, where most of the under-five deaths occur, the leading cause of death is pneumonia and children under the age of 2 years are the most affected [3, 4].

The Democratic Republic of the Congo (DR Congo) is one of the countries with the highest mortality due to childhood pneumonia; in 2015, pneumonia was the leading cause of death under 5 years of age, killing 46,000 Congolese children [5, 6].

Many risk factors, including malnutrition, lack of pneumococcal immunisation, parental smoking and crowded living conditions, [7, 8], as well as exposure to smoke due to the household use of solid fuels has been associated with an increased risk of pneumonia in children [9, 10]. Women and children living in severe poverty have the greatest exposure to household air pollution [11]. In DR Congo, open fires are commonly used in rural villages, while charcoal stoves and electricity are more often used in the cities.

To lower the burden of severe pneumococcal infections among children, pneumococcal conjugate vaccines, covering up to 13 of 98 known pneumococcal serotypes [12], have been introduced in the infant vaccination programmes in many countries. The 13-valent conjugate pneumococcal vaccine (PCV13), containing the serotypes 1, 3, 4, 5, 6A, 6B, 7F, 9 V, 14, 18C, 19A, 19F and 23F, was introduced in DR Congo in 2013. A recent study from Kenya showed that the prevalence of vaccine serotypes was reduced by two-thirds in children younger than 5 years of age after the introduction of PCV10, suggesting that the conjugate vaccines will have substantial effects in reducing invasive pneumococcal disease in Africa [13]. However, in many countries, pneumococcal disease caused by non-vaccine serotypes has increased after the start of vaccination [14] and, in the Gambia, an increase in non-typeable serotypes was noted after the introduction of PCV13; the clinical significance of this finding is not known [15].

There are some reports on the carriage rate and serotype distribution of pneumococci in healthy sub-Saharan children before and after PCV13 vaccination [13, 16, 17], but there are no available data on the child population in DR Congo, either before or after the introduction of PCV13.

According to recommendations revised by the World Health Organisation (WHO) in 2014, oral amoxicillin is the drug of choice for children with pneumonia, while parenteral ampicillin (or penicillin) together with gentamicin should be used in severe cases. Ceftriaxone is recommended as the second-line treatment in children with severe pneumonia who have failed with the first-line treatment. There might, however, be a delay of several years before these recommendations are implemented in local treatment guidelines. Since December 2016, the national policy in DR Congo recommends amoxicillin rather than trimethoprim-sulphamethoxazole (TMP-SMX) for the treatment of pneumonia at community level. As in many other low-income countries, the prescription of antibiotics is, however, not restricted solely to physicians, and children may be treated by people other than educated health workers [18]. Children hospitalised in the South-Kivu province, in eastern DR Congo, due to pneumonia are currently treated with ceftriaxone or ampicillin, together with gentamicin, according to local guidelines, while a combination of ceftriaxone and cloxacillin is used after 48 h without clinical improvement [19].

Resistance to antibiotics is a worldwide concern and the proportion of pneumococci that are not susceptible to penicillin even exceeds 50% in some countries [20]. Before the introduction of the conjugate vaccine, more than two thirds of the pneumococci detected in healthy children in Dar Es Salaam, Tanzania, were non-susceptible to penicillin [21], while the rate was 45% in Gambia [22]. A Peruvian study showed no changes in antibiotic resistance in colonising pneumococci after the introduction of the vaccine, suggesting significant antibiotic resistance in non–PCV7 strains [23], while other studies from South Africa

[24], the United States of America [25] and Canada [26] have shown a decrease in the antibiotic resistance of invasive pneumococci.

Here, we report on the first study of nasopharyngeal carriage and predisposing conditions for pneumococcal colonisation in healthy Congolese children after the introduction of PCV13. The profiles of the circulating pneumococcal serotypes/serogroups and the antibiotic susceptibility of the carried pneumococci were also assessed.

Methods

Study population

From January 2014 to June 2015, 794 healthy children aged one to 60 months attending one of seven health centres in the South-Kivu province in the eastern part of DR Congo for immunisation or growth monitoring were included in the study. The health centres were located in the city of Bukavu ($n = 3$), in the suburban area ($n = 1$), or in the surrounding rural area (n = 3) (Additional file 1).

Written questionnaires about immunisation status and demographic factors were completed by trained final-year medical students or nurses in the presence of a paediatrician and a basic physical examination of the children was performed to monitor current signs of a respiratory tract infection. When available, the immunisation card was checked to confirm the vaccination status of the child. For the 284 healthy children enrolled in 2015, another questionnaire containing questions about socio-economic conditions and previous illness was added. The weight and height were measured and standardised for age using the Emergency Nutrition Assessment (ENA) software 2011 [27].

Signed informed consent was obtained from the parent or guardian of each included child. The study was approved by the Ethics Committees at the Université Catholique de Bukavu, DR Congo, and at the University of Gothenburg, Sweden.

Specimen collection

A nasopharyngeal specimen was obtained from all participating children using an Eswab (Copan Diagnostics Inc., Murrieta, CA). A single trained investigator at each centre obtained the sample following a standardised procedure. The head of the child was tipped backwards and gently immobilised. The bent swab was inserted into the nostril and then passed into the nasopharynx to a distance equal to that from the nose to the tip of the ear and kept in that position for 5 s. The samples were shipped to the Clinical Laboratory at Panzi Hospital within two to 6 h for subsequent pneumococcal culture.

Culture and antibiotic susceptibility testing of pneumococci

The samples were cultured for *Streptococcus pneumoniae* on 5% human blood agar plates (Oxoid Columbia Blood Agar Base – Thermo Fisher Scientific, Waltham, MA), incubated overnight at 34–36 °C in closed jars (Oxoid Limited, Thermo Fisher Scientific, Hampshire, UK) supplied with CO_2 paper sachets (BD GasPak™ EZ CO_2 Container System, Becton, Dickinson and Company, Franklin Lakes, New Jersey) and CO_2 indicators (BD CO_2 Indicator 0.5 mL, Becton, Dickinson and Company).

Suspected pneumococci were identified by a positive optochin test (diameter ≥ 14 mm) and were further tested for antibiotic susceptibility using a disc diffusion test against oxacillin (1 µg) (screening for beta-lactam resistance), trimethoprim-sulphamethoxazole (TMP-SMX) (1.25/23.75 µg), norfloxacin (10 µg) (screening for fluoroquinolone resistance, i.e. levofloxacin and moxifloxacin), tetracycline (30 µg), erythromycin (15 µg) and clindamycin (2 µg) (all from Oxoid Limited), using breakpoints according to the European Committee on Antimicrobial Susceptibility Testing, 2017 [28]. The bacteria and antibiotic discs were applied to Muller Hinton agar plates (Oxoid Limited) supplied with 5% sheep blood (Thermo Fisher Scientific) and 20 mg/L β-Nicotinamide adenine dinucleotide (NAD) (AppliChem GmbH, Darmstadt, Germany) that were incubated over night at 34–36 °C in a CO_2 environment as described above. Pneumococcal isolates with reduced sensitivity to oxacillin (diameter < 20 mm) were further tested using minimal inhibitory concentration (MIC) determination against penicillin G, ampicillin and ceftriaxone (all 0.016–256 µg/mL, bioMérieux, Marcy l'Etoile, France). Pneumococci with an MIC of > 0.06 mg/L were defined as having reduced susceptibility to benzylpenicillin. Multi-drug resistant (MDR) isolates were defined as those that were non-susceptible (intermediate or resistant) to at least one drug from three or more different classes of antimicrobial agents, including the beta-lactams (the penicillins benzylpenicillin and ampicillin and the cephalosporin ceftriaxone) [29]. Apart from the beta-lactams, all drugs tested belong to different classes, namely fluoroquinolones (norfloxacin), lincosamides (clindamycin), macrolides (erythromycin), folate pathway inhibitors (trimethoprim-sulphamethoxazole) and tetracyclines (tetracycline) [29]. The isolates were frozen (– 20 °C) in STGG storage medium [30] before being transported to Gothenburg, Sweden, for further analyses.

Reproducibility of the antibiotic susceptibility results

Out of the 163 pneumococcal strains isolated at the Clinical Laboratory at Panzi Hospital in Bukavu, 151 isolates were transported frozen in STGG medium to Gothenburg. Of these, 32 isolates could be re-cultured after storage and transport, and were tested for antibiotic susceptibility at the Department of Infectious Diseases, University of Gothenburg, Sweden, as well (Fig. 1). When the results were compared with those obtained at the laboratory in Bukavu for the same isolates, the diameter zones for all the tested antibiotic discs varied by 6 mm or less in at least 75% of the cases (Table 1). The resulting interpretation into Sensitive (S), Intermediate (I) or Resistant (R) was similar in both groups (Table 1).

The distributions of MIC values were also compared between the analyses performed in Bukavu and Gothenburg, respectively (Additional file 2). There was an even distribution of MIC values between the two sites for all of penicillin G, ampicillin and ceftriaxone. When interpreting the MIC values for penicillin G, all the isolates were categorised in the same SIR category. For ampicillin, one isolate was differently categorised into sensitive and intermediate, respectively, and the same was true in two cases for ceftriaxone. We also compared the MIC distributions between 2014 and 2015 for all the isolates tested in Bukavu and found an even distribution of the MIC values between the 2 years for ampicillin (Additional file 3). We concluded that the reproducibility was satisfactory for both the disc diffusion tests and the MIC determinations performed in Bukavu and all the results shown in the results section are therefore from the antibiotic susceptibility tests performed in Bukavu.

Nucleic acid extraction and multiplex real-time PCR

The pneumococcal isolates were further analysed by molecular methods in Gothenburg for confirmation of species identification, and for determination of serotypes/serogroups. For those isolates that could be re-cultured after storage and transport ($n = 32$), one colony of each isolate was suspended in 1 mL of PBS prior to the extraction of nucleic acids. For unculturable isolates, 100 µL of STGG storage medium containing non-viable bacteria was diluted in 900 µL of phosphate buffered saline (PBS). DNA was extracted from 200 µL of the suspended isolates or diluted non-viable isolates using a MagNA Pure LC instrument (Roche Diagnostics, Mannheim, Germany) and the Total Nucleic acid Isolation kit (Roche Diagnostic). The extracted nucleic acids were eluted in 100 µL elution buffer. The samples were stored at – 20 °C until further analysis.

A multiplex real-time PCR, able to detect 40 different serotypes, was used according to a protocol published by Centers for Disease Control and Prevention (CDC) using previously published primers with slight modifications (preprint available at https://www.biorxiv.org/content/early/2018/09/12/415422).

The multiplex real-time PCR assays were performed using the Quant Studio 6 Flex with a 384-well system (Applied Biosystems, Carlsbad, CA). Each reaction consisted of a 20 µL reaction volume, including 4 µL of template nucleic acid, along with 1 µM of each of the forward and reverse primers, 0.85 µM of the probe,

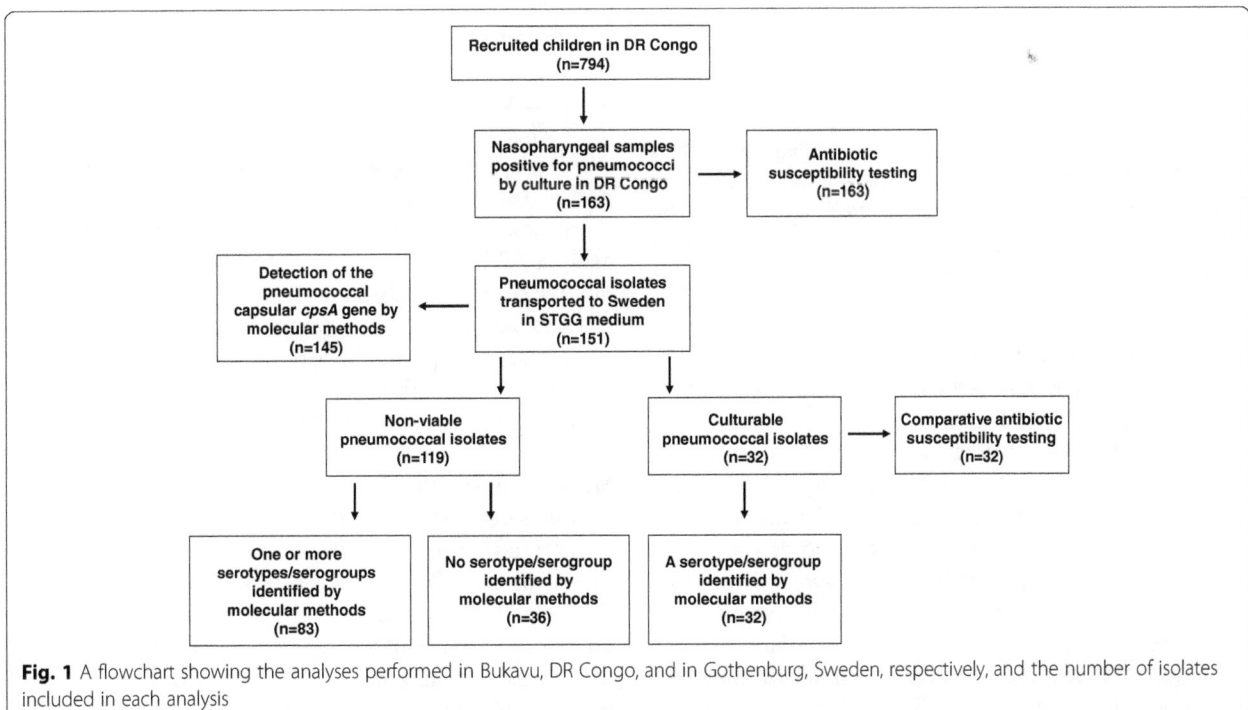

Fig. 1 A flowchart showing the analyses performed in Bukavu, DR Congo, and in Gothenburg, Sweden, respectively, and the number of isolates included in each analysis

Table 1 Comparison of disc diffusion tests on pneumococcal isolates performed in Bukavu and in Gothenburg, respectively (n = 32)

	Oxacillin[a] N (%)	TMP-SMX[b] N (%)	Erythromycin N (%)	Clindamycin N (%)	Norfloxacin[c] N (%)	Tetracycline N (%)
Difference in disc diffusion test (mm)						
≤ 3	23 (73)	29 (91)	22 (69)	23 (73)	25 (79)	14 (44)
4–6	5 (15)	1 (3)	3 (11)	3 (11)	5 (15)	10 (31)
> 6	4 (12)	2 (6)	7 (32)	6 (18)	2 (6)	8 (25)
Difference in SIR[d] interpretation[e]	0	0	0	0	0	0

[a] Screening disc for beta-lactam resistance
[b] *TMP-SMX* Trimethoprim-sulphamethoxazole
[c] Screening disc for fluoroquionolone resistance, i.e. levofloxacin and moxifloxacin
[d] *SIR* Sensitive, Intermediate, Resistant
[e] Breakpoints used according to EUCAST 2017

10 μl of 2X Universal Master Mix for DNA targets (Applied Biosystems) [31] and RNAase free water. The Tecan Freedom EVO PCR setup workstation (Tecan Group Ltd., Männedorf, Switzerland) was used to prepare the PCR reactions in a 384-well plate. The PCR reaction conditions were as follows: one initial cycle at 46 °C for 2 min, followed by denaturation at 95 °C for 10 min and 45 amplification cycles of 95 °C for 15 s and 58 °C for 1 min. Each multiplex performance was evaluated using an internal control (*CpsA*) to verify the presence of pneumococcal DNA in the sample, as well as two pUC57 plasmids containing each PCR target amplicon for all serotype systems.

Sequetyping

For eight out of the 32 pneumococcal isolates that could be re-cultured after storage and transport to Gothenburg, Sweden, and in which the multiplex PCR serotyping method was inconclusive, the serotypes/serogroups were determined using a modified Sequetyping protocol (https://www.biorxiv.org/content/early/2018/09/12/415422). Briefly, two PCR reactions were set up to amplified the whole cpsB gene. The PCR products were sent to GATC Biotech (Cologne, Germany) for purification and sequencing using the four PCR primers. The 1006 bp sequence product was matched to a reference database for determination of the serotype.

Data management and statistical analysis

Descriptive analysis was performed using the SPSS package (version 24.0) for logistic regression to analyse the relationship between carriage and socio-demographic or medical factors. Prevalence rates and the 95% CI were calculated. Potential variables associated with pneumococcal carriage were assessed by odds ratios (OR) with 95% CI and tested by univariate analysis with the Pearson chi-square or Fisher's exact test (n < 5). Associations with p < 0.05 were re-analysed by multivariate analysis. A p-value of < 0.05 was considered significant. Malnutrition was defined as the weight for age or weight for

height as a Z score ≤ − 2 standard deviations, determined by ENA for smart software 2011.

Results

Characteristics of the included children

From seven health care centres located in the city of Bukavu, in the suburban area or in the surrounding rural area, 794 children (age range one to 60 months, median 9.0 months) were included in the study and sampled from the nasopharynx. The background health data and living conditions of the children are shown in Additional file 1.

Socio-demographic risk factors for pneumococcal carriage

Overall, 163 (20.5%) of the children were culture positive for *S. pneumoniae* in the nasopharynx. The detection rate was associated with age but not with sex. Children aged 24–60 months had a more than three times higher rate of pneumococcal carriage that children below 6 months of age (p-value < 0.0001) (Table 2).

A higher frequency of pneumococcal carriage was observed in children living in the rural area as compared with the urban sites (28% versus 13%) and among children who lived in a house with an enclosed kitchen, i.e. with an open fire located inside the house, directly connected to the living room and/or the bedrooms, and these associations remained significant in multivariate analysis (Table 2). The type of stove and fuel for cooking did not correlate with carriage. Nor were there any associations between pneumococcal carriage and the number of rooms, having siblings, parents smoking tobacco, type of building material in the walls or the roof of the house, or having an animal in the household (Additional file 4).

Medical risk factors

Immunisation with PCV13 was strongly associated with lower rates of pneumococcal carriage, which was observed in only 3% of children who had received two or three doses of PCV13 as compared with approximately 30% of the unvaccinated children (p < 0.0001) (Table 2). Malnourished children, children with current fever and those who had had recent antibiotic treatment were

Table 2 Socio-demographic and medical factors related to nasopharyngeal carriage of pneumococci in children living in eastern DR Congo

Socio-demographic factors:	N carrier/N (%)	Univariate analysis		Multivariate analysis	
		OR (95% CI)	p-value	OR (95% CI)	p-value
Age in months					
< 6	29/302 (9.6)	1.00			
6–12	46/184 (25)	1.41 (0.85–2.36)	0.170	0.14 (0.08–0.26)	0.750
> 12–24	32/125 (26)	2.12 (1.25–3.62)	0.005	0.77 (0.44–1.36)	0.381
> 24–60	56/183 (31)	3.45 (2.19–5.44)	< 0.0001	0.90 (0.48–1.68)	< 0.0001
Sex, male	91/402 (23)	1.30 (0.92–1.84)	0.13	1.17 (0.78–1.77)	0.437
Living in rural area	98/355 (28)	2.51 (1.67–3.77)	< 0.0001	0.57 (0.33–0.97)	0.039
No of people sleeping in the same room as the child					
< 3	3/31 (9.7)	1.00			
≥ 3	74/253 (29)		0.018	1.27 (0.45–3.55)	0.644
Enclosed kitchen[a] (N = 77)	43/77 (56)	6.47 (3.62–11.56)	< 0.0001	10.18 (4.93–21.02)	< 0.0001
Medical factors					
Undernutrition[b] (N = 286)	83/286 (29)	2.18 (1.54–3.10)	< 0.0001	0.48 (0.32–0.73)	0.001
Current fever[c] (N = 22)	14/22 (64)	5.52 (2.21–13.78)	< 0.0001	7.96 (2.38–26.58)	0.001
Previous hospitalisation (N = 74)	27/74 (36)	1.83 (1.04–3.25)	0.035	1.61 (0.72–3.59)	0.244
Antibiotics last month (N = 55)	23/55 (42)	2.32 (1.25–4.31)	0.006	2.42 (1.07–5.45)	0.033
Neonatal problems[d] (n = 284)	22/51 (43.1)	2.45 (1.30–4.61)	0.004	1.27 (0.53–3.02)	0.580
PCV13 immunisation					
2 or 3 doses (n = 646[e])	9/283 (3.2)	1.00			
1 dose (n = 773)	46/159 (29)	12.39 (5.87–26.16)	< 0.0001	30.12 (14.36–63)	< 0.0001
0 dose (n = 773)	108/331 (33)	13.47 (6.68–27.17)	< 0.0001	20.57 (9.41–44.96)	< 0.0001

[a]Enclosed kitchen = Kitchen with an open fire located inside the house directly connected to the living room and/or the bedrooms
[b]Undernutrition = weight for age or weight for height as a Z score ≤ −2 standard deviations, determined by ENA for smart software 2011
[c]Fever = 37.5–39.0 °C
[d]Neonatal problems = neonatal hospitalisation, neonatal asphyxia or neonatal resuscitation
[e]645 = the number of children that were supposed to be given ≥2 doses of PCV13 when they were older than 10 weeks or two and a half months

more commonly colonised with pneumococci than children without these factors (*p* < 0.05). In contrast, neonatal problems, asthma, a recent history of malaria or gastroenteritis, or immunisation against measles, tuberculosis or *Hemophilus influenzae* type B were not associated with carriage, nor were symptoms of upper respiratory airway infection, such as a runny nose or cough (Table 2 and Additional file 5).

Taken together, age, living in a household with an enclosed kitchen, living in a rural area, undernutrition, current fever and antibiotic treatment during the last month were significantly associated with a higher, and vaccination with PCV13 with a lower, frequency of pneumococcal detection (Table 2).

Antimicrobial susceptibility of S. pneumoniae isolates

The antimicrobial susceptibility pattern was determined at the Clinical Laboratory, Panzi Hospital, Bukavu, for the 163 pneumococcal strains that were isolated from the children (Fig. 2). Using disc diffusion tests, 145 (89%) of the isolates were shown to be non-susceptible to oxacillin and they were therefore regarded as resistant to phenoxymethylpenicillin. These 145 strains were further tested by MIC determination against penicillin G and 101 (62%) strains were categorised as intermediate (MIC 0.06–2 mg/L), while 30 (18%) were resistant (MIC > 2 mg/L). Taken together, 131/163 (80%) of the strains showed reduced susceptibility to benzylpenicillin, as confirmed by MIC determination (Fig. 2). Sixty-eight isolates (42%) had reduced susceptibility to ampicillin, of which 18 were resistant (MIC > 2 mg/L), and 61 isolates (37%) had reduced susceptibility to ceftriaxone (Fig. 2). High rates of non-susceptibility were also found for tetracycline and as many as 94% of the isolates were resistant to trimethoprim-sulphamethoxazole (TMP-SMX), also known as co-trimoxazole (Fig. 2). Notably, 70 (43%) of the pneumococci were multidrug resistant (non-susceptible to ≥3 classes of antimicrobial agents, including the beta-lactams).

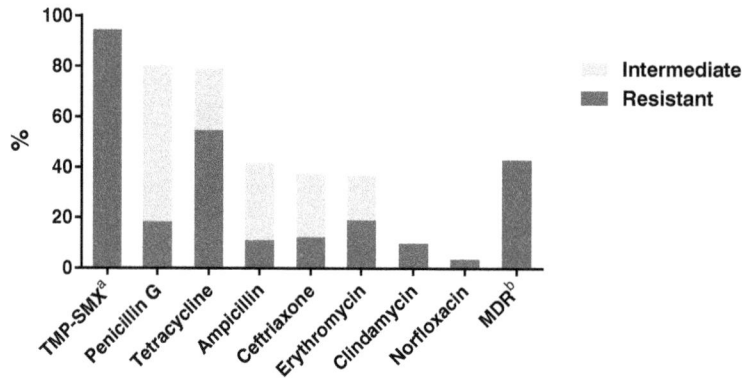

Fig. 2 The antimicrobial susceptibility pattern was determined in Bukavu, DR Congo for 163 pneumococcal strains isolated from healthy Congolese children. Disc diffusion tests were performed to detect reduced susceptibility to oxacillin, trimethoprim-sulfamethoxazole (TMP-SMX), tetracycline, erythromycin, clindamycin or norfloxacin (screening for fluoroquinolone resistance, i.e. levofloxacin and moxifloxacin). For oxacillin non-susceptible isolates, the minimal inhibitory concentration (MIC) was determined for penicillin G, ampicillin and ceftriaxone. [a]TMP-SMX = trimethoprim-sulfamethoxazole, [b]MDR = multi-drug resistant, i.e. non-susceptible to ≥3 classes of antibiotics including the beta-lactams

Serotype distribution

The serotypes or serogroups of the isolated pneumococci were determined by multiplex real-time PCR or by the modified Sequetyping protocol, both performed in Gothenburg, Sweden. Among the 32 living isolates the most common serotype was 19F ($n = 11$), followed by 11A/D ($n = 5$) and 35B/35C (n = 5). The pneumococcal capsular *cpsA* gene was detected in all viable isolates, confirming their species identification.

The serotypes/serogroups of the pneumococci that could not be re-cultured were determined by multiplex PCR after isolation of genomic material from the non-viable isolates

in the STGG storage medium ($n = 119$). In 62/119 cases (52%), one serotype/serogroup could be identified, whereas in 21 cases more than one serotype/serogroup was detected. Of these, two serotypes/groups were determined in 17 cases, three serotypes/groups in three cases, while one tube contained four serotypes/groups. In 36/119 cases (30%), no serotype or group could be determined by multiplex real-time PCR. The combined results for all 141serotypes/serogroups that were identified in the viable and non-viable pneumococcal isolates are shown in Fig. 3.

Hence, out of the 141 identified serotypes/serogroups, 76 (54%) belonged to a serotype/serogroup included in

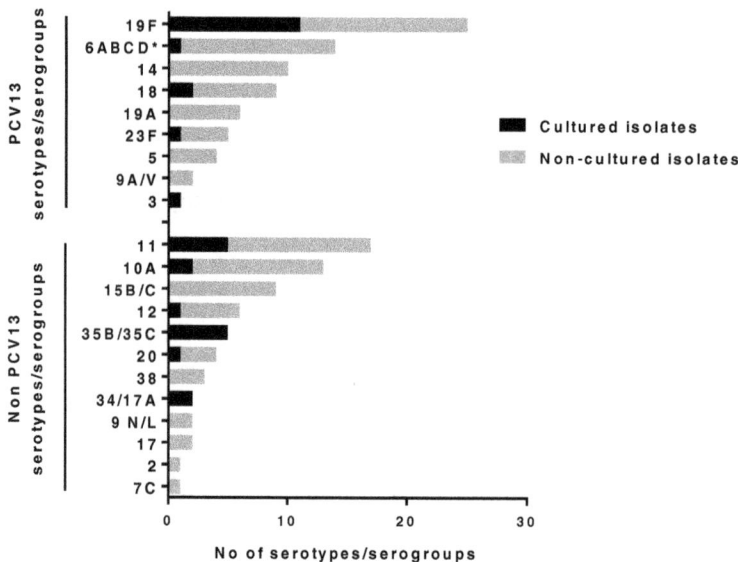

Fig. 3 The combined results of the 141 serotypes/serogroups identified by multiplex PCR or Sequetyping in the cultured, living pneumococcal isolates ($n = 32$) and by multiplex PCR in the non-viable pneumococcal isolates stored in tubes containing bacteria and STGG medium ($n = 83$). In 21 of these tubes containing non-viable bacteria, two or more serotypes/serogroups could be detected (two serotypes/serogroups in 17 cases; three serotypes/groups in three cases and four serotypes/groups in one case). * One culturable isolate could be determined by Sequetyping as 6B

High rate of antibiotic resistance among pneumococci carried by healthy children in the eastern...

225

PCV13. However, these 76 included 13 pneumococcal strains that could not be distinguished between 6A, 6B, 6C and 6D, of which only 6A and 6B are included in PCV13. Two further strains could not be separated between 9A and 9 V, of which only 9 V is included. Sixty-five (46%) of the identified serotypes/serogroups could, however, be categorised as non-PCV13-containing types/groups. Thus, the proportion of identified serotypes/serogroups belonging to PCV13 was similar to those not belonging to the vaccine. In the nine children who had received two or three doses of PCV13, vaccine serotypes/groups (*n* = 9) were as commonly detected as were serotypes/groups not included in the vaccine (*n* = 7). There was no significant difference in the distribution of penicillin non-susceptibility between strains whose serotypes/serogroups are included in the PCV13 compared to strains with non-vaccine serotypes/groups (Additional file 6).

In 113/119 non-viable isolates, the pneumococcal capsule gene, *CpsA*, could be detected in the STGG medium.

In the 36 samples, in which no serotype/serogroup could be identified using the multiplex real-time PCR method, the capsule gene, *CpsA*, was detected in 34 cases, verifying the presence of pneumococcal genomic material in the samples, and excluding a complete pneumococcal degradation during transport and storage.

Discussion

This is the first study to report the prevalence, serotype distribution and antimicrobial susceptibility of *Streptococcus pneumoniae* carried by healthy children in DR Congo.

By using culture for pneumococcal detection, we found that the prevalence of nasopharyngeal carriage was 21%. Generally higher levels of carriage have been reported from several other African countries, but there is also a great deal of variation between different regions [21, 32–35].

Differences in carriage rates can be due to geographical and regional variations, or to methodological differences. Limitations of the culture procedures in the present study include use of human blood in the agar plates. The pneumococci were initially identified in Bukavu, DR Congo, using the optochin test, which is not recommended as single test for *S. pneumoniae* identification [36]. However, molecular methods performed in Sweden confirmed the species identification in all but two isolates, either by detection of the pneumococcal capsular gene *CpsA*, or by serotype/serogroup determination. The low rate of positive culture in Sweden after storage and transport could be due to activation of the pneumococcal enzyme autolysin, LytA, which causes the bacterium to lyse and die. If activation of the autolysin also had an impact on the initial cultures performed in Bukavu can only be speculated upon. Apart from

potential methodological limitations, our relatively low detection rate could indeed reflect an early effect of the newly introduced pneumococcal conjugate vaccine. To our knowledge, only a few studies have determined the carrier rate of pneumococci among sub-Saharan children after the introduction of the pneumococcal conjugate vaccine [13, 16].

Our study showed that living in a rural area was associated with a higher rate of pneumococcal carriage than in an urban area, in agreement with other studies showing the socio-economic and geographical disparity of pneumococcal carriage [37, 38]. We also found a strong association between pneumococcal carriage and living in a house with an enclosed kitchen, i.e. with an open fire located inside the house, similar to what has been reported before [39]. Many studies have shown that an increased risk of pneumonia and other lower respiratory infections correlates with household air pollution and poverty, but few have studied the association with pneumococcal carriage. Hussey et al. have reported that air pollution alters pneumococcal biofilms, antibiotic tolerance and colonisation [40]. Here, we also confirm the relationship between malnutrition and pneumococcal carriage, as described before [37, 41, 42].

We found an increased prevalence of pneumococci with age, in agreement with the results from Niger [33], while other studies in Africa showed the contrary [38, 43, 44]. One explanation of this could be that the sampling started a few months after the introduction of a PCV13 vaccine programme in DR Congo. Since the children are given vaccine doses when they are six, ten and 14 weeks old, without a catch-up programme, most of the under 2 year olds were vaccinated, while most of the children older than 2 years of age were not. The majority of the children under 6 months of age had already received three doses of PCV13.

Although the vaccination status could not be confirmed by checking the immunisation child cards in all cases, but instead relied on self-reports of the caretakers, we found that PCV13 immunisation was highly protective against pneumococcal carriage. Only 3% of the children that had received two or three doses of PCV13 carried pneumococci, compared with approximately 30% in those that were unvaccinated or had only been given one dose. Among the 141 serotypes/serogroups that were identified, approximately half belonged to a serotype/serogroup included in PCV13, which is similar to other studies [38, 44–47]. Since 24% of the isolates could not be identified to serotype/serogroup and the fact that the multiplex PCR was developed mainly to cover PCV-containing serotypes, it is possible that the number of non-vaccine serotypes/serogroups could be even higher. In Kenya, the prevalence of vaccine serotypes was reduced from 34 to 13% after the introduction of PCV10 [13]. The predominant serotype circulating in the eastern part of DR Congo was found to be the vaccine-type 19F, corroborating the results from Mozambique [48] and Ghana [22]. We detected equally numbers of vaccine- and non-vaccine-serotypes/groups in the nine children who had received two or more doses of PCV13. The distribution of penicillin non-susceptible strains was also similar between the identified vaccine- and non-vaccine serotypes/groups, indicating a limited effect of PCV13 on the carriage of antibiotic resistant strains in the area shortly after introduction of the vaccine.

The relatively high prevalence of serotype 11A/D and 35B/35C, which are not included in the PCV13 vaccine, among the living isolates was unexpected and has not been reported in other African studies [21, 38, 49]. As there are no studies of pneumococcal carriage in DR Congo prior to the introduction of PCV13, no evaluation of serotype replacement can be performed.

In some of the samples containing non-viable pneumococci, we unexpectedly detected more than one serotype/serogroup, although the STGG medium was supposed to contain only one pure cultured pneumococcal isolate. This might reflect the difficulties to visually separate different pneumococcal strains according to their colony morphology on the agar plate, and also confirms other observations that children often carry more than one pneumococcal strain in nasopharynx [50, 51].

We found an association between antibiotic treatment within 1 month prior to sampling and pneumococcal carriage among the children, similar to a study from Iran [39], but contrary to the results from Kenya [52] and Niger [33]. This finding indicates the carriage of pneumococci resistant to antibiotics used in the area and we were in fact able to show alarmingly high resistance rates to the antibiotics commonly used in the eastern part of DR Congo. Amoxicillin (or intravenous ampicillin in severe cases) is recommended by the WHO as the first-line treatment for pneumonia. We found that 42% of the isolated pneumococci had reduced susceptibility to ampicillin, while the rate of non-susceptibility to benzylpenicillin was 80%. High rates of pneumococcal non-susceptibility to ampicillin and/or penicillin have been reported in other sub-Saharan countries [53, 54], but lower rates have also been observed [21, 22, 33]. There is some reported high resistance to TMP-SMX, as we found in this study (94%) [44, 55]. One of the rare post-PCV studies in sub-Saharan Africa reported a limited impact on antibiotic resistance [56]. TMP-SMX or co-trimoxazole and penicillin are the two most available and accessible antibiotics in DR Congo [57]. Self-medication is fairly common in the country, due to inadequate access to formal health care and the wide availability of antibiotics without prescription [57].

Due to the absence of a national antibiotic use policy in DR Congo, non-governmental organisations have introduced their guidelines on empirical antibiotic treatment recommendations, without having enough data on local antibiotic resistance rates. Until recently, co-trimoxazole was recommended as empirical treatment for acute lower respiratory infections in DR Congo, instead of amoxicillin, as recommended by the WHO, and the use of this antibiotic is still widespread in the country. In addition, in many cases, HIV-positive children are likely to be administered TMP-SMX as prophylaxis for *Pneumocystis jirovecii* infections, which might contribute to the development of TMP-SMX-resistant pneumococci.

In DR Congo, the cephalosporin ceftriaxone is the most commonly used antimicrobial drug for severe pneumococcal infections like meningitis. Here, we demonstrate a higher level of resistance (37%), compared with previous studies from Botswana [58] and Tanzania [21].

Moreover, many isolated pneumococcal strains also had reduced susceptibility to erythromycin, tetracycline and clindamycin. Notably, a large proportion of pneumococcal isolates (43%) were multi-drug resistant, i.e. non-susceptible to ≥3 classes of antimicrobial agents, in contrast to the situation in other countries close to DR Congo [21, 44, 53].

The high level of antimicrobial resistance found in our study can be explained by the absence of regulation for the use of antibiotics and no national guidelines for the management of frequent diseases in DR Congo. Moreover, there is an urgent need for microbiological competence and knowledge, as well as well-equipped laboratories, capable of clinical diagnostics and antibiotic resistance surveillance.

Conclusions

To conclude, this study was performed on healthy children below 5 years of age in the eastern part of DR Congo after the introduction of PCV13. Living in rural areas, having an enclosed kitchen with an open fire and undernutrition correlated with higher pneumococcal carriage and PCV13 vaccination with a lower carriage rate. Moreover, it highlights an alarmingly high level of reduced susceptibility to commonly used antibiotics, especially ampicillin and ceftriaxone, among the isolated pneumococcal strains. This underlines the need for new antibiotic treatment guidelines, as well as necessitating local and national antibiotic resistance surveillance programmes.

Abbreviations
CARe: Center for Antibiotic Resistance ResearchGothenburg; CDC: Centers for Disease Control and Prevention; CI: Confidence interval; DR Congo: Democratic Republic of the Congo; ENA: Emergency Nutrition Assessment; EUCAST: European committee on antimicrobial susceptibility testing; HIV: Human immunodeficiency virus; MIC: Minimum inhibitory concentration; MSF: Médecins Sans Frontières; OR: Odds ratio; PCV: Pneumococcal conjugate vaccine; PCV10: 10 valent pneumococcal conjugate vaccine; PCV13: 13 valent pneumococcal conjugate vaccine; PCV7: 7-valent pneumococcal conjugate vaccine; TMP-SMX: Trimethoprim-sulphamethoxazole; WHO: World Health Organisation

Acknowledgements
Acknowledgments to the Gothenburg University Research Fund for starting up research in global health.

Our sincere appreciation is also due to all the staff at Panzi Hospital, Kaziba Hospital, the Malkiya Wa Amani health centre, the Muhanzi health centre, the Kadutu BDOM health centre, the Muku health centre and the Nyantende health centre for their co-operation and collaboration in this study.

We thank the staff at the Clinical Laboratory, Microbiology Department, at Panzi Hospital, especially Maombi Chibashimba Ezekiel and Mugisho Muhandule David, for assisting Balthazar and Erick in performing excellent lab work.

Funding
This study was supported by the Sahlgrenska Academy, University of Gothenburg. The funding body had no role in the design of the study, the collection, analysis, interpretation of data, nor in writing of the manuscript.

Authors' contributions
SS, RA and RN designed and supervised the study. AMB, JM1, DC, LM, BM2, JM2 and NK obtained consent from the parents/guardians to participate, acquired information for the questionnaires and collected the samples. Further, AMB, BM1, TK, EM assisted by local lab-technicians performed the lab-work in DR Congo and ME, LG, ES, AMB and SG performed the lab-work in Sweden. AMB analysed the data with close communication with SS, RA and RN under the orientation of statistician at Goteborg University. AMB was mainly responsible for writing the manuscript which was critically revised by SS, RA, RN, and ML. All authors read and approved of the final manuscript.

Competing interests
The authors declare that they have no competing interests.

Author details
[1]Department of Infectious Diseases, Institute of Biomedicine, University of Gothenburg, Gothenburg, Sweden. [2]Panzi Hospital, Bukavu, Democratic Republic of the Congo. [3]Université Evangélique en Afrique, Bukavu, Democratic Republic of the Congo. [4]CARe – Center for Antibiotic Resistance Research, Gothenburg University, Gothenburg, Sweden. [5]Hôpital Général de Référence de Panzi, BP: 266 Bukavu, DR, Congo.

References
1. Zar HJ, Ferkol TW. The global burden of respiratory disease-impact on child health. Pediatr Pulmonol. 2014;49(5):430–4.
2. Rudan I, Boschi-Pinto C, Biloglav Z, Mulholland K, Campbell H. Epidemiology and etiology of childhood pneumonia. Bull World Health Organ. 2008;86(5): 408–16.
3. Hea W. Global, regional, national, and selected subnational levels of stillbirths, neonatal, infant, and under-5 mortality, 1980–2015: a systematic analysis for the Global Burden of Disease Study 2015. Lancet. 2017;388(Issue 10053):1725–74.
4. Lea L. Global, regional, and national causes of under-5 mortality in 2000–15: an updated systematic analysis with implications for the sustainable development goals. Lancet. 2016;388(Issue 10063):3027–35.
5. Amouzou A, Velez L, Tarekegn H, Young M. One is too many: ending child deaths from pneumonia and diarrhoea; 2016.
6. Troeger C, Forouzanfar M, Rao PC, Khalil I, Brown A, Swartz S, Fullman N, Mosser J, Thompson RL, Reiner RC Jr. Estimates of the global, regional, and national morbidity, mortality, and aetiologies of lower respiratory tract infections in 195 countries: a systematic analysis for the global burden of disease study 2015. Lancet Infect Dis. 2017;17(11):1133 61.
7. Ram PK, Dutt D, Silk BJ, Doshi S, Rudra CB, Abedin J, Goswami D, Fry AM, Brooks WA, Luby SP, et al. Household air quality risk factors associated with childhood pneumonia in urban Dhaka, Bangladesh. Am J Trop Med Hyg. 2014;90(5):968–75.
8. Shibata T, Wilson JL, Watson LM, LeDuc A, Meng C, Ansariadi LAR, Manyullei S, Maidin A. Childhood acute respiratory infections and household environment in an eastern Indonesian urban setting. Int J Environ Res Public Health. 2014;11(12):12190–203.
9. Karki S, Fitzpatrick AL, Shrestha S. Risk factors for pneumonia in children under 5 years in a teaching Hospital in Nepal. Kathmandu Univ Med J (KUMJ). 2014;12(48):247–52.
10. Panosian Dunavan C. From cookstoves to oxygen concentrators: a few important tools can help tackle global respiratory disparities. Am J Respir Crit Care Med. 2012;186(9):811–2.
11. SBea G. Respiratory risks from household air pollution in low and middle income countries. Lancet Respir Med. 2014;2(10):823–60.
12. Geno KA, Saad JS, Nahm MH. Discovery of novel pneumococcal serotype 35D, a natural WciG-deficient variant of serotype 35B. J Clin Microbiol. 2017; 55(5):1416–25.
13. Hammitt LL, Akech DO, Morpeth SC, Karani A, Kihuha N, Nyongesa S, Bwanaali T, Mumbo E, Kamau T, Sharif SK, et al. Population effect of 10-valent pneumococcal conjugate vaccine on nasopharyngeal carriage of Streptococcus pneumoniae and non-typeable Haemophilus influenzae in Kilifi, Kenya: findings from cross-sectional carriage studies. Lancet Glob Health. 2014;2(7):e397–405.
14. DMea W. Serotype replacement in disease after pneumococcal vaccination. Lancet. 2011;378(9807):1962–73.
15. Roca A, Bojang A, Bottomley C, Gladstone RA, Adetifa JU, Egere U, Burr S, Antonio M, Bentley S, Kampmann B. Effect on nasopharyngeal pneumococcal carriage of replacing PCV7 with PCV13 in the expanded Programme of immunization in the Gambia. Vaccine. 2015;33(51):7144–51.
16. Klugman KP. Herd protection induced by pneumococcal conjugate vaccine. Lancet Glob Health. 2014;2(7):e365–6.
17. Roca A, Hill PC, Townend J, Egere U, Antonio M, Bojang A, Akisanya A, Litchfield T, Nsekpong DE, Oluwalana C, et al. Effects of community-wide vaccination with PCV-7 on pneumococcal nasopharyngeal carriage in the Gambia: a cluster-randomized trial. PLoS Med. 2011;8(10):e1001107.
18. Van Boeckel TP, Gandra S, Ashok A, Caudron Q, Grenfell BT, Levin SA, Laxminarayan R. Global antibiotic consumption 2000 to 2010: an analysis of national pharmaceutical sales data. Lancet Infect Dis. 2014;14(8):742–50.
19. Grouzard V, Rigal J, Sutton M. Clinical guidelines: Diagnosis and treatment manual for curative programmes in hospitals and dispensaries: guidance for prescribing. 7th revised ed. Medecins Sans Frontieres. 2007. ISBN 978-2-37585-029-9. http://www.refbooks.msf.org/.
20. World Health Organization. Antimicrobial resistance: global report on surveillance. World Health Organization; 2014. www.who.int/drugresistance/documents/surveillancereport/en/.
21. Moyo SJ, Steinbakk M, Aboud S, Mkopi N, Kasubi M, Blomberg B, Manji K, Lyamuya EF, Maselle SY, Langeland N. Penicillin resistance and serotype distribution of Streptococcus pneumoniae in nasopharyngeal carrier children under 5 years of age in Dar Es Salaam, Tanzania. J Med Microbiol. 2012;61(7):952–9.
22. Dayie NT, Arhin RE, Newman MJ, Dalsgaard A, Bisgaard M, Frimodt-Moller N, Slotved HC. Penicillin resistance and serotype distribution of Streptococcus pneumoniae in Ghanaian children less than six years of age. BMC Infect Dis. 2013;13:490.
23. Hanke CR, Grijalva CG, Chochua S, Pletz MW, Hornberg C, Edwards KM, Griffin MR, Verastegui H, Gil AI, Lanata CF, et al. Bacterial density, serotype distribution and antibiotic resistance of pneumococcal strains from the nasopharynx of Peruvian children before and after pneumococcal conjugate vaccine 7. Pediatr Infect Dis J. 2016;35(4):432–9.
24. Klugman KP, Madhi SA, Huebner RE, Kohberger R, Mbelle N, Pierce N. A trial of a 9-valent pneumococcal conjugate vaccine in children with and those without HIV infection. N Engl J Med. 2003;349(14):1341–8.
25. Tomczyk S, Lynfield R, Schaffner W, Reingold A, Miller L, Petit S, Holtzman C, Zansky SM, Thomas A, Baumbach J. Prevention of antibiotic-nonsusceptible invasive pneumococcal disease with the 13-valent pneumococcal conjugate vaccine. Clin Infect Dis. 2016;62(9):1119–25.
26. Tyrrell GJ, Lovgren M, Chui N, Minion J, Garg S, Kellner JD, Marrie TJ. Serotypes and antimicrobial susceptibilities of invasive Streptococcus pneumoniae pre-and post-seven valent pneumococcal conjugate vaccine introduction in Alberta, Canada, 2000–2006. Vaccine. 2009;27(27):3553–60.
27. ENA 2011(july 9: *smartmethodologyorg//smart-emergency-nutrition-assessment/e.*

28. http://www.eucast.org/clinical_breakpoints/: *wwweucastorg/clinical_breakpoints/* Accessed 29 Sept 2017.

29. Neves FP, Cardoso NT, Souza AR, Snyder RE, Marlow MM, Pinto TC, Teixeira LM, Riley LW. Population structure of Streptococcus pneumoniae colonizing children before and after universal use of pneumococcal conjugate vaccines in Brazil: emergence and expansion of the MDR serotype 6C-CC386 lineage. J Antimicrob Chemother. 2018;73(5):1206–12.

30. O'Brien KL, Bronsdon MA, Dagan R, Yagupsky P, Janco J, Elliott J, Whitney CG, Yang Y-H, Robinson L-GE, Schwartz B. Evaluation of a medium (STGG) for transport and optimal recovery of Streptococcus pneumoniae from nasopharyngeal secretions collected during field studies. J Clin Microbiol. 2001;39(3):1021–4.

31. Heid CA, Stevens J, Livak KJ, Williams PM. Real time quantitative PCR. Genome Res. 1996;6(10):986–94.

32. Usuf E, Bojang A, Camara B, et al. Maternal pneumococcal nasopharyngeal carriage and risk factors for neonatal carriage after the introduction of pneumococcal conjugate vaccines in The Gambia. Clinical microbiology and infection. 2018;24(4):389-95.

33. Ousmane S, Diallo BA, Ouedraogo R, Sanda AA, Soussou AM, Collard JM. Serotype distribution and antimicrobial sensitivity profile of Streptococcus pneumoniae carried in healthy toddlers before PCV13 introduction in Niamey, Niger. PLoS One. 2017;12(1):e0169547.

34. Usuf E, Bottomley C, Adegbola RA, Hall A. Pneumococcal carriage in sub-Saharan Africa--a systematic review. PLoS One. 2014;9(1):e85001.

35. Rutebemberwa E, Mpeka B, Pariyo G, Peterson S, Mworozi E, Bwanga F, Kallander K. High prevalence of antibiotic resistance in nasopharyngeal bacterial isolates from healthy children in rural Uganda: a cross-sectional study. Ups J Med Sci. 2015;120(4):249–56.

36. Satzke C, Turner P, Virolainen-Julkunen A, Adrian PV, Antonio M, Hare KM, Henao-Restrepo AM, Leach AJ, Klugman KP, Porter BD, et al. Standard method for detecting upper respiratory carriage of Streptococcus pneumoniae: updated recommendations from the World Health Organization pneumococcal carriage working group. Vaccine. 2013;32(1):165–79.

37. Coles CL, Rahmathullah L, Kanungo R, Katz J, Sandiford D, Devi S, Thulasiraj RD, Tielsch JM. Pneumococcal carriage at age 2 months is associated with growth deficits at age 6 months among infants in South India. J Nutr. 2012;142(6):1088–94.

38. Usuf E, Badji H, Bojang A, Jarju S, Ikumapayi UN, Antonio M, Mackenzie G, Bottomley C. Pneumococcal carriage in rural Gambia prior to the introduction of pneumococcal conjugate vaccine: a population-based survey. Trop Med Int Health : TM & IH. 2015;20(7):871–9.

39. Mirzaei Ghazikalayeh H, Moniri R, Moosavi SG, Rezaei M, Yasini M, Valipour M. Serotyping, antibiotic susceptibility and related risk factors aspects of nasopharyngeal carriage of Streptococcus pneumoniae in healthy school students. Iran J Public Health. 2014;43(9):1284–90.

40. Hussey S, Purves J, Allcock N, Fernandes VE, Monks PS, Ketley JM, Andrew PW, Morrissey JA. Air pollution alters Staphylococcus aureus and Streptococcus pneumoniae biofilms, antibiotic tolerance and colonisation. Environ Microbiol. 2017;19(5):1868–80.

41. Verhagen LM, Hermsen M, Rivera-Olivero IA, Sisco MC, de Jonge MI, Hermans PWM, de Waard JH. Nasopharyngeal carriage of respiratory pathogens: significant relationship with stunting. Tropical Med Int Health. 2017;22(4):407–14.

42. Rylance J, Kankwatira A, Nelson DE, Toh E, Day RB, Lin H, Gao X, Dong Q, Sodergren E, Weinstock GM. Household air pollution and the lung microbiome of healthy adults in Malawi: a cross-sectional study. BMC Microbiol. 2016;16(1):182.

43. Adetifa IM, Antonio M, Okoromah CA, Ebruke C, Inem V, Nsekpong D, Bojang A, Adegbola RA. Pre-vaccination nasopharyngeal pneumococcal carriage in a Nigerian population: epidemiology and population biology. PLoS One. 2012;7:e30548.

44. Assefa A, Gelaw B, Shiferaw Y, Tigabu Z. Nasopharyngeal carriage and antimicrobial susceptibility pattern of Streptococcus pneumoniae among pediatric outpatients at Gondar University hospital, north West Ethiopia. Pediatr Neonatol. 2013;54(5):315–21.

45. Kamng'ona AW, Hinds J, Bar-Zeev N, Gould KA, Chaguza C, Msefula C, Cornick JE, Kulohoma BW, Gray K, Bentley SD, et al. High multiple carriage and emergence of Streptococcus pneumoniae vaccine serotype variants in Malawian children. BMC Infect Dis. 2015;15:234.

46. Kandasamy RGM, Thapa A, Ndimah S, Adhikari N, Murdoch DR, et al. Multi-Serotype Pneumococcal Nasopharyngeal Carriage Prevalence in Vaccine Naïve Nepalese Children, Assessed Using Molecular Serotyping. PloS one. 2015;10(2):e0114286 doi:10.1371/journal. pone.0114286(PLoS ONE 10(2): e0114286. doi:10.1371/journal. pone.0114286):PLoS ONE 10(12): e0114286. doi:0114210.0111371/journal. pone.0114286.

47. Kellner JD, McGeer A, Cetron MS, Low DE, Butler JC, Matlow A, Talbot J, Ford-Jones EL. The use of Streptococcus pneumoniae nasopharyngeal isolates from healthy children to predict features of invasive disease. Pediatr Infect Dis J. 1998;17(4):279–86.

48. Vallès X, Flannery B, Roca A, Mandomando I, Sigaúque B, Sanz S, Schuchat A, Levine M, Soriano-Gabarró M, Alonso P. Serotype distribution and antibiotic susceptibility of invasive and nasopharyngeal isolates of Streptococcus pneumoniae among children in rural Mozambique. Tropical Med Int Health. 2006;11(3):358–66.

49. Adegbola RA, Hill PC, Secka O, Ikumapayi UN, Lahai G, Greenwood BM, Corrah T. Serotype and antimicrobial susceptibility patterns of isolates of Streptococcus pneumoniae causing invasive disease in the Gambia 1996–2003. Tropical Med Int Health. 2006;11(7):1128–35.

50. Rivera-Olivero IA, Blommaart M, Bogaert D, Hermans PW, de Waard JH. Multiplex PCR reveals a high rate of nasopharyngeal pneumococcal 7-valent conjugate vaccine serotypes co-colonizing indigenous Warao children in Venezuela. J Med Microbiol. 2009;58(Pt 5):584–7.

51. Brugger SD, Frey P, Aebi S, Hinds J, Muhlemann K. Multiple colonization with S. pneumoniae before and after introduction of the seven-valent conjugated pneumococcal polysaccharide vaccine. PLoS One. 2010;5(7):e11638.

52. Abdullahi O, Karani A, Tigoi CC, Mugo D, Kungu S, Wanjiru E, Jomo J, Musyimi R, Lipsitch M, Scott JA. The prevalence and risk factors for pneumococcal colonization of the nasopharynx among children in Kilifi District, Kenya. PLoS One. 2012;7(2):e30787.

53. Kobayashi M, Conklin LM, Bigogo G, et al. Pneumococcal carriage and antibiotic susceptibility patterns from two crosssectional colonization surveys among children aged <5 years prior to the introduction of 10-valent pneumococcal conjugate vaccine — Kenya, 2009–2010. BMC Infect Dis. 2017;17:25 10.1186/s12879-016-2103-0(10.1186/s12879-016-2103-0):10.1186/s12879-12016-12103-12870.

54. Joloba ML, Bajaksouzian S, Palavecino E, Whalen C, Jacobs MR. High prevalence of carriage of antibiotic-resistant Streptococcus pneumoniae in children in Kampala Uganda. Int J Antimicrob Agents. 2001;17:395–400.

55. Mills RO, Twum-Danso K, Owusu-Agyei S, Donkor ES. Epidemiology of pneumococcal carriage in children under five years of age in Accra, Ghana. Infect Dis (Lond). 2015;47(5):326–31.

56. Cheung Y-B, Zaman SM, Nsekpong ED, Van Beneden CA, Adegbola RA, Greenwood B, Cutts FT. Nasopharyngeal carriage of Streptococcus pneumoniae in Gambian children who participated in a 9-valent pneumococcal conjugate vaccine trial and in their younger siblings. Pediatr Infect Dis J. 2009;28(11):990–1.

57. Tsakala T, Tona G, Mesia K, Mboma J, Vangu J, Voso S, Kanja G, Kodondi K, Mabela M, Walo R. Évaluation des prescriptions dans le traitement du paludisme et de la gastroentérite en milieu hospitalier: Cas des hôpitaux Bondeko et St Joseph à Kinshasa (République démocratique du Congo). Cahiers d'études et de recherches francophones/Santé. 2005;15(2):119–24.

58. Huebner RE, Wasas A, Mushi A, Mazhani L, Klugman K. Nasopharyngeal carriage and antimicrobial resistance in isolates of Streptococcus pneumoniae and Haemophilus influenzae type b in children under 5 years of age in Botswana. Int J Infect Dis. 1998;3(1):18–25.

24

A formative study exploring perceptions of physical activity and physical activity monitoring among children and young people with cystic fibrosis and health care professionals

James Shelley[1]* , Stuart J Fairclough[1,4], Zoe R Knowles[1], Kevin W Southern[2], Pamela McCormack[3], Ellen A Dawson[1], Lee E F Graves[1] and Claire Hanlon[1]

Abstract

Background: Physical activity (PA) is associated with reduced hospitalisations and maintenance of lung function in patients with Cystic Fibrosis (CF). PA is therefore recommended as part of standard care. Despite this, there is no consensus for monitoring of PA and little is known about perceptions of PA monitoring among children and young people with CF. Therefore, the research aimed to explore patients' perceptions of PA and the acceptability of using PA monitoring devices with children and young people with CF.

Methods: An action research approach was utilised, whereby findings from earlier research phases informed subsequent phases. Four phases were utilised, including patient interviews, PA monitoring, follow-up patient interviews and health care professional (HCP) interviews. Subsequently, an expert panel discussed the study to develop recommendations for practice and future research.

Results: Findings suggest that experiences of PA in children and young people with CF are largely comparable to their non-CF peers, with individuals engaging in a variety of activities. CF was not perceived as a barrier per se, although participants acknowledged that they could be limited by their symptoms. Maintenance of health emerged as a key facilitator, in some cases PA offered patients the opportunity to 'normalise' their condition. Participants reported enjoying wearing the monitoring devices and had good compliance. Wrist-worn devices and devices providing feedback were preferred. HCPs recognised the potential benefits of the devices in clinical practice.
Recommendations based on these findings are that interventions to promote PA in children and young people with CF should be individualised and involve families to promote PA as part of an active lifestyle. Patients should receive support alongside the PA data obtained from monitoring devices.

Conclusions: PA monitoring devices appear to be an acceptable method for objective assessment of PA among children and young people with CF and their clinicians. Wrist-worn devices, which are unobtrusive and can display feedback, were perceived as most acceptable. By understanding the factors impacting PA, CF health professionals will be better placed to support patients and improve health outcomes.

Keywords: Youth physical activity promotion, Fitbit, GENEActiv, ActiGraph, Qualitative

* Correspondence: J.Shelley@2016.ljmu.ac.uk
[1]Physical Activity Exchange, Research Institute for Sport and Exercise Sciences, Liverpool John Moores University, 62 Great Crosshall Street, Liverpool L3 2AT, England
Full list of author information is available at the end of the article

Background

Cystic Fibrosis (CF) affects approximately 11,000 individuals in the United Kingdom (UK), with median predicted survival reported as 45 years of age [1]. CF is an autosomal recessive disorder caused by mutation of the CF Transmembrane Conductance Regulator (*CFTR*) gene. The CFTR protein has an important role in co-ordinating transepithelial salt transport, which impacts on a number of important physiological functions [2]. Most importantly, the salt transport defect impairs mucociliary airway clearance by disrupting the airway surface liquid and predisposing the airway to a build-up of excess and viscous mucus. Subsequent chronic airway infection and inflammation lead to airway damage and eventual respiratory failure as the primary cause of early death [1]. In addition, the CF defect impacts on other epithelial surfaces, such as the sweat gland, pancreas and liver [3].

CF is also characterised by reduced exercise capacity [4] and, although the exact mechanisms are not yet fully understood, physical inactivity, pulmonary, cardiac, and peripheral skeletal muscle function all contribute [5]. Critically, higher aerobic fitness is associated with reduced mortality in patients with CF and therefore provides useful prognostic information [4]. Furthermore, physical activity (PA) is related to aerobic fitness, independent of sex, lung function, body size and muscle power [6], with higher PA associated with a slower decline in lung function [7] and fewer hospitalisations [8]. There is good evidence that PA has a positive impact on bone mineral density [9], glycaemic control [10] and mucociliary clearance [11], all of which contribute to wellbeing for a person with CF.

PA promotion and exercise prescription are currently recommended as part of standard CF care, alongside chest physiotherapy [12]. Despite the documented benefits and clinical recommendations there is some evidence to suggest that children with CF engage in less strenuous PA than age-matched controls [13]. The reduction in PA has been attributed to a number of perceived barriers including progressive lung function decline, symptoms of breathlessness, coughing and fatigue [14] as well as the burdensome treatment regimen associated with CF [15]. High treatment burden may influence the acceptability of additional measures such as PA monitoring. Additionally, patients with CF are experts in their condition and are typically very engaged in their medical care and self-care. They would need to value PA monitoring to make PA assessment feasible.

In order to provide guidance on PA, clinicians require knowledge of population specific barriers and facilitators for PA as perceived by children and young people with CF. Despite PA assessment and advice being perceived as important by clinicians, PA assessment is not common or consistent in CF centres [16]. Moreover, there is no consensus for monitoring or reporting of PA in CF [16]. There is little known about perceptions and acceptability of PA monitoring among children and young people with CF. Previous research has highlighted the need to better understand self-efficacy for PA and suggests that self-monitoring is central to all PA behaviours [17]. Though this research does not specifically refer to self-monitoring via monitoring devices it is possible that PA monitoring devices may feed into this self-monitoring process. Accordingly, exploring clinicians' knowledge and perceptions of PA monitoring as well as those of the patients is needed to move towards the utilisation of PA monitoring devices as part of routine clinical care.

Methods
Ethical considerations

Ethical approval was sought and granted by South West Cornwall and Plymouth National Health Service (NHS) Research Ethics Committee and Liverpool John Moores University Ethics Committee prior to data collection. NHS Caldicott principles were strictly adhered to throughout, all data were anonymised and all personal details kept confidential. Parents/carers written consent and participants' written assent were obtained. Parents/carers were also invited to be present during their child's interviews.

The Medicines for Children Research Network Clinical Trials Network (MCRN) consultative group situated at Alder Hey Children's NHS Foundation Trust, were consulted to appraise the 'appropriateness' of the language used in the study participant information sheets, consent forms and interview schedule. To ensure face validity, the interview schedule was reviewed during development, prior to phase one commencement.

Aims

The overarching aim of the research was to explore the use of PA monitoring devices with children and young people with CF. As part of this, our objectives were to: (1) explore barriers, facilitators and perceptions of PA among children and young people with CF; (2) explore the acceptability of a range of PA monitoring devices; (3) explore clinicians' existing knowledge and perceptions of PA monitoring, and; (4) explore the clinical application of PA monitoring as part of routine clinical care as well as identifying any disease specific limitations to PA monitoring.

Design

An action research approach was utilised to achieve the study objectives whereby an iterative approach was used with findings from earlier research phases informing subsequent phases, of which there were four in total (see Additional file 1). The first included patient interviews to explore perceptions of PA. The second phase included the allocation of PA monitoring devices. Phase three had two components which ran simultaneously. The first included follow-up patient interviews informed by phases one and two. The second included health care professional interviews. Phase four included an adapted consensus approach, involving an expert panel to discuss the study findings, to develop recommendations and to inform future research directions. A researcher trained in qualitative research methods (CH) conducted all interviews and subsequent analysis.

Participants

Participants were recruited from the CF clinic at Alder Hey Children's Hospital. Potential participants were identified by members of the usual care team from the clinic database. Inclusion criteria included participants aged between 8 and 16 years, with a confirmed diagnosis of CF. Initially, potential participants were approached during their routine clinical appointments by a member of their CF care team, who briefly explained the purpose of the study. Parents/carers of children and young people who expressed an informal interest were later formally invited to participate in the study by a researcher via telephone. From 13 potential participants initially identified, 9 formally agreed to participate (5 female; mean age 12 ± 3 years). The remaining 4 either verbalised they were no longer willing to participate or the researcher was unable contact their parents/carers.

Procedure

Phase 1

An open-ended, semi-structured interview protocol was devised using the principal enabling, reinforcing and predisposing factors of the Youth Physical Activity Promotion Model (YPAPM) [18]. The YPAPM is consistent with the socio-ecological model of health promotion and describes the hypothesised influences of diverse correlates on children's and young people's PA participation. Use of the YPAPM facilitated the development of a theory-driven interview schedule that would elicit beliefs and attitudes towards PA and reveal psychological enablers and barriers of PA as perceived by each individual, whilst allowing the researcher to explore individual nuances relating to the experience of PA in children and young people with CF.

Semi-structured interviews were conducted between children and young people with CF and the researcher (CH). It was felt that parent/carer presence would be reassuring for the participants, creating a positive and comfortable interview environment. In the interest of inclusivity some interview questions were directed specifically towards the parent/carer, however these questions were separated before analysis. Parents/carers were also asked, where appropriate, to prompt their child only to expand upon examples given when explaining their experiences of PA and not to respond directly for them. Interviews were arranged to take place at a time and place most convenient to the participants parents/carers, the majority were in the participants own home, with one at Alder Hey Children's NHS Foundation Trust Hospital.

Data analysis Participants were assigned a participant number (P1–P9) to protect participant confidentiality. Data analysis utilised a broad model of interpretative phenomenology as described by Fereday et al. [19]. Identification of emerging themes at the manifest level were discussed and coded between two researchers (CH & ZK) following each interview. Resultant themes were further discussed with reference to the interview data until final themes were determined and clustered around the YPAPM. As a result, no new themes were identified following interview with P9. Transcripts were deductively and inductively coded, illustrative quotes were extracted and clustered around emergent themes anchored according to the main factors of the YPAPM.

Phase 2

Phase 2 commenced midway through phase 1 and the two phases ran concurrently until the final participant interview was completed.

Each of the 9 participants were allocated PA monitoring devices to assess their acceptability in children and young people with CF. Allocation ensured that each participant received a research grade device alongside a consumer level device. Participants wore either a GENEActiv (ActivInsights Ltd., Cambs, UK) or ActiGraph GT3X+ (ActiGraph, Pensacola, FL) triaxial accelerometer on the non-dominant wrist or left hip, respectively. Both devices have demonstrated acceptable validity and reliability for use with children and young people [20]. In addition to the accelerometers participants were allocated either a Yamax Digiwalker pedometer (Yamax UK and Europe, Tasley UK) or one of two consumer level PA trackers; 'Fitbit Flex' or 'Moves' smartphone application (Table 2). Unfortunately, only one participant was able to trial the 'Moves' application, as it required participants to have a compatible smartphone. Participants were asked to wear the devices for seven consecutive days and were provided with instructions for how to wear the devices as well as an information sheet. Participants were asked to wear the devices during waking hours, unless engaging in water-based activity. Participants were instructed to clip the pedometer onto the waistband of their clothing or to wear the Fitbit on their wrist like a watch. The participant using the 'Moves' application was informed that the application is always running and that they should keep their phone on their possession throughout the day and to use it as usual. Additionally, participants allocated a Fitbit device were shown how to access the Fitbit dashboard, although were not given specific instructions about how to use the available features, as the researchers did not want to influence how participants explored such features.

After trialling each device participants were asked to complete a short questionnaire to obtain a self-reported measure of satisfaction of using the devices (see Additional file 2). This comprised of 10 statements, which required participants to rate their response along a 5-point Likert scale. The 'Moves' application questionnaire only comprised of 9 of the relevant statements and Likert scales, excluding a question relating to the comfort of wearing a device. The questionnaire served to provide preliminary information to inform subsequent interviews.

Data analysis Both the GENEActiv and ActiGraph tri-axial accelerometers were initialised to record data at a frequency of 100 Hz using GENEActiv PC software (version 2.2, Activinsights, Cambs, UK) and ActiLife software (version 6.11.0, ActiGraph corp, Pensacola, FL) respectively. The raw ActiGraph and GENEActiv data files were processed in R (http://cran.r-project.org) using the GGIR package (version 1.5–7) which autocalibrated the raw triaxial accelerometer signals [21]. Accelerometer wear time inclusion criteria were a minimum of 600 min·day^{-1} for at least any 3 days [22]. Non-wear was estimated on the basis of the standard deviation and value range of each accelerometer axis, calculated for moving windows of 60 min with 15 min increments [23], which has been applied previously in studies involving children [24]. For each 15 min period detected as non-wear time over the valid days, missing data were replaced by the mean value calculated from measurement on other days at the same time of day [21].

The self-report questionnaires were analysed to assess compliance with the remaining devices and to inform Phase 3. The questionnaire also provided information relating to the experience of wearing each device, which were explored further in phase 3.

Phase 3
Following the action research approach, phase 1 and 2 findings were formative to the methodology used during phase 3. Phase 3 consisted of patient follow-up interviews and health care professional (HCP) interviews.

Participant interviews The remaining participants were invited to participate in the follow-up semi-structured interviews with the PA data collected in phase 2 reported back to patients as part of the interview. Interview questions focussed upon the experiences and

opinions of each participant's acceptability of the PA devices allocated during phase 2. Individualised interview schedules were designed for each participant, informed by participant's individual responses to the phase 2 feedback questionnaires, and also their activity and sedentary levels as measured by their allocated accelerometry device. In addition, related themes of acceptability pertaining to the influence of others (family and peers) and change in PA (attitudes and behaviours) were explored.

Health care professional interviews During phase 1 participants identified the Clinical Lead Consultant for CF (HCP-C), a Dietitian with special interest in CF (HCP-D) and a Specialist Physiotherapist in CF (HCP-P) as key members of the multi-disciplinary CF team. Therefore, during phase 3, three one-to-one semi-structured interviews were conducted to explore the clinicians' perceptions of PA monitoring in children and young people with CF. The semi-structured interview schedule consisted of 15 open-ended questions to explore opinions, existing knowledge and experience of using PA monitoring devices, including, the perceived benefits and barriers of using PA monitoring devices and acceptability of using PA monitoring devices as part of routine clinical practice (see Additional file 3). In addition to the HCP interviews, an online survey was disseminated to Physiotherapists across the UK, via regional CF representatives. The survey consisted of 5 questions designed to explore issues concerning the promotion of PA and the feasibility of using PA monitoring in clinical practice. The results of which converged with data from the HCP interviews and are therefore discussed together throughout.

Phase 4
A single round consensus technique was used to examine the findings of previous phases, to develop evidence-based recommendations and to direct future research. To reflect on the findings in the context of a real-world clinical setting participation of the HCPs was essential. However, due to their clinical duties, it was not feasible to follow the iterative process representative of the Delphi consensus technique in its entirety, hence the single round technique was adopted. An expert focus group was developed, consisting of five expert-members including HCPs and researchers. The Clinical Lead Consultant and Specialist Physiotherapist in CF who participated in the earlier phases of the research participated in the focus group, unfortunately the Dietitian was unable to accept the invitation to participate in the focus group due to clinical commitments. Two researchers from within the PA field also participated in the focus group, one with expertise in PA monitoring and exercise prescription in children and a second with expertise as a

Sports and Exercise Psychologist. The focus group was facilitated by an additional researcher (CH). In total, 5-expert-members attended the meeting, which was recorded using a Dictaphone and transcribed verbatim (Additional file 4).

Members were provided with a working document (see Additional file 5) in advance of the focus-group meeting. The document outlined the session structure and summarised the key findings from phases 1–3. Members independently reviewed the summary to formulate their own opinions concerning PA monitoring among children and young people with CF ahead of the meeting.

Principles of the nominal consensus technique were applied to develop a structured session for the expert-members panel (see Additional file 6). Drawing upon their respective expertise, each member was invited to present 2 or 3 relevant questions and/or statements which they perceived to be priority issues in the use of PA monitoring among children and young people with CF. Once each member had explicitly stated their ideas, a discussion between panel members was initiated to explore and expand upon the issues identified. Equal attention was given to areas of consensus and non-consensus, areas of agreement and non-agreement were each discussed. Priority issues were noted and organised into themes. Panel members also independently ranked each issue, according to their perceived priority

significance within the relevant theme and collectively. This was completed after the meeting via email, which allowed members privacy to reflect upon and consider the key priorities and discussion points (see Additional file 7). This was returned to the facilitator who organised the emerging issues (Table 3).Qualitative data are reported following the consolidated criteria for reporting qualitative research (COREQ) checklist (see Additional file 8).

Results
Phase 1
Nine interviews were conducted, recorded using a Dictaphone and transcribed verbatim. Interviews lasted between 39 and 94 min (mean = 61.5 min), generating 247 pages (Arial font, size 12 double spaced) and 554 min of audio data. Barriers and facilitators to PA are outlined in (Table 1). Individuals with CF engage in a variety of activities and enjoy PA. Maintenance of health and improved fitness emerged as a key facilitator of PA, with participants recognising the prospective long-term benefits of PA. Participants acknowledged the reinforcing influence that parents/carers, peers and coaches have on PA engagement, in promoting family cohesiveness and normalising the condition. Further to this, the CF Physiotherapist was highlighted as being the most influential member of the CF team in reinforcing PA engagement.

Table 1 Illustrative quotes exploring PA perceptions among children and young people with CF

Physical activity participation	Enabling factors		Perceived barrier	Perceived enabler
			Limited PA facilities available locally	Community activities facilitated by private clubs (Thai boxing, football, dance, table tennis, gymnastics) and/or local authorities.
			"A few more different clubs that do different sports that are around, because there isn't many." (P4, pg7, lines 306–307).	The swimming centre up the road, and out there is a big Astro Turf…so I'll usually go there, and the other places are sports clubs and stuff." (P2, pg7, lines 301–302).
			Limited time available to introduce and explore new activities	Curricular physical education (PE) and additional non-structured activities such as walking to and from school and play during recess.
			"Maybe if I'd seen a game or something on the telly, or one of my mates was going to somewhere and said that "it's good". "You should come and try it". I might have a go, but I probably wouldn't, because I don't really have time…" (P7, pg10, lines 431–440).	"I don't do any out of school, but in school, apart from PE I do football at breaks and dinners." (P3, pg3, lines 120–121).
				Autonomy promoted by independent travel
				"I can do it [travel] on my own. It's like I'm not dependent on everyone else to do it for me." (P7, pg9, lines 361–362).
				"It's either a lift or, because it's across the [name of local] field across the road, so I can just walk over to that…" (P6, pg8, lines 326–327).
	Predisposing factors	Am I able?	Participants attributed poor PA-related performance to CF related symptoms, such as breathlessness, fatigue and pain.	CF was not perceived as a barrier to PA per se.

Table 1 Illustrative quotes exploring PA perceptions among children and young people with CF *(Continued)*

"I can do it [PA], but not as good as other people…I get tired quicker than them, or out of breath more quicker. I can do it to a certain point, but then I have to stop." (P3, pg13, lines 573–579).

For some this results in frustration, anger and boredom;

"Well, it's a bit annoying, because they're all doing it, and I'm sat at the side, and it winds me up that I should be able to do it, but I just can't." (P3, pg13, lines 584–585).

CF- related illness can render participants incapable of engaging in PA.

"…Like when I'm ill I feel like I can't do anything. I'm sitting on the couch and watching TV, and I'm not doing much." (P9, pg23, lines 1004–1005).

Is it worth it? Some participants reported disliking the experience of pain, fatigue and breathlessness associated with PA;

"(I dislike) The way you get tired and out of breath sometimes." (P3, pg23, line 1025).

"That now and then it gives you the pains the next day. Like you're dragging your legs up the stairs the next day." (P9, pg35, lines 1517–1518).

Reinforcing factors Parental support can generate a negative affect;

"I did a mile on the treadmill the other day, and Dad was like, "No, you're going to do another one… (I feel like) I'm going to slap him. Push him off his bike. You do another mile!" (P7, pg12, lines 493–503).

"…there's nothing really…wrong with me I can still do it…I'm not stuck like at home or in hospital. I'm out, like able to do anything, really." (P1, pg12, lines 515–525).

"I know just because I've got CF doesn't mean I can't do it [PA]." (P3, pg23, lines 1020–1021).

"… I have to do twice as much as my mate, to do what my mates do, so then when I can do what my mates are doing I just feel better, because I know that it doesn't show that it's affecting me, and I can keep up with my mates and just do all the exercise and everything." (P6, pg20, lines 846–849).

Perceptions of current well-being

"…'cos I am generally quite well, I can do it." (P7, pg16, line 702).

"I tend to have quite a high lung function, and I don't really get ill a lot…" (P7, pg17, line 707).

All participants report enjoying PA. Enjoyment also appears to be inextricably linked to physical benefits gained through PA

"I like it [PA] because it helps my chest and stuff." (P2, pg19, line 864)

Participants also recognise health benefits associated with PA, both in the short and long term.

"…it [PA] keeps you active and your lungs clear, and instead of just sitting in hospital or something." (P1, pg14, lines 631–632).

Engaging in PA becomes a normaliser;

"It's just like you're doing it because you can, and you want to. You kind of feel the same as everyone else for an hour and a half…" (p7, pg19, lines 803–804).

Family support and encouragement

…my Mum always like, not makes me go, but if like I'm just too tired, I don't want to, she'd be like, "Oh no, come on, let's get out or something." (P1, pg14, lines 641–643).

Peer support

"…my friends who knock on for me, they are dead nice because they always ask if I'm ok if I'm out of breath and stuff when I'm out playing footy and stuff." (P2, pg21, lines 942–944).

"Like one of us wins a race or wins a game or something, I can go, "Oh yes, well, I've got CF", and then it's like pulling a CF card…I just find it funny, because they're like, "Aaaaaaah! She's done it again"…we have a laugh about it…." (P7, pg13–14, lines 565–574).

Significant coaches (conventional and novel, including PE teachers) influence

"Well, a mixture of everyone. There isn't really anyone that influences me any more than

A formative study exploring perceptions of physical activity and physical activity monitoring among...

235

Table 1 Illustrative quotes exploring PA perceptions among children and young people with CF *(Continued)*

someone else… Family, people in the CF team, my PE teachers." (P4, pg11, lines 498–503).
The CF specialist physiotherapist was identified by participants (P2, 3 and 9) as the CF clinician who most encourages them to be physically active. Participants also perceive health-related information and advice to be trustworthy and reliable;
"I think that it's good advice, and that I should take it." (P1, pg11, line 482).
Family facilitating activity (e.g. driving to sports clubs or engaging in family activities)
"My Mum or Dad would usually take me." (P4, pg7, line 279).

Illustrative quotes anchored to the Youth Physical Activity Promotion Model [18]. *'Enabling factors'* allow individuals to engage in PA, including environmental factors (access to facilities, weather and safety), levels of fitness and skill which are impacted by perceived competence. *'Predisposing factors'* increase the likelihood of an individual engaging in PA: *'Is it worth it?* (Benefits and costs associated with PA) which includes attitudes and beliefs and interests and enjoyment of PA. *'Am I able?'* (Perceived competence and self-efficacy). *'Reinforcing factors'* reinforce an individual's PA behaviour (e.g. parents/carers, peers and coaches influence PA behaviour directly and indirectly).

Phase 2

Participant 3 was hospitalised during the period that they were asked to wear the ActiGraph, and subsequently withdrew from the study. Due to data files being corrupted, data for P2, P5 and P6 was not available for analysis. Compliance and mean wear time were generally good (Table 2).

Phase 3

Participant interviews

Eight interviews were conducted, recorded using a Dictaphone and transcribed verbatim. Interviews lasted between 27 min and 75 min (mean = 40.6 min), generating 130 pages and 324.5 min of audio data (Additional file 9). Transcripts were deductively and inductively coded, illustrative quotes were extracted and clustered around emergent themes.

Exploration of participant's opinions, experiences and acceptability of the allocated devices resulted in the emergence of a number of themes including wear-ability, device feedback and compliance.

Wear-ability

Wear-ability of the research-based devices proved to be problematic for many participants. Participants reported finding the "watch-like" designs easier to wear, with some participants citing issues with the fitting, positioning and comfort of the ActiGraph hip-worn device.

Table 2 Reporting participant characteristics, compliance and wear time from GENEActiv and ActiGraph accelerometers

P	Age Group (Years)	Gender	Allocated device(s)	Compliance (Days worn)	Valid days included (≥10 h·day)	Mean wear time (h)
1	≤10	Female	ActiGraph & Pedometer	6	4	12.5
2	> 10	Male	ActiGraph & Fitbit			
3	> 10	Male	ActiGraph & Pedometer			
4	> 10	Male	GENEActiv	7	6	16.3
5	≤10	Female	ActiGraph & Pedometer			
6	> 10	Male	GENEActiv & Smartphone			
7	> 10	Female	GENEActiv	6	6	13.3
8	≤10	Male	GENEActiv & Fitbit	7	4	23.3
9	> 10	Female	GENEActiv & Fitbit	7	6	14.8

The data presented are from the research devices which are able to provide objective data. A self-report questionnaire was used to assess compliance of the consumer level devices and acceptability, which is further explored in Phase 3

"The Fitbit was basically just like wearing a watch, but the ActiGraph kept getting in the way of when I'd be doing my PE and stuff" (P2, pg4, lines 145–146).

"Well, I liked wearing the wrist one because I just liked it more than the other [ActiGraph]...it didn't have anything for me to do on it, but it kept falling down at my waist and then making my waist really itchy and stuff." (P2, pg1, lines 36–45).

"because, do you know when you put it on the side, it hurts...it did hurt when I was doing some jogging" (P5, pg2–3, lines 62–70).

Participants trialling the GENEActiv commented on the thickness of the wrist strap, some finding it interfered with activities

"It was just a bit thick, and it got in my way of doing general activities I do every day, and I had to be careful that I didn't knock it and stuff like that, and it was quite thick. People noticed it a lot more, and was asking me about it, thinking it was a watch, and then when they actually saw it there was no watch... I was just a bit like, oh..." (P9, pg1, lines 27–30).

whilst others found it didn't interfere with activities.

"it didn't get in the way of me doing anything, or didn't prevent me from doing anything either..." (P4, pg1, lines 35–36).

The visual appearance of the devices often attracted attention from others. This was not perceived to be an issue by some participants, though for some older participants this attention was unwanted, with one opting to tell inquisitive others that the device was a broken watch.

"They just asked what it was and what it did, and someone asked what the time was with the GENEActiv, and I had to say, "Oh no, it's not a watch, it's a blah, blah, blah..." (P7, pg4, lines 180–182).

"They'd just ask for the time and I'd get my phone out, and they'd be like, "Why didn't you just use your watch?" I'd be like, "because it's this monitoring thing for the hospital", or like my Mum said, "It's broke." (P6, pg5, lines 142–144).

The consumer level Fitbit with a smaller rubber strap was perceived to be more comfortable than the research-based device and proved favourable.

"It was a lot more comfortable, the Fitbit. It looks 'slicker', it looks smarter than a big bulky thing." (P8, pg2, lines 74–75).

P6 did not encounter any problems having their smartphone on their person whilst engaging in PA.

"Well I usually carry my phone everywhere anyway, so it didn't really affect me." (P6, pg12, line 382).

Device feedback

The LED display of the consumer devices was reported as a desirable feature, with participants enjoying the interactive nature of these devices.

"It was fun to know that I could look back and see how much I was doing...how many calories I've burned, how many steps I took, which was good." (P4, pg1, lines 25–31).

The information provided by these devices also facilitated self-monitoring for some participants assuring them they had achieved adequate levels of PA.

"I suppose it taught me that what I was doing, I was doing it right. Like playing table tennis, I was actually doing the right amount of activity that I should be" (P4, pg13, lines 566–567).

Other participants found the level of information available and interactive dashboard to be overwhelming and complicated, with some opting not to use it at all.

"It was a bit confusing with too much going on, so it was hard to use." (P7, pg13, line 581).

P6 reported that the smartphone based application provided sufficient PA-related information and was simple to use.

"I didn't really dislike anything, because it was so simple, and showed you what you wanted to see." (P6, pg12, lines 376–377).

The research-based devices do not provide participants with PA-related information or feature a display.

Compliance

Some compliance issues were highlighted when discussing results derived from the accelerometry data. Exploration of whether participants remembered to wear their devices or used any strategies to do so revealed that wearing the devices became integrated into their daily routines.

"I just think it feels like a natural thing, like say you're getting ready for school in a morning, it's like you get your t-shirt on, and you put it on basically, like natural." (P1, pg4, lines 107–108).

Leaving their device close to where they slept acted as an adequate prompt for participants.

"Well, I kept it next to where I sleep, so as soon as I woke up I'd put it on." (P4, pg3, line 132).

Although, one participant found that despite leaving it by their bedside, they forgot to wear their GENEActiv device.

"I didn't forget with the Fitbit, but I could just keep it on all the time...I think I forgot with the GENEActiv because you have to take it off at night, so I might forget to put it on in the morning." (P7, pg4, lines 148–151).

Participants opted to remove the devices during activities due to concerns about damaging the devices and/or causing injury to others.

"Well, usually when we go on the field, we always just run after each other, like taking each other out...but I wouldn't go too mad on doing that compared to what I normally do... If I take someone down, I won't just damage whatever it is." (P2, pg6, lines 255–258).

"so you actually might hurt someone else, and you might hurt yourself in gymnastics" (P7, pg4, lines 140–141).

Summary
Overall, participants reported that they enjoyed testing the devices, stating a preference for wrist-worn devices and devices that allowed interaction and feedback. Compliance was generally good, suggesting that the devices were not a significant burden, although P5 did not provide sufficient wear time.

Health care professional interviews
Three interviews were conducted, recorded using a Dictaphone and transcribed verbatim. Interviews lasted between 46 min and 55 min (mean = 51.3 min), generating 38 pages and 154 min of audio data. Transcripts were deductively and inductively coded, illustrative quotes were extracted and clustered around emergent themes.

The online Physiotherapist survey had 30 respondents, 93% (*n* = 28) of respondents agreed that PA monitoring devices could influence their clinical practice. Qualitative data provided are consolidated and discussed with data obtained from the HCP interviews.

Exploration of HCP's opinions, experiences and acceptability of the PA devices for PA monitoring also resulted in the emergence of a number of themes including, perceived benefits, perceived barriers, and patient and families' acceptability.

Existing knowledge
None of the HCP's had previously used PA monitoring as part of their clinical practice. HCP-C and HCP-P reported using consumer devices and applications to assess their personal PA levels, though HCP-P did acknowledge concerns about the validity of these devices.

PA is not formally measured as part of routine clinical practice, however an exercise test is administered as part of a patient's annual review. Whilst the exercise test offers clinically relevant and prognostic information, it does not provide information about daily PA, which was perceived to be a limitation.

"...the once a year test will prove what they do on that day, and it doesn't tell us how they do their normal week, cope on a day-to-day week, so we don't have any kind of measure about what they do, other than subjective, them telling us, "I do, and I'm fine". You don't have that information, so I suppose this just gives you over a period of time, if it's a week or whatever, or two weeks if they were an in-patient, it would give us kind of better understanding of how they're functioning on a day-to-day level." (HCP-P, pg11, lines 411–416).

PA was reported to be informally discussed on an individual basis and advice may be given accordingly although this is not standardised.

"I will ask them what they do, what sports they do, and how active they are, particularly if we're having problems with weight gain or weight loss, so say for example you have somebody present to you who's maybe lost a significant amount of weight, so part of that discussion will be about are you doing more activity, have you joined any other groups, are you doing more planned activity, trying to look at reasons why they might have lost weight. We don't formally measure how much activity they've done and what the energy cost of that is..." (HCP-D, pg4, lines 128–140).

This reveals that, for these practitioners, current assessments are not sufficient in providing information about habitual PA, therefore individualised interventions to promote PA are limited to informal discussions and generic PA advice.

Perceived benefits

Although experience of using PA measurement devices in clinical practice was limited, there was consensus among HCP's that PA monitoring devices offered a number of potential benefits.

It was perceived that PA monitoring could provide an *'objective'* measure of PA, which would allow HCP's and patients to track PA alongside markers of health over a given period.

> *"I think, I suppose, trying to help young people to see that actually being physically inactive is potentially having an impact on their health and on their respiratory function, and helping them to see that if they can just increase their activity a bit, then that might have a positive impact on their respiratory health." (HCP-D, pg5, lines 185–188).*

Objective PA measurement is often used to inform development and evaluation of interventions to promote PA [25, 26] and was highlighted by HCP-C as missing from current practice.

> *"...I think we need a more consistent approach across the team, so it will help that. We can formalise more of our interventions with the patients, but we don't know what those interventions should be, but we can be a bit more robust about it, a bit more sort of systematic, as opposed to just making it up as we go along, which is kind of what we do at the moment." (HCP-C, pg9, lines 312–315).*

The potential for using the devices as an intervention in themselves was also acknowledged particularly in respect of a motivational aid.

> *"I think it would be maybe even a realism about what they do, or how little they do, or it reassures them that they're doing enough, if they're doing a lot. Certainly from our experience of monitoring when they do their nebulisers, they have been very very, surprised when they know what they've done, compared to what they think they've done. So I think that the effect might be, "Oh my God, I thought I was doing lots more than that", or it might motivate them to do better, to improve." (HCP-P, pg8, lines 293–298).*

HCP-C concedes that informing a patient of their low PA may have a detrimental effect, rather than encourage PA.

> *"...the ones we need to target are the ones who hate physical activity, who find gymnasiums an abomination. And we have a significant number of patients like that, and also quite a large proportion of our young women who are fourteen, fifteen, sixteen, exercise seems to be a non-cool thing for young girls particularly, to do. So those are the challenges we face. Now I've absolutely no hesitation to feel that our well-motivated patients will completely embrace this and will love it, and will get a lot out of it, and actually use it in their lives, and that'll be great for them. But I have extreme anxieties how [sedentary patients] will not in any way be helped by this kind of monitoring. I don't know. That might not be true. I don't know what the answer is. If you monitor somebody and show them that the level of activity they're doing is woeful, then that may motivate them to take a step forward themselves, and try and sort it out. I suspect not, but I don't know." (HCP-C, pg5, lines 151–161).*

Acceptability

Owing to the perceived benefits of the devices, there was strong acceptability amongst the HCP's that devices could become part of their routine care, progressing the service and moving with innovation.

> *"we could very easily fit it into what we do. We have a very good relationship with our families, a respectful relationship, and we have the capacity within our care programme to sort of slot it in. We have plenty of time. We see them regularly in clinic every two to three months. We do annual review, obviously every year, and we see them in between times. Our families are very engaged, they're very empowered, they want to do things for the better, on the whole, and they're very keen to take on, to embrace new developments and new technologies." (HCP-C, pg4, lines 132–137).*

It was reported that use of the devices would be the responsibility of the CF Physiotherapist, (HCP-P, pg10, lines 386–390) and although some scepticism was anticipated from more established members of the CF team, it was felt that the importance of PA would supersede any resistance to the acceptability of the devices.

> *"I think generally everyone can appreciate the importance of exercise, but there is some definite variability amongst the team as to how we do that, and how important people feel it is." (HCP-C, pg11, lines 394–396).*

Aside from the acceptability among HCP's, the importance of working in partnership with patient families was highlighted.

"I think we would really need to have families on board in partnership, and it would be something that they would need to see as a routine part of their CF care rather than just something that is a bit different and a bit special." (HCP-C, pg4, lines 116–119).

Nevertheless, HCP-C felt that patients and families would embrace the integration of technology-based strategies to improve the management of CF, as demonstrated by the acceptance of other medical device such as the I-neb.

"Well, I think that the relationship you have with your team, your CF team, is a very close relationship. It's not always a relationship based on the greatest amount of honesty, and in those cases it's just a bit tricky, but we've kind of dealt with a lot of these issues with a lot of our aerosol delivery devices, and are now able to incorporate data logging, so we have dealt with these issues with the i-neb, and we've been able to sort of sit down with the families and the young person in a very open way, and say...'Just looking over the course of three months, we've seen you've gone from being a hundred per cent adherent to what you're doing, to sort of just doing it once a day or whatever, and they're going, "Yes, it's a real struggle. Maybe we could go down to once a day". So working in that open way has worked, I think, and we've been able to do some really good stuff in improving adherence in our patients with CF, and support them with treatments that they might be finding difficult or impossible.'" (HCP-C, pg10, lines 356–374).

In order to maintain standards of patient care a number of considerations were suggested as needing to be addressed prior to the implementation of PA monitoring devices including; cost-effectiveness, available resources, staffing, cross-contamination and accuracy of the devices.

"I think handling data is the key thing, and making sure that the data is readily available in a way that's readily understood, both professionals and the family." (HCP-D, pg11, lines 413–414).

"I think we need to know what monitors and which are the best...We need to decide what information we need from them as to what benefit they're going to be. So I think that's one of the key issues, and I think they also need to be relatively affordable...And cleanable,

and from that aspect, so that they can be wiped down." (HCP-P, pg11, lines 394–398).

Summary

HCP's acknowledged that overall their current practice does not include adequate measurement of PA or sufficient interventions to promote PA engagement. HCP's recognised the potential benefits that PA monitoring devices could have in clinical monitoring, informing interventions and motivating patients on an individual basis. Acceptability among the CF team was good, with the Physiotherapist deemed as the individual most likely to be responsible for using the devices. A number of potential barriers will require consideration prior to use as part of routine care.

Phase 4

Priority issues emerging from the focus group were organised into three themes, patient-related issues, clinical practice issues and research issues as outlined in Table 3.

Patient-related issues

The theme of a 'lifestyle based approach to PA' centred on parental influences on PA through their reinforcement and facilitating of PA to promote PA engagement as a *'part of normal life'*. This was viewed by the expert members as an important patient-related issue, which should form part of any recommendations and may warrant further research, for example HCP-P noted;

"Really important is to continue ongoing education on the exercise with the patients and the families, throughout all ages and stages of disease progression, with discussion concerning expectations of the patient, the family and the therapist, and to reinforce that exercise and activity as a lifestyle choice rather than prescription, in order to improve compliance." (P3, pg3, lines 92–96).

The 'motivation is a key issue' theme included issues relating to the use of goal setting to promote PA and the impact that device feedback may have on motivation, either positively or negatively.

"You might get that instant feedback, but you don't know how to interpret that information correctly. That could have a negative impact on your motivation, or a positive impact, or no impact." (P4, pg18, lines 691–693).

Clinical practice issues

'Education (for practitioners, parents/carers and children and young people)' was identified as a key

Table 3 Displaying ranking of priority issues identified during phase 4

		Individual priority ranking				Sum total	Collective ranking
		HCP-C (P5)	HCP-P (P3)	Researcher 1 (P4)	Researcher 2 (P2)		
Part 1: Patient-Related Issues							
1	Lifestyle based approach to physical activity	5th	1st	2nd	1st	9	1st
5	Motivation is a key issue	2nd	2nd	1st	6th	11	2nd
6	Perceived importance of physical activity and the data retrieved by the devices	4th	5th	3rd	3rd	15	3rd
3	Experience of CF symptoms during physical activity	6th	3rd	4th	4th	17	4th
7	Importance of fitness over physical activity	3rd	7th	5th	2nd	17	5th
2	Decline of Physical activity	1st	4th	7th	8th	20	6th
4	Importance of clinical versus "field" testing of physical activity levels	7th	8th	6th	5th	26	7th
8	Structured vs. non-structured activity	8th	6th	8th	7th	29	8th
Part 2: Clinical Practice Issues							
2	Education (for practitioners, parents/carers and children and young people)	1st	1st	7th	2nd	11	1st
4	Importance of meaningful feedback	5th	5th	3rd	3rd	16	2nd
1	Role of feedback provided by devices	4th	6th	2nd	5th	17	3rd
9	Clinical barriers identified (cost, resources, time)	10th	2nd	4th	1st	17	4th
8	Issues of compliance raised	3rd	4th	5th	7th	19	5th
6	Sustainability of the physical activity engendered by the tool used in terms of:	2nd	7th	9th	6th	24	6th
7	Importance of accruing 7 days worth of physical activity data:	7th	8th	6th	4th	25	7th
10	Team message is important	6th	3rd	8th	8th	25	8th
3	Testing vs. Monitoring	8th	9th	1st	9th	27	9th
5	Distinction between the use of physical activity monitoring devices as a research tool vs. commercial tool	9th	10th	10th	10th	39	10th
Part 3: Research Issues							
1	Cost	5th	1st	1st	1st	8	1st
4	Children and young people involvement required to inform the research process	1st	2nd	3rd	4th	10	2nd
3	Type of data produced by research vs. commercial devices	2nd	3rd	2nd	5th	12	3rd
5	Literacy and understanding	3rd	4th	5th	3rd	15	4th
2	Issues of compliance	4th	N/A	4th	2nd	N/A	N/A

Expert members of the phase 4 focus group were asked to rank the issues discussed during the focus group meeting in order of priority

clinical practice issue and included education around physical activity monitoring and promotion. It was also suggested that this education could encompass an element of counselling.

"In terms of the education, I think that kind of counselling, it doesn't have to be a psychologist. It can be, that type of support can be offered in different ways through different roles, through training, through educating parents. It's not necessarily about parachuting a specific practitioner in. I guess it's looking for that opportunity, capacity, and the willingness to sort of take on board some of that, in the same way that exercise professionals who work in gyms, they're not exercise psychologists, but they are very much at the front end of applying principles of

exercise psychology in order to make sure that the people they address, whether it's the cardiac rehab plan or reducing obesity, whatever it is, they're sort of applying the technique." (P2, pg19, lines 698–706).

It was also viewed as important that both clinicians and patients are able to view and interpret the feedback obtained from the devices. This will have implications for the choice of device used and the balance between research data and feedback from consumer devices.

Research issues

A priority research issue that emerged was 'Cost', with members of the focus group stating that funding would be required to support further research in the area and the clinical use of PA monitoring devices.

> *"We need some funding to be able to do this."* (P2, pg23, line 855).

'Children and young people involvement required to inform the research processes' emerged as a recommendation from the focus group discussion.

> *"...they are very articulate and able to talk about these devices, and therefore in any future research we should make sure that it's not just research on children, it's research with, and alongside, and involve them in the design."* (P2, pg24, lines 896–898).

Summary
The focus group discussion, emergent themes and prioritisation of key issues were consolidated into a number of agreed recommendations and areas for consideration concerning the application of PA monitoring in clinical practice.

Recommendations from phase 4
Interventions to promote PA engagement in children and young people with CF should be individualised and involve family members to promote PA as part of an active lifestyle, as opposed to that referred to as prescribed exercise.

Patients should receive education and support alongside the PA data obtained from monitoring devices.

The process of developing interventions and their subsequent evaluations should involve patients and their families throughout the research process who, from the outcomes of this study, are well informed and able to contribute to such matters effectively.

Future research considerations
Consideration should be given to the impact that device feedback may have on motivation. It is acknowledged that patients and their parents/carers may respond to device feedback on an individual basis with some having a negative response.

The choice of device will influence a number of key issues identified including, motivation, meaningful feedback, cost and clinical application.

Discussion
Phase 1
We employed a socio-ecological model (YPAPM) [17] to facilitate a theory-driven, comprehensive approach to understanding the perceived enablers and barriers among this cohort. Collectively, findings indicate that

children and young people with CF engage in a variety of physical activities comparable to their non-CF peers. CF was not perceived as a barrier per se, although reduced exercise capacity and exercise related symptoms were reported to have a detrimental impact on PA engagement, as previously reported in children and young people with CF [27]. As in previous research, there was no evidence of PA avoidance as a result of CF related symptoms in the current study [19]. Rather, PA engagement offered an opportunity to *'normalise'* their condition by attaining PA levels similar to their non-CF peers. Whilst social comparison in this way can encourage PA engagement it can also be detrimental to PA engagement depending on the level of self-monitoring and perception of differences/similarities in PA ability [17].

Key facilitators of PA engagement were health and improved fitness. Key reinforcing factors were the influence of parents/carers, peers and HCPs who influence PA directly and indirectly. Direct influences include facilitating engagement through pursuing activities together, transport to activities or encouragement [17]. Indirect influences may include affecting predisposing factors, such as attitudes and beliefs (Is it worth it?) or perceived confidence and self-efficacy (Am I able?) [17]. Individuals who report positive PA experiences also report receiving family support and encouragement [14].

Phase 2 and phase 3
Findings suggest that children and young people with CF are mostly compliant with wearing a range of PA monitoring devices, which is further explored in phase 3.

When determining the feasibility of using PA monitors in clinical practice, guidelines set by Bowen et al. [28] were utilised, the primary areas of evaluation were acceptability, implementation, practicality and integration. Qualitative data supported the acceptability of PA monitoring devices among both patients and clinicians. A number of issues relating to the visual appearance and comfort of some of the devices were identified, with better acceptability reported for wrist-worn devices. Qualitative data obtained from HCPs suggests that implementation of PA monitoring into routine clinical care may be feasible. The data collected from the current study suggests that PA monitoring in clinical care may be limited by practicality. The number of devices which did not provide data due to technical faults was high (4 out of 9), which may limit the feasibility of using these device in clinical practice. However, accelerometers are widely used in clinical research and typically device failure is much lower than reported in the current study [29]. Data from the five devices which did not experience any malfunctions provided usable PA data, demonstrating good participant compliance, as indicated by valid wear time. Demand was not specifically assessed as PA monitoring formed part of a wider researcher study, therefore it was not possible to determine if patients' decision to not take part was a result of PA monitoring specifically or the study more broadly. Of the 13 participants screened only 9 (70%) were willing to participate, which may suggest moderate demand.

From the follow-up interviews three themes were identified; wear-ability, device feedback and compliance. The visual appearance and comfort of the devices was perceived as important, with wrist-worn devices reported to be more favourable. A combination of these factors may contribute to improving compliance to wrist-worn devices [24, 30]. Feedback from devices was also preferred, as it allowed self-monitoring and provided motivation. Monitoring devices may have a role in clinical practice as a motivation tool, and though there remains a lack of evidence to support clinical use [31], acceptability of the devices was high among HCPs who felt that devices have the potential to provide clinically relevant information which could improve current practice. The data from the current study does not allow comparisons to be made between the acceptability of the consumer level devices and the research grade devices, though only the research grade devices are supported by evidence of reliability and validity [16]. The CF Physiotherapist was identified as best placed to implement the use of PA monitoring devices, although the wider CF team also have a role in promoting PA and supporting monitoring. In addition to Physiotherapists, CF centres are increasingly employing members of staff specifically to deliver exercise testing and prescription [32, 33] and may have additional interest and/or qualifications in exercise-related fields, making them well placed to utilise PA monitoring in the clinical setting.

Phase 4

Patient related priority issues included a lifestyle-based approach to increase PA and the importance of motivation and family involvement. Clinical priorities included education alongside PA monitoring (for clinicians, patients and parents/carers), and the requirement for meaningful feedback. A wrist-worn device capable of providing research level data, which can be interpreted and analysed by clinicians, whilst also featuring a display for time or user feedback if desired would appear to be acceptable amongst both patients and clinicians (e.g. the ActiGraph GT9X Link, although there are a number of devices available).

The cost of using monitoring devices in clinical practice was also identified as a priority issue. Consumer level devices may offer a lower cost alternative to research based devices and may be perceived to be more 'stylish' and less obtrusive. Although beyond the scope of the current paper, the clinimetric properties (reliability, validity and responsiveness) of research grade devices has been reviewed elsewhere [16], providing evidence for their use. Consumer level technology is constantly improving, and a number of devices have become commercially available since this research was conducted which may offer validity comparable to research grade devices, with further improvements anticipated in future [34]. Though agreement with research grade devices is good, validity of consumer devices remains highly variable, which may cause concern for clinical use [34]. A third party software package 'Fitabase' (Small Steps Labs LLC, San Diego, CA) has recently become available, which allows Fitbit data to be analysed in a similar manor to the research devices. The choice of device may ultimately be determined by the requirement for user feedback and whilst user feedback is avoided in observational research to control for the risk of participant reactivity, it may be appealing for PA interventions as users can view a range of variables (steps, activity, energy expenditure etc.) [34]. However, HCPs expressed concern that device feedback may be demotivating in some children and young people with CF, suggesting feedback would be best given as part of a package of care delivered from with the CF team, which also included education and support.

Limitations

A number of limitations are present in the study. Whilst there is a small sample collected form a single centre, the study design allowed for the collection of in depth qualitative data taking a broad perspective with representatives of patients and clinicians. Participants were active and well at the time of recruitment and the self-selecting nature of recruitment perhaps resulted in a sample of patients already motivated to be physically active. It is not known if similar findings would be seen in patients with more severe disease or at the time of an exacerbation. However, HCPs are experienced working with a variety of patients through periods of fluctuating health, which will have informed their responses during the interviews and prioritisation of key issues. Not all participants approached agreed to partake in the study and we did not explore their reasons for refusal. A number of technical malfunctions occurred with the PA monitoring devices, although this is a risk associated with monitoring PA in free-living, the number of issues in the present study was greater than anticipated.

Conclusions

PA monitoring devices appear to be an acceptable method for the objective assessment of PA among children and young people with CF and their clinical team, though further research is required to determine the validity and reliability of consumer level devices. Wrist-worn devices that are unobtrusive and can display feedback are most acceptable for patients and clinicians.

Experiences of PA among children and young people with CF are largely comparable to their non-CF peers, with individuals engaging in a variety of activities. CF was not perceived as a barrier per se, although participants acknowledged that they could be limited by their symptoms.

HCPs perceive monitoring devices to be a beneficial addition to routine clinical care, although education for clinicians, patients and families is required. Health professionals expressed enthusiasm for PA monitoring, but caution that the information is processed in a positive manner in partnership with the young people.

Future considerations

This study highlights that whilst PA monitoring has potential as a clinical tool, future work is required to develop a programme of education and support to allow clinicians to utilise the devices, followed by support for patients and families with the aim to understand and use the data obtained for the devices to promote PA engagement as part of an active lifestyle.

A variety of PA monitoring devices are widely available, with each offering a range of different features. Careful consideration should be given to the purpose of monitoring PA in order to select an appropriate device. A device which can be bespoke for individual patients is required to control the use of feedback as a motivational tool to allow for self-monitoring whilst avoiding negative impact.

Further exploration of perceptions of PA throughout childhood and adolescents will improve understanding of how children and young people with CF conceptualise PA. By understanding the factors impacting on PA, CF health care professionals will be better placed to support patients and improve health outcomes. Further research exploring children and young people's perceptions of PA monitoring devices being used as part of routine CF care may also be warranted.

Abbreviations

CF: Cystic fibrosis; CFTR: Cystic Fibrosis Transmembrane Conductance regulator; HCP: Health care professional; MCRN: Medicines for Children Research Network Clinical Trials Network; MVPA: Moderate-Vigorous physical activity; NHS: National Health Service; PA: Physical activity; UK: United Kingdom; YPAPM: Youth Physical Activity Promotion Model

Acknowledgements

The authors would like to thank the patients and families who volunteered to participate in the study, the CF team at Alder Hey Children's NHS Foundation Trust Hospital and the Medicines for Children Research Network Clinical Trials Network (MCRN) for their assistance throughout the study.

Funding

Funding was provided by the British United Provident Association (BUPA) UK foundation Seed Corn fund, which was awarded to Prof. Stuart Fairclough. The funding body were not involved in any aspect of the study design, data collection, data analysis or manuscript preparation/review.

Authors' contributions

Conception and design, SJF, ZRK, KWS, PM, LEFG and CH; Acquisition of data, SJF, ZRK, KWS, PM, LEFG and CH; Analysis and interpretation of data, JS, SJF, ZRK, EAD and CH; Manuscript preparation, JS; Manuscript review, JS, SJF, ZRK, KWS, PM, EAD, LEFG and CH. All authors read and approved the final manuscript.

Competing interests

The authors declare that they have no competing interests.

Author details

[1]Physical Activity Exchange, Research Institute for Sport and Exercise Sciences, Liverpool John Moores University, 62 Great Crosshall Street, Liverpool L3 2AT, England. [2]Department of Women's and Children's Health, University of Liverpool, Institute in the Park, Alder Hey Children's Hospital, Eaton Road, L12 2AP Liverpool, England. [3]Respiratory Department, Alder Hey NHS Foundation Trust Children's Hospital, Eaton Road, Liverpool L12 2AP, England. [4]Edge Hill University, St Helens Road, Ormskirk, Lancashire L39 4QP, England.

References

1. Jeffery A, Charman S, Cosgriff R, Carr S. UK Cystic Fibrosis Registry Annual Data Report 2016; 2017. p. 80.
2. Zielenski J. Genotype and phenotype in cystic fibrosis. Respiration. 2000;67: 117–33.
3. Davies JC, Alton EWFW, Bush A. Cystic fibrosis. BMJ. 2007;335:1255–9.
4. Nixon PA, Orenstein DM, Kelsey SF, Doershuk CF. The prognostic value of exercise testing in patients with cystic fibrosis. N Engl J Med. 1992;327: 1785–8.
5. Almajed A, Lands LC. The evolution of exercise capacity and its limiting factors in cystic fibrosis. Paediatr Respir Rev. 2012;13:195–9.
6. Hebestreit H, Kieser S, Rüdiger S, Schenk T, Junge S, Hebestreit A, et al. Physical activity is independently related to aerobic capacity in cystic fibrosis. Eur Respir J. 2006;28:734–9.
7. Schneiderman JE, Wilkes DL, Atenafu EG, Nguyen T, Wells GD, Alarie N, et al. Longitudinal relationship between physical activity and lung health in patients with cystic fibrosis. Eur Respir J. 2014;43:817–23.
8. Cox NS, Alison JA, Button BM, Wilson JW, Morton JM, Holland AE. Physical activity participation by adults with cystic fibrosis: an observational study. Respirology. 2016;21:511–8.
9. Tejero García S, Giráldez Sánchez MA, Cejudo P, Quintana Gallego F, Dapena J, García Jiménez R, et al. Bone health, daily physical activity, and exercise tolerance in patients with cystic fibrosis. Chest. 2011;140:475–81.
10. Beaudoin N, Bouvet GF, Coriati A, Rabasa-Lhoret R, Berthiaume Y. Combined exercise training improves glycemic control in adult with cystic fibrosis. Med Sci Sports Exerc. 2016;49:231–7.
11. Dwyer TJ, Alison JA, McKeough ZJ, Daviskas E, Bye PTP. Effects of exercise on respiratory flow and sputum properties in patients with cystic fibrosis. Chest. 2011;139:870–7.
12. Swisher AK, Hebestreit H, Mejia-downs A, Lowman JD. Exercise and habitual physical activity for people with cystic fibrosis : An Expert Consensus-Based Guide for Advising Patients. Cardiopulm Phys Ther J. 2015;26:85–98.
13. Jantzen A, Opoku-Pare M, Bieli C, Ruf K, Hebestreit H, Moeller A. Perspective on cystic fibrosis and physical activity: is there a difference compared to healthy individuals? Pediatr Pulmonol. 2016;51:1020–30.
14. Moola FJ, Faulkner GE, Schneiderman J. "No time to play": perceptions toward physical activity in youth with cystic fibrosis. Adapt Phys Act Q. 2012;29:44–62.
15. Prasad SA, Cerny FJ. Factors that influence adherence to exercise and their effectiveness: application to cystic fibrosis. Pediatr Pulmonol. 2002;34:66–72.
16. Bradley J, O'Neill B, Kent L, Hulzebos E, Arets B, Hebestreit H, et al. Physical activity assessment in cystic fibrosis: a position statement. J Cyst Fibros. 2015;14:e25–32.

17. Street R, Mercer J, Mills-Bennett R, O Leary C, Thirlaway K. Experiences of physical activity: a phenomenological study of individuals with fibrosis. J Health Psychol. 2014;21:261–70.

18. Welk GJ. The youth physical activity promotion model: a conceptual bridge between theory and practice. Quest. 1999;51:5–23.

19. Fereday J, MacDougall C, Spizzo M, Darbyshire P, Schiller W. "There's nothing I can't do I just put my mind to anything and I can do it": a qualitative analysis of how children with chronic disease and their parents account for and manage physical activity. BMC Pediatr. 2009;9:1.

20. Hildebrand M, Van Hees VT, Hansen BH, Ekelund U. Age group comparability of raw accelerometer output from wrist-and hip-worn monitors. Med Sci Sports Exerc. 2014;46:1816–24.

21. Van Hees VT, Fang Z, Langford J, Assah F, Mohammad A, da Silva IC, et al. Autocalibration of accelerometer data for free-living physical activity assessment using local gravity and temperature: an evaluation on four continents. J Appl Physiol. 2014;117:738–44.

22. Rich C, Geraci M, Griffiths L, Sera F, Dezateux C, Cortina-Borja M. Quality control methods in accelerometer data processing: defining minimum Wear time. PLoS One. 2013;8:1–8.

23. Van Hees VT, Gorzelniak L, Dean León EC, Eder M, Pias M, Taherian S, et al. Separating movement and gravity components in an acceleration signal and implications for the assessment of human daily physical activity. PLoS One. 2013;8:e61691.

24. Fairclough SJ, Noonan R, Rowlands AV, Van Hees V, Knowles Z, Boddy LM. Wear compliance and activity in children wearing wrist- and hip-mounted accelerometers. Med Sci Sports Exerc. 2016;48:245–53.

25. Borde R, Smith JJ, Sutherland R, Nathan N, Lubans DR. Methodological considerations and impact of school-based interventions on objectively measured physical activity in adolescents: a systematic review and meta-analysis. Obes Rev. 2017;18:476–90.

26. Verloigne M, Bere E, Van Lippevelde W, Maes L, Lien N, Vik FN, et al. The effect of the UP4FUN pilot intervention on objectively measured sedentary time and physical activity in 10–12 year old children in Belgium: the ENERGY-project. BMC Public Health. 2012;12:805.

27. Moola FJ. "CF chatters": the development of a theoretically informed physical activity intervention for youth with cystic fibrosis. Open J Prev Med. 2011;01:109–24.

28. Bowen DJ, Kreuter M, Spring B, Linnan L, Weiner D, Bakken S, et al. How we design feasibility studies. Am J Prev Med. 2010;36:452–7.

29. Rich C, Geraci M, Griffiths L, Sera F, Dezateux C, Cortina-borja M. Quality Control Methods in Accelerometer Data Processing : Identifying Extreme Counts. PLoS One. 2014;9:e85134.

30. Freedson PS, John D. Comment on "estimating activity and sedentary behavior from an accelerometer on the hip and wrist". Med Sci Sport Exerc. 2013;45:962–3.

31. Bradley JM, Kent L, Elborn JS, O'Neill B, Kent L, et al. Motion sensors for monitoring physical activity in cystic fibrosis: what is the next step? Phys Ther Rev. 2010;15:197–203.

32. Stevens D, Oades PJ, Armstrong N, Williams CA. A survey of exercise testing and training in UK cystic fibrosis clinics. J Cyst Fibros. 2010;9:302–6.

33. Cystic Fibrosis Trust. Standards of care and good clinical practice for the physiotherapy management of cystic fibrosis. 3rd ed; 2017.

34. Ferguson T, Rowlands AV, Olds T, Maher C. The validity of consumer-level, activity monitors in healthy adults worn in free-living conditions: a cross-sectional study. Int J Behav Nutr Phys Act. 2015;12:42.

25

Human immunodeficiency virus infection disclosure status to infected school aged children and associated factors in bale zone, Southeast Ethiopia: cross sectional study

Bikila Lencha[1], Gemehu Ameya[2]*[iD], Zanebe Minda[1], Feyissa Lamessa[3] and Jiregna Darega[4]

Abstract

Background: Human immunodeficiency virus (HIV) positive status disclosure is an essential component of Pediatric care and long term disease management. Children have a right to know their HIV diagnosis result. However, Pediatric HIV disclosure is complex and varies in different communities. This study aimed to assess the prevalence of HIV-positive status disclosure to infected children and associated factors among caregivers of infected children.

Methodology: A facility based mixed methods research design study was conducted in Bale Zone of South East Ethiopia. Randomly selected caregivers of HIV-positive children were interviewed using structured questionnaires for quantitative study and 17 in-depth interviews of health care workers and caregivers were conducted for qualitative data. Content analysis was done for qualitative data and logistic regression analysis was used to see the association between different variables and HIV-positive disclosure status. Odds ratio with 95% CI was computed to determine the presence and strength of the associated factors.

Results: A total of 200 caregivers of school aged (6–14 years) children participated in the study. Only 57 (28.5%) of the care givers disclosed HIV-positive status to the child for whom they were caring. The main reason for disclosure delay was due to fear of negative consequences, perception on maturity of the child, and fear of social rejection and stigma. Having social support [AOR = 2.7, 95% CI: (1.1–6.4)], caring for a child between 10 and 14 years with HIV [AOR = 6.5, 95% CI: (2.1–20.2)], a child diagnosed with HIV at age > 5 years [AOR = 2.8, 95% CI: (1.1–7.1)], and children on antiretroviral therapy (ART) with follow-up for > 5 years [AOR = 4.7, 95% CI: (1.8–11.2)] had significant association with HIV- positive status disclosure to infected children.

Conclusion: The frequency of HIV infection disclosure to infected children was very low in our cohort. Having social support, having an older child with HIV, a long period of ART follow-up and HIV diagnosis after age of five years were positively associated with HIV-positive status disclosure to infected children. Giving age appropriate counselling to children, social support to the caregivers and working on related factors are very important to improve the observed low disclosure status.

Keywords: Caregivers, Health care workers, HIV-positive status disclosure, School aged children

* Correspondence: gemechuameya@gmail.com
[2]Department of Medical Laboratory Science, College of Medicine and Health Sciences, Arba Minch University, P.O. Box: 21, Arba Minch, Ethiopia
Full list of author information is available at the end of the article

Background

Globally, Pediatric human immunodeficiency virus (HIV) infection continues to be a major problem. A 2013 WHO report showed that approximately 3.3 million children younger than 15 years are living with HIV, with about 88% of them living in sub-Saharan Africa [1]. The annual number of new infections among children was almost halved since 2010. Regardless of this significant reduction, the number of children newly infected with HIV remains unacceptably high. According to 2017 global HIV statistics, there are 1.8 million children living with HIV. Among these about 10% of them were new infections. Of newly infected Pediatric cases, more than half of them were from eastern and southern Africa. The majority of pediatric HIV was acquired from their infected mothers vertically or during breast feeding [2]. The pediatric HIV-positive population in Ethiopia is mostly an older age group that probably vertically transmitted in earlier years when mother to child HIV transmission prevention coverage was not well established [3]. The current expansion of ART plays a significant role in reducing mortality of infected children. Studies revealed that many HIV-positive children on ART do not know their HIV status [4, 5].

The American Academy of Pediatrics strongly encourages disclosure of HIV-positive status to school-age children [6]. It is believed that disclosure of HIV status to infected children has tremendous benefit in improving the treatment outcome. The disclosure resulted in mental relief for caregivers from the burden of keeping a secret [7]. It is belived that children have the right to know their HIV status. Further more, disclosure of HIV-positive status following the child's diagnosis is very important to ensuring child wellbeing. Different factors may be associated with lack of disclosure of HIV status to infected children. The depth of HIV status information to be shared with children, the manner and time of disclosure are things to be considered by caregivers and healthcare workers [8].

Early disclosure is more appropriate than immediate and unplanned disclosure upon entrance into the adult clinic, and also helps to reduce HIV transmission [9]. The prevalence of pediatric HIV disclosure to infected children varies widely throughout the world. In developed countries such as the United States, HIV diagnosis disclosure was reported to be up to 100% according to a study conducted in 2009 [10]. In developing countries, caregivers often do not disclose HIV-positive status to infected children. Vreeman et al. showed that the disclosure of HIV-positive status was as low as 1.6% in Kenya [11]. HIV disclosure practices in sub-Saharan African countries remain complex due to the immense influence of politics, culture and HIV surveillance limitation [12]. Studies of HIV disclosure in children are

very limited in Ethiopia, and available studies are more prevalent in Addis Ababa and the Northern part of the country. In Ethiopia, studies showed that the prevalence of disclosure among caregivers' of children varies from 16.3 to 39.5% [13–15]. In addition to the low frequency of disclosure in Ethiopia, little is known about the associated factors of HIV disclosure in school-aged children.

In previous studies which were conducted in other areas, factors like a child's age, the age of diagnosis, being on antiretroviral therapy (ART), caregiver-reported child depression symptoms, caregivers relation with the child and loss of a family member were found to be associated with HIV infection disclosure. Children with a deceased father tended to be more likely to know their status than non-orphans [16, 17]. These factors may vary depending on factors like sociodemographic characteristics, sociocultural aspects, awareness of care givers and knowledge of health professionals. Therefore, it is important to know the frequency of disclosure, its associated factors, the opinion and experience of caregivers and health care workers (HCWs) to design an appropriate intervention suitable with specific living and the cultural context of the society. Thus, this study aimed to assess the prevalence of HIV-positive status disclosure and associated factors among caregivers of HIV-infected children in Bale Zone, South East Ethiopia.

Methods

Study setting and period

The study was conducted in Bale Zone of south east Ethiopia at a distance of 430 km from Addis Abeba. The zone has four hospitals (Goba, Ginnir, Robe and Dallomana) and five health centers (Gasara, Goro, Agarfa, Dinsho and Barbare) that were giving pediatric ART service during the data collection period. Bale zone was selected as no studies on pediatric HIV-positive disclosure have been conducted there. There are also a large number of children followed in the ART clinic in the governmental health facility in the zone.

Study design and population

An institutional based mixed methods research design was conducted. Both qualitative and quantitative methods were used to collect the data. The caregivers of children aged between 6 and 14 years who were on ART were included from selected pediatric ART clinics for quantitative study. The caregivers were randomly selected for quantitative study. For those children who came by themselves, their caregivers were contacted with the help of pediatric ART service providers. Health care workers (HCWs) working in the pediatric ART clinics and caregivers were purposively included in the study for the in-depth interviews. The health care workers working in ART clinics during data collection and caregivers coming with their children were selected for in-depth interviews.

Sample size determination and sampling methods

The sample size was calculated using a single population proportion formula with estimated proportion of disclosure among school-aged children to be 50% due to a lack of previous studies conducted in the same areas. Marginal error was assumed to be 5 and 95% confidence interval. The estimated sample size was 384 subjects, and a population correction formula was used because of the low number (< 10,000) of school-age children on ART in the study area. Finally, after adding 10% non-response rate, the sample size was estimated to be 201. Two hospitals and two health centers were randomly selected by lottery method from those institutions giving pediatric ART service. The total sample size was allocated proportionally to the total number of children on treatment in each of the selected ART clinics. The children were selected by simple random sampling technique using sample frames recorded on computer data after excluding drop-out, transfer-out and lost to follow-up. The children's corresponding caregivers were interviewed in a separate room while they came for follow-up to the ART clinic. For the qualitative study, purposive sampling was used and 17 in-depth interviews were conducted.

Data collection methods and instruments

Data were collected using the structured interviewer administered questionnaire which was adapted after reviewing related literature [14, 15, 18]. The questionnaire was first prepared in English (Additional file 1) and then translated into local languages (Amharic and Afaan Oromo) by language experts and back translated into English to check its consistency. Data were collected by 6 health professionals working in the pediatric ART clinics. Medical records of HIV-positive children were reviewed for date of HIV diagnosis, current WHO treatment stage and the most recent CD4 count.

For the in-depth interview, a semi-structured interview guide (Additional file 1) was developed from pertinent literature [7, 18] and held with caregivers and HCWs to explore and understand perceptions and experiences towards disclosure of HIV-positive status to infected children. The interview was facilitated by investigators using a guide and it was tape recorded. Notes were taken by one of the investigators. Seventeen in-depth interviews were conducted until thematic saturation was reached.

Data quality control

Training was given for data collectors for two days on the objectives, contents, and procedures of the data collection. The questionnaire was pretested on 5% of the sample in non-selected hospitals before the actual data collection and revised prior to data collection. Data was checked for completeness during the data collection by supervisors and investigators. The realiablity of the questionnaire was checked using cronbach's alpha and it was above 0.7. Qualitative data was transcribed on the same day after data collection and appropriate corrections were made for the next day.

Data processing and analysis

Data were entered using Epi info version 7.0 and exported to Statistical Package for Social Sciences (SPSS) version 21 for analysis. Descriptive statistics were used to assess the socio-demographic characteristics of caregivers and children. HIV-positive status disclosure to infected children was dichotomized to 'yes' and 'no' based on caregivers' self-report.

Bivariable and multivariable logistic regression analyses were used to determine factors associated with HIV infection disclosure status to children. Variables with a p-value of ≤ 0.25 in univariate logistic regression were included in a multiple logistic regression model to control for potential confounders. The stepwise backward variable selection method was used in the multivariable analysis. P-values < 0.05 were considered to declare statistical significance in the models.

For the qualitative data, the recorded data was transcribed verbatim and then translated into English word-for-word. The content analysis was used by sorting information, looking for similarities and differences, and developing appropriate codes. Then, similar codes were used to make categories. Finally, the qualitative data was summarized and direct quotations were used to present the data along with the quantitative findings.

Results

Socio-demographic characteristics of HIV-positive school aged Children's caregivers

A total of 200 caregivers of children aged from 6 to 14 years participated in the study with a response rate of 99.5%. About two-thirds of the respondents were female and nearly half of the respondents were within the age group from 31 to 40 years. About 70% of the respondents were married and 27% of them were unemployed. A majority of the respondents (68%) were urban residents and nearly three-fourths of the caregivers were biological parents of the children for which they cared (Table 1).

Socio-demographic characteristics of the HIV-positive school aged children

More than half of the HIV-positive children were boys. The mean age of the children was 9.9 years

Table 1 Socio-demographic characteristics of the HIV-positive school aged children's caregivers of Bale Zone, Southeast Ethiopia

Variables	Categories	No.	%
Age (years)	19–30	52	26.0
	31–40	93	46.5
	>40	55	27. 5
Sex	Male	66	33.0
	Female	134	67.0
Religion	Orthodox	102	51.0
	Muslim	68	34.0
	Protestant	30	15.0
Marital status	Single	21	10.5
	Married	139	69.5
	Divorced	10	5.0
	Widowed	30	15.0
Occupation	Unemployed	54	27.0
	Government Employee	32	16.0
	Merchant	38	19.0
	Farmer	52	26.0
	Others[a]	24	12.0
Income (Birr)	≤500	60	30.0
	501–1000	78	39.0
	≥1000	62	31.0
Educational status	Unable to read and write	64	32.0
	Able to read and write	62	31.0
	Primary (1–8)	20	10.0
	Secondary (9–12)	40	20.0
	Tertiary (12 and above)	14	7.0
Residence	Urban	136	68.0
	Rural	64	32.0
Relation of caregiver to the child	Biological parents	143	71.5
	Non-biological parents	41	20.5
	Others[b]	16	8.0

Others[a] students and pensioners, Others[b] caregivers from the camp (foster parents)

Table 2 Socio demographic characteristics of the HIV-positive school aged children in Bale Zone, Southeast Ethiopia

Variable	Categories	No.	%
Age of the child	6–9 years	91	45.5
	10–14 years	109	54.5
Sex of the child	Male	108	54.0
	Female	92	46.0
Age at diagnosis of HIV	1–5 years	113	56.5
	6–11 years	87	43.5
Age when ART was initiated	1–5 years	95	47.5
	6–11 years	105	52.5
Duration on ART	1–5 years	136	68.0
	6–12 years	64	32.0
Responsible to take ART	Yes	86	43.0
	No	114	57.0
Schooling	Yes	164	82
	No	36	18
With whom the child is currently living?	Biological parents	142	71.0
	Non-biological parents	46	23.0
	Foster parents (camp)	12	6.0
Did the child lose any of their biological parents?	Yes	104	52.0
	No	96	48.0

Magnitude and reasons of disclosure of HIV-positive result to infected school aged children

Based on caregiver reports, only 28.5% of the children were disclosed their HIV-positive status. About 91% of the disclosed children were in the age range from 10 to 14 years while the remaining were from 6 to 9 years. The mean age at disclosure was 10.7 ± 1.8 years. More than half of the caregivers' children in the age range between 10 and 14 years were not disclosed about their HIV-positive status.

The major reasons for disclosure were repeated questions from the children to know why they took the drugs, followed by positive perception on child maturation and ability of understanding the information. In-depth interview of the caregivers also supports this idea. The caregiver believed that the appropriate age for disclosure is 10 years or above. In qualitative study, the age of children and their ability to understand were important issues to consider regarding disclosure of HIV-positive status to infected children. Health care workers had almost similar opinions concerning the preferred age of disclosure. The majority of caregivers (70.5%) preferred the age group between 10 and 14 years to disclose HIV-positive status, whereas about 27% of them preferred children aged 15 years and above. However, a 32-year-old health worker with 2-years work

with ±2.6 years standard deviation (SD). About 55% of children were between 10 and 14 years. The mean age at which the children were diagnosed was 5.6 ± 2.4 years SD. All the children were on ART during the time of the caregivers' interview, and the mean duration of stay on ART was 4.4 ± 2.4 years. The majority of the children (82%) were attending school. About 43% of the children on ART were taking the drug by their own initiative. According to caregivers report, more than half of the children were cared for by single parents (Table 2).

experience in ART mentioned that a 14-year-old female who was not disclosed started a relationship with her boyfriend and infected him with the virus.

Of the 57 children to whom the HIV-positive result was disclosed, nearly two-thirds of them were disclosed by their biological parents followed by health worker (16%) and relatives (9%). In the in-depth interview, the HCWs said that willingness of the family is important to disclose the HIV-positive status to the infected children. In addition, HCWs said that the families have the responsibility to start the process of disclosure at home because they stay with the child for a long time. HCWs also said that their role is to support the caregiver's disclosure, teach the process and help caregivers with the day to day challenges about disclosure.

Reasons for non-disclosure of HIV-positive status

Out of the total study participants, 143 (71.5%) of the caregivers did not disclose the diagnosis result of HIV infection to their children. Of these participants, 91 (64%) of the care-givers delayed disclosure for fear of negative consequences for the child (fear of emotional distress), 81 (56.6%) reported that the child was too young to understand the diagnosis, and 51 (35.6%) of them replied the child would be socially rejected (fear of stigma and discrimination) (Fig. 1).

In in-depth interviews, all the caregivers mentioned that the age of the children is the main factor hindering disclosure. The participants also mentioned that the child could not understand the information and may disclose to other people. And health care workers also shared their ideas. A 42 year old female HCW with

4-years experiences in ART clinic said that *"Families believe that they are the cases for themselves and feel guilty and ashamed. Fear of stigma and age of the child were also another problem. Family believe that the child couldn't understand at this age and disclosure leads to emotional abuse."*

Health care workers were asked for their experience about disclosure, and they responded that a sudden disclosure of infection status to HIV-infected children in the school and from families other than biological parents ended up with bad consequences. Children became emotional when they heard their diagnosis from the person they did not expect and in an unexpected situation. One of the HCWs said that *"Once upon a time the foster father of a child comes home after drinking alcohol and said 'keep silent and take your long life medication' to the child. Then the child went to the kitchen and took insecticide medication and died. Therefore, sudden disclosure has bad consequences"* (34-year-old HCW with 2 years expriance).

All the HCWs and caregivers were also asked about the way of disclosure. The participants responded that disclosure should be a process, not a one-time activity. They said 'How much does the child understand about HIV/AIDS?' is the main question that should be addressed. One of the HCWs said *"Those 10 years and above should be told about the diagnosis step by step. The child will understand you through time. It needs time. The HCW will stay with the child not more than 1hr. If the health worker discloses within this short time, the child will become emotional. Therefore, it should be at home by taking time and convincing the child slowly"* (42-year-old HCW with 4 years experience).

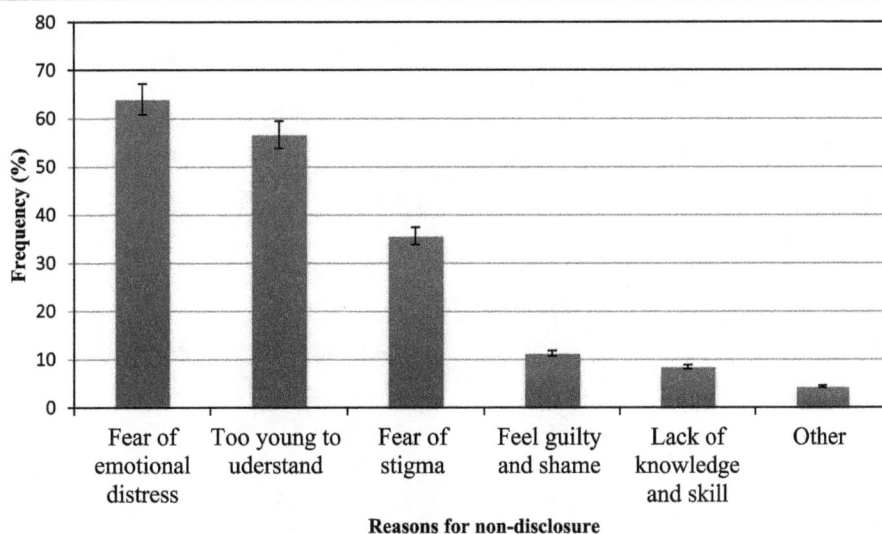

Fig. 1 Caregivers' reasons for non-disclosure of HIV infection to their children in Bale Zone, Southeast Ethiopia

Factors associated with disclosure of HIV-positive status to HIV-infected children

Factors associated with disclosure of HIV-positive status to infected children was assessed by binary logistic regression. In univariate analysis, gender of caregivers with whom the children were living, HIV status of care giver, respondent residence, presence of social support, age of the children, schooling status of the children, age at which the child was diagnosed with HIV and duration of ART had p-values less than 0.25 and the variables were selected for multivariate analysis. In multivariate analysis, presence of social support for caregiver, age of children, age at which children were diagnosed with HIV and duration of ART were independently associated with disclosure of HIV-positive status to infected children.

Caregivers who had social support were about three times more likely to disclose HIV-positive status to the infected children than those caregivers without social support [AOR = 2.7, 95% CI: (1.1–6.4)]. HIV-positive status disclosure was 6.5 times higher in those caregivers who had HIV-positive children in the age group of 10–14 years than those caregivers who had HIV-positive children less than 10 years of age [AOR = 6.5, 95% CI: (2.1–20.2)]. Children diagnosed with HIV in age of 6–11 years had about three times more disclosure than children diagnosed at age less than six years [AOR = 2.8, 95% CI: (1.1–7.1)]. Duration of ART was also a factor that affects the disclosure of HIV-positive status to infected children. Caregivers who have HIV-positive children > 5 years on ART follow-up had about 5 times more chance of disclosure than those who have ART follow-up for five and less years [AOR = 4.7, 95% CI: (1.8–11.2)] (Table 3).

Discussion

In this study, only about a quarter of the HIV-infected children were allowed to know their diagnosis result. Disclosing HIV status to children has a number of benefits for children, however, due to different factors, caregivers abstain from revealing their status. This finding is in line with studies done in 2013 and 2014 in northern Ethiopia which showed a prevalence of 31.5 and 33.3%, respectively [15, 19]. In contrary to our study finding, low prevalence of disclosure was reported from Kenya [9, 11], and Addis Ababa (17%) in 2012 [13]. The probable reason for the better prevalence (28.5%) of disclosure in our study could be due to a higher number of older school aged children in the study (mean age of 9.9 years). In addition, the study conducted in Addis Ababa included all pediatric patients whereas our study only focused on school aged children. The time difference between the studies could be another possible reason for observed difference. As the time passes, an awareness is created and different stakehoders work on areas to improve the disclosure status. Still the disclosure in the study area was unacceptably low.

Age of the child was found to be one of the factors independently associated with HIV-positive status disclosure to

Table 3 Associated factors of disclosure of HIV-positive status of school aged children in Bale, Southeast Ethiopia

Variables	Categories	Disclosed n (%)	Non-disclosed n (%)	COR (95% CI)	AOR (95% CI)	p-Value
Sex of caregivers	Male	25 (43.9)	41 (28.7)	Ref.	Ref.	
	Female	32 (56.1)	102 (71.3)	.73 (0.3, 1.9)	–	
With whom children is living	Biological parent	35 (61.4)	107 (74.8)	Ref.	Ref.	
	None biological parent	22 (38.6)	36 (25.2)	0.10 (0.01, 1.0)	–	
HIV status of care giver	Positive	34 (59.6)	102 (71.3)	Ref.	Ref.	
	Negative	23 (40.4)	41 (28.7)	0.6 (0.3, 1.2)	–	
Residence	Urban	44 (77.2)	92 (64.3)	Ref.	Ref.	
	Rural	13 (22.8)	51 (35.6)	0.7 (0.3, 1.6)	–	
Presence of social support	Present	19 (33.3)	29 (20.3)	Ref.	Ref.	
	Absent	38 (66.7)	114 (79.7)		2.7 (1.1, 6.4)	0.028[a]
Age of children	6–9	5 (8.7)	86 (60.1)	Ref.	Ref.	
	10–14	52 (91.2)	57 (39.9)		6.5 (2.1, 20.2)	0.001[a]
Schooling status of children	Enrolled	55 (96.5)	109 (76.2)	Ref.	Ref.	
	Non-enrolled	2 (3.5)	34 (23.8)	3.2 (1.3, 7.7)	–	
Age at which children were diagnosed with HIV	≤5 year	21 (36.8)	92 (64.3)	Ref.	Ref.	
	6–11	36 (63.2)	51 (35.6)		2.8 (1.1, 7.1)	0.027[a]
Duration of ART	≤5 year	22	114	Ref.	Ref.	
	6–12	35	29		4.7 (1.8, 11.2)	0.001[a]

Ref Reference, *AOR* Adjusted Odd Ratio, *COR* Crude Odd Ratio, [a] independently associated with disclosure of HIV positive status of children

infected children. Those children in the age group 10–14 years were about seven times more likely to be disclosed of their HIV-positive status as compared to those children whose age was from 6 to 9 years. This could be due to the older children repeatedly asking the reason why they were taking medication. Furthermore, a majority of older children were also in school, and they may have had a chance to learn about HIV. This finding was in agreement with studies conducted in central and northwest Ethiopia where children of the same age were more likely to be disclosed than their counterparts not in school [13, 15]. Similar findings in other African countries reported that children were more likely to know their HIV diagnosis result when older [9, 17]. This result was also supported by qualitative findings of this study.

In this study, more than half of children in the age group 10–14 years were still not disclosed their HIV-positive status. This implies that the majority of HIV-positive children entering secondary sexual characteristics were still unaware of their HIV status. This may result in unknowingly transmitting the virus to others and challenging the strategy of reducing the new HIV infection to zero. This idea was also supported by one of the health care worker participated in in-depth interview. In the HCW in-depth interview, she maintioned that a 14-year-old female infected her boyfriend with the virus unknowingly due to lack of early discloser.

Duration of stay on ART was another factor associated with disclosure of HIV status to children. Those children who were on ART from 6 to 12 years were about five times more likely to be disclosed their HIV status than their counterparts. This finding was in agreement with studies done in developing countries including Ethiopia [19, 20]. The study in Bahirdar reported that children who have taken ART for more than five years were 5 times more likely to be disclosed their status [15]. When the children stay on ART for a long period of time, they might have a chance to ask questions about their HIV medications. The children might ask why they take the medication while they apparently seem healthy. This is also the issue discussed in in-depth interviews.

The age at which children were diagnosed with HIV infection was also associated with disclosure of HIV infection. Childeren who diagnosed with HIV at age above 5 years were about three times more likely to be disclosed their status than those diagnosed at age 5 and less. This may be due to older children asking their caregiver about their diagnosis result. This finding was also supported by qualitative study conducted on the HCWs and caregivers in which they belived that disclosure of HIV status needs maturity of children. Those caregivers who got social support from any source were more likely to disclose the HIV status to infected children than those

who didn't have social support. This may be due to encouragement and social acceptance of the children's positive status [21].

Limitations of the study
Clinical characteristics of both children and caregivers were not assessed. Secondary data was used for the children's information. There may be social desirability bias, and recall bias that might have affected this study. The cross-sectional nature of the study may also have its own limitations. To mimimize this, secondary data was used to cross check some information.

Conclusions
The prevalence of HIV-positive status disclosure to infected children in Bale zone of Ethiopia was low. Having social support, caring for an older age HIV-positive child, ART follow up for long duration, and HIV diagnosis after age of five years were positively associated with the disclosure of HIV-positive status to infected children. The main reasons for non disclosure were fear of negative consequences for the child, children were too young to understand about HIV, and fear of stigma and discrimination. Health care workers should give age-appropriate counseling, support, and work together with caregivers on the processes of disclosing their diagnostic result to infected children. Non-governmental organizations should strengthen and continue their support for the caregivers on the care of children. Further research should be conducted to address the relationship between disclosure to HIV-infected children and variables like depression, stigma, and adherence involving both children and caregivers.

Abbreviations
AIDS: Acquired Immune Deficiency Syndrome; ART: Anti-Retroviral Therapy; HAART: Highly Active Anti-Retroviral Therapy; HCW: Health Care Workers; HIV: Human Immunodeficiency Virus

Acknowledgements
We would like to thank Maddawalabu University Research and Community Service Directorate for supporting this study. We also thank data collectors for their work and support. Caregivers have also great thanks because of their time to give information. Finally the Bale Zone Health Office has also great thanks for providing us with all necessary information.

Authors' contributions
BL and FL designed and conceived the study. BL, GA, FL, JD, and ZM enriched the methodology. BL, JD, and ZM supervised. BL, GA, JD, and FL analyzed the data and interpreted the results. BL, GA, ZM, and FL wrote the original draft. All the authors read and approved the manuscript.

Competing interests
The authors declare that they have no any competing interests.

Author details
[1]Department of Public Health, Goba Referral Hospital, Maddawalabu University, Bale-Goba, Addis Ababa, Ethiopia. [2]Department of Medical Laboratory Science, College of Medicine and Health Sciences, Arba Minch

University, P.O. Box: 21, Arba Minch, Ethiopia. [3]Department of Nursing, Goba Referral Hospital, Maddawalabu University, Bale-Goba, Addis Ababa, Ethiopia. [4]Department of Nursing, College of Medicine and Health sciences, Ambo University, Ambo, Ethiopia.

References

1. World Health Organization, UNICEF, and UNAIDS. Global update on HIV treatment: Results, impact, and opportunities. Global AIDS Response Progress Reporting. WHO/UNICEF/UNAIDS. HIV treatment. 2013. Available on: http://www.who.int/hiv/data/global_treatment_report_presentation_2013.pdf Accessed 25 Aug 2017.

2. UNAIDS. Global HIV & AIDS statistics - 2018 fact sheet. 2018. Available on:http://www.unaids.org/en/resources/fact-sheet, Accessed on 12th October, 2018

3. Federal HIV/AIDS prevention and Control office. Country progress report on HIV/AIDS response. Addis Ababa: FHAPCO; 2014.

4. Lorenz R, Grant E, Muyindike W, Maling S, Card C, Henry C, et al. Caregivers' attitudes towards HIV testing and disclosure of HIV statusto at risk children in rural Uganda. PLoSONE. 2016;11(2):e0148950.

5. Vaz L, Corneli A, Dulyx J, Rennie S, Omba S, Kitetele F, et al. The process of HIV status disclosure to HIV-positive youth in Kinshasa, Democratic Republic of the Congo. AIDS Care. 2008;20(7):842–52.

6. American Academy of Pediatrics. Disclosure of illness status to children and adolescents with HIV infection pediatrics. Pediatrics. 1999;103(1):164–6. https://doi.org/10.1542/peds.103.1.164.

7. Motshome P, Madiba S. Perceptions, reasons and experiences of disclosing HIV diagnosis to infected children in Kweneng District, Botswana. Int J Health Sci Res. 2014;4(2):129–39.

8. Kyaddondo D, Wanyenze RK, Kinsman J, Hardon A. Disclosure of HIV status between parents and children in Uganda in the context of greater access to treatment. SAHARA J. 2013;10(I):S37–45.

9. Turissini ML, Nyandiko MW, Ayaya SO, Marete I, Mwangi A, Chemboi V, et al. The prevalence of disclosure of HIV status to HIV-infected children in Western Kenya. J Pediatric Infect Dis Soc. 2013;2(2):136–43. https://doi.org/10.1093/jpids/pit024.

10. Butler AM, Williams PL, Howland LC, Storm D, Hutton N, Seage GR, et al. Impact of disclosure of HIV infection on health related quality of life among children and adolescents with HIV infection. Pediatrics. 2009;123:935–43.

11. Vreeman RC, Nyandiko WM, Ayaya SO, Walumbe EG, Marrero DG, Inui TS. The perceived impact of disclosure of pediatric HIV status on pediatric antiretroviral therapy adherence, child well-being and social relationships in a resource limited setting. AIDS Patient Care STDs. 2010;24:639–49.

12. Aderomilehin O, Hanciles-Amu A, Ozoya OO. Perspectives and practice of HIV disclosure to children and adolescents by health-care providers and caregivers in sub-Saharan Africa: a systematic review. Front Public Health. 2016;4:166. https://doi.org/10.3389/fpubh.2016.00166.

13. Abebe W, Teferra S. Disclosure of diagnosis by parents and caregivers to children infected with HIV: prevalence associated factors and perceived barriers in Addis Ababa, Ethiopia. AIDS Care. 2012;24:1097–102.

14. Negese D, Addis K, Awoke A, Birhanu Z, Muluye D, Yifru S, et al. HIV-positive status disclosure and associated factors among children in North Gondar, Northwest Ethiopia. ISRN AIDS. 2012;2012:485720. https://doi.org/10.5402/2012/485720 7.

15. Alemu A, Berhanu B, Emishaw S. Challenges of caregivers to disclose their Children's HIV-positive status receiving highly active anti retroviral therapy at pediatric anti-retroviral therapy clinics in Bahir Dar, North West Ethiopia. J AIDS Clin Res. 2013;4:253. https://doi.org/10.4172/2155-6113.1000253.

16. Binagwaho A, Murekatete I, Rukundo A, Mugwaneza P, Hinda R, Lyambabaje A, et al. Factors associated with disclosure of HIV status among HIV-positive children in Rwanda. Rwanda Medical Journal. 2012;69(3):987–4.

17. Vreeman RC, Scanlon ML, Mwangi A, Turissini M, Ayaya SO, Tenge C, et al. A cross-sectional study of disclosure of HIV status to children and adolescents in Western Kenya. PLoS One. 2014;9(1):e86616.

18. Madiba S. Patterns of HIV diagnosis disclosure to infected children and family members: data from a pediatric antiretroviral program in South Africa. World J of AIDS. 2012;2(3):212–21.

19. Tamir Y, Aychiluhem M, Jara D. Disclosure status and associated factors among children living with HIV in east Gojjam, northwest of Ethiopia. Qual Prim Care. 2014;23(4):223–30.

20. Kallem S, Renner L, Ghebremichael M, Paintsil E. Prevalence and pattern of disclosure of HIV status in HIV-infected children in Ghana. AIDS Behav. 2011; 15:1121–7.

21. Vreeman RC, Gramelspacher AM, Gisore PO, Scanlon ML, Nyandiko WM. Disclosure of HIV status to children in resource-limited settings: a systematic review. J Int AIDS Soc. 2013;16(1):18466. https://doi.org/10.7448/IAS.16.1.18466.

26

Pre-lacteal feeding practice and associated factors among mothers having children less than two years of age in Aksum town, Tigray, Ethiopia, 2017: a cross-sectional study

Girmay Tekaly[1*], Mekuria Kassa[2], Tilahun Belete[2], Hagos Tasew[1], Tekelwoini Mariye[3] and Tsega Teshale[4]

Abstract

Background: Pre-lacteal feeding has continued as a deep-rooted nutritional malpractice in developing countries. Pre-lacteal feeding is a barrier to the implementation of optimal breastfeeding practices and increases the risk of neonatal early-life diseases and mortality. Therefore, the aim of this study was to assess pre-lacteal feeding practice and associated factors among mothers having children less than 2 years of age in Aksum town, central Tigray, Ethiopia.

Methods: A community-based cross-sectional study was conducted to interview 477 mother-child pairs by systematic random sampling technique. Data were collected through interviewer-administered semi-structured questionnaires. Data were coded, entered, cleaned and edited using EPIDATA version 3.1 and export to SPSS Version 22.0 for analysis. To identify the significant variables binary logistic regression were employed. Variables with p-value < 0.05 at 95% CI in multivariate logistic regression were considered statistically significant.

Result: The prevalence of pre-lacteal feeding in Aksum town was 10.1% (95% CI: 7.3%, 13%). Mothers with no previous birth (AOR: 2.93(95% CI:1.21,7.09)), birth spacing less than 24 (AOR: 2.88(95% CI: 1.15,7.25)), colostrum discarding (AOR: 6.72 (95% CI: 2.49,18.12)), less than four anti natal care follow up (AOR: 10.55 (95% CI: 4.78,23.40)), those who underwent cesarean section (AOR: 4.38 (95% CI:1.72,11.12)) and maternal believe on purported advantage of pre-lacteal feeding (AOR: 3.36 (95%CI: 1.62,6.96)) were more likely to practice pre-lacteal feeding to their infants.

Conclusions: Pre-lacteal feeding is still practiced in the study area. Childbirth spacing, colostrum discarding, antenatal Care follow up, maternal belief in pre-lacteal feeding was contributing factors for practicing of pre-lacteal feeding. Coordination and sustaining the existing strategies and approaches are recommended to give emphasis on the nutritional value of colostrum and anti-natal care follow up.

Keywords: Pre-lacteal feeding, Mothers, Children less than two years, Aksum town

* Correspondence: girmeat@gmail.com
[1]Department of Pediatrics and Child Health Nursing, School of Nursing, College of Health Science, Aksum University, Aksum, Ethiopia
Full list of author information is available at the end of the article

Background

Globally, it is estimated that every day about 4000 infants and young children die worldwide because they don't breastfeed [1]. Of around 3 million neonatal deaths every year, two-thirds occur in South-East Asia and sub-Saharan Africa [2]. Sub -Saharan Africa, still with the highest neonatal mortality rates in the world [3].

A pre-lacteal feeding (PLF) is any food except mother's milk provided to a newborn before initiating breastfeeding in the first 3 days of life [4, 5]. The most common pre-lacteal foods given to infants in many low-middle income countries could be grouped into three: water only, water-based (rice water, herbal mixture, juice), and milk-based (animal milk, infant formula) [6]. Water is dangerous pre-lacteal feed in terms of the detrimental effect on the nutritional aspect and makes the neonate more prone for early risk of severe gastrointestinal infections [7].

Pre-lacteal feeding is a major barrier to first fundamental rights of exclusive breastfeeding (EBF) [8, 9]. The practice of giving other substances (pre-lacteal feeding) to the newborn babies even before lactation is a common cultural practice and this practice also delays the initiation of breastfeeding [10]. pre-lacteal feeding is a risk indicator for infant morbidity and mortality especially during the neonatal period and Some of the practices of pre-lacteal feeding are associated with different belief, misconceptions, faith, and advice by the senior family members or priests of some religions [7].

The child is vulnerable in nutrition, socioeconomic and health factors, which causes malnutrition [11]. Malnutrition is an underlying factor in more than 50% of the major cause of infant mortality and the risk of malnutrition in children during the first 2 years of life is an indication of poor infant feeding practices [12]. Poor feeding practices are chief challenges to the social and economic development of one country [11].

Pre-lacteal feeding practice deprives newborns of colostrum rich in nutrients and immunoglobulins—thus, causing a reduction of the priming of the gastrointestinal tract, and increases the risk of infant morbidity and mortality [13]. Colostrum deprivation was the major cause of stunting in children [14].

Pre-lacteal feeding and its consequences contribute to significant health problems, poor intellectual, physical development and lowered resistance to diseases [15]. In addition, mother-baby bonding may be interrupted by pre-lacteal feeding as it decreases skin-to-skin contact. Thus, this feeding process reduces the practice of exclusive breastfeeding which can be dangerous to the child and may even result in death [16].

Even though, Ethiopia has developed the National Infant and Young Child Feeding (IYCF) Guideline [17] and acknowledged gains of Baby Friendly Hospital Initiative (BFHI) that discourages pre-lacteal feeding practices on newborns to achieve optimal breastfeeding [18], a wide range of harmful newborn feeding practices are documented.

This study will help to health care service provider in their counseling/health education session. This also helps for policymakers, Non-Governmental Organizations (NGOs) and other stakeholders to formulate appropriate implementation tool for achieving sustainable development goal. Moreover, the finding of this study will also help as a baseline data for researchers for further research with this regard. The purpose of the study was to assess pre-lacteal feeding practice and associated factor among mothers having children less than 2 years of age in Aksum town, Central Tigray, Ethiopia.

Methods
Study design and setting

A community-based cross-sectional study design was employed in Aksum town of northern Ethiopia from March 1 to 30/ 2017. Aksum town is located 1024 Km north of Addis Ababa and 241 Km far from Mekelle which is the capital city of Tigray region. According to the Central Statistical Agency of Ethiopia (CSA), the population of the town was 56,576 [19, 20]. According to Aksum town health office, the town has one general hospital, one referral hospital, two health center and seven private clinics.

Sample size determination

The sample size was determined based on the formula used to estimate a single population proportion by using 24.4% prevalence of PLF in Fitche town, north Showa, Ethiopia [21] and a 5% margin of error with 95% confidence level.

$$n = \frac{(z/2\,a)^2 p\,(1\text{-}p)}{d^2} = \frac{(1.96)^2 0.244(1\text{-}0.244)}{(0.05)^2} = 283$$

The required final sample size with and a design effect of 1.5 and adjustment for non-response rate (15%) was 489.

Study population

Mothers having children less than 2 years of age who were living for ≥6 months in the selected kebeles of Aksum town were considered as the study population. Mothers who live < 6 months in the town and non-biological mothers were excluded from the study.

Sampling technique

Multi-stage sampling technique was employed to select 489 study participants. A pre-survey was conducted before the actual day of data collection and 5629 mother-child pairs were targeted in the selected five kebeles (the smallest administrative unit in Ethiopia). From the total of 5 Kebeles of Aksum town, 3 Kebeles were selected by lottery method. To obtain the sample size from every 3 kebeles proportional allocation to sample size was done. Participating households from the selected Kebele's were identified using a systematic random sampling technique. Finally, every 9th mother from each Kebeles was identified until the required sample size fulfilled and the starting mother was selected using a lottery method by using the house number.

Data collection tools and procedure

Data was collected using interviewer-administered semi-structured questionnaires by six diploma midwives and three Bachelor of Science degree holder as supervisors. Data were adapted from Ethiopian Demographic and Health Survey [22], Ethiopian National Nutrition Program [16], from the research done in Raya kobo district [23], Harari region [13], Mizan Aman town [24] and Fitche town [21]. The questionnaire was adapted and contextualized to fit the research objective and the local condition.

Study variables

In this study, the outcome variable was pre-lacteal feeding practice among mothers of children aged less than 24 months. The independent variables were maternal and child Socio-demographic variable (number of children, family size, birth order, maternal age, educational status, occupation, religion), feeding practice (colostrum avoidance, breastfeeding initiation), health care service utilization (ANC utilization, place of delivery and mode of delivery) and maternal level of information on the risk of pre-lacteal feeding.

Operational definitions
Antenatal care utilization
Having at least one visit to a health institution for checkup purpose during the pregnancy of the index child [25].

Good level of information about breastfeeding
Those mothers who told two or more components of breastfeeding counseling during their ANC visit (1. Benefits of breastfeeding 2. positioning of the baby 3. Exclusive breastfeeding 4. Management of breast problem 5. expression of breast milk) [26].

Poor level of information about breastfeeding
Those mothers who told one or none components of breastfeeding counseling during their ANC visit (1. Benefits of breastfeeding 2. Positioning of the baby 3. Exclusive breastfeeding 4. Management of breast problem 5. expression of breast milk) [26].

Postnatal care utilization
Receiving the care provided to the woman and the index child at least once during the 6 weeks' period following delivery [26].

Pre-lacteal feeding
Defined as giving fluid or semisolid food before breastfeeding to an infant during the first 3 days after birth. A mother who gives any food/fluid without the breastmilk regardless of the frequency is considered as pre-lacteal feeding [7].

Data quality assurance
To ensure data quality, training and orientation were given for 1 day to data collectors and supervisors by the primary investigator. The questionnaire was initially prepared in English and then translated into Tigrigna version (local language) by different experts of both languages to check its consistency. The questionnaire was pre-tested 2 weeks prior to the actual data collection on 5 % of the sample size in shire town and the necessary amendment was done on the questionnaire per pre-test result. The collected data was reviewed and checked for completeness and consistency by the supervisor and principal investigator on a daily bases at the spot during the data collection time. Finally, data collectors were closely followed by the supervisors and principal investigator.

Data processing and analysis
The Data was coded, entered, cleaned edited using EPIDATA version 3.1, and then exported to SPSS Version 22.0 for analysis. Binary logistic regression analysis was employed to examine the statistical association between the outcome variable and every single independent variable. Variables which showed statistical significance during bivariate analysis at $\leq 25\%$ (p-value ≤ 0.25) were entered into multivariate logistic regression to isolate an independent effect of the predictors by using the backward elimination method. The Hosmer-Lemeshow test was used to check the appropriateness of the model for analysis. Results were presented using tables, figures, and texts. Adjusted odds ratios (AOR) with 95% CI, were estimated to assess the strength of associations and statistical significance was declared at a p-value < 0.05.

Results
Socio-demographic characteristics
About 477 mothers having children less than 24 months of age were consented to participate in the study with 97.5%% of response rate. Out of the total respondent, 202(42.3%) were aged from 25 to 29 years old, 319(66.9%) had ≥4 family number.

About 291(61%) were housewife by occupation and 393(82.4%) of the mothers were had ≤3 children in number. Out of the total children, about 145(30.4%) were aged less than 6 months with 212(44.4%) birth spacing of greater than 24 months (Table 1).

Feeding practice in the study population

In this study, about 48 (10.1% (95% CI: 7.3%, 13%)) respondents give pre-lacteal feeding within 3 days before giving breastfeeding to their child. The most common type of pre-lacteal feeding given to the child was formula milk 15 (31.3%). About 16 (33.3%) of the respondents were given pre-lacteal feeding to their child due to breastfeeding problem at the time of childbirth. Regarding the influence/advise to provide such kind of pre-lacteal feeding, mothers own decision was more dominant factor 31 (64.6%). About 271(56.8%) mothers were initiate breastfeeding within 1 h (Table 2).

Maternal health care service utilization

From the total 461(96.6%) respondent mothers who were attended ANC visit; 341(71.5%) utilized four times and above (which is internationally recommended) and 467(97.9%) had gotten breastfeeding counseling at ANC clinic. From these who had gotten breastfeeding counseling at ANC clinic, 228(48%) of them were counseled about the benefit of breastfeeding. Four hundred fifty-three (95%) mothers were delivered their child at governmental institutions with 436(91.4%) of them were delivered through normal spontaneous delivery and all facility delivery was assisted by a health professional. About 412(86.4%) mothers had at least one visit of PNC and all of them were got breastfeeding counseling in the post-natal clinic (Table 3).

Maternal level of information on pre-lacteal feeding

Of the total 477 respondents, 447 (93.7%) respondent mothers had information on the advantage of colostrum giving to their child. About 434 (91%) mothers were at the good level of information by which they were able to mention two or more components of breastfeeding counseling during their ANC visit. In this study 165 (34.6%) mothers believe in the purported advantage of pre-lacteal feeding. Of these 101 (61.2%) respondents believe that pre-lacteal feeding was important for child health and growth. About 376 (78.8%) mothers were having information on the risk associated with giving of pre-lacteal feeding to the infant. The problems associated with pre-lacteal feeding includes 343 (72.4%) diarrhea and vomiting and 274 (41.5%) (Table 4).

Factors associated with pre-lacteal feeding practice

In the binary logistic regression at p-value of ≤0.25 maternal education, age of the child, birth order, birth spacing, family size, colostrum discarding, number of ANC visit, breastfeeding counseling during ANC visit, place of delivery, mode of delivery, PNC follow up, maternal belief on the purported advantage of pre-lacteal feeding and information on risk associated with pre-lacteal feeding were statistically associated with pre-lacteal feeding.

In multiple logistic regression by using backward elimination method, mothers with no previousthe birth was about three times higher to introduce pre-lacteal feeding than those mothers who with a birth spacing of greater than or equal to 24 months (AOR: 2.93; 95%CI (1.21, 7.09)). A child who born with a birth spacing of less than 24 months were almost three times more likely to practice pre-lacteal feeding than those who born with a birth spacing of greater than or equal to 24 months (AOR:2.89; 95% CI (1.15,7.25)). A child whose mother discarded her colostrum was about seven times higher to receive pre-lacteal feeding (AOR: 6.72; 95% CI (2.49, 18.12)) than those who gave colostrum to their child. Mothers who have an ANC follow up of less than four times were about 11 times higher to give pre-lacteal feeding than mothers who have four and above ANC follow up (AOR: 10.55; 95%CI (4.76, 23.40)). Mothers who underwent cesarean section were about four times higher to practice pre-lacteal feeding as compared to those who delivered through spontaneous vaginal delivery (AOR:4.38 95% CI (1.72,11.12)). Mothers who believe on the purported advantage of pre-lacteal feeding were three times more to give pre-lacteal feeding than those who didn't believe the advantage of pre-lacteal feeding (AOR:3.36;95%CI (1.62,6.96)) (Table 5).

Discussion

With the existing strategies and approaches which increase the awareness of mothers, there is has poor maternal knowledge of the advantage of pre-lacteal feeding. Generally, there is a relationship between ANC follow up, colostrum discarding, childbirth spacing and mode of delivery with the introduction of pre-lacteal feeding.

This study revealed that the prevalence of pre-lacteal feeding was 10.1%. This is lower than the national prevalence which was 27% [22]. This result was also lower than the study done in selected regions of Ethiopia, which was 28.9% [27]. This could be due to the study participant were from the town and nearby to health institution, they would have more information on the advantage of visiting

Table 1 Socio-demographic characteristics mothers and child, in Aksum town, central zone of Tigray. Ethiopia 2017

Demographic variables	Frequency	Percentage
Age of the mother (n = 477)		
≤ 19	18	3.8
20–24	97	20.3
25–29	202	42.3
30–34	85	17.8
35–39	53	11.1
40–44	17	3.6
≥ 45	5	1
Family size (n = 477)		
≤ 3	158	33.1
≥ 4	319	66.9
Level of educational (n = 477)		
No education	161	33.8
Primary school (1–8)	120	25.2
Secondary school and above	196	41.1
Marital status (n = 477)		
Single	17	3.6
Married	407	85.3
Widowed	43	9
Divorced	10	2.1
Religion (n = 477)		
Orthodox	396	83
Muslim	81	17
Ethnicity (n = 477)		
Tigrian	473	99.2
Amhara	4	0.8
Occupation (n = 477)		
Housewife	291	61
Governmental employee	59	12.4
Private employee	91	19.1
Daily labor	35	7.3
Other	1	0.2
Number of children (n = 477)		
≤ 3	393	82.4
≥ 4	84	17.6
Age of the child (n = 477)		
< 6 months	145	30.4
6–11 months	141	29.6
12–17 months	89	18.7
18–24 months	102	21.4
Sex of the child (n = 477)		
Male	254	53.2
Female	223	46.8

Table 1 Socio-demographic characteristics mothers and child, in Aksum town, central zone of Tigray. Ethiopia 2017 *(Continued)*

Demographic variables	Frequency	Percentage
Birth order (n = 477)		
Birth order one	150	31.4
Birth order 2–3	239	50.1
Birth order ≥4	88	18.4
Birth spacing (n = 477)		
No previous child	150	31.4
< 24 months	115	24.1
≥ 24 months	212	44.4

antenatal/maternal and child health (MCH) clinics and may have better access to health education materials supportive to decrease the pre-lacteal feeding practice [6]. This could be due to the expansion of community health education in the town through the effective information, education and communication (IEC) strategies. The other possible reasons could be due to the difference in year of the study and sample size difference.

This study is also lower than studies done in different corners of Ethiopia. Eastern Ethiopia, which was 45.4% [13], Raya Kobo district 38.8% [23], northwest Ethiopia 26.8% [26], southern Ethiopia 41% [28], north Showa 24.4% [21], South-west Ethiopia 21.9% [24] and Jimma zone 17% [15]. The difference between these studies might be due to the difference in traditional practice between ethnic groups. This difference might also be due to the difference in the study setting, in the case of the Raya Kobo district 86% of the study subjects were from rural areas, whereas in this study the study participants were from the urban part of Aksum town. This might have been the result of key messages on infant feeding being delivered to pregnant women by healthcare workers during the mothers' attendance at antenatal care. Hence, mothers who reside in the towns have better access to maternal and child health services. Mothers who live in urban has a good coverage of television and newspapers for access to health education and information. The result of this study was comparable with the study done in northeastern Ethiopia 11.1% [29], in Nigeria 11.7% [30] and in India in Gautam Nagori 10.2% [31].

The current finding is also lower than reports from other developing countries (26.5% in Nepal [6], 31.3%, in Uganda [32], 58% Egypt [33] and 88% in India [34]). This could be due to the difference in contextual regions and health policy, our country currently implementing which is mainly focused on prevention

Table 2 Feeding practice of mothers, in Aksum town, central zone of Tigray, 2017

Variables	Frequency	Percentage
Pre-lacteal feeding practice for the index child ($n = 477$)		
Yes	48	10.1
No	429	89.9
Type of pre-lacteal ($n = 48$)		
Formula milk	15	31.3
Plain water	13	27.1
Sugar/glucose water	9	18.8
Caw milk	6	12.5
Butter	3	6.3
Other[a]	2	4.2
Reason to give pre-lacteal ($n = 48$)		
Breast problem	16	33.3
Breast feed for infant will cause thirsty	13	27.1
Maternal medical illness	10	20.8
For child growth	3	6.3
Infant feeding problem	3	6.3
Inadequate breast milk secretion	2	4.2
Cultural practice	1	2.1
Influence to give pre-lacteal feeding ($n = 48$)		
Mothers own decision	31	64.6
Health professional	13	27.1
Traditional birth attendant	3	6.3
Grand mothers	1	2.1
Colostrum giving ($n = 477$)		
Yes	447	93.7
No	30	6.3
Reason for discarding colostrum (30)		
Maternal medical illness	12	40
My breast has no milk	12	40
For the child growth	4	13.3
Cause abdominal discomfort and diarrhea	2	6.7
Breast feeding initiation (477)		
Within 1 h	271	56.8
Greater than 1 h	206	43.2

[a]Tenadam with water

Table 3 Maternal health care service utilization of mothers, in Aksum town, Tigray, Ethiopia 2017

Variables	Frequency	Percentage
ANC visit ($n = 477$)		
Yes	461	96.6
No	16	3.4
How many ($n = 477$)		
$>=4$	341	71.5
<4	120	25.2
Not at all	16	3.4
Breast feeding counseling ($n = 477$)		
Yes	467	97.9
No	10	2.1
Place of giving birth ($n = 477$)		
Health facility	453	95
At home	24	5
Mode of delivery ($n = 477$)		
C/S delivery	41	8.6
Normal spontaneous	436	91.4
The person who assisted you during delivery ($n = 477$)		
Health profession	453	95
Traditional birth attendant	24	5
PNC follow ($n = 477$)		
Yes	412	86.4
No	65	13.6

with community involvement on different health issues (with special attention to mothers and infants) through implementing a health extension program that works with the health development army and women networking comprised of the community.

Colostrum feeding provides newborns with immunity to infection. Mothers who discard colostrum in the first 5 days were about seven times more likely to practice pre-lacteal feeding than those who give colostrum to their index child. This result is consistent with the study done in northeastern Ethiopia [29]. This might be because those mothers may believe that pre-lacteal feeding has some advantages and/or have cultural practice to feed other than breast milk, thus more likely to feed pre-lacteals. Lack of full information on the advantages of giving newborn colostrum and the disadvantage of pre-lacteal feeding could lead to mothers discarding the first milk [35]. A cesarean section may also hamper immediate colostrum feeding due to post anesthesia or postoperative effects [36]. There are also many women say that they have breastfeeding problems. During this interval, babies are likely to feed pre-lacteal feeding.

Antenatal care visit is a best opportunity to promote skilled attendance at birth and to counsel and educate mothers on essential healthy behaviors like newborn feeding. The result of this study revealed that mothers with less than four ANC visit were about 11 times more likely to introduce pre-lacteal feeding than those

Pre-lacteal feeding practice and associated factors among mothers having children less than two years...

259

Table 4 Maternal level of information on pre-lacteal feeding among mothers having children less than 24 months, in Aksum town, Tigray, Ethiopia, 2017

Variables	Frequency	Percentage
Advantage of Colostrum (n = 477)		
Yes	447	93.7
No	30	6.3
Level of information (n = 477)		
Poor level	43	9
Good level	434	91
Believe on purported PLF advantage (n = 477)[a]		
Yes	165	34.6
No	312	65.4
Reason for believing on purported advantages (n = 165)[b]		
For child health and growth	101	61.2
Breast feed to child cause thirty	53	32.1
To calm the baby	21	12.7
To clean infant's bowel/throat/mouth	7	4.2
Other[c]	1	0.6
Risk of PLF (n = 477)		
Yes	376	78.8
No	101	21.2
Information on risks of PLF (n = 376)[b]		
Diarrhea & vomiting	343	72.4
Poor growth	278	41.5
Infection	303	36.6

[a]The medical community defines pre-lacteal feeding as (potentially) dangerous which had no any recognized benefits [39], [b]multiple answer were possible, [c]culture

who had greater than four ANC follow up. This may be due to the fact that those mothers who follow ANC get information on feeding practice of the newborn and infant from the health workers. This is similar to the studies done in the Harari region [13] and south Ethiopia [28]. This is also consistent with the study done in sub-Saharan Africa [37] and in Nepal [6]. This result was inconsistent with the study done in the selected regions Ethiopian [27]. This could be due to the different sample size difference in which our sample size was smaller than the study done in selected regions Ethiopian. Therefore, Coordination, strengthening and sustaining of the existing strategies and approaches to give more emphasize on the nutritional value of colostrum and ANC services utilization is recommended to reduce health problems associated with the introduction of pre-lacteal feeding.

Furthermore, first time mothers were more likely to introduce pre-lacteal feeds in this study. The first-time mothers could have less skill and knowledge of newborn care and proper infant feeding practice. They may also rely more on the older women in the household and community who follow the traditional practice [38]. In this study mothers with no previous birth were about three times higher to practice introduction of pre-lacteal feeding. Moreover, pre-lacteal feeding was almost three times higher among mothers who gave birth within 24 years. Short inter-pregnancy intervals are associated with a higher risk of low birth weight, preterm birth and a higher risk of cesarean section. During that time, the neonate may be admitted to an intensive care unit which may hamper the exclusive breastfeeding and leads to practice pre-lacteal feeding.

In this study, pre-lacteal feeding was about four times higher in mothers who delivered through the cesarean section as compared to those who had vaginal delivered. This is consistent with the studies done in Egypt [33], in Uganda [32] and in India [36]. Use of general or spinal anesthesia for cesarean delivery and the trauma during surgery may delay the recovery of mothers. The caretakers then tend to provide alternative feeding to the baby during this period, often on the suggestion of the hospital staff.

The medical community defines pre-lacteal feeding as (potentially)dangerous which had no any recognized benefits [39]. In this study mothers who believe in the purported advantage of pre-lacteal feeding was about three times higher to provide pre-lacteal feeding to their index child. This implies they have poor knowledge of the risk associated with pre-lacteal feeding [23]. This finding is similar to the study done in northwest Ethiopia [26]. Boosting a mother's knowledge of IYCF is a cornerstone for implementing sustainable strategies to improve appropriate feeding practices [35].

Findings from this study have a substantial contribution to the promotion of optimal breastfeeding practices and the achievement of the sustainable development goal in reducing child mortality in Ethiopia. However, the limitation of this study was that the information obtained from mothers might be subjected to recall bias. Lack of support with qualitative data is also another limitation. Therefore, further follow up research with qualitative support is recommended to understand the relationship between (cesarean delivery, colostrum discarding) and pre-lacteal feeding. The study also shares the limitation of the cross-sectional study design.

Conclusions

Although Ethiopia has set breastfeeding policies consistent with international recommendations, there are still neonates who receiving pre-lacteal feeding in Aksum town, which leads to decrease exclusive breastfeeding

Table 5 Factors associated with pre-lacteal feeding practices among mothers, in Aksum town, Tigray, Ethiopia 2017

Variables	Pre-lacteal feeding		Crude OR (CI: 95%)	Adjusted OR (CI: 95%)
	Yes	No		
Level of education				
No education	29(18%)	132(82%)	3.695(1.78,7.66)	2.4 (0.95,5.93)
Primary school	8 (6.7%)	112(93.3%)	1.2(0.47,3.08)	1.145(0.39,3.38)
Secondary and above	11(5.6%)	185(94.4%)	1	1
Child age				
< 6 months	16(11.3%)	126(88.7%)	1	1
6–11 months	12(8.7%)	126(91.3%)	0.75(0.34,1.65)	0.43(0.16,1.19)
12-17 months	5(5.8%)	81(94.2%)	0.48(0.17,1.36)	0.434(0.13,1.41)
18–24 months	15(14.9%)	86(85.1%)	1.39(0.65,2.96)	0.843(0.31,2.25)
Birth spacing				
No previous child	19(12.7%)	131(87.3%)	2.417(1.14,5.15)	2.931(1.21,7.09) *
< 24 months	17(14.8%)		2.891(1.33, 6.29)	2.887(1.15,7.25) *
≥ 24 months	12(5.7%)	200(94.3%)	1	1
Colostrum giving				
Yes	32(7%)	425(93%)	1	1
No	16(80%)	4(20%)	10.629(4.78, 23.61)	6.724(2.49,18.12) *
Number of ANC visit				
≥ 4	10(2.9%)	331(97.1%)	1	1
< 4	38(27.9%)	98(72.1%)	11.529 (5.44, 24.41)	10.549 (4.76, 23.40) *
Breast feeding counseling[a]				
Yes	45(9.6%)	422(90.4%)	1	1
No	3(30%)	7(70%)	4.019(1.00, 16.09)	0.648(0.07,6.2)
Place of delivery[a]				
Heath facility	40(8.7%)	418(91.3%)	1	1
At home	8(42.1%)	11(57.9%)	5.162(2.08, 12.81)	1.192(0.03,4.77)
Mode of delivery				
Normal	37(8.5%)	399(91.5%)	1	1
C/S	11(26.8%)	30(73.2%)	3.954(1.83,8.53)	4.377 (1.72,11.12) *
PNC follow up[a]				
Yes	36(8.7%)	376(91.3%)	1	1
No	12(18.5%)	53(81.5%)	2.365(1.16, 4.83)	1.323(0.47,3.70)
Believe on purported advantage of PLF				
Yes	30(18.2%)	135(81.8%)	3.63(1.95, 6.81)	3.359 (1.62,6.96) *
No	18(5.8%)	294(94.2%)	1	1
Risk of PLF[a]				
Yes	28(7.4%)	348(92.6%)	1	1
No	20(19.8%)	81(80.2%)	3.069(1.65, 5.72)	1.454(0.58,3.64)
Family size[a]				
< =3	21(13.3%)	137(86.7%)	1	1
> =4	27(8.5%)	292(91.5%)	0.603(0.33,1.10)	1.403(0.35,5.67)

*Statistically significant variables at *p*-value of < 0.05
[a]Variable excluded after adjusting them in multivariate logistic regression

practices in the town. The current study showed that the prevalence of pre-lacteal feeding is still high that remained a challenge for optimal breastfeeding in the town. Childbirth spacing and maternal-related factors were contributing factors for practicing of pre-lacteal feeding.

Abbreviations
ANC: Antenatal care; AOR: Adjusted odds ratio; COR: Crude odds ratio; IEC: Information Education and Communication; PLF: Pre-lacteal feeding

Acknowledgments
Authors thanks to Mekelle University, data collectors, supervisors and study subjects.

Authors' contributions
GT: Conceived and designed the study, supervised the data collection, performed the analysis, interpretation of data and drafted the manuscript. MK: Assisted in analysis, interpretation and reviewed the manuscript critically. TB: Assisted in the study design, analysis, and interpretation and reviewed the manuscript critically. HT: Assisted in designing the study, data interpretation and critically reviewed the manuscript. TM: Assisted in data interpretation and reviewed the manuscript critically. TS: Assisted in analysis, interpretation and reviewed the manuscript critically. All authors were read and approved the final manuscript.

Competing interests
The authors declare that they have no competing interests.

Author details
[1]Department of Pediatrics and Child Health Nursing, School of Nursing, College of Health Science, Aksum University, Aksum, Ethiopia. [2]Department of Nursing, College of Health Science, Mekelle University, Mekelle, Ethiopia. [3]Department of Adult Health Nursing, School of Nursing, College of Health Science, Aksum University, Aksum, Ethiopia. [4]Department of Medical Laboratory, College of Health Science, Aksum University, Aksum, Ethiopia.

References
1. Marriott BP, et al. World Health Organization (WHO) infant and young child feeding indicators: associations with growth measures in 14 low-income countries. Matern Child Nutr. 2012;8(3):354–70.
2. You, D., N.R. Jin, and T. Wardlaw, Levels & trends in child mortality. 2012.
3. UNICEF. Committing to child survival: a promise renewed. Progress report 2013. New York: UNICEF; 2013. p. 2014.
4. Laroia N, Sharma D. The religious and cultural bases for breastfeeding practices among the Hindus. Breastfeed Med. 2006;1(2):94–8.
5. Federal Democratic Republic of Ethiopia. Ethiopia demographic and health survey, 2016. Addis Ababa: Central Statistical Agency; 2019.
6. Khanal V, et al. Factors associated with the introduction of prelacteal feeds in Nepal: findings from the Nepal demographic and health survey 2011. Int Breastfeed J. 2013;8(1):9.
7. McKenna KM, Shankar RT. The practice of prelacteal feeding to newborns among Hindu and Muslim families. J Midwifery Womens Health. 2009;54(1): 78–81.
8. Chandrashekhar T, et al. Breast-feeding initiation and determinants of exclusive breastfeeding–a questionnaire survey in an urban population of western Nepal. Public Health Nutr. 2007;10(2):192–7.
9. Nguyen PH, et al. Prelacteal feeding practices in Vietnam: challenges and associated factors. BMC Public Health. 2013;13(1):932.
10. Sadhasivam M, Kanagasabapathy S. Pre-lacteal feeding practice among rural mothers in Tamilnadu-a questionnaire-based study. Int J Biomed Adv Res. 2015;6(6):484–7.
11. Sriram S, et al. Knowledge, attitude, and practices of mothers regarding infant feeding practices. Natl J Commun Med. 2013;3(2).
12. Onah S, et al. Infant feeding practices and maternal socio-demographic factors that influence the practice of exclusive breastfeeding among mothers in Nnewi south-East Nigeria: a cross-sectional and analytical study. Int Breastfeed J. 2014;9(1):6.
13. Bekele Y, Mengistie B, Mesfine F. Prelacteal feeding practice and associated factors among mothers attending immunization clinic in Harari region public health facilities, eastern Ethiopia. Open J Prev Med. 2014;2014.
14. Kogi-Makau, W., et al., Magnitude and determinants of stunting in children under five years of age in food surplus region of Ethiopia: the case of west Gojam zone. 2009.
15. Beyene TT. Predictors of nutritional status of children visiting health facilities in Jimma Zone, South West Ethiopia. Int J Adv Nurs Sci Pract. 2012;1(1):1–13.
16. Ethiopian Health and Nutrition Institute (EHNRI)., Nutritional Baseline Survey Report for the National Nutrition Program of Ethiopia. 2010. Available at www.ephi.gov.et/images/nutrition/nutrition%20baseline%20survey%20reportpdf.
17. Agency, C.S. ETHIOPIA demographic and health survey, key indicators report. Rockville: The DHS Program ICF; 2016.
18. Disha A, et al. Infant and young child feeding (IYCF) practices in Ethiopia and Zambia and their association with child nutrition: analysis of demographic and health survey data. Afr J Food Agric Nutr Dev. 2012;12(2): 5895–914.
19. De Sousa, B.J.S., Aksum (አክሱም). 2010.
20. Gerensea, H. and R. Murugan, Is there significant difference between digital and glass mercury thermometer? Advances in nursing, 2016. 2016.
21. Hailu D. Assessment of pre-lacteal feeding practice and its associated factors among mothers having children less than 24 months of age in Fitche town, North Showa, Ethiopia: AAU; 2016.
22. Ethiopian central statistics agency (ECSA). Ethiopian demographic and health survey 2011. Addis Ababa: Central Statistical Agency and ICF International; 2012.
23. Legesse M, et al. Prelacteal feeding practices and associated factors among mothers of children aged less than 24 months in Raya kobo district, north eastern Ethiopia: a cross-sectional study. Int Breastfeed J. 2014;9(1):189.
24. Muluken A. Assessment of the prevalence of pre-lacteal feeding and associated factors among mothers of children less than one year of age in Mizan-Aman town bench-Maji zone, Southwest Ethiopia: AAU; 2015.
25. Alemayehu T, Haidar J, Habte D. Determinants of exclusive breastfeeding practices in Ethiopia. Ethiop J Health Dev. 2009;23(1).
26. Tariku A, et al. Factors associated with pre-lacteal feeding in the rural population of Northwest Ethiopia: a community cross-sectional study. Int Breastfeed J. 2016;11(1):14.
27. Belachew AB, Kahsay AB, Abebe YG. Individual and community-level factors associated with the introduction of pre-lacteal feeding in Ethiopia. Arch Public Health. 2016;74(1):6.
28. Tessema M, Belachew T, Ersino G. Feeding patterns and stunting during early childhood in rural communities of Sidama, South Ethiopia. Pan Afr Med J. 2013;14(1).
29. Bililign N, et al. Factors associated with pre-lacteal feeding in north eastern Ethiopia: a community based cross-sectional study. Int Breastfeed J. 2016;11(1):13.
30. Ibadin OM, et al. Prelacteal feeding practices among lactating mothers in Benin City, Nigeria. Niger J Paediatr. 2013;40(2):139–44.
31. Gupta RK, Nagori G. A study on changing trends and impact of ante-natal education and mother's educational status on pre-lacteal feeding practices. J Pharm Biomed Sci©(JPBMS). 2012;19(19).
32. Ogah A, et al. A cross-sectional study of pre-lacteal feeding practice among women attending Kampala International University teaching hospital maternal and child health clinic, Bushenyi, Western Uganda. Asian J Med Sci. 2012;4(3):79–85.
33. El-Gilany A-H, Abdel-Hady DM. Newborn first feed and pre-lacteal feed in Mansoura, Egypt. Biomed Res Int. 2014;2014.
34. Raina SK, Mengi V, Singh G. Determinants of pre-lacteal feeding among infants of RS Pura block of Jammu and Kashmir, India. J Fam Med Prim Care. 2012;1(1):27.

35. Katepa-Bwalya M, et al. Infants and young children feeding practices and nutritional status in two districts in Zambia. Int Breastfeed J. 2015;10(1):5.
36. Patel A, Banerjee A, Kaletwad A. Factors associated with pre-lacteal feeding and timely initiation of breastfeeding in hospital-delivered infants in India. J Hum Lact. 2013;29(4):572–8.
37. Berde AS, Ozcebe H. Risk factors for pre-lacteal feeding in sub-Saharan Africa: a multilevel analysis of population data from twenty-two countries. Public Health Nutr. 2017:1–10.
38. Dawal S, et al. Study of pre-lacteal feeding practices and its determinants in a rural area of Maharashtra. Sch J App Med Sci. 2014;2(4):1422–7.
39. Saadeh R, Casanovas C. Implementing and revitalizing the baby-friendly hospital initiative. Food Nutr Bull. 2009;30(2_suppl2):S225–9.

27

Prognostic value of early, conventional proton magnetic resonance spectroscopy in cooled asphyxiated infants

Hajnalka Barta[1]*(iD), Agnes Jermendy[1], Marton Kolossvary[2], Lajos R. Kozak[3], Andrea Lakatos[3], Unoke Meder[1], Miklos Szabo[1†] and Gabor Rudas[3†]

Abstract

Background: Neonatal hypoxic-ischemic encephalopathy (HIE) commonly leads to neurodevelopmental impairment, raising the need for prognostic tools which may guide future therapies in time. Prognostic value of proton MR spectroscopy (H-MRS) between 1 and 46 days of age has been extensively studied; however, the reproducibility and generalizability of these methods are controversial in a general clinical setting. Therefore, we investigated the prognostic performance of conventional H-MRS during first 96 postnatal hours in hypothermia-treated asphyxiated neonates.

Methods: Fifty-one consecutive hypothermia-treated HIE neonates were examined by H-MRS at three echo-times (TE = 35, 144, 288 ms) between 6 and 96 h of age, depending on clinical stability. Patients were divided into favorable (n = 35) and unfavorable (n = 16) outcome groups based on psychomotor and mental developmental index (PDI and MDI, Bayley Scales of Infant Development II) scores ($\geq$ 70 versus < 70 or death, respectively), assessed at 18–26 months of age. Associations between 36 routinely measured metabolite ratios and outcome were studied. Age-dependency of metabolite ratios in whole patient population was assessed. Prognostic performance of metabolite ratios was evaluated by Receiver Operating Characteristics (ROC) analysis.

Results: Three metabolite ratios showed significant difference between outcome groups after correction for multiple testing ($p < 0.0014$): myo-inositol (mIns)/N-acetyl-aspartate (NAA) height, mIns/creatine (Cr) height, both at TE = 35 ms, and NAA/Cr height at TE = 144 ms. Assessment of age-dependency showed that all 3 metabolite ratios (mIns/NAA, NAA/Cr and mIns/Cr) stayed constant during first 96 postnatal hours, rendering them optimal for prediction. ROC analysis revealed that mIns/NAA gives better prediction for outcome than NAA/Cr and mIns/Cr with cut-off values 0. 6798 0.6274 and 0.7798, respectively, (AUC 0.9084, 0.8396 and 0.8462, respectively, $p < 0.00001$); mIns/NAA had the highest specificity (95.24%) and sensitivity (84.62%) for predicting outcome of neonates with HIE any time during the first 96 postnatal hours.

Conclusions: Our findings suggest that during first 96 h of age even conventional H-MRS could be a useful prognostic tool in predicting the outcome of asphyxiated neonates; mIns/NAA was found to be the best and age-independent predictor.

Keywords: Perinatal asphyxia, Hypoxic-ischemic encephalopathy, Proton magnetic resonance spectroscopy, Conventional sequence, Neurodevelopmental outcome

---

* Correspondence: barta.hajnalka@med.semmelweis-univ.hu
†Miklos Szabo and Gabor Rudas contributed equally to this work.
[1]1st Department of Paediatrics, Semmelweis University, Budapest, Hungary
Full list of author information is available at the end of the article

Background

Perinatal asphyxia and consequential hypoxic-ischemic encephalopathy (HIE) remains one of the leading causes of perinatal brain injury, affecting more than two million neonates yearly worldwide [1]. Although full recovery is possible, HIE can also lead to permanent mental or psychomotor disability [2].

Currently, therapeutic hypothermia is the one and only neuroprotective method proven effective to reduce mortality and long-term morbidity in HIE [3]. However, mortality or moderate to severe developmental delay still affects over 40% of cooled infants, demanding future therapeutic approaches additional to hypothermia [4, 5]. In theory, the key to successful neuroprotection is the earliest possible initiation regardless of the therapy chosen [6]. This in turn requires proper and timely diagnosis and early establishment of prognosis [7].

This underscores the need for an appropriate and as-early-as-possible prognostic tool for the selection of infants who are most likely to suffer moderate to severe disability and would thus benefit from future personalized neuroprotective protocols.

Proton magnetic resonance spectroscopy (H-MRS) is one of the tools proposed for such a biomarker [8]. This examination is becoming increasingly widespread in various medical fields, i.e. tumor diagnosis or neurodegenerative diseases. H-MRS usually accompanies brain magnetic resonance imaging (MRI) scans, and is capable of registering the spectra of various metabolites present in the examined volume of interest (VOI). Since water is the molecule most abundantly present in brain tissue, its acquired spectrum would be several orders of magnitude higher than those of other metabolites; consequently, acquisition of H-MRS requires suppression of the water signal. This can be achieved by several acquisition protocols [9]. The analysis of the acquired spectrum informs the clinician of the metabolic state of the examined tissue, providing valuable functional information in a non-invasive way. To acquire motionless images during brain MR scans, most infants require sufficient sedation and intravenous access, not all; however, no administration of contrast material is necessary.

Several studies investigated the prognostic power of H-MRS in neonatal asphyxia, between 4 h and 46 days of age [10–19], often covering a wide age range, given the need for earliest possible prognosis.

Establishing the reproducibility of H-MRS as a prognostic biomarker also poses a problem [20], as previous studies used a wide range of data-optimizing equipment, software, or absolute quantification approaches to improve data quality. Taken together, there is no universal agreement regarding how H-MRS should be applied in the daily clinical practice.

Aim

The purpose of our study was to determine the prognostic value of a completely conventional H-MRS sequence (i.e. without special equipment and post-processing techniques other than basic vendor-provided analysis), performed before the 96th hour of life in infants with HIE, analyzing various metabolite ratios, their age-dependence and association with long-term neurodevelopmental outcome.

Methods

Patient selection

In our retrospective descriptive analysis, we reviewed all 283 patients with suspected HIE born between January 2006 and December 2010 and admitted to the regional cooling center, the Neonatal Intensive Care Unit (NICU) of the 1st Department of Paediatrics, Semmelweis University, Budapest, Hungary.

From this patient pool, we only included patients who (A) fulfilled the diagnostic criteria for moderate to severe HIE according to the international TOBY trial [21], being as follows: (i) at least one of the following: continued need for resuscitation/ventilation at 10 min after birth, OR Apgar score ≤ 5 at 5 min after birth OR pH < 7.0 or BE ≤ – 16 mmol/L within 60 min after birth AND (ii) altered level of consciousness (lethargy, stupor or coma) AND hypotonia or abnormal reflexes or seizures AND (iii) abnormal brain background activity registered on amplitude-integrated electroencephalography (aEEG). Additional inclusion criteria were (B) brain H-MRS scan performed before the 96th postnatal hour AND (C) having a neurodevelopmental follow-up examination using the Bayley Scales of Infant Development II between 18 and 26 months of age, as detailed below OR death (< 28 days of age OR > 28 days associated with HIE).

We excluded all patients who (a) had other underlying conditions, which could be responsible for encephalopathy besides asphyxia (i.e. stroke, intracranial hemorrhage, congenital malformation or metabolic disease). As only early onset (< 6 postnatal hours) hypothermia treatment was thought to be neuroprotective at the time of the study, we excluded patients who (b) did not receive hypothermia treatment due to delayed admission. Further exclusion criteria were: (c) gestational age < 36 weeks and (d) low quality brain H-MRS.

Altogether, 51 patients met inclusion criteria and were included in the analysis (Fig. 1).

Clinical care

Whole-body hypothermia treatment was initiated as soon as possible but within 6 h after delivery, using a water-filled mattress (Tecotherm©; TecCom, Halle, Germany). The target rectal temperature was between 33 and 34 °C, maintained for 72 h. In the rewarming phase, temperature

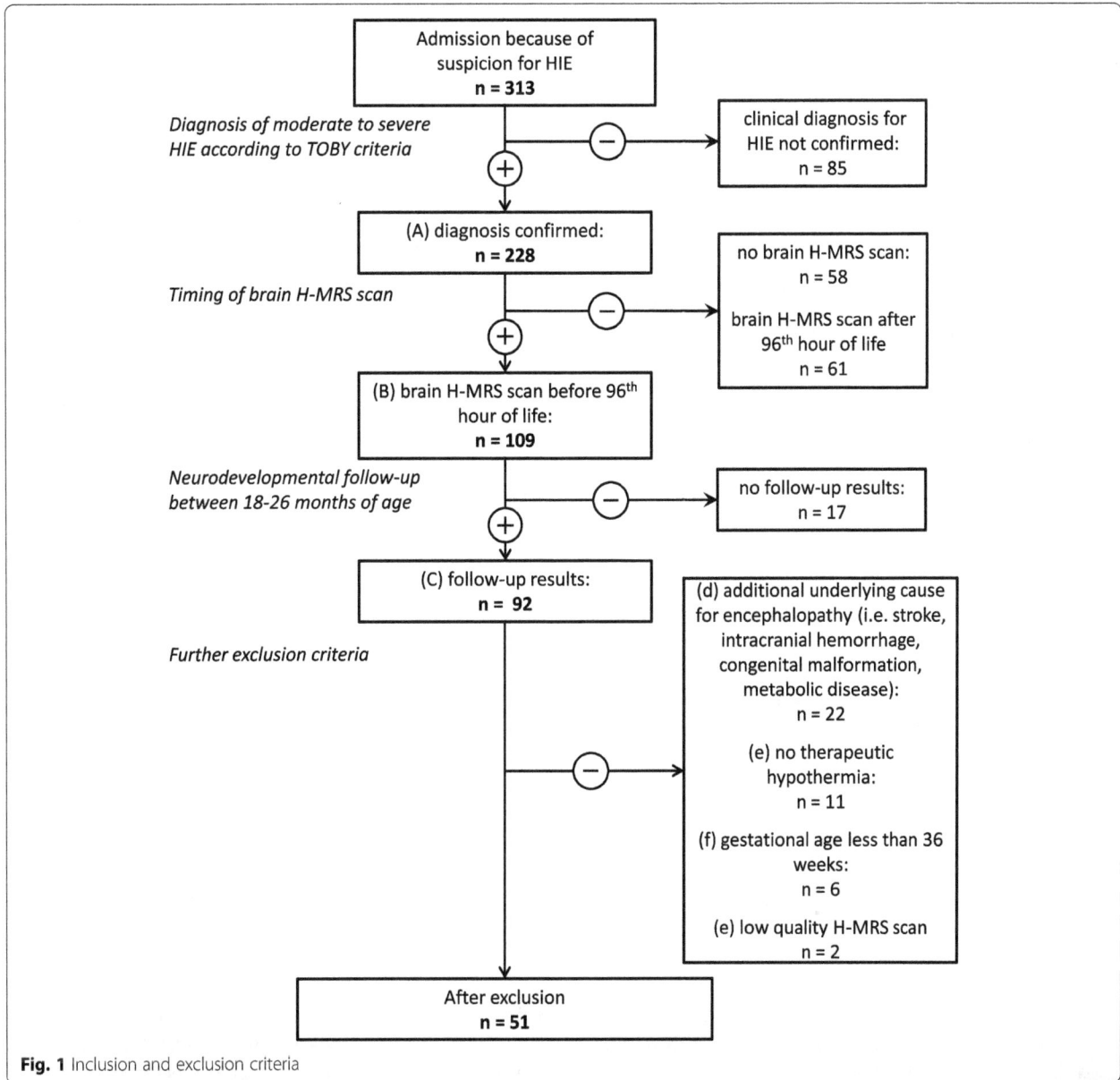

Fig. 1 Inclusion and exclusion criteria

increase velocity was 0.5 °C/h. All infants were ventilated throughout the cooling and rewarming phase.

Continuous morphine (Morph. hydrochlor. 10 mg/mL; TEVA Magyarország Zrt., Gödöllő, Hungary) sedation (10 μg/kg BW/h) was started following the loading dose (0.1 mg/kg BW) administered when the cooling was initiated. Phenobarbitone (Gardenal 40 mg; Aventis, Maisons-Alfort, France, 20 mg/kg BW) was given as the first line of anticonvulsant therapy if clinical or electrophysiological seizures were detected. In case of noncontrolled seizures, the phenobarbitone loading dose was repeated, or midazolam (Midazolam Torrex 5 mg/ml; Chiesi Pharmaceuticals GmbH, Vienna, Austria) was given in single or repeated doses (0.1 mg/kg BW) or in continuous infusion (0.1 mg/kg BW/h). In some cases, newborns received lidocain, phenytoin, diazepam or chloral hydrate alternatively, according to the attending clinician's decision.

The severity of encephalopathy was determined based on a combination of aEEG background activity at 6 h of age and Sarnat staging at admission [22]. Infants with abnormal aEEG pattern by 6 h of age (burst suppression (BS), low voltage (LV) or flat trace (FT)) OR meeting Sarnat stage 3 criteria were considered having severe encephalopathy. A normal aEEG pattern (continuous normal voltage (CNV) or discontinuous normal voltage (DNV)) AND Sarnat stage 1–2 constituted moderate encephalopathy.

H-MRS examination

Proton MR spectroscopy studies were carried out on a 3 Tesla Philips Achieva MRI scanner (Philips Medical Systems,

Best, The Netherlands), at the MR Research Center of Semmelweis University, as early as the infant reached clinical stability and was suitable for transport. All MR scans were performed between 6th and 96th postnatal hours (median 25th postnatal hour). The Neonatal Emergency & Transport Services of the Peter Cerny Foundation provided the neonatal transport and the critical care, including hypothermia treatment. For the time of the examination, the infants were removed from the incubator and received continuous morphine sedation. In case of intubated infants, skilled personnel provided manual ventilation with an AMBU bag throughout the MR examination. Continuous monitoring of transcutaneous oxygen saturation and capnography was provided for all neonates during the MR scan, using Medrad Veris MR Monitoring System (Bayer Healthcare LLC, Whippany, NJ).

Ethical considerations

Patients enrolled did not undergo procedures or interventions for the purposes of the study. Brain MRI and H-MRS are part of routine diagnostic imaging in our unit as a center practice, and are performed on all neonates with suspected moderate-to-severe HIE. Use of these imaging tools aid in confirming the diagnosis, determining the timing of and nature of the hypoxic-ischemic insult (chronic intrauterine or intrapartum), and ruling out other etiologies. Finally, H-MRS measurements are not used to redirect clinical care of infants with HIE.

Acquisition protocols

MR spectra were acquired using the PRESS (Point RE-Solved Spectroscopy) single voxel localization sequence, at echo-times TE = 35 ms, 144 ms and 288 ms, repetition time TR = 2000, number of acquisitions NSA = 128. Duration of scan was approximatively 30 min. The analyzed VOI was a $1 \times 1 \times 1$ cm voxel in the left thalamus of infants, localized based on gradient echo survey images acquired with TE = 5 ms, TR = 75 ms and 30° flipangle.

Registered metabolites

The most frequently determined and analyzed metabolites in the H-MRS spectra are N-acetyl-aspartate (NAA), creatine (Cr), choline (Cho), myo-inositol (mIns) and lactate (Lac).

There are different TE optima for the different metabolites, due to their acquisition-dependent signal-to-noise characteristics, e.g. the Lac's optimum is at TE = 288 ms, while for mI either TE = 35 ms or TE = 144 ms suffices. We recorded peak height, and peak area for all the above-listed metabolites (Fig. 2).

MR data analysis

We used the vendor-provided data-processing software on the MR console for analysis without any specific equipment or tool for data-optimization, in order to obtain results applicable to a general clinical setting. In order to reproduce basic, non-research center hospital level circumstances, no data-optimizing equipment or further post-processing methods were used to ameliorate the registered spectra.

Since we did not use absolute quantification protocols due to their high technical requirements, statistical analysis was carried out on all possible ratios of metabolite spectral peak heights and peak areas-under-curve, recorded at same TE. This resulted in the determination of overall 36 metabolite ratios (Table 1).

To improve the accuracy of our analyses, we excluded metabolite ratios derived from metabolite spectra with signal-to-noise ratio (SNR) below 1, i.e. where noise intensity exceeded signal intensity [23, 24].

Follow-up

Neurodevelopmental follow-up was measured by Bayley Scales of Infant Development II tool-kit, performed between 18 and 26 months of age by trained personnel, blinded to the H-MRS results. We defined poor outcome as either death (< 28 days of age OR > 28 days associated with HIE) OR moderately/severely delayed development (Mental Developmental Index (MDI) or Psychomotor Developmental Index (PDI) < 70). All other outcomes were considered as good outcome.

Statistical analysis

Categorical variables are reported as absolute numbers and percentages while continuous variables as mean ± standard deviation or median [25th to 75th interquartile range] depending on the distribution of the parameters. Shapiro-Wilk test was used to assess normality. Categorical variables were compared with the Fisher's exact test, while continuous variables were compared with the Student t-test or Mann-Whitney U-test for parametric and non-parametric comparisons, respectively.

To select the best metabolite ratios for prognostication, a three-step statistical procedure was implemented. First, we tested the association between the metabolite ratios and outcome. To adjust for multiple testing, we used Bonferroni-correction, that is to say, due to 36 examined metabolite ratios, we considered statistical results significant at $p < 0.0014$ (0.05/36 = 0.0014).

Second, we considered the fact that in the early hours after hypoxic insult, the brain metabolic activity shows extreme variations in time-dependent fashion [25, 26]. Therefore, metabolite ratios measured by H-MRS may also vary significantly depending on timing of data acquisition. Considering that these metabolic changes are still not fully understood and described, we aimed to select metabolite ratios with low or no variability during the first 96 postnatal hours, in order to ensure generalizability of

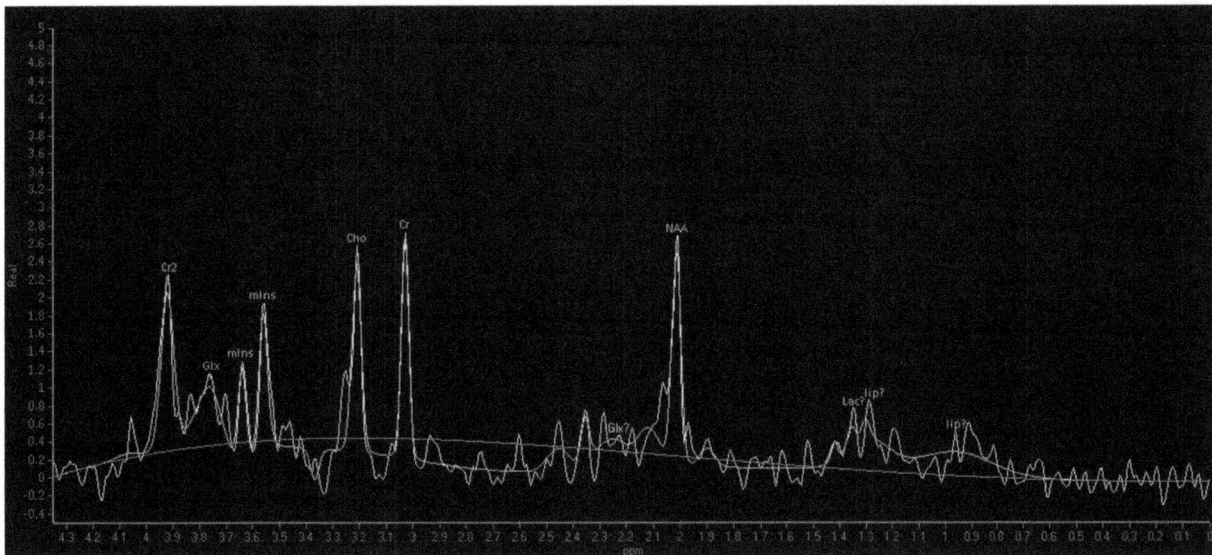

Fig. 2 Spectrum acquired by H-MRS at echo time (TE) = 35 ms. The registered metabolites are from left to right: Cr2: secondary creatine peak, Glx: glutamine/glutamate (multiple peaks, here, double peaks), mIns: myo-inositol (double peaks), Cho: choline, Cr: primary creatine peak, NAA: N-acetyl-aspartate, Lac: lactate, lip: lipid (double peaks). In HIE, metabolites considered to have clinical significance are mIns, Cho, Cr, NAA and Lac.? represent low (< 1) signal-to-noise ratio (SNR). NB: at TE = 35 ms, the Lac peak is difficult to differentiate from the overlapping lip peaks

our results for all infants within this period, irrespective of timing of the MR examination. We tested postnatal age-dependence of metabolite ratios using Spearman rank-correlation analysis.

Third, we evaluated the prognostic performance of metabolite ratios using Receiver Operating Characteristics (ROC) curve analysis to establish the potential cut-off-value (corresponding to the highest likelihood ratio of ROC curves), as well as to determine the sensitivity, specificity, positive and negative predictive values of the proposed markers. Moreover, we compared the metabolite ratios as diagnostic tests using the area under the ROC curve (AUC) using the method described by Hanley and McNeil [27].

Demographic, clinical and spectral data were analyzed and plotted using the GraphPad Prism software version 6.0 (GraphPad Software Inc., San Diego, California, USA).

Results

Fifty-one neonates with moderate-to-severe HIE met the inclusion criteria, and were enrolled in our study.

Hypothermia treatment was initiated before the 6th postnatal hour for all 51 neonates, with median [IQR] 2 [1.4; 3.1] hours. Forty-five out of the 51 patients had the H–MRS examination performed while receiving whole-body hypothermia. The remaining 6 patients had the examination done before the initiation or after the completion of hypothermia treatment. Nevertheless, all scans were performed within 96 h of age.

Clinical characteristics and MRI findings of these patients are shown in Tables 2 and 3, accordingly, categorized by long-term outcome. Of the 51 patients, 16 infants were considered to have poor outcome, including the 9 patients that died in the perinatal period (i.e. first 28 days), and the 7 patients who had moderately/severely delayed development (Mental Developmental Index (MDI) or Psychomotor Developmental Index (PDI) < 70). Of these 7 patients, 4 infants were diagnosed with cerebral palsy (2 associated with mental retardation and one with epilepsy), 2 had mental retardation and one patient suffered from neuronal hearing loss and epilepsy. None of our patients died between 28 days and the follow-up examination. Good and poor outcome

Table 1 List of ratios of peak heights and peak areas of the analyzed metabolites: (NAA: N-acetyl-aspartate, Cho: choline, Cr: creatine, mIns: myo-inositol and Lac: lactate), determined at echo-times TE = 35 ms, 144 ms and 288 ms

TE = 35 ms	TE = 144 ms	TE = 288 ms
• NAA/Cho height and area	• NAA/Cho height and area	• NAA/Cho height and area
• NAA/Cr height and area	• NAA/Cr height and area	• NAA/Cr height and area
• Cho/Cr height and area	• Cho/Cr height and area	• Cho/Cr height and area
• mIns/NAA height and area	• mIns/NAA height and area	• Lac/NAA height and area
• mIns/Cho height and area	• mIns/Cho height and area	• Lac/Cho height and area
• mIns/Cr height and area	• mIns/Cr height and area	• Lac/Cr height and area

Table 2 Clinical characteristics of newborns enrolled in the study ($n = 51$)

Variable	Good outcome ($n = 35$)	Poor outcome ($n = 16$)	p value
Male sex	19 (51%)	12 (75%)	0.1365
Gestational age (weeks)	39 [38; 40]	38 [37; 40]	0.0536
Birth weight (g)	3261 ± 577	3128 ± 537	0.4379
Apgar 1'	2 [1; 4]	1 [0; 2]	0.0091
Apgar 5'	5 [4; 7]	3 [2; 4]	0.0002*
Apgar 10'	6 [5; 8]	4 [2; 4]	0.0005*
Lowest pH < 1 h of age	7.21 [6.98; 7.28]	7.10 [7.00; 7.20]	0.1643
Highest BD < 1 h of age	14.1 ± 5.9	17.1 ± 4.6	0.0860
Onset of hypothermia (h)	1.8 [1.4; 3.1]	2.1 [1.4; 3.3]	0.6309
Severity of encephalopathy (severe)[#]	31 (89%)	15 (94%)	> 0.9999
Clinical or aEEG seizures (< 24 h)	28 (80%)	14 (88%)	0.7012
Abnormal aEEG pattern (BS, LV, FT)	31 (88%)	12 (75%)	0.2396
aEEG normalization (CNV, DNV) < 72 h	22 (63%)	5 (31%)	0.0681
aEEG normalization time (h)	30 [12; 47]	60 [42; 68]	0.1381
Age at MR scan (h)	25 [14; 49]	30 [16; 54]	0.6625
Abnormalities on MR Imaging (T1/T2 weighted imaging or DWI)	13 (37%)	11 (69%)	0.0681
Death	0	9 (56%)	NA[†]

Data shown as median [IQR], mean ± SD or percentage. Good outcome is defined as both MDI (Mental Developmental Index) and PDI (Psychomotor Developmental Index) ≥ 70 achieved on Bayley II test, poor outcome is defined as either MDI or PDI < 70 OR death (< 28 days of age OR > 28 days of age associated with HIE)

BD base deficit, aEEG amplitude-integrated electroencephalography, CNV continuous normal voltage, DNV discontinuous normal voltage, BS burst suppression, LV low voltage, FT flat trace, DWI diffusion weighted imaging

* represents significant results surviving Bonferroni-correction ($p < 0.0014$)

moderate encephalopathy: 6 h normal aEEG pattern (CNV, DNV) AND Sarnat stage 1–2, severe encephalopathy: 6 h abnormal aEEG pattern (BS, LV, FT) OR Sarnat stage 3 [21]

NA[†] (not applicable) represents statistical significance not applicable as death was included in the definition of the poor outcome group

groups only differed significantly in their 5' and 10' Apgar scores, as well as occurrence of stage 3 HIE seen on MR images.

Of the 36 metabolite ratios evaluated in the first 96 postnatal hours for prognostication of good or poor neurodevelopmental outcome, 3 metabolite ratios differed significantly between the good and poor outcome groups, rendering them candidates for further analysis (Table 4): mIns/NAA height (TE = 35 ms), NAA/Cr height (TE = 144 ms) and mIns/Cr height (TE = 35 ms).

Next, we tested the age-dependence of these 3 metabolite ratios during the first 96 postnatal hours among all 51 patients, as it has been described that the brain metabolic activity shows extreme time dependent variations

Table 3 Location and severity of observed MR Imaging abnormalities in newborns with good versus poor outcome

	MRI abnormality and good outcome ($n = 13$)	MRI abnormality and poor outcome ($n = 11$)	p value
Location of injury			
Basal ganglia and thalami	6 (46%)	8 (72%)	0.2397
Internal capsule	5 (38%)	6 (54%)	0.6824
White matter	5 (38%)	0 (0%)	0.0411
Cortex	1 (8%)	1 (9%)	> 0.9999
Severity of injury (MRI score)			
HIE score 1	3 (23%)	2 (18%)	> 0.9999
HIE score 2	6 (46%)	3 (27%)	0.4225
HIE score 3	0 (0%)	8 (72%)	0.0002*

Abnormalities are described as signal intensity abnormality on T1/T2 weighted images, or diffusion abnormality. Severity of injury is described as MR imaging score of HIE [35], assigned by our neuroradiologist blinded to the newborns' clinical condition

* represents significant results surviving Bonferroni-correction ($p < 0.0014$)

Table 4 Metabolite ratios differing significantly between the outcome groups ($p < 0.0014$)

Assessed metabolite ratio	value of metabolite ratio (median [IQR])		p value
	good outcome ($n = 35$)	poor outcome ($n = 16$)	
mIns/NAA height (TE = 35 ms)	0.534 [0.440; 0.601]	0.780 [0.694; 0.894]	< 0.0001
NAA/Cr height (TE = 144 ms)	0.990 [0.897; 1.096]	0.808 [0.690; 0.863]	<0.0001
mIns/Cr height (TE = 35 ms)	0.471 [0.387; 0.530]	0.640 [0.528; 0.724]	0.0005

For all other metabolite ratios, see Additional file 1

in the early hours after hypoxic insult. We aimed to search for a uniformly detectable metabolite ratio that would be suitable for prognostication any time during the first 4 postnatal days. Assessment of age-dependence did not show significant correlation between either of the 3 metabolite ratios and age at the H-MRS examination. All 3 metabolite ratios showed weak correlation with the timing of the examination, hence might be considered relatively stable during the first 96 postnatal hours (Fig. 3).

Finally, comparing the prognostic performance of these 3 relatively age-independent metabolite ratios, mIns/NAA height at TE = 35 ms had a better discriminative power than NAA/Cr height at TE = 144 ms and mIns/Cr height at TE = 35 ms to identify patients with good versus poor outcome (cut-off-values 0.6798, 0.6274 and 0.7798, respectively, AUC: 0.9084, 0.8396 and 0.8462, respectively, difference between ROC curves $p < 0.00001$). Thus, out of the 36 evaluated metabolite ratios within the first 96 h of age, mIns/NAA height at TE = 35 ms seems to give the best prediction of outcome, with 84.6% sensitivity and 95.2% specificity, irrespective of the timing of the MR examination (Fig. 4 and Table 5).

Discussion

To the best of our knowledge, this preliminary study with a relatively small sample size is the first one that investigated the prognostic accuracy of conventional H-MRS examination performed during the first 4 postnatal days in a group of infants with moderate to severe HIE in the era of hypothermia treatment. We found that myo-inositol/

N-acetyl-aspartate height ratio (TE = 35 ms) was the best predictor of neurodevelopmental outcome at 2 years of age. This metabolite ratio proved to have low correlation with age at MR scan during the first 4 postnatal days and showed a specificity of 95.2% and a sensitivity of 84.6% for discriminating between good and poor outcome.

Previously, several studies investigated the prognostic power of H-MRS in asphyxiated neonates using various methods, protocols and equipment [10–19]. Nevertheless, it is problematic to draw an overarching conclusion applicable for the general clinical practice, due to the difference of the methods, findings and conclusions. Indeed, a wide range of H-MRS derived metabolites were suggested as potential biomarkers, e.g. some studies concluded that absolute Lac levels and/or Lac-containing metabolite ratios (Lac/NAA, Lac/Cho, Lac/Cr) were the most accurate in prediction of outcome [11–14, 16–19], while others showed that NAA/Cr, NAA/Cho, absolute NAA and/or Cho levels had promising prognostic powers [10, 11, 15, 17, 18], but only few studies investigated glutamate (Glx) or glutamate-containing metabolite ratios (Glx/Cr) [16], and/or mIns [17].

Interpretation and generalizability of these results are hindered by the fact that there was a marked variability regarding the methods used, some studies applied various data-optimizing software [15, 18] methods for absolute metabolite quantification [14, 15], or special head-coils [14, 17] in order to ameliorate the information acquired from the metabolite spectra. These methods may indeed improve data quality; however, they are not generally applicable in standard clinical settings [20].

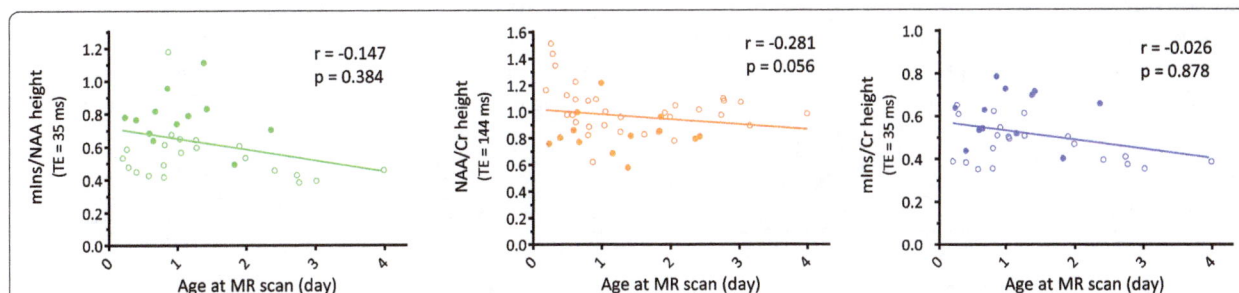

Fig. 3 Age-correlation diagrams of the 3 metabolite ratios showing strong association with outcome. Measurements from good outcome group are marked by empty bullet (o), measurements from poor outcome group are marked by circle bullet (•)

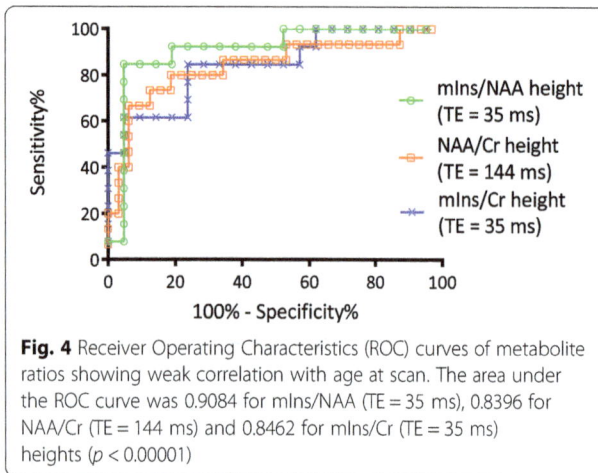

Fig. 4 Receiver Operating Characteristics (ROC) curves of metabolite ratios showing weak correlation with age at scan. The area under the ROC curve was 0.9084 for mIns/NAA (TE = 35 ms), 0.8396 for NAA/Cr (TE = 144 ms) and 0.8462 for mIns/Cr (TE = 35 ms) heights ($p < 0.00001$)

Therefore, our intent was to prove the clinical utility of conventional H-MRS sequence with vendor-provided analysis tools in the diagnostic workup of neonatal asphyxial encephalopathy.

Despite their limitations, existing evidence largely supports the use of peak areas as prognostic markers in patients with neonatal encephalopathy. A meta-analysis concluded that deep gray matter Lac/NAA peak area ratio is the most accurate predictor of adverse outcome [28]. Based on Bottomley's comprehensive review of MR spectroscopy [29] however, without post-processing techniques, the use of peak height and peak area has certain challenges. While peak height provides an acceptable measure for non-overlapping peaks, it is affected by patient motion and inhomogeneous widening of spectrum widths. Peak areas are relatively immune to motion artefacts and spectrum widening. However, since most of the integrated area of a peak resides near its base, noise and overlapping of other peaks can significantly affect the measurements. Taking these factors into consideration, we assessed the prognostic value of both peak heights and peak areas. Based on our findings, it seems that without the use of post-processing, peak height may have an appropriate predictive value and might be useful in the common clinical setting without the use of specialized imaging and post-processing techniques.

We set out to find markers that have similar or possibly even higher value for prognostication than markers published earlier.

To this end, we targeted our investigation on H-MRS scans performed the earliest possible, within 96 postnatal hours, presuming that the earlier the accurate prognostic information, the higher its clinical importance. The majority of the above-listed studies investigated H-MRS scans that were performed significantly later and in a wider range of infant age (3 to 45 days of age) [10, 11, 15–19], with only three papers focusing on early infant ages similar to our study [12–14], all three analyzing considerably small patient cohorts. One of them investigated infants during their first day of life (31 neonates of 4–18 postnatal hours); however, considering the unstable clinical status of many severely asphyxiated infants, this may be unfeasible in the clinical practice [12]. The second paper (11 neonates of 12–48 postnatal hours) concluded that only combined H-MRS and diffusion-weighted imaging is capable of accurate prediction of outcome [13], while the third one (17 neonates of 48–96 postnatal hours) used absolute quantification and a custom-made head-coil to optimize data acquisition [14]. Nevertheless, none of these early-acquisition studies examined neonates while undergoing therapeutic hypothermia.

In addition, although a recent study examined 88 infants with perinatal asphyxia who underwent therapeutic hypothermia, MR scans and H-MRS were acquired only within the first 7 postnatal days [30].

In the era of therapeutic hypothermia, the effect of cooling on brain metabolites is an important issue. Existing evidence suggests that hypothermia increases the clearance of lactate upon cerebral reperfusion [31] and increases overall lactate and myo-inositol levels in the cortex, while increasing the level of taurine and decreasing the level of choline in the thalamus [32]. Even though further studies are needed to outline the hypothermia-induced changes in metabolites detected by H-MRS, these findings suggest that thalamic myo-inositol/N-acetyl-aspartate values are not affected by cooling.

As an essential step in our analysis, we searched for metabolite ratios independent from postnatal age at the MR examination. It is well-known that in the early hours after hypoxic insult, the brain has an extremely dynamic metabolic profile [25, 26], so theoretically, metabolite ratios measured by H-MRS may vary significantly depending on the timing of the MR examination. In addition, the timing of the MR scan is influenced by the clinical stability of newborns. Based on these considerations, the acquisition of a single cut-off value for the proposed biomarker suitable

Table 5 Results of Receiver Operating Characteristics (ROC) analysis

Assessed metabolite ratio	Cut-off-value	Area under curve (AUC)	Sensitivity	Specificity	Positive predictive value	Negative predictive value
mIns/NAA height (TE = 35 ms)	0.6798	0.9084	84.62%	95.24%	91.67%	90.91%
NAA/Cr height (TE = 144 ms)	0.7798	0.8396	70.59%	85.29%	75,00%	75,61%
mIns/Cr height (TE = 35 ms)	0.6274	0.8462	61.54%	95.24%	88.89%	80.00%

Difference between ROC curves was significantly different ($p < 0.00001$)

for differentiation between outcomes may be extremely complex, given that the time-dependent metabolite changes are still not fully understood and described. Subsequently, the prognostic markers that vary depending on patient age may show false negative or false positive results, if performed too early or too late in the examined time period, so would require a dynamic range of cut-off-values (cut-off-curve) which calls for considerably larger population and/or repeated measures. Conclusively, until the precise kinetics of brain metabolites are described, the cut-off-value of the proposed prognostic marker should ideally not change with time but should only be determined by severity of encephalopathy and potential outcome. None of the existing studies contemplated the possible postnatal age dependence of the observed metabolites or metabolite ratios. Therefore, we aimed to investigate the stability of metabolite ratios, and found that none of the 3 metabolite ratios associated with outcome showed correlation with timing of the examination in the investigated time window, hence could be potentially independent of postnatal age. We consider the contemplation of the time-dependence of brain metabolites as one of the strengths of our analysis, even though further dependence analyses in repeated measures and larger population are needed to confirm our findings.

Existing evidence suggests that the role of both myo-inositol and N-acetyl-aspartate is complex. Myo-inositol is a pentose sugar, precursor for inositol-derived lipid synthesis and part of the intracellular second-messenger system [33]. To date, studies suggest that myo-inositol could be the breakdown product of abnormal cerebral inositol-polyphosphate metabolism and the cell membrane component myelin [34], implementing that increased myo-inositol levels signal cell death.

N-acetyl-aspartate is the second most abundant amino acid in the brain, functioning as an osmolite with multiple functions, e.g. molecular water pump for neurons to help osmotic regulation, as well as source, storage and transport of acetyl-group, aspartate and amino-nitrogen, for protein and lipid synthesis [33]. Studies suggest that NAA levels decrease after neuronal injury or dysfunction, even in the absence of cell death [34].

Conclusively, neuronal injury induced by hypoxia-ischemia is considered to raise myo-inositol levels and decrease N-acetyl-aspartate levels, thus increasing myo-inositol/N-acetyl-aspartate ratio and providing scientific background for our findings.

It is surprising that none of the lactate-containing metabolite ratios met the strict significance requirements of Bonferroni-correction. One of the reasons for this finding might be the low quality of lactate spectral data. In our measurements, signal-to-noise ratio of lactate peaks were extremely low, with a median [IQR] signal-to-noise ratio of 1.0 [0.7; 1.6] without selection, and 1.6 [1.1; 2.5]

after selection based on SNR = 1 criterion. However, low spectral data quality only affected peaks of lactate, since all other metabolites showed significantly more favorable signal-noise characteristics, with a median [IQR] signal-to-noise ratio of 10.8 [8.0; 12.8] for N-acetyl-aspartate, 11.9 [8.8; 14.5] for choline, 11.4 [7.3; 13.9] for creatine and 5.7 [4.8; 7.5] for myo-inositol, reflecting significantly better data quality. Based on these findings, spectral peak of lactate cannot be accurately assessed and interpreted in the general clinical setting and in the absence of post-processing techniques, despite its widespread use in previous studies.

In our study, the volume of interest was a $1 \times 1 \times 1$ cm voxel in the left thalamus. In this cohort, only one patient presented with watershed injury in the left parieto-occipital region, and one patient with widespread cortical lesion. Due to the low prevalence of watershed lesions, we were unable to assess the prognostic value of H-MRS in this type of neuronal injury.

Our study also has a number of limitations. Even though we outlined our methodology to eliminate all possible errors, there are certain points that still might have given way to inaccuracy in our conclusions. First, our study is retrospective in nature, therefore we could not control for factors possibly affecting the findings such as the imaging process and the clinical parameters. This may be considered a limitation compared to a prospective clinical study, where imaging and clinical parameters would have been fine-tuned for the purpose of the study. On the other hand, this could be viewed as a strength from a clinical standpoint, since we had to rely on data that could have been obtained in any MR facility imaging asphyxiated neonates. Therefore, our findings might have more relevance in the general clinical practice. The small sample size of our population is another limitation decreasing the accuracy and reliability of the statistical analysis. The difference between the sizes of the outcome groups (35 good versus 16 poor) might also be considered as a limitation, as our analysis might have been underpowered. Moreover, some may criticize our approach, and may state that all neonates should be examined at the exact same age, which would enable prognostic results to be as accurate as possible. However, considering that infants cannot be assessed before reaching certain clinical stability, this would not be a realistic expectation in the clinical practice.

Obviously, our results must be verified in prospective trials on larger populations and on different MR scanners to corroborate the prognostic power of the proposed H-MRS metabolite ratios.

Conclusions

In summary, we propose that H-MRS performed before 96 h of age is a potentially promising tool for early prediction of outcome in asphyxiated neonates. The use of

H-MRS may add valuable information for the clinicians to assess the severity of the hypoxic insult and potentially utilize additional neuroprotective therapies. Furthermore, our results suggest that even conventional H-MRS might have a high enough prognostic accuracy to be used in routine clinical practice.

Abbreviations

aEEG: amplitude-integrated electroencephalography; AUC: Area-under-curve; BD: Base deficit; BS: Burst suppression; Cho: Choline; CNV: Continuous normal voltage; Cr: Creatine; DNV: Discontinuous normal voltage; DWI: Diffusion weighted imaging; FT: Flat trace; Glx: Glutamate; HIE: Hypoxic-ischemia encephalopathy; H-MRS: Proton magnetic resonance spectroscopy; Lac: Lactate; lip: Lipid; LV: Low voltage; MDI: Mental Developmental Index; mIns: myo-inositol; MR: Magnetic resonance; MRI: Magnetic resonance imaging; NAA: N-acetyl-aspartate; PDI: Psychomotor Developmental Index; ROC: Receiver Operating Characteristics; SNR: Signal-to-noise intensity; TE: echo-time; VOI: Volume of interest

Acknowledgements

We would like to acknowledge the important contribution of Istvan Seri MD, PhD, HonD, Professor of Pediatrics, Children's Hospital Los Angeles and USC Keck School of Medicine, Los Angeles, CA and Honorary Member at Hungarian Academy of Sciences, Budapest, Hungary. We would also like to acknowledge the technical contributions of Adam Gyorgy Szabo MD, MR Research Center, Semmelweis University, Budapest, Hungary.

Funding

AJ was supported by Hungarian Academy of Science, Premium Postdoctoral Fellowship (PPD460004). LRK was supported by the Bolyai Research Fellowship program of the Hungarian Academy of Sciences. The funders had no role in the design and conduct of the study; collection, management, analysis, and interpretation of the data; and preparation, review, or approval of the manuscript.

Authors' contributions

HB acquired clinical and radiological patient information, finalized and interpreted the analysis of data, as well as drafted the manuscript. ÁJ participated in the conception of the study, outlined the statistical analysis and critically revised the statistical analysis and the manuscript language. MK participated in the acquisition of clinical data and critically revised the statistical analysis. LRK participated in acquisition of H-MRS data, and critically revised the statistical analysis and the manuscript language. AL contributed to the acquisition and interpretation of MRI for required exclusions. UM analyzed and interpreted the patient data regarding the clinical care of neonates. MSz outlined the methods and aims of the study, and participated in the analysis and interpretation of results. GR was responsible for the conception, analysis and interpretation of data for the work. All authors read and approved the final manuscript.

Competing interests

The authors declare that they have no competing interests.

Author details

[1]1st Department of Paediatrics, Semmelweis University, Budapest, Hungary. [2]MTA-SE Cardiovascular Imaging Research Group, Heart and Vascular Center, Semmelweis University, Budapest, Hungary. [3]MR Research Center, Semmelweis University, Budapest, Hungary.

References

1. Kurinczuk JJ, White-Koning M, Badawi N. Epidemiology of neonatal encephalopathy and hypoxic-ischaemic encephalopathy. Early Hum Dev. 2010;86:329–38.
2. Mwaniki MK, Atieno M, Lawn JE, Newton CRJC. Long-term neurodevelopmental outcomes after intrauterine and neonatal insults: a systematic review. Lancet. 2012;379:445–52.
3. Edwards AD, Brocklehurst P, Gunn AJ, Halliday H, Juszczak E, Levene M, et al. Neurological outcomes at 18 months of age after moderate hypothermia for perinatal hypoxic ischaemic encephalopathy: synthesis and meta-analysis of trial data. BMJ. 2010;340:c363.
4. Rogers EE, Bonifacio SL, Glass HC, Juul SE, Chang T, Mayock DE, et al. Erythropoietin and hypothermia for hypoxic-ischemic encephalopathy. Pediatr Neurol. 2014;51:657–62.
5. Aly H, Elmahdy H, El-Dib M, Rowisha M, Awny M, El-Gohary T, et al. Melatonin use for neuroprotection in perinatal asphyxia: a randomized controlled pilot study. J Perinatol. 2015;35:186–91.
6. Sabir H, Scull-Brown E, Liu X, Thoresen M. Immediate hypothermia is not neuroprotective after severe hypoxia-ischemia and is deleterious when delayed by 12 hours in neonatal rats. Stroke. 2012;43:3364–70.
7. The American College of Obstetricians and Gynecologists. Neonatal encephalopathy and neurologic outcome, second edition. Obstet Gynecol. 2014;123:896–901.
8. Douglas-Escobar M, Weiss MD. Hypoxic-ischemic encephalopathy: a review for the clinician. JAMA Pediatr. 2015;169:397–403.
9. Barker PB, Lin DDM. In vivo proton MR spectroscopy of the human brain. Prog Nucl Magn Reson Spectrosc. 2006;49:99–128.0.
10. Peden CJ, Rutherford MA, Sargentoni J, Cox IJ, Bryant DJ, Dubowitz LM. Proton spectroscopy of the neonatal brain following hypoxic-ischaemic injury. Dev Med Child Neurol. 1993;35:502–10.
11. Groenendaal F, Veenhoven RH, van der Grond J, Jansen GH, Witkamp TD, de Vries LS. Cerebral lactate and N-acetyl-aspartate/choline ratios in asphyxiated full-term neonates demonstrated in vivo using proton magnetic resonance spectroscopy. Pediatr Res. 1994;35:148–51.
12. Hanrahan JD, Cox IJ, Azzopardi D, Cowan FM, Sargentoni J, Bell JD, et al. Relation between proton magnetic resonance spectroscopy within 18 hours of birth asphyxia and neurodevelopment at 1 year of age. Dev Med Child Neurol. 1999;41:76–82.
13. L'Abee C, de Vries LS, van der Grond J, Groenendaal F. Early diffusion-weighted MRI and 1H-magnetic resonance spectroscopy in asphyxiated full-term neonates. Biol Neonate. 2005;88:306–12.
14. Cheong JLY, Cady EB, Penrice J, Wyatt JS, Cox IJ, Robertson NJ. Proton MR spectroscopy in neonates with perinatal cerebral hypoxic-ischemic injury: metabolite peak-area ratios, relaxation times, and absolute concentrations. Am J Neuroradiol. 2006;27:1546–54.
15. Boichot C, Walker PM, Durand C, Grimaldi M, Chapuis S, Gouyon JB, et al. Term neonate prognoses after perinatal asphyxia: contributions of MR imaging, MR spectroscopy, relaxation times, and apparent diffusion coefficients. Radiology. 2006;239:839–48.
16. Zhu W, Zhong W, Qi J, Yin P, Wang C, Chang L. Proton magnetic resonance spectroscopy in neonates with hypoxic-ischemic injury and its prognostic value. Transl Res. 2008;152:225–32.
17. Ancora G, Soffritti S, Lodi R, Tonon C, Grandi S, Locatelli C, et al. A combined a-EEG and MR spectroscopy study in term newborns with hypoxic-ischemic encephalopathy. Brain and Development. 2010;32:835–42.
18. van Doormaal PJ, Meiners LC, ter Horst HJ, van der Veere CN, Sijens PE. The prognostic value of multivoxel magnetic resonance spectroscopy determined metabolite levels in white and grey matter brain tissue for adverse outcome in term newborns following perinatal asphyxia. Eur Radiol. 2012;22:772–8.
19. Alderliesten T, de Vries LS, Staats L, van Haastert IC, Weeke L, Benders MJNL, et al. MRI and spectroscopy in (near) term neonates with perinatal asphyxia and therapeutic hypothermia. Arch Dis Child - Fetal Neonatal Ed 2016; fetalneonatal-2016-310514.
20. Wilkinson D. MRI and withdrawal of life support from newborn infants with hypoxic-ischemic encephalopathy. Pediatrics. 2010;126:e451–8.
21. Azzopardi DV, Strohm B, Edwards a D, Dyet L, Halliday HL, Juszczak E, et al. Moderate hypothermia to treat perinatal asphyxial encephalopathy. N Engl J Med. 2009;361:1349–58.
22. Shalak LF, Laptook AR, Velaphi SC, Perlman JM. Amplitude-integrated electroencephalography coupled with an early neurologic examination enhances prediction of term infants at risk for persistent encephalopathy. Pediatrics. 2003;111(2):351–7.
23. Blüml S. Magnetic resonance spectroscopy: basics. In: MR spectroscopy of pediatric brain disorders. New York, NY: Springer New York; 2013. p. 11–23.
24. Holmes D. Basic practical NMR concepts: a guide for the modern. Laboratory. 2004:1–42.
25. Vannucci RC, Towfighi J, Vannucci SJ. Secondary energy failure after cerebral hypoxia-ischemia in the immature rat. J Cereb Blood Flow Metab. 2004;24: 1090–7.

26. Hassell KJ, Ezzati M, Alonso-Alconada D, Hausenloy DJ, Robertson NJ. New horizons for newborn brain protection: enhancing endogenous neuroprotection. Arch Dis Child Fetal Neonatal Ed. 2015;100:F541–52.
27. Hanley JA, McNeil BJ. A method of comparing the areas under receiver operating characteristic curves derived from the same cases. Radiology. 1983;148:839–43.
28. Thayyil S, Chandrasekaran M, Taylor A, Bainbridge A, et al. Pediatrics. 2010;125:e382–95.
29. Bottomley P. The trouble with spectroscopy papers. Radiology. 1991;181: 344–50.
30. Alderliesten T, De Vries LS, Staats L, Van Haastert IC, et al. Arch Dis Child Fetal Neonatal Ed. 2017;102:F147–52.
31. Lei H, Peeling J. Effect of temperature on the kinetics of lactate production and clearance in a rat model of forebrain ischemia. Biochem Cell Biol. 1998;76:503–9.
32. Chan KWY, Chow AM, Chan KC, Yang J, Wu EX. Magnetic resonance spectroscopy of the brain under mild hypothermia indicates changes in neuroprotection-related metabolites. Neurosci Lett. 2010;475:150–5.
33. Brighina E, Bresolin N, Pardi G, Rango M. Human fetal brain chemistry as detected by proton magnetic resonance spectroscopy. Pediatr Neurol. 2009;40:327–42.
34. Macrì MA, D'Alessandro N, Di Giulio C, Di Iorio P, Di Luzio S, Giuliani P, et al. Regional changes in the metabolite profile after long-term hypoxia-ischemia in brains of young and aged rats: a quantitative proton MRS study. Neurobiol Aging. 2006;27:98–104.
35. Barkovich AJ, Hajnal BL, Vigneron D, et al. Prediction of neuromotor outcome in perinatal asphyxia: evaluation of MR scoring systems. Am J Neuroradiol. 1998;19(1):143–9.

Permissions

All chapters in this book were first published in PEDIATRICS, by BioMed Central; hereby published with permission under the Creative Commons Attribution License or equivalent. Every chapter published in this book has been scrutinized by our experts. Their significance has been extensively debated. The topics covered herein carry significant findings which will fuel the growth of the discipline. They may even be implemented as practical applications or may be referred to as a beginning point for another development.

The contributors of this book come from diverse backgrounds, making this book a truly international effort. This book will bring forth new frontiers with its revolutionizing research information and detailed analysis of the nascent developments around the world.

We would like to thank all the contributing authors for lending their expertise to make the book truly unique. They have played a crucial role in the development of this book. Without their invaluable contributions this book wouldn't have been possible. They have made vital efforts to compile up to date information on the varied aspects of this subject to make this book a valuable addition to the collection of many professionals and students.

This book was conceptualized with the vision of imparting up-to-date information and advanced data in this field. To ensure the same, a matchless editorial board was set up. Every individual on the board went through rigorous rounds of assessment to prove their worth. After which they invested a large part of their time researching and compiling the most relevant data for our readers.

The editorial board has been involved in producing this book since its inception. They have spent rigorous hours researching and exploring the diverse topics which have resulted in the successful publishing of this book. They have passed on their knowledge of decades through this book. To expedite this challenging task, the publisher supported the team at every step. A small team of assistant editors was also appointed to further simplify the editing procedure and attain best results for the readers.

Apart from the editorial board, the designing team has also invested a significant amount of their time in understanding the subject and creating the most relevant covers. They scrutinized every image to scout for the most suitable representation of the subject and create an appropriate cover for the book.

The publishing team has been an ardent support to the editorial, designing and production team. Their endless efforts to recruit the best for this project, has resulted in the accomplishment of this book. They are a veteran in the field of academics and their pool of knowledge is as vast as their experience in printing. Their expertise and guidance has proved useful at every step. Their uncompromising quality standards have made this book an exceptional effort. Their encouragement from time to time has been an inspiration for everyone.

The publisher and the editorial board hope that this book will prove to be a valuable piece of knowledge for researchers, students, practitioners and scholars across the globe.

List of Contributors

Duncan N. Shikuku, Elizabeth Ayebare and Gorrette Nalwadda
Department of Nursing, Makerere University, School of Health Sciences, Kampala, Uganda

Benson Milimo
Department of Midwifery and Gender, Moi University, School of Nursing, Eldoret, Kenya

Peter Gisore
Department of Child Health and Pediatrics, Moi University, School of Medicine, Eldoret, Kenya

C. Aydemir
Department of Pediatrics, Medical Faculty, Division of Neonatology, Bülent Ecevit University, Zonguldak, Turkey

H. Aydemir
Department of Infectious Diseases and Clinical Microbiology, Medical Faculty, Bulent Ecevit University, 67600 Zonguldak, Turkey

F. Kokturk
Department of Biostatistics, Medical Faculty, Bulent Ecevit University, Zonguldak, Turkey

C. Kulah
Department of Microbiology, Medical Faculty, Bulent Ecevit University, Zonguldak, Turkey

A. G. Mungan
Department of Biochemistry, Medical Faculty, Bulent Ecevit University, Zonguldak, Turkey

M. Trip-Hoving, J. Landier, T. J. Prins, C. Po, C. Beau, M. Mu and V. I. Carrara
Shoklo Malaria Research Unit, Mahidol-Oxford Tropical Medicine Research Unit, Faculty of Tropical Medicine, Mahidol University, Mae Sot, Thailand

L. Thielemans
Shoklo Malaria Research Unit, Mahidol-Oxford Tropical Medicine Research Unit, Faculty of Tropical Medicine, Mahidol University, Mae Sot, Thailand
Neonatology-Pediatrics, Cliniques Universitaires de Bruxelles – Hôspital Erasme, Université Libre de Bruxelles, Brussels, Belgium

F. Nosten and R. McGready
Shoklo Malaria Research Unit, Mahidol-Oxford Tropical Medicine Research Unit, Faculty of Tropical Medicine, Mahidol University, Mae Sot, Thailand
Centre for Tropical Medicine and Global Health, Nuffield Department of Medicine, University of Oxford, Oxford, UK

E. M. N. Wouda
Shoklo Malaria Research Unit, Mahidol-Oxford Tropical Medicine Research Unit, Faculty of Tropical Medicine, Mahidol University, Mae Sot, Thailand
University of Groningen, Groningen, The Netherlands

B. Van Overmeire
Neonatology-Pediatrics, Cliniques Universitaires de Bruxelles – Hôspital Erasme, Université Libre de Bruxelles, Brussels, Belgium

C. Turner
Centre for Tropical Medicine and Global Health, Nuffield Department of Medicine, University of Oxford, Oxford, UK
Cambodia-Oxford Medical Research Unit, Angkor Hospital for Children, Siem Reap, Cambodia
Angkor Hospital for Children, Siem Reap, Cambodia

B. Hanboonkunupakarn
Mahidol-Oxford Tropical Medicine Research Unit (MORU), Faculty of Tropical Medicine, Mahidol University, Salaya, Thailand

T. Hannay
University of Glasgow, Glasgow, Scotland, UK

Bhishma Pokhrel, Ganesh Shah and Suchita Joshi
Department of Pediatrics, Patan Academy of Health Sciences, Lagankhel, Lalitpur, Nepal

Tapendra Koirala
School of Medicine, Patan Academy of Health Sciences, Lagankhel, Lalitpur, Nepal

Pinky Baral
School of Health and Allied Sciences, Pokhara University, Lekhnath-12, Kaski, Nepal

Temitayo Famoroti
Department of Virology, National Health Laboratory Service, Nelson R Mandela School of Medicine, University of KwaZulu-Natal, Durban, KwaZulu-Natal, South Africa

Wilbert Sibanda
Biostatistics Unit, School of Nursing and Public Health, College of Health Sciences, University of KwaZulu-Natal, Durban, KwaZulu-Natal, South Africa

Thumbi Ndung'u
HIV Pathogenesis Programme, Doris Duke Medical Research Institute, Nelson R Mandela School of Medicine, University of KwaZulu-Natal, Durban, KwaZulu-Natal, South Africa

Michaela Mathes, Christoph Maas, Christine Bleeker, Julia Vek, Wolfgang Bernhard and Christian F. Poets
Department of Neonatology, University Children's Hospital, Tübingen University Hospital, Calwerstr. 7, Tübingen, Germany

Axel R. Franz
Department of Neonatology, University Children's Hospital, Tübingen University Hospital, Calwerstr. 7, Tübingen, Germany
Center for Pediatric Clinical Studies, University Children's Hospital, Tübingen University Hospital, Tübingen, Germany

Andreas Peter
Department of Internal Medicine IV, Division of Endocrinology, Diabetology, Vascular Medicine, Nephrology and Clinical Chemistry and Pathobiochemistry, University of Tuebingen, Tübingen, Germany
Institute of Diabetes Research and Metabolic Diseases (IDM) of the Helmholtz Center Munich at the University of Tuebingen, Tübingen, Germany
German Center for Diabetes Research (DZD), Muenchen-Neuherberg, Germany

Birhanu Wondimeneh Demissie and Tesfaye Yitna Chichiabellu
Department of Nursing, College of Health Sciences and Medicine, Wolaita Sodo University, Sodo, Ethiopia

Balcha Berhanu Abera
School of Nursing and Midwifery, College of Health Science, Addis Ababa University, Addis Ababa, Ethiopia

Feleke Hailemichael Astawesegn
School of Public Health, College of Medicine and Health Sciences, Hawassa University, Hawassa, Ethiopia

Shuby Puthussery, Muhammad Chutiyami and Pei-Ching Tseng
Maternal and Child Health Research Centre, Institute for Health Research, University of Bedfordshire, Putteridge Bury, Hitchin Road, Luton, Bedfordshire LU2 8LE, UK

Lesley Kilby and Jogesh Kapadia
Neonatal Unit, Luton and Dunstable Hospital, Lewsey Rd, Luton LU4 0DZ, UK

Ranmali Rodrigo
Department of Paediatrics, University of Kelaniya, 6 Thalagolla Road, Ragama 11010, Sri Lanka
Judith Lumley Centre, La Trobe University, 215 Franklin Street, Melbourne, VIC 3000, Australia

Lisa H. Amir
Judith Lumley Centre, La Trobe University, 215 Franklin Street, Melbourne, VIC 3000, Australia

Della A. Forster
Judith Lumley Centre, La Trobe University, 215 Franklin Street, Melbourne, VIC 3000, Australia
Royal Women's Hospital, Locked Bag 300, Parkville, VIC 3052, Australia

Anh Thi Nguyet Nguyen, Muneko Nishijo, Nghi Ngoc Tran and Yoshikazu Nishino
Department of Public Health and Epidemiology, Kanazawa Medical University, 1-1, Daigaku, Uchinada, Ishikawa 920-0293, Japan

Tai The Pham, Anh Hai Tran and Luong Van Hoang
Biomedical and Pharmaceutical Research Center, Vietnam Military Medical University, Ha Noi, Vietnam

Hitomi Boda and Yuko Morikawa
School of Nursing, Kanazawa Medical University, 1-1 Daigaku, Uchinada, Ishikawa 920-0293, Japan

Hisao Nishijo
System Emotional Science, Graduate School of Medicine and Pharmaceutical Sciences, University of Toyama, 2630 Sugitani, Toyama 930-0194, Japan

Annika Kruse and Markus Tilp
Institute of Sports Science, University of Graz, Mozartgasse 14, 8010 Graz, Austria

Christian Schranz and Martin Svehlik
Department of Paediatric Surgery, Medical University of Graz, Auenbruggerplatz 34, 8036 Graz, Austria

Brennan Vail
Department of Pediatrics, University of California San Francisco, 550 16th Street, 4th Floor, San Francisco, CA 94158, USA

Melissa C. Morgan
Department of Pediatrics, University of California San Francisco, 550 16th Street, 4th Floor, San Francisco, CA 94158, USA
Maternal, Adolescent, Reproductive, and Child Health Centre, London School of Hygiene and Tropical Medicine, Keppel Street, London WC1E 7HT, UK
Institute for Global Health Sciences, University of California San Francisco, 550 16th Street, San Francisco, CA 94158, USA

Hilary Spindler
Institute for Global Health Sciences, University of California San Francisco, 550 16th Street, San Francisco, CA 94158, USA

Dilys M. Walker
Institute for Global Health Sciences, University of California San Francisco, 550 16th Street, San Francisco, CA 94158, USA
Department of Obstetrics and Gynecology and Reproductive Services, University of California San Francisco, 1001 Potrero Ave, San Francisco, CA 94110, USA
PRONTO International, 1820 E. Thomas Street APT 16, Seattle, WA 98112, USA

Amelia Christmas
PRONTO International, State RMNCH+A Unit, C-16 Krishi Nagar, A.G. Colony, Patna, Bihar 80002, India

Susanna R. Cohen
College of Nursing, University of Utah, 10 South 2000 East, Salt Lake City, UT 84112, USA

Chidiebere D. I. Osuorah
Child Survival Unit, Medical Research Council UK, The Gambia Unit, Fajara, Banjul, Gambia

Uchenna Ekwochi and Isaac N. Asinobi
Department of Paediatrics, Enugu State University of Science and Technology, Enugu, Enugu State, Nigeria

Amy Sweeny
Department of Emergency Medicine, Gold Coast University Hospital, 1 Hospital Boulevard, Southport, QLD 4215, Australia

Gerben Keijzers
Department of Emergency Medicine, Gold Coast University Hospital, 1 Hospital Boulevard, Southport, QLD 4215, Australia
School of Medicine, Bond University, Gold Coast, QLD, Australia
School of Medicine, Griffith University, Gold Coast, QLD, Australia

Julia Crilly
Department of Emergency Medicine, Gold Coast Health, Gold Coast, QLD, Australia
Menzies Health Institute, Gold Coast, QLD, Australia

Norm Good
CSIRO Digitial Productivity/ Australian e-Health Research Centre, Royal Women's and Children's Hospital, Brisbane, QLD, Australia

Cate M. Cameron
Jamieson Trauma Institute, Royal Brisbane and Women's Hospital, Metro North Hospital and Health Service, Herston, QLD, Australia
Menzies Health Institute Queensland, Griffith University, Meadowbrook, QLD, Australia

Rani Scott
Menzies Health Institute Queensland, Griffith University, Meadowbrook, QLD, Australia

Gabor Mihala and Paul A. Scuffham
Menzies Health Institute Queensland, Griffith University, Nathan, QLD, Australia

Daniele Kedy Koum
Clinical sciences department, Faculty of Medicine and Pharmaceutical Sciences, University of Douala, Douala, Cameroon

Calixte Ida Penda
Clinical sciences department, Faculty of Medicine and Pharmaceutical Sciences, University of Douala, Douala, Cameroon

HIV Care and Treatment Centre, Laquintinie Hospital of Douala, Douala, Cameroon

Carole Else Eboumbou Moukoko and Cedric Anatole Zambo Meyong
HIV Care and Treatment Centre, Laquintinie Hospital of Douala, Douala, Cameroon

Joseph Fokam
Virology Laboratory, Chantal Biya International Reference Centre for research on HIV/AIDS prevention and management, Yaoundé, Cameroon
Faculty of Medicine and Biomedical Sciences, University of Yaoundé I, Yaoundé, Cameroon

Paul Koki Ndombo
Faculty of Medicine and Biomedical Sciences, University of Yaoundé I, Yaoundé, Cameroon
Mother-Child Centre, Chantal BIYA Foundation, Yaoundé, Cameroon

Sandrine Talla
Technical office, Elizabeth Glaser Pediatric AIDS Foundation, LDH, Douala, Cameroon

Michiko Nakamura, Kimihiko Moriya, Yoko Nishimura, Yukiko Kanno, Takeya Kitta, Masafumi Kon and Nobuo Shinohara
Department of Renal and Genitourinary Surgery, Hokkaido University Graduate School of Medicine, North-15, West-7, Kita-Ku, Sapporo 060-8638, Japan

Mutsumi Nishida and Yusuke Kudo
Diagnostic Center for Sonography, Hokkaido University Hospital, Sapporo, Japan
Division of Laboratory and Transfusion Medicine, Hokkaido University Hospital, Sapporo, Japan

Nihad A. Almasri and Maysoun Saleh
Department of Physiotherapy, School of Rehabilitation Sciences, The University of Jordan, Queen Rania Al Abdallah St, Amman 11942, Jordan

Sana Abu-Dahab and Somaya H. Malkawi
Department of occupational therapy, School of Rehabilitation Sciences, The University of Jordan, Queen Rania Al Abdallah St, Amman 11942, Jordan

Eva Nordmark
Faculty of Medicine, Lund university, P.0. 157, SE-221 00 Lund, Sweden

Emma Olsson
Department of Pediatrics, Faculty of Medicine and Health, Örebro University Hospital, S-701 85 Örebro, Sweden
Faculty of Medicine and Health, School of Medical Sciences, Örebro University, Örebro, Sweden

Agneta Anderzén-Carlsson
University Health Care Research Center, Faculty of Medicine and Health, Örebro University, Örebro, Sweden

Sigríður María Atladótti and Guðrún Kristjánsdóttir
Faculty of Nursing, University of Iceland, Reykjavik, Iceland
Neonatal Intensive Care Unit, Lanspitali University Children's Hospital, Reykjavik, Iceland

Anna Axelin and Emilia Peltonen
Department of Nursing Science, University of Turku, Turku, Finland

Marsha Campbell-Yeo
School of Nursing, Faculty of Health Professions and Departments of Pediatrics, Psychology and Neuroscience, Dalhousie University, Halifax, Canada
Centre for Pediatric Pain Research, IWK Health Centre, Halifax, Canada

Mats Eriksson
Faculty of Medicine and Health, School of Health Sciences, Örebro University, Örebro, Sweden

Bonnie Stevens
Lawrence S Bloomberg, Faculty of Nursing, University of Toronto, Toronto, Canada
Department of Nursing, The Hospital for Sick Children, Toronto, Canada

Bente Vederhus
Department of Pediatrics, Haukeland University Hospital, Bergen, Norway

Randi Dovland Andersen
Department of Child and Adolescent Health Services, Telemark Hospital, Skien, Norway
Department of Neurobiology, Care Sciences and Society, Karolinska Institutet, Stockholm, Sweden

Bella Monse
Deutsche Gesellschaft für Internationale Zusammenarbeit (GIZ), L.P. Leviste corner Rufino Street, Makati City, Metro Manila, Philippines

Jed Dimaisip-Nabuab
Deutsche Gesellschaft für Internationale Zusammenarbeit (GIZ), L.P. Leviste corner Rufino Street, Makati City, Metro Manila, Philippines
Department of Epidemiology and Biostatistics, College of Public Health, University of the Philippines, 625 Pedro Gil St, Ermita, Manila, Philippines

Denise Duijster
Department of Social Dentistry, Academic Centre for Dentistry Amsterdam, Gustav Mahlerlaan 3004, 1081LA Amsterdam, The Netherlands
Department of Epidemiology and Public Health, University College London, Torrington Place 1-19, London WC1E 6BT, UK

Habib Benzian
Department of Epidemiology and Health Promotion, WHO Collaborating Center for Quality Improvement and Evidence-based Dentistry, College of Dentistry, New York University, 433 First Avenue, New York, NY 10010, USA

Roswitha Heinrich-Weltzien
Department of Preventive Dentistry and Pediatric Dentistry, University Hospital Jena, Friedrich Schiller University Jena, Bachstraße 18, 07743 Jena, Germany

Amphayvan Homsavath
Faculty of Dentistry, University of Health Sciences Ministry of Health, 7444 Mahosot Rd, Vientiane, Lao People's Democratic Republic

Hak Sithan
Department of Preventive Medicine, Ministry of Health, 151-153 Kampuchea Krom Avenue, Phnom Penh, Cambodia

Nicole Stauf
The Health Bureau Ltd., Whiteleaf Business Center, 11 Little Balmer, Buckingham MK18 1TF, UK

Sri Susilawati
Department of Dental Public Health, Faculty of Dentistry, Padjadjaran University, Sekelda Selatan I, Bandung, Indonesia

Katrin Kromeyer-Hauschild
Institute of Human Genetics, University Hospital Jena, Friedrich Schiller University Jena, Am Klinikum 1, 07740 Jena, Germany

Midori Ishikawa and Tetsuji Yokoyama
Department of Health Promotion, National Institute of Public Health, 2-3-6 Minami, Wako, Saitama 351-0197, Japan

Noriko Kato
Department of Health Promotion, National Institute of Public Health, 2-3-6 Minami, Wako, Saitama 351-0197, Japan
Present Address: Department of Early Childhood Care and Education, Jumonji University, 2-1-28 Sugasawa, Niizashi, Saitama 352-8510, Japan

Kumi Eto
Faculty of Nutrition, Kagawa Nutrition University, 3-9-21 Chiyoda, Sakado, Saitama 350-0288, Japan

Mayu Haraikawa
Department of Child Studies, Faculty of Child Studies, Seitoku University, 550 Iwase, Matsudo, Chiba 271-8555, Japan

Yoshihisa Yamazaki
Child Health Center, Aichi Children's Health and Medical Center, 426-7, Morioka, Obu, Aichi 474-8710, Japan

Kemal Sasaki
Department of Food and Health Sciences, Jissen Women's University, 4-1-1 Osakaue, Hino, Tokyo 191-8510, Japan

Zentaro Yamagata
Faculty of Medicine, University of Yamanashi, 1110 Shimokato, Chuo, Yamanashi 409-3898, Japan

Yumiko Morinaga
Faculty of Medicine, School of Nursing Public Health Nursing, Kagawa University, 1750-1, Ikenobe, Miki, Kita, Kagawa 761-0793, Japan

Leena Dhande
Department of Pediatrics, Indira Gandhi Government Medical College, Nagpur, Maharashtra 440018, India

Archana Patel
Department of Pediatrics, Indira Gandhi Government Medical College, Nagpur, Maharashtra 440018, India

Lata Medical Research Foundation, Nagpur, Maharashtra 440022, India

Priyanka Kuhite, Amrita Puranik, Samreen Sadaf Khan and Jitesh Borkar
Lata Medical Research Foundation, Nagpur, Maharashtra 440022, India

Angeline Tangiora, Raymond Jones and Barry J. Taylor
Department of Women's and Children's Health, Dunedin School of Medicine, University of Otago, Dunedin, New Zealand

Kathy M. Manhire and David Tipene-Leach
Department of Women's and Children's Health, Dunedin School of Medicine, University of Otago, Dunedin, New Zealand
Faculty of Education, Humanities and Health Sciences, Eastern Institute of Technology, Hawke's Bay, New Zealand

Sheila M. Williams
Department of Preventive and Social Medicine, Dunedin School of Medicine, University of Otago, Dunedin, New Zealand

Sally A. Baddock
School of Midwifery, Otago Polytechnic, Dunedin, New Zealand

Sally Abel
Kaupapa Consulting Ltd, Napier, Napier, New Zealand

Matilda Emgård, Rickard Nordén, Ebba Samuelsson, Shadi Geravandi, Lucia Gonzales-Siles, Magnus Lindh and Susann Skovbjerg
Department of Infectious Diseases, Institute of Biomedicine, University of Gothenburg, Gothenburg, Sweden

Rune Andersson
Department of Infectious Diseases, Institute of Biomedicine, University of Gothenburg, Gothenburg, Sweden
CARe – Center for Antibiotic Resistance Research, Gothenburg University, Gothenburg, Sweden

Archippe M. Birindwa
Department of Infectious Diseases, Institute of Biomedicine, University of Gothenburg, Gothenburg, Sweden

Panzi Hospital, Bukavu, Democratic Republic of the Congo
Université Evangélique en Afrique, Bukavu, Democratic Republic of the Congo
Hôpital Général de Référence de Panzi, BP: 266 Bukavu, DR, Congo

Balthazar Muhigirwa, Eric Munguakonkwa, Jeanière T. Manegabe, Didace Cibicabene, Lambert Morisho, Benjamin Mwambanyi, Jacques Mirindi and Nadine Kabeza
Panzi Hospital, Bukavu, Democratic Republic of the Congo

Théophile Kashosi
Université Evangélique en Afrique, Bukavu, Democratic Republic of the Congo

James Shelley, Zoe R Knowles, Ellen A Dawson, Lee E F Graves and Claire Hanlon
Physical Activity Exchange, Research Institute for Sport and Exercise Sciences, Liverpool John Moores University, 62 Great Crosshall Street, Liverpool L3 2AT, England

Stuart J Fairclough
Physical Activity Exchange, Research Institute for Sport and Exercise Sciences, Liverpool John Moores University, 62 Great Crosshall Street, Liverpool L3 2AT, England
Edge Hill University, St Helens Road, Ormskirk, Lancashire L39 4QP, England

Kevin W Southern
Department of Women's and Children's Health, University of Liverpool, Institute in the Park, Alder Hey Children's Hospital, Eaton Road, L12 2AP Liverpool, England

Pamela McCormack
Respiratory Department, Alder Hey NHS Foundation Trust Children's Hospital, Eaton Road, Liverpool L12 2AP, England

Bikila Lencha and Zanebe Minda
Department of Public Health, Goba Referral Hospital, Maddawalabu University, Bale-Goba, Addis Ababa, Ethiopia

Gemehu Ameya
Department of Medical Laboratory Science, College of Medicine and Health Sciences, Arba Minch University, Arba Minch, Ethiopia

Feyissa Lamessa
Department of Nursing, Goba Referral Hospital, Maddawalabu University, Bale-Goba, Addis Ababa, Ethiopia

Jiregna Darega
Department of Nursing, College of Medicine and Health sciences, Ambo University, Ambo, Ethiopia

Girmay Tekaly and Hagos Tasew
Department of Pediatrics and Child Health Nursing, School of Nursing, College of Health Science, Aksum University, Aksum, Ethiopia

Mekuria Kassa and Tilahun Belete
Department of Nursing, College of Health Science, Mekelle University, Mekelle, Ethiopia

Tekelwoini Mariye
Department of Adult Health Nursing, School of Nursing, College of Health Science, Aksum University, Aksum, Ethiopia

Tsega Teshale
Department of Medical Laboratory, College of Health Science, Aksum University, Aksum, Ethiopia

Hajnalka Barta, Agnes Jermendy, Unoke Meder and Miklos Szabo
1st Department of Paediatrics, Semmelweis University, Budapest, Hungary

Marton Kolossvary
MTA-SE Cardiovascular Imaging Research Group, Heart and Vascular Center, Semmelweis University, Budapest, Hungary

Lajos R. Kozak, Andrea Lakatos and Gabor Rudas
MR Research Center, Semmelweis University, Budapest, Hungary

Index